Aldeen and Rosenbaum's

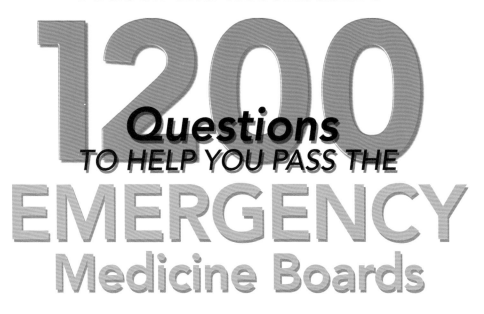

1200 Questions

TO HELP YOU PASS THE

EMERGENCY
Medicine Boards

THIRD EDITION

Aldeen and Rosenbaum's

1200 Questions TO HELP YOU PASS THE EMERGENCY Medicine Boards

THIRD EDITION

Amer Z. Aldeen, MD, FACEP

Executive Medical Director
Center for Emergency Medical Education
Vice Chair
National Clinical Governance Board
US Acute Care Solutions
Chicago, Illinois

David H. Rosenbaum, MD, FACEP, FAAEM

Wake Emergency Physicians, P.A.
WakeMed Health and Hospitals
Raleigh, North Carolina
Adjunct Professor of Emergency Medicine
University of North Carolina at Chapel Hill
Chapel Hill, North Carolina

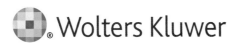

. Wolters Kluwer

Philadelphia • Baltimore • New York • London
Buenos Aires • Hong Kong • Sydney • Tokyo

Acquisitions Editor: Sharon Zinner
Product Development Editor: Ashley Fischer
Editorial Assistant: Brian Convery
Marketing Manager: Rachel Mante Leung
Production Project Manager: Bridgett Dougherty
Design Coordinator: Stephen Druding
Manufacturing Coordinator: Beth Welsh
Prepress Vendor: Aptara, Inc.

Third edition

Library of Congress Cataloging-in-Publication Data

Names: Aldeen, Amer Z., author. | Rosenbaum, David H., author.
Title: Aldeen and Rosenbaum's 1200 questions to help you pass the emergency
   medicine boards / Amer Z. Aldeen, David H. Rosenbaum.
Other titles: 1200 questions to help you pass the emergency medicine boards
Description: Third edition. | Philadelphia : Wolters Kluwer, [2017] |
   Preceded by 1200 questions to help you pass the emergency medicine boards /
   Amer Z. Aldeen, David H. Rosenbaum. 2nd ed. 2012.
Identifiers: LCCN 2016049471 | ISBN 9781496343260
Subjects: | MESH: Emergency Treatment–methods | Emergency Medicine–methods |
   Examination Questions
Classification: LCC RC86.9 | NLM WB 18.2 | DDC 616.02/5076–dc23
LC record available at https://lccn.loc.gov/2016049471

To our three beautiful daughters, Arissa, Rania, and Nyla,
You are the light of our lives. May you create a more tolerant and peaceful world with your knowledge, creativity, and dedication. Ameen.

—AMER Z. ALDEEN

To Sophie and Lucie,
May your joy, energy, and excitement remain untempered, even by your sometimes impatient dad.

—DAVID H. ROSENBAUM

Preface

The goal of this text is to help prepare you for the American Board of Emergency Medicine's (ABEM) Written Qualifying Examination. The book's content is based on the ABEM Model of the Clinical Practice of Emergency Medicine. This document, which ABEM systematically updates every 2 years to reflect changes and advancements, serves as the blueprint for ABEM's In-Training, Written Qualifying, Oral Certification, and Continuous Certification (ConCert) examinations.

In addition to ensuring that we addressed the breadth of ABEM's Model, we deliberately designed most of our questions to be slightly more difficult than the average question in ABEM's Written Qualifying Examination. As a result, most readers will agree that the questions in this book are moderately hard. In our view, it is better to overprepare than be falsely reassured by a bank of practice questions that does not adequately challenge (and add to) the reader's existing knowledge.

In this third edition of our work, we added 200 new, mostly case-based questions, many with images. We also updated many of our existing questions in response to valuable feedback from readers. The pace of new knowledge development in emergency medicine is rapid, and we have attempted to incorporate as much cutting edge information as possible.

We actively invite your feedback, both positive and critical, to help improve the quality of this work. Please do not hesitate to contact us via email (ameraldeen@gmail.com or david.h.rosenbaum@gmail.com) should you have any comments or questions.

Amer Z. Aldeen, MD, FACEP
David H. Rosenbaum, MD, FACEP, FAAEM

Acknowledgments

I would like to thank my colleagues at US Acute Care Solutions for supporting my interest in education. In particular, I am indebted to Drs. Tim Corvino, Dominic Bagnoli, Anita Gage, and Jim Augustine. I would also like to thank the resident physicians of the Northwestern Department of Emergency Medicine—academic discussions with them while on shift contributed greatly to the genesis of this work. Lastly, and most importantly, I owe a debt of gratitude to my wife, Farheen Aldeen, for managing our lives' many tasks, allowing me time and energy to produce this work.

Amer Z. Aldeen, MD, FACEP

I am indebted to my colleagues, Drs. Fernando Guarderas, Skylar Lentz, and Robert Sackmann, for their thoughtful editorial comments that helped improve this book. I am also grateful to the many inquisitive emergency medicine residents at the University of North Carolina, whose curiosity, passion, and drive not only push me to keep learning, but awaken the joy in it. Finally, I would like to thank my many wonderful colleagues at Wake Emergency Physicians—I am fortunate to be part of a practice with so many gifted clinicians.

David H. Rosenbaum, MD, FACEP, FAAEM

Contents

TEST 1

1. A 33-year-old female presents with numbness and weakness in the right side of her face for several days as shown (Fig. 1-1). The remainder of her examination is normal and she has no other symptoms. Which of the following is the next best step in management?

   A. Valacyclovir
   B. Prednisone
   C. Tissue plasminogen activator
   D. Sour candy
   E. Amoxicillin–clavulanic acid

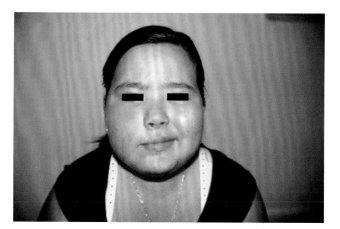

Figure 1-1

2. A 23-year-old female presents with 2 days of fever and severe right ankle pain and swelling. She denies a history of trauma. Past medical history is unremarkable. Physical examination reveals significant edema, effusion, tenderness, and pain on range of motion in the right ankle. Which of the following is the most likely etiology?

   A. S. aureus
   B. S. pneumoniae
   C. S. pyogenes
   D. Salmonella
   E. N. gonorrhoeae

3. A 77-year-old male with Parkinson disease is brought to the hospital with obstipation. His abdomen is distended and mildly tender with decreased bowel sounds. His abdominal x-ray is shown in Figure 1-2. Which of the following is the most likely diagnosis?

   A. Small bowel ischemia
   B. Viscus perforation
   C. Sigmoid volvulus
   D. Swallowed air
   E. Gastric outlet obstruction

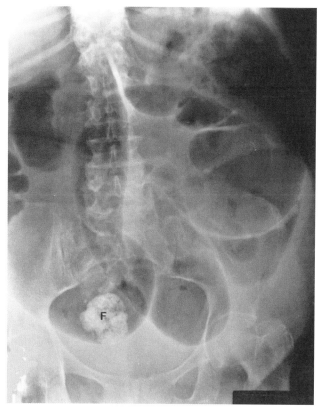

Figure 1-2

4. A 27-year-old female without past medical history presents with 2 days of pain in her right ear. The patient notes that the symptoms started with an itchy ear which progressed to pain, discharge, and hearing loss. Examination reveals an afebrile patient who is nontoxic, with moderate tenderness on manipulation of the auricle, erythema and edema of the tympanic canal, and no external rash. Cranial nerve examination is normal. Which of the following will be most helpful in treating this condition?

   A. Antihistamines
   B. Tympanostomy tubes
   C. Systemic antivirals
   D. Adenoidectomy
   E. Acetic acid otic washes

5. A 35-year-old female without any past medical history presents with a red, painful region on her right arm where she had a bug bite 3 days before. She denies fever. She is allergic to penicillin. Vital signs are normal. Physical examination is remarkable for a 10×6 cm^2 area on her right arm that is red, warm, tender, and sharply demarcated. There is no lymphangitic streaking or axillary lymphadenopathy. You diagnose her with cellulitis. Which of the following is the most appropriate choice of antibiotic?

   A. Clindamycin
   B. Doxycycline
   C. Dicloxacillin
   D. Linezolid
   E. Metronidazole

6. Clinically significant hypermagnesemia almost always occurs in the setting of:

   A. Renal insufficiency
   B. Pancreatitis
   C. Trauma
   D. Laxative abuse
   E. Alcoholism

7. Which of the following is true about myasthenia gravis (MG)?

   A. Incidence peaks in the eighth decade of life.
   B. Sensory deficits are most severe in the lower extremities.
   C. The most frequent initial symptom is dysarthria.
   D. Cooling decreases symptoms.
   E. Muscle weakness tends to worsen after long periods of rest.

8. A 57-year-old female with a history of hypertension presents with headache, mild confusion, and vomiting. She describes an acutely worsening global headache over the last several hours with nausea and vomiting. A family member states she is confused. She admits to noncompliance with her blood pressure medications for the last

week. Vital signs are: T 98.4, HR 92, BP 220/130, RR 20, SpO$_2$ 97%. Examination reveals a patient in moderate discomfort, papilledema, hypertensive retinopathy, and a nonfocal neurologic examination. Laboratory studies, EKG, and noncontrast CT brain are all normal. Which of the following is the most appropriate next step in management?

   A. Neurosurgical consultation
   B. Reduction of blood pressure by 25%
   C. Lumbar puncture
   D. Corticosteroids
   E. Noncontrast MRI of the brain

9. The hallmark of rubella is:

   A. Generalized lymphadenopathy
   B. Tonsillar exudates
   C. Koplik spots
   D. Febrile seizures
   E. Pastia lines

10. A 24-year-old male presents with bloody diarrhea for 2 days. Which of the following antibiotics is considered first-line therapy to treat all of the following organisms: *Salmonella*, *Shigella*, *Yersinia*, *Vibrio*, and enterotoxigenic *E. coli* (ETEC)?

    A. Trimethoprim–sulfamethoxazole
    B. Doxycycline
    C. Metronidazole
    D. Ciprofloxacin
    E. Erythromycin

11. A 34-year-old female presents to the ED with increasing low abdominal pain. She was seen by a colleague a week ago and diagnosed with an early ectopic pregnancy in her left fallopian tube. Her OB was consulted at that time and the patient was started on methotrexate therapy. What is the *most likely* cause of her abdominal pain?

    A. Treatment failure and increasing size of the ectopic pregnancy
    B. Tubal rupture
    C. Appendicitis
    D. "Separation pain" from methotrexate use
    E. Pelvic inflammatory disease (PID)

12. A 28-year-old female presents with fever and painful oral lesions for 2 days as shown in Figure 1-3. Which of the following is the most likely cause?

    A. HSV-1
    B. HSV-2
    C. Epstein–Barr virus
    D. Coxsackievirus
    E. Group A streptococcus

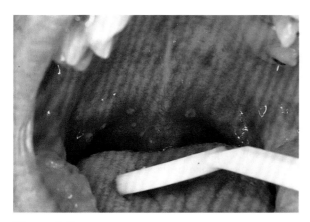

Figure 1-3

13. Which of the following is the optimal vascular access for adult trauma patients?

A. Single 14-g peripheral IV
B. Double 16-g peripheral IVs
C. Double 18-g peripheral IVs
D. Single triple-lumen catheter
E. Intraosseous catheter

14. A 34-year-old male presents after a high-speed motor vehicle collision with shortness of breath. A large flail segment is noted on his right lateral chest. Which of the following is the most appropriate therapy at this time?

A. Place the patient in the right lateral decubitus position
B. Place the patient in the left lateral decubitus position
C. Place a heavy weight on the flail segment
D. Administer 100% oxygen by nonrebreather mask
E. Perform rapid sequence intubation

15. A 68-year-old female presents with a 2-day history of left lower quadrant pain. CT reveals diverticulitis. Which of the following is true?

A. The recurrence rate of diverticulitis after a single, uncomplicated episode is 75%.
B. Avoiding nuts, seeds, and corn has not been shown to decrease recurrence.
C. Patients younger than 40 years with diverticulitis should have resection of the diseased segment of colon.
D. She should be admitted for colonoscopy to exclude colon cancer.
E. The mortality rate of hospitalized patients with acute diverticulitis is 35%.

16. Which of the following is true regarding botulism?

A. It is not contagious.
B. It usually causes an ascending paralysis.
C. It usually spares the cranial nerves.
D. It stimulates presynaptic acetylcholine release.
E. Broad-spectrum antibiotic therapy significantly improves survival.

17. Which of the following has the highest sensitivity for ruling out testicular torsion?

A. Normal cremasteric reflex
B. Presence of Prehn sign (relief of scrotal pain upon elevating the scrotum)
C. Normal urinalysis
D. Absence of fever
E. Absence of vomiting

18. A 61-year-old male presents to the ED with a chief complaint of chest pain. His EKG is shown (Fig. 1-4). Which of the following is the most likely explanation?

A. Ectopic atrial rhythm in the low atria
B. Limb lead reversal
C. Acute ischemia
D. Complete heart block
E. Undiagnosed tetralogy of Fallot

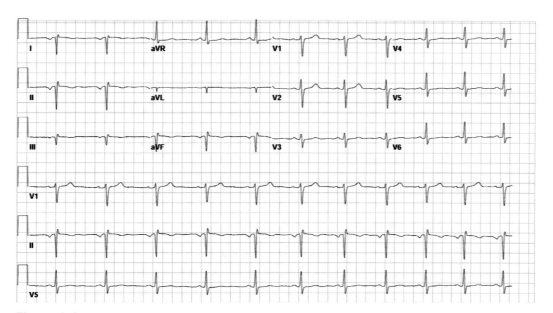

Figure 1-4

19. A 29-year-old female with a history of gout presents with a diffuse rash consisting of erythematous target lesions as well as oral sores for several days (Fig. 1-5). She recently started a course of medication for a urinary tract infection the week prior but cannot remember the name. Which of the following is the most likely cause?

    A. Ciprofloxacin
    B. Cefdinir
    C. Cephalexin
    D. Trimethoprim–sulfamethoxazole
    E. Macrodantin

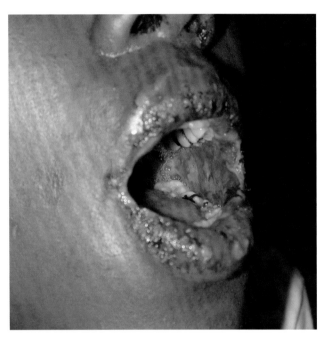

Figure 1-5

20. Which of the following is true regarding the treatment of a peritonsillar abscess (PTA)?

    A. Incision and drainage is superior to needle aspiration.
    B. Recurrent PTAs typically occur >1 year after the initial episode.
    C. Antibiotic therapy is as effective as surgical incision and drainage.
    D. Antibiotic coverage directed at Strep, Staph, and anaerobic species is necessary.
    E. Clinically, it is easy to distinguish a PTA from peritonsillar cellulitis.

21. Bites from which of the following snakes would most likely result in respiratory failure and death?

    A. Rattlesnake
    B. Cottonmouth (water moccasin)
    C. Coral snake
    D. Copperhead snake
    E. All of the above

22. A first-time mother presents with her 13-day-old infant with a chief complaint of seizures. The infant had an uncomplicated term delivery, is afebrile and had been well until the day of presentation. Which of the following is the most likely cause of this infant's seizures?

    A. Hypokalemia
    B. Hyponatremia
    C. Hypocalcemia
    D. Hypomagnesemia
    E. Maple syrup urine disease

23. Which of the following is true regarding candidiasis?

    A. Cutaneous candidiasis is the most common manifestation of infection.
    B. *Candida* is part of the normal oral flora in most humans.
    C. Thrush in otherwise healthy newborns is self-limited and does not require treatment.
    D. *Candida* is the most common cause of jock itch (tinea cruris).
    E. Maceration and lichenification with thick scale is the hallmark of cutaneous candidiasis.

24. Which of the following is true regarding the focused assessment of sonography in trauma (FAST) scan for evaluation of blunt abdominal trauma?

    A. Higher accuracy for penetrating trauma than blunt trauma
    B. Can distinguish between blood and urine
    C. Not associated with reductions in time to surgery or CT utilization
    D. More accurate than any single element of history or physical examination
    E. Sensitivity is much higher than specificity

25. A 26-year-old previously healthy male presents to the ED in January with a chief complaint of a 2-day history of fever, cough, diffuse body aches, and general malaise. He reports no history of influenza vaccination. His vital signs are P 110, BP 130/75, RR 18, SaO2 97% RA. Which of the following is true?

    A. Oseltamivir reduces the risk of serious complications of influenza
    B. Immunizing the patient with the influenza vaccine in the ED will hasten recovery
    C. Oseltamivir may cause nausea and vomiting
    D. Oseltamivir reduces spread of influenza to unaffected patients
    E. All of the above

26. A 34-year-old male with a history of HIV presents with headache. Contrast CT scan of the brain is shown in Figure 1-6. Which of the following is the most appropriate therapy?

   A. Surgical excision
   B. Mebendazole
   C. Sulfadiazine and pyrimethamine
   D. Methylprednisolone
   E. Clindamycin plus cefotaxime

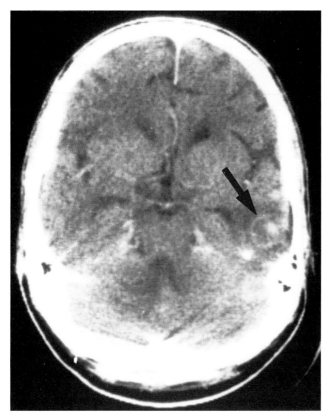

Figure 1-6

27. Delayed sequence intubation (DSI) is best used for which of the following patients?

   A. An elderly chronic obstructive pulmonary disease (COPD) patient with hypoxia, CO_2 retention, and excessive somnolence
   B. A 23-year-old trauma patient with hypoxia and a large hemothorax after a rollover motor vehicle collision (MVC)
   C. An agitated asthmatic patient, who persistently pulls off his oxygen mask exclaiming he can't breathe

   D. A 14-year-old comatose male with an intracranial hemorrhage after a biking injury
   E. A middle-aged congestive heart failure (CHF) patient with hypoxia and severe hypertension

28. Which of the following is the most appropriate suture to be used for gaping intraoral lacerations involving the mucosal surface?

   A. 6-0 nylon
   B. 6-0 polyglactin 910 (Vicryl)
   C. 4-0 nylon
   D. 4-0 polyglactin 910 (Vicryl)
   E. 2-0 silk

29. Which of the following is the most common cause of acute respiratory distress syndrome (ARDS)?

   A. Sepsis
   B. Near drowning
   C. Multiple blood transfusions
   D. Multiple blunt trauma
   E. Pancreatitis

30. A 5-year-old male presents with confirmed rotavirus diarrhea. He is tachycardic and lethargic with sunken eyes, poor skin turgor, and dry mucous membranes. Which of the following is the most appropriate next step in management?

   A. 0.45 NS 100 mL/hour drip
   B. D5 0.45 NS 20 mL/kg bolus
   C. 0.9 NS 100 mL/hour drip
   D. 0.9 NS 10 mL/kg bolus
   E. 0.9 NS 20 mL/kg bolus

31. Which of the following is true regarding gastroesophageal reflux disease (GERD) in infants?

   A. Ranitidine and metoclopramide are often required and are the mainstays of medical therapy.
   B. Vomiting is typically nonbilious and progressive, resulting in projectile emesis.
   C. Most infants respond to conservative measures such as smaller, thickened feedings and frequent burpings.
   D. Most infants with GERD ultimately suffer from failure to thrive.
   E. Infant GERD typically persists into adulthood.

32. A 6-year-old male presents with left hip pain and a limp. There is no history of trauma. The pain is relieved by rest. Plain radiographs are shown in Figure 1-7. Which of the following is true regarding this condition?

    A. It is much more common in boys than in girls.
    B. It is usually bilateral.
    C. It most commonly occurs in obese children.
    D. Almost all patients require surgical fixation.
    E. Joint aspiration confirms the diagnosis.

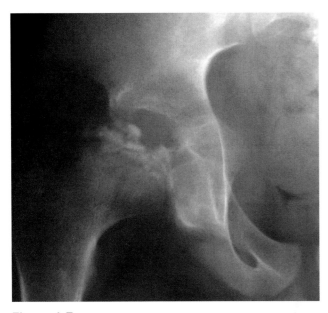

Figure 1-7

33. A 78-year-old male presents with sudden onset of right-sided arm and leg weakness. He was brought in by private car by his son, who states that the patient was totally normal 20 minutes prior to arrival. You immediately recognize the potential for acute stroke and initiate your stroke protocol, which involves immediate noncontrast CT brain. His blood pressure is 169/95. As the CT scan is being cleared, performance of which of the following diagnostic maneuvers is of paramount importance?

    A. EKG
    B. Temperature
    C. Blood glucose
    D. Prolactin
    E. PO challenge

34. Which of the following patients with a febrile seizure most likely requires further evaluation with a lumbar puncture (LP) to look for an infectious source?

    A. A fully vaccinated 10-month-old
    B. An 18-month-old with a recent "cold"
    C. A 9-month-old currently receiving antibiotics for otitis media
    D. A 4-year-old with a history of epilepsy
    E. An unvaccinated 5-year-old

35. Which of the following is true regarding reduction of an anterior shoulder dislocation?

    A. The Kocher maneuver is the most reliable method.
    B. Adequate muscle relaxation is the most important factor in successful reduction.
    C. The Hippocratic method should be the first one attempted.
    D. Scapular manipulation in the prone position is the method of choice in third-trimester pregnant patients.
    E. Intra-articular anesthetic injection is contraindicated.

36. Which of the following is the best modality to diagnose posterior sternoclavicular dislocation?

    A. Anteroposterior chest x-ray
    B. Lateral chest x-ray
    C. Anteroposterior clavicle x-ray
    D. CT chest
    E. Thoracic ultrasound

37. A 62-year-old female presents with left lower quadrant abdominal pain. You suspect acute sigmoid diverticulitis. Which of the following symptoms is likely to also be present?

    A. Vomiting
    B. Hematochezia
    C. Dysuria
    D. Change in bowel habits
    E. Anorexia

38. Which of the following is true regarding nitroprusside?

    A. Cyanide toxicity is common.
    B. Extravasation causes severe local skin necrosis.
    C. It decreases intracranial pressure (ICP).
    D. It is safe for use during pregnancy.
    E. It has a delayed onset of action compared with other IV antihypertensive agents.

39. Which of the following is true regarding the potential space between the labeled structures (Fig. 1-8)?

A. It is known as the pouch of Douglas
B. It is the most posterior part of the peritoneal cavity
C. It is the most anterior part of the retroperitoneum
D. It is the first view performed on the FAST scan
E. It is more sensitive when the patient is in Trendelenburg position

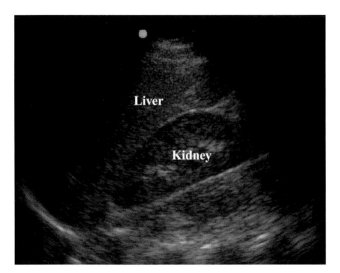

Figure 1-8

40. A third-year medical student presents to the ED with diffuse arthralgias of the hands, wrists, and knees. She has been taking isoniazid (INH) because she was exposed to a patient with active tuberculosis and subsequently had a positive purified protein derivative (PPD) test. She is most likely suffering from a syndrome mimicking:

A. Systemic sclerosis
B. Systemic lupus erythematosus (SLE)
C. Gouty arthritis
D. Rheumatoid arthritis
E. Sjögren syndrome

41. A 48-year-old male presents to the emergency department with abdominal pain 4 months after an uncomplicated Roux-en-Y gastric bypass. The patient's initial postoperative course was uncomplicated and he has been losing weight as expected. However, over the past few weeks, he has noted intermittent, crampy, and diffuse abdominal pain that appears unrelated to eating. In the ED, his vital signs, blood tests, and CT are normal. What's the likely explanation for the patient's symptoms?

A. Drug seeking
B. Internal hernia

C. Gastrogastric fistula
D. Postoperative gastroesophageal reflux
E. Cholelithiasis

42. A 24-year-old male presents with abdominal fullness. He is very nervous, but in no acute distress. Vital signs and physical examination are normal. An obstructive radiography series is ordered. Which of the following is the most appropriate next step in management (see Fig. 1-9)?

A. MRI abdomen
B. Surgery
C. Polyethylene glycol
D. NG aspiration
E. Endotracheal intubation

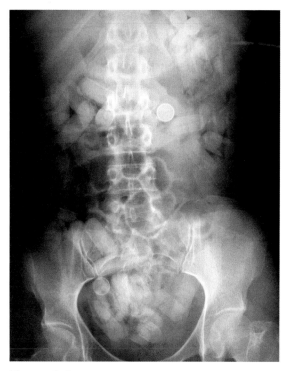

Figure 1-9

43. Which of the following is true regarding the Ottawa ankle rules (OAR)?

A. Patients who do not meet the OAR criteria never have an ankle fracture.
B. The OAR should not be applied to intoxicated patients.
C. The OAR criteria include a positive "squeeze" test.
D. The OAR can be applied to pediatric patients older than 8 years.
E. The specificity of the OAR is roughly 90%.

44. A concerned mother brings her 15-year-old daughter to the ED with a chief complaint of irregular vaginal bleeding. The patient experienced menarche at age 13 and has never had regular periods. Recently, the bleeding has been heavier and more irregular than normal. She reports no history of easy bruising and has no petechiae on examination. Her hemoglobin is 11 g/dL. Which of the following is the most likely cause of her symptoms?

    A. Hyperthyroidism
    B. Anovulation
    C. Endometriosis
    D. Asymptomatic *Chlamydia* infection
    E. Polycystic ovarian syndrome

45. A 35-year-old male with a history of sickle cell disease presents with acute onset of fever, malaise, fatigue, and lightheadedness. Physical examination demonstrates a tachycardic patient with pale conjunctivae. You suspect aplastic crisis and draw a complete blood count with reticulocyte count. You review his old records and note that the patient's baseline hemoglobin level is 8 g/dL. Which of the following laboratory abnormalities is most consistent with an aplastic crisis?

    A. Hemoglobin 8 g/dL, reticulocyte count 6%
    B. Hemoglobin 8 g/dL, reticulocyte count 1%
    C. Hemoglobin 6 g/dL, reticulocyte count 6%
    D. Hemoglobin 6 g/dL, reticulocyte count 1%
    E. Hemoglobin 4 g/dL, reticulocyte count 6%

46. A 22-year-old male presents with rash, lightheadedness, and generalized malaise. He denies fever or pruritus. A few hours before presentation, he was seen in another emergency department (ED) and received treatment for syphilis. He denies any medication allergies. His vital signs are 99.2, 94, 16, 134/65, 99% RA. His physical examination demonstrates a normal uvula, no pulmonary wheezes, and a faint macular rash on his trunk and abdomen, which he states was there before he received the treatment today. Which of the following is the most appropriate next step in management?

    A. Immediate endotracheal intubation
    B. IM epinephrine
    C. Diphenhydramine and famotidine
    D. Prednisone
    E. Acetaminophen and observation

47. What is the most common cause of traveler's diarrhea?

    A. *Shigella* spp.
    B. *Giardia lamblia*
    C. *Salmonella* spp.
    D. Rotavirus
    E. Enterotoxigenic *Escherichia coli* (ETEC)

48. A 72-year-old male arrives at the hospital with acute right-sided facial droop and right arm and leg weakness. He is immediately sent to the CT scanner where he has a generalized seizure lasting just over a minute. While the seizure terminates without intervention, the patient is brought back to the emergency department immediately because of severe bradycardia and ventricular escape beats. In addition to atropine, what other measures will most likely be helpful?

    A. Dopamine
    B. Continuous albuterol
    C. Epinephrine
    D. Bicarbonate
    E. Calcium

49. Which of the following is true regarding gonococcal septic arthritis?

    A. Open surgical drainage is usually required.
    B. It is more common in men than in women.
    C. Genitourinary symptoms occur in most patients.
    D. Synovial fluid Gram stain is positive more often than culture.
    E. The hip is the most common joint affected.

50. Which of the following parenteral agents is the initial preferred agent for blood pressure management in patients with acute aortic dissection?

    A. Hydralazine
    B. Enalapril
    C. Labetalol
    D. Diltiazem
    E. Nicardipine

51. A 23-year-old female with sickle cell disease presents with pain in her right shin and fevers for 2 weeks. She never has leg pain with her sickle cell pain crises. An x-ray demonstrates evidence of osteomyelitis. Which of the following is the most likely etiologic agent?

    A. *S. aureus*
    B. *Salmonella*
    C. *Aspergillus*
    D. *Neisseria gonorrhoeae*
    E. *Pseudomonas*

52. A 64-year-old male with a history of hypertension presents to the ED with a painful rash on the right side of his back spreading to his trunk (see Fig. 1-10). Which of the following underlying diseases should be suspected?

    A. Chronic lymphocytic leukemia
    B. Human immunodeficiency virus (HIV)
    C. Asplenia
    D. Rheumatoid arthritis
    E. He is most likely to be healthy

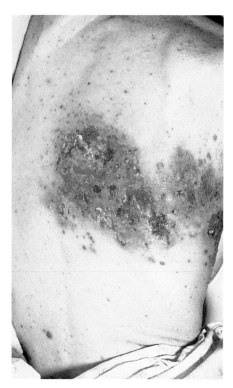

Figure 1-10

53. A 57-year-old female with a history of hypertension presents for evaluation of a 1-day history of pleuritic right-sided chest pain. She has no leg pain or swelling. She is afebrile with a P 82, RR 14, SaO_2 97% on room air. Which of the following is true?

   A. The pulmonary embolism (PE) rule-out criteria ("PERC rule") can be used to exclude pulmonary embolism
   B. A d-dimer with an age-adjusted cutoff could be used to determine if imaging is needed
   C. A CT pulmonary angiogram (CTA) of the chest should be performed to exclude pulmonary embolism
   D. No further testing is needed because the patient is low-risk by Wells criteria
   E. Negative Doppler venous imaging of the patient's legs excludes a pulmonary embolism

54. The most common sexually transmitted organism in the United States is:

   A. *T. pallidum*
   B. *C. trachomatis*
   C. *Neisseria gonorrhoeae*
   D. HSV
   E. *H. ducreyi*

55. A 22-year-old G1 female at 28 weeks gestational age presents to the ED after a motor vehicle collision. She has right-sided pneumothorax and a unilateral pubic ramus fracture, for which she is being treated. Review of records indicates that her blood type is A negative.

Which of the following is the most appropriate next step in management?

   A. Transfusion of one unit packed red blood cells
   B. Transfusion of six units of fresh frozen plasma (FFP)
   C. Administration of 50 mcg RhIG
   D. Administration of 300 mcg RhIG
   E. No specific management

56. A 65-year-old male presents with acute onset of back pain and bilateral leg weakness after a recent diagnosis of prostate cancer. Physical examination demonstrates 3/5 strength in both of his lower extremities and tenderness to palpation of his lower back. An emergent MRI demonstrates epidural lumbar spinal cord compression secondary to metastasis. Which of the following is the most appropriate initial consultation?

   A. Radiation oncology
   B. General surgery
   C. Urology
   D. Neurology
   E. Neurosurgery

57. A 23-year-old female presents with pain in her right lateral chest after a low-speed motor vehicle collision. She is most tender in the fifth rib at the posterior axillary line. Her vital signs are normal. Which of the following is the most appropriate next step in evaluation?

   A. Chest x-ray
   B. Rib x-rays
   C. CT abdomen/pelvis
   D. CT brain
   E. Cervical spine radiographs

58. A 35-year-old female presents in a coma (Glasgow Coma Scale 3) after a motor vehicle crash and is intubated for airway protection. Further evaluation reveals no life-threatening chest, abdomen, or pelvic injuries. Vital signs are normal. A computed tomography (CT) scan of the head is normal. Which of the following is the most likely diagnosis?

   A. Epidural hematoma
   B. Subdural hematoma
   C. Diffuse axonal injury (DAI)
   D. Cerebral contusion
   E. Intraparenchymal hematoma

59. Which of the following correctly matches the vasculitic syndrome to its primary clinical manifestations?

   A. Polyarteritis nodosa (PAN) and peripheral neuropathy and bowel ischemia
   B. Takayasu arteritis and oral and genital ulcerations
   C. Wegener granulomatosis and cardiac ischemia
   D. Behçet disease and sinusitis, otitis, and nasal congestion
   E. Churg–Strauss syndrome and glomerulonephritis

60. A 52-year-old previously healthy female collapses while coaching her daughter's soccer team and bystanders initiate chest compressions. When EMS arrives, they find the patient in ventricular fibrillation. EMS immediately defibrillates the patient and initiates ACLS. They also placed a temporary supraglottic airway. After following ACLS algorithms for 14 minutes including three defibrillation attempts, the patient experiences a return of spontaneous circulation (ROSC). Shortly after arrival in the emergency department (ED), a definitive airway is obtained and placement is confirmed by x-ray. The patient is noted to be comatose, with a GCS of 3, and has the following vital signs: T 95.8°F, P 115, BP 79/40 (mean arterial pressure [MAP] = 53), SaO$_2$ 97% on the ventilator. Which of the following is true?

    A. The patient is not a candidate for therapeutic hypothermia because her GCS score is too low.
    B. The patient should undergo immediate cooling with a specialized intravenous cooling catheter.
    C. The patient is not likely to benefit from cooling because her core temperature is already low.
    D. Vasopressors are needed to raise her blood pressure prior to the initiation of cooling.
    E. Shivering is an expected, benign side effect of therapy, and does not require treatment.

61. Which of the following is the most common cause of death among African-American adolescents?

    A. Infection
    B. Cancer
    C. Motor vehicle collision
    D. Gunshot wound
    E. Drug overdose

62. Which of the following is true about appendicitis in adult women?

    A. Pregnant women are twice as likely as nonpregnant women to develop appendicitis.
    B. Cervical motion tenderness (CMT) rules out appendicitis.
    C. Even in the third trimester, most pregnant women still have pain in the right lower quadrant.
    D. Due to anatomic changes, appendicitis in pregnant women occurs most often in the third trimester.
    E. Fetal abortion occurs in 50% of pregnant women with perforated appendicitis.

63. A 44-year-old male presents with hypotension after a motor vehicle collision. His chest x-ray is normal. Pelvis x-ray is shown in Figure 1-11. Which of the following is the most important next step in management?

    A. Foley catheterization
    B. CT scan of the abdomen and pelvis
    C. Tightening a bedsheet around the pelvis
    D. ED thoracotomy
    E. Inlet and outlet radiographs of the pelvis

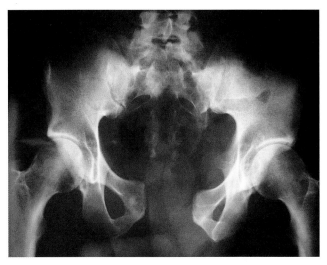

Figure 1-11

64. When compared to younger adults, which of the following traumatic injuries is more common in elderly patients?

    A. Subdural hematoma
    B. Odontoid fracture
    C. Flail chest
    D. Central cord syndrome
    E. All of the above

65. Which of the following is true regarding the role of ipratropium in asthma management?

    A. The main benefit of ipratropium, instead of atropine or other anticholinergic drugs, is ipratropium has a more rapid onset of action.
    B. Ipratropium is useful as a sole bronchodilator in the treatment of acute asthma exacerbations.
    C. Ipratropium is most useful as an adjunct for patients with severe asthma exacerbations.
    D. Ipratropium has never been proven to be of benefit in patients with acute asthma exacerbations.
    E. None of the above

66. A 22-year-old female presents with intermittent fever and chills for 2 weeks. She has no past medical history, but reports using intravenous heroin several times a week. Physical examination reveals a febrile, ill-appearing woman with a heart murmur. Blood cultures are most likely to reveal which of the following organisms?

    A. *S. aureus*
    B. *Streptococcus pneumoniae*
    C. *Streptococcus viridans*
    D. *Pseudomonas aeruginosa*
    E. *Candida albicans*

67. A 67-year-old female with diabetes, hypertension, and a history of an aortoiliac bypass graft presents with abdominal pain and dark, "funny-smelling" stools. She states the symptoms started 2 days ago and seem to have gone away as she had a "nearnormal" bowel movement this morning and no longer has pain. On examination, she has guaiac positive, dark brown, but not melenic stool. Which of the following must be excluded as a cause of hemorrhage?

A. Acute mesenteric ischemia
B. Abdominal aortic aneurysm (AAA)
C. Aortoenteric fistula
D. Duodenal ulcer
E. Ischemic colitis

68. A 26-year-old female presents with dyspnea and pleuritic chest pain and is subsequently diagnosed with a PE. She is not pregnant, takes no oral contraceptive therapy, and is a nonsmoker, but she notes that her mother has had two PEs. Which of the following is the most likely cause of this patient's PE?

A. Plasminogen deficiency
B. Nephrotic syndrome
C. Cervical cancer
D. Factor V Leiden
E. Protein S deficiency

69. A 34-year-old male is brought into the emergency department (ED) after a motor vehicle collision. Which of the following findings is an indication to perform a computed tomography (CT) of the abdomen/pelvis with IV contrast to look for renal injury in this patient?

A. Microscopic hematuria
B. Gross hematuria
C. Flank pain
D. Flank ecchymosis
E. Penile hematoma

70. A 42-year-old female who is a self-described "seafood fanatic" presents with a chief complaint of an "allergic reaction." Thirty minutes after eating tuna at a local restaurant she developed a severe headache, palpitations, nausea, abdominal cramping, and remarkable facial flushing. She has eaten fish for her entire life without incident. Which of the following is true?

A. She should be given subcutaneous epinephrine and parenteral corticosteroids.
B. Perioral paresthesias are typically a classic feature of this illness.
C. Upon discharge, the patient should be advised to avoid all seafood products in the future.

D. The patient should expect symptoms to resolve slowly over the course of 1 week.
E. The symptoms are due to excessive histamine levels in the fish.

71. Which of the following is true regarding posterior shoulder dislocations?

A. External rotation is usually intact.
B. Neurovascular injury is more common than in anterior dislocations.
C. The absence of pain excludes the diagnosis.
D. Seizures are a common mechanism of injury.
E. Recurrent injury is more common than in anterior dislocations.

72. In a perilunate dislocation, which bone is dorsally dislocated?

A. Lunate
B. Scaphoid
C. Capitate
D. Hamate
E. Pisiform

73. Which of the following is true with respect to carditis caused by Lyme disease?

A. Patients most commonly experience initial symptoms several years after the initial tick bite.
B. Patients most commonly present with variable degrees of atrioventricular (AV) block.
C. Patients most commonly suffer from symptoms of CHF.
D. The prognosis of patients with Lyme carditis is poor, as almost one-third of patients ultimately require a heart transplant.
E. Most patients are sero-negative for anti-Borrelia antibodies at the time of presentation.

74. A 76-year-old female with a history of hypertension, diabetes, and hyperlipidemia presents with rapid palpitations that started one day prior to her ED evaluation. They have waxed and waned in intensity but seemed more persistent on the day of presentation. Her EKG is shown (Fig. 1-12). Aside from tachycardia, her vital signs are stable. Which of the following is true?

A. The two pads for cardioversion should both be placed on the front of the chest
B. Electrical cardioversion is the treatment of choice
C. The primary ED treatment goal should be controlling the heart rate
D. If the patient converts to normal sinus rhythm, no anticoagulation is needed
E. In patients with heart failure, digoxin is the preferred agent

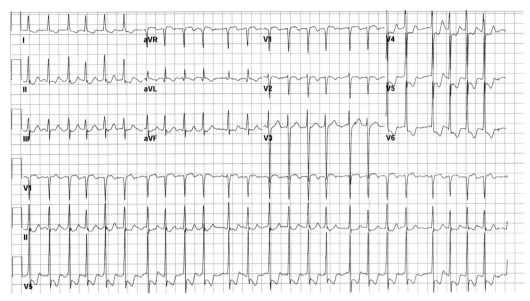

Figure 1-12

75. A 23-year-old female presents with fever, chills, and right flank pain. She just completed treatment for pyelonephritis with a 2-week course of ciprofloxacin. The patient states that the symptoms are very similar to when she had pyelonephritis and she cannot understand why she did not get better with the antibiotics. She admits to having waited "longer than usual" before seeking care for the pyelonephritis during the first visit, but swears that she took all the antibiotics as directed. The initial urine culture revealed *E. coli* that was sensitive to ciprofloxacin. Which of the following is the most appropriate next step in management?

   A. Switch to cefpodoxime for 10 days
   B. Continue ciprofloxacin for 7 more days
   C. Switch to trimethoprim–sulfamethoxazole (TMP-SMX) for 3 days
   D. Switch to metronidazole for 3 days
   E. CT scan of the abdomen/pelvis

76. A 26-year-old female involved in an MVC has persistent abdominal tenderness after a negative CT of the abdomen and pelvis. Her vital signs are normal and there is no seatbelt sign. Which of the following is true?

   A. She should be admitted for further observation and serial physical examinations
   B. She should undergo ED observation with repeat CT imaging in 6 hours if her tenderness persists
   C. A FAST scan should be performed to detect intraperitoneal bleeding that may have been missed by CT

   D. She may be discharged with close outpatient follow-up
   E. She should be under repeat CT testing with oral contrast to further investigate possible bowel injuries

77. A 22-year-old male presents with acute onset of right scrotal pain for 2 hours. He has severe, colicky pain with nausea and vomiting but no fevers, chills, or dysuria. Vital signs are normal, but the patient is in extreme discomfort. Abdominal examination is normal. Testicular examination reveals a tender right testis with an absent ipsilateral cremasteric reflex. Which of the following is the most appropriate next step in evaluation?

   A. CT scan of the abdomen and pelvis
   B. MRI of the abdomen and pelvis
   C. Color Doppler ultrasonography of the scrotum
   D. Retrograde urethrogram
   E. Elicitation of the bulbocavernosus reflex

78. A 29-year-old male is sent by his primary care doctor's office for evaluation of an abnormal EKG. He is asymptomatic and his physical examination is normal. The EKG is shown in Figure 1-13. Which of the following is the most appropriate next step in management?

   A. No acute therapy
   B. Atropine 1 mg IV
   C. Amiodarone 150 mg IV
   D. Transcutaneous pacing
   E. Synchronized cardioversion at 50 J

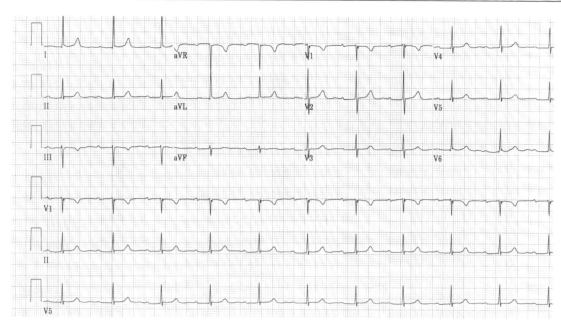

Figure 1-13

79. Which of the following sleeping positions is the best method to reduce the risk of sudden infant death syndrome (SIDS)?

   A. Prone
   B. Supine
   C. Side
   D. Standing
   E. Head down

80. A 32-year-old male presents to the ED with headache and fever for 2 days. He also reports a stiff neck and photophobia. Past medical history is unremarkable. Physical examination reveals a febrile patient with nuchal rigidity, no papilledema, and no focal neurologic deficits. Which of the following is the most appropriate next step in management?

   A. Antibiotic therapy
   B. Antibiotic therapy with corticosteroids
   C. CT brain with IV contrast
   D. MRI brain with gadolinium contrast
   E. Lumbar puncture

81. A 78-year-old male presents with marked left foot weakness and hypoesthesia. In addition, his family states that he is not acting himself and seems to be having difficulty making decisions. Which of the following arteries is most likely affected?

   A. Vertebrobasilar artery
   B. Posterior cerebral artery
   C. Middle cerebral artery
   D. Anterior cerebral artery
   E. None of the above

82. A 37-year-old male presents with left eye pain and redness after rubbing his eye the day before. Slit lamp evaluation with fluorescein stain is shown in Figure 1-14. Which of the following is the most appropriate next step in management?

   A. Topical antivirals
   B. Topical steroids
   C. Topical antibiotics
   D. Intravenous acetazolamide
   E. Emergent ophthalmologic consultation

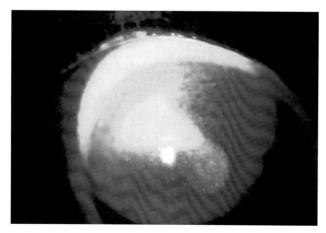

Figure 1-14

83. A 34-year-old male complaining of neck pain and leg pain is brought in by EMS after hitting a tree while driving his car. A cervical spine CT is negative and x-rays of his foot reveal no fracture. He has no neurologic complaints and his neurologic examination is normal. However, he has persistent cervical spine tenderness on examination. Which of the following is true?

    A. A cervical spine MRI should be performed
    B. Flexion and extension views of the spine are needed
    C. Either MRI or flexion–extension plain films should be performed to diagnose ligamentous injury
    D. Cervical spine CT may miss 15% of cervical spine fractures
    E. Injuries found on MRI are unlikely to require surgical intervention

84. A 29-year-old female with a history of multiple sclerosis (MS) presents to the ED with a chief complaint of a 2-day history of right arm weakness and clumsiness. She reports that these symptoms are similar to a past "MS flare." Her examination reveals proximal and distal right arm weakness but no other findings. Which of the following is the best next step?

    A. CT to exclude a stroke
    B. Admission for plasma exchange
    C. Neurology consult
    D. MRI to verify a demyelinating plaque is causing the symptoms
    E. 1,000 mg IV methylprednisolone

85. A 37-year-old male presents with eye pain and redness as shown (Fig. 1-15). He has experienced no trauma. Which of the following is the most likely diagnosis?

    A. Corneal abrasion
    B. Anterior uveitis
    C. Acute angle closure glaucoma
    D. Pinguecula
    E. Pterygium

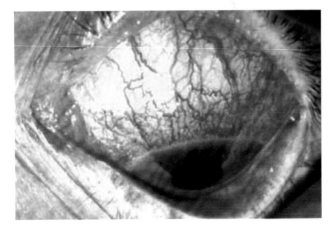

Figure 1-15

86. An 11-year-old male hit the curb while riding his bicycle and was thrown forward into his handlebars. The classic injury associated with this accident is:

    A. Myocardial contusion
    B. Pancreatic injury
    C. Liver contusion
    D. Splenic contusion
    E. Diaphragmatic rupture

87. The best indicator of successful neonatal resuscitation is:

    A. Improved skin color
    B. Improved oxygen saturation
    C. Improved respiratory rate
    D. Improved heart rate
    E. Improved muscle tone

88. A 62-year-old healthy male presents with a 1-day history of painful, partially crusted vesicular rash over his left flank radiating to his left hemiabdomen that appears most consistent with shingles. Which of the following is true?

    A. Prednisone is a useful adjunct to reduce the incidence of postherpetic neuralgia
    B. Antiviral therapy decreases the rate of postherpetic neuralgia with or without steroids
    C. Antiviral therapy speeds healing from the rash
    D. The shingles vaccine may help hasten recovery from the rash and acute neuritis
    E. All of the above

89. Which of the following is the most frequently affected structure in thoracic outlet syndrome?

    A. Subclavian artery
    B. Subclavian vein
    C. Ulnar nerve
    D. Radial nerve
    E. Median nerve

90. A 25-year-old female presents with acute onset of a severe occipital headache. CT reveals a subarachnoid hemorrhage (SAH). Which of the following clinical findings is likely present?

    A. Focal neurologic deficit
    B. Exertional activity immediately before symptoms
    C. Seizure
    D. Nausea
    E. Intraocular hemorrhage

91. When compared with patients with deep venous thrombosis (DVT) of the lower extremities, patients with an upper extremity DVT

    A. Tend to be older
    B. Are more likely to have an underlying diagnosis of cancer

C. More often have an inherited or acquired hypercoagulable state

D. Do not require anticoagulation

E. More commonly experience complications as a result of the DVT

92. Thirty minutes after a 35-year-old female presents to the ED with a severe asthma exacerbation, you intubate her because she is showing signs of fatigue and ventilatory failure. You use ketamine and succinylcholine, and pass the endotracheal through the vocal cords without difficulty. A colleague who is assisting you aggressively "bags" the patient until the respiratory therapist connects the mechanical ventilator. Thirty seconds after intubation, the nurse reports that the patient's blood pressure (BP) has dropped to 93/46. Her BP before intubation was 138/80. The patient has an 18-gauge peripheral intravenous (IV) line in her left antecubital fossa and her trachea appears midline. What is the best course of action?

A. Ask the nurses to place a second large-bore peripheral IV and immediately bolus the patient with 2 L of normal saline.

B. Extubate the patient and deliver breaths using a bag–valve mask.

C. Disconnect the ventilator but keep the endotracheal tube (ETT) in place and allow the patient to exhale.

D. Ask the nurses to start a dopamine drip at 5 µg/kg/minute.

E. Perform an immediate needle thoracostomy.

93. A 55-year-old female presents with 1 to 2 days of palpitations, anxiety, agitation, tachycardia, and hypertension. Her thyroid-stimulating hormone level is very low and her free T_4 and free T_3 levels are elevated. Which of the following is the most appropriate sequence in which to administer ideal therapies?

A. Potassium iodide → Propranolol → Propylthiouracil → Dexamethasone

B. Potassium iodide → Propylthiouracil → Dexamethasone → Propranolol

C. Dexamethasone → Propranolol → Propylthiouracil → Potassium iodide

D. Propylthiouracil → Potassium iodide → Propranolol → Dexamethasone

E. Propranolol → Potassium iodide → Dexamethasone → Propylthiouracil

94. The most common cause of hypomagnesemia in the ED is likely

A. Alcoholism

B. Diuretic therapy

C. Acute tubular necrosis

D. Chronic diarrhea

E. Diabetic ketoacidosis (DKA)

95. A 3-year-old previously healthy female is brought to the emergency room after ingesting three of her mother's 2.5 mg glyburide tablets, believing they were candy. Her mother estimates that the ingestion occurred almost 2 hours before presenting, but she only noticed the open box shortly before arrival. She states her daughter seems "ok" but has been a bit more tired and irritable than normal. The patient's initial blood glucose is 58. Which of the following is the best next step?

A. Administration of ½ an ampule of intravenous D50W and observation in the emergency room for 4 hours.

B. Administration of 5 mL/kg of intravenous D25W and observation in the emergency room for 4 hours.

C. Administration of 5 mL/kg of intravenous D10W and admission for overnight observation.

D. Administration of 10 mL/kg of intravenous D10W and observation in the emergency room for 4 hours.

E. Administration of 5 mL/kg of intravenous D10W, subcutaneous octreotide at 1 mcg/kg, and observation in the emergency room for 4 hours.

96. Which of the following is the most common cause of dysuria?

A. Bacterial infection

B. Viral infection

C. Fungal infection

D. Parasitic infection

E. Allergic urethritis

97. The most widely used critical care ventilatory strategy in acute asthmatic patients aims to accomplish which of the following objectives?

A. Patients are purposefully hypoventilated, maintaining elevated $Paco_2$ values, to keep their airway pressures at safe levels to avoid barotrauma.

B. Patients are purposefully hyperventilated to bring their $Paco_2$ levels back to normal because ventilatory failure is the primary reason for intubating patients in status asthmaticus.

C. The initial ventilator settings are no different than for a patient intubated for airway protection due to altered mental status.

D. Inspiratory flow rates are set very low to avoid causing very high peak airway pressures due to bronchoconstriction.

E. The inspiratory flow curve should be a ramp-style wave instead of a square-style wave to maximize expiratory time.

98. A 65-year-old female pedestrian presents after being struck by a car moving at about 20 mph. She has an obvious, open, deformed leg fracture and was unable to walk at the scene. Her prehospital vital signs are P 105, 85/55, and 100% RA. She is awake and alert and in significant pain. You confirm that her airway, breathing, and pulses are intact. On visual inspection, she has an open tibial shaft fracture and has decreased sensation distal to the fracture. Which of the following is the most important next step in management?

    A. Splint application to leg
    B. Irrigation of leg wound
    C. IV gentamicin and cefazolin
    D. Tetanus immunization
    E. Chest and pelvis x-rays

99. A 65-year-old female presents with right eye pain, irritation, foreign body sensation, and tearing. Skin lesions are seen on the right side of the forehead and the conjunctivae are injected. Slit lamp examination reveals pseudodendrites. Which of the following is true?

    A. Patients with associated nasal vesicles should not receive topical ophthalmic steroids.
    B. A prodrome is uncommon.
    C. Cranial nerve VII is most commonly involved.
    D. Anterior uveal involvement is dependent upon severity of corneal disease.
    E. Systemic antivirals are more effective than topical antivirals.

100. Which of the following is true regarding the management and prognosis of trigeminal neuralgia?

    A. Remission, with or without treatment, rarely occurs.
    B. Antiviral medications directed at herpes and corticosteroids have been shown to reduce the duration of pain and prevent recurrence.
    C. In addition to medical treatment, all patients should be referred to a neurologist for further evaluation by MRI.
    D. Fifty percent of patients will eventually require neurosurgical ablation of the trigeminal nerve.
    E. All patients should be loaded with phenytoin and prescribed an outpatient regimen.

1. **Answer B.** With unilateral upper and lower facial weakness and the absence of other concerning neurologic features, the diagnosis is very likely idiopathic facial nerve palsy, also known as Bell palsy. Steroid therapy (prednisone 60 mg daily for 1 week) has been shown to improve outcomes in Bell palsy, but antiviral therapy in the absence of steroids appears to have no effect. Tissue plasminogen activator would be indicated for an acute ischemic stroke within 3 hours of presentation, but would not be appropriate in this case. Sour candy can be used to treat sialolithiasis, but there is no observable swelling to suggest this. Antibiotics are not indicated for the management of Bell palsy. (Figure from Salimpour RR, Salimpour P, Salimpour P. *Photographic Atlas of Pediatric Disorders and Diagnosis.* 1st ed. Philadelphia, PA: Wolters Kluwer; 2013.)

2. **Answer E.** The patient has evidence of acute monoarticular arthritis. In a young, sexually active patient without prior history of arthritis, the most likely bacterial cause is gonococcus. The overall most common cause of septic arthritis is *S. aureus*. Choices B, C, and D are less common causes. Septic arthritis is a joint-threatening infection diagnosed by synovial fluid analysis. It must be aggressively treated with intravenous antibiotics and possible surgical irrigation, even though gonococcal arthritis rarely requires surgical management.

3. **Answer C.** The image indicates sigmoid volvulus. Abdominal radiography lacks sensitivity for small bowel ischemia and signs such as thumbprinting and pneumatosis are rare. Viscus perforation would be suspected if there were free air seen under the diaphragm, but abdominal radiography is incompletely sensitive for evaluation of perforation. Swallowed air would be unlikely to cause abdominal distention and obstipation. Gastric outlet obstruction might not demonstrate any findings on x-ray. Of all the answer choices, sigmoid volvulus is the only diagnosis that can be made solely relying on abdominal radiography. (Figure from Daffner RH. *Clinical Radiology: The Essentials.* 3rd ed. Philadelphia, PA: Lippincott Williams & Wilkins; 2007.)

4. **Answer E.** The patient has otitis externa, inflammation of the external ear, and tympanic canal almost always because of infection. Trauma and excessive moisture are commonly implicated in the development of the condition. Patients generally present with otalgia and otorrhea. Debridement of the external ear canal is the most important aspect of treatment. In nontoxic patients, this is achieved with topical acetic acid washes with or without topical antibiotics and steroids. A cotton or methylcellulose wick for drainage of the tympanic canal may be placed 1 cm deep in the ear and stays for 2 days. Systemically ill patients or diabetic patients require systemic antibiotics and sometimes admission. Antihistamines can be used for symptomatic relief but do not affect the duration of illness. Tympanostomy tubes and adenoidectomy may be indicated for prevention of chronic/recurrent otitis media but have no effect on acute management of otitis externa. Herpes zoster can occur in the ear and is referred to as Ramsay Hunt syndrome. This condition requires antivirals and is associated with a vesicular rash and sometimes cranial nerve palsies.

5. **Answer A.** Cellulitis in the healthy patient is most often caused by *Streptococci* and *Staphylococci*. In most communities, methicillin-resistant *Staphylococcus aureus* (MRSA) accounts for a significant number of staphylococcal infections. Thus, initial antibiotic therapy is usually with a penicillinase-resistant penicillin or first-generation cephalosporin to treat streptococci plus TMP-SMX to treat MRSA. Doxycycline covers MRSA but is inadequate against streptococci, so it should be combined with amoxicillin (or cephalexin). Clindamycin can be used as monotherapy, but there is significant resistance to clindamycin among MRSA isolates in many communities. This patient has an allergy to penicillin, and dicloxacillin is therefore contraindicated. In addition, dicloxacillin is ineffective against MRSA. Linezolid is an effective, relatively new treatment that is generally reserved for infections that are not amenable to treatment with the other options listed above. Metronidazole covers anaerobes only and would not be appropriate as monotherapy for cellulitis. Note that in its most recent guidelines (2011), the Infectious Disease Society of America differentiates between purulent and nonpurulent cellulitis. The rationale behind this division is to illustrate that MRSA is typically responsible for abscess formation and the development of purulent drainage. Thus, in cases in which both cellulitis and an abscess are present (or forming), empiric therapy directed only at MRSA is appropriate, and dual therapy is unnecessary. Clindamycin, doxycycline, TMP-SMX, and linezolid are all useful for monotherapy in this setting.

6. **Answer A.** The kidneys are almost wholly responsible for magnesium excretion and are able to enhance excretion in the setting of a magnesium load. Therefore, in the absence of renal insufficiency, hypermagnesemia rarely occurs. Abuse of magnesium-containing laxatives may cause a transient increase in magnesium levels but

will not persist in the setting of normal renal function. Trauma could feasibly lead to hypermagnesemia if associated with rhabdomyolysis.

7. **Answer D.** The fact that cooling improves the symptoms of MG is the basis for the "ice test." When ptosis is present, an ice pack is placed over the affected eye for 2 minutes. It is thought that the local cooling results in a slowing of the kinetics of the acetylcholine receptor, allowing for a prolonged effect of acetylcholine and an improvement in symptoms. In clinical studies, 80% of patients with ptosis due to MG experienced some improvement with a locally applied ice pack. MG has a bimodal peak of incidence with the first peak in the 20s and the second peak in the 50s. Interestingly, women are more commonly affected during the first peak, but men are more commonly affected in the second peak. Sensory loss is not a feature of MG. The most frequent initial symptoms of MG are ptosis and diplopia due to ocular muscular weakness or weakness of the levator palpebrae superioris.

8. **Answer B.** The patient has hypertensive encephalopathy. The history of acute headache with vomiting and confusion in the setting of severely elevated blood pressure is characteristic. Neuroimaging with CT scan is often normal. The treatment is immediate reduction of blood pressure by as much as 30%. By definition, hypertensive encephalopathy is reversible when blood pressure is reduced. Neurosurgical consultation may be indicated later in the course, but blood pressure management should be instituted early. Lumbar puncture would be contraindicated in this circumstance due to the papilledema indicating increased intracranial pressure. Corticosteroids are indicated in cases of temporal arteritis, which is on the differential diagnosis but is far less common than hypertensive encephalopathy and requires the presence of an elevated erythrocyte sedimentation rate. MRI of the brain can add important structural information but is not indicated emergently.

9. **Answer A.** In children, rubella (German measles) is characterized by a minimal prodromal illness (as opposed to adults), a "3-day rash," and generalized lymphadenopathy. Forchheimer spots, pinpoint or larger erythematous spots on the soft palate, may also be found. However, similar lesions may also be seen in measles and scarlet fever, so the presence of Forschheimer spots is not pathognomonic for rubella. The rash is a pink-red maculopapular eruption that first appears on the face and rapidly spreads downward to the neck, arms, trunk, and legs. On the second day, it begins to disappear from the face and the entire rash typically disappears by the end of the third day. Lymphadenopathy is generalized but most commonly involves the suboccipital, postauricular, and cervical nodes. Although lymph node tenderness typically subsides after 1 to 2 days, lymphadenopathy may persist for several weeks. Tonsillar exudates are present in several causes of pharyngitis. Koplik spots are pathognomonic for measles. Febrile seizures classically occur in patients with roseola infantum (exanthem subitum). Pastia lines occur in scarlet fever.

10. **Answer D.** Ciprofloxacin is the drug of choice for most causes of invasive bacterial diarrhea. The one exception to this is *Campylobacter* diarrhea, which has a high resistance to ciprofloxacin, especially in strains from Southeast Asia. Treatment with macrolides is preferred with *Campylobacter* infections. Trimethoprim–sulfamethoxazole can be used to treat *Yersinia*, *Vibrio*, ETEC, and certain parasites. Doxycycline is used as alternate therapy for *Vibrio*. Metronidazole is the drug of choice to treat *C. difficile* and *Giardia*.

11. **Answer D.** A large percentage of women, estimated to be from 30% to 60%, experience abdominal pain approximately 1 week after starting methotrexate for ectopic pregnancy. This is known as *separation pain* as it is thought to result from tubal distension as a result of tubal abortion or hematoma formation. However, all women with a history of methotrexate treatment for ectopic pregnancy who present with abdominal pain merit further investigation by ultrasonography to explore the possibility of tubal rupture. Interestingly, the size of the ectopic mass may actually increase before involution, but this finding has not been shown to be associated with treatment failure. However, if patients have an increase in the amount of pelvic free fluid or a decrease in their hemoglobin, a presumptive diagnosis of tubal rupture should be made and an OB should be urgently consulted. Although it is a risk factor for ectopic pregnancy, active PID at the same time as pregnancy (ectopic or intrauterine) is extremely rare.

12. **Answer D.** The patient has vesicular lesions on the soft palate consistent with herpangina, caused by coxsackievirus. In children, this often presents as hand–foot–mouth disease. Management is supportive, with special emphasis on pain control, as lesions are extremely painful and can limit oral intake. HSV-1 can cause herpetic gingivostomatitis, which causes lesions on the hard palate and gums and can be treated with valacyclovir. HSV-2 usually causes genital herpes rather than oral lesions. Epstein–Barr virus causes infectious mononucleosis, resulting in pharyngitis usually without discrete lesions. Group A streptococcus causes strep throat, a pharyngitis with exudate on the tonsils but without discrete oral ulcers. (Figure from Stedman's Medical Dictionary. 28th edition. Philadelphia, PA: Wolters Kluwer; 2005.)

13. **Answer B.** Trauma patients require rapid access with large-bore peripheral IVs to optimize fluid administration. Two 14-g or 16-g IVs are ideal. Rate of fluid flow is inversely proportional to the length of the vessel and directly proportional to the radius of the vessel to the

fourth power. Therefore, short, wide-bore catheters are preferred over long, narrow-bore catheters. A single IV is not adequate, given the risk of expulsion from patient movement during trauma resuscitation. Triple-lumen catheters, though generally large-bore lines, are limited in their fluid passage rates by their length, which can be up to 10 times that of a peripheral line. Cordis catheters are shorter than triple-lumens, and they are large-bore (8.5 Fr). Thus they can achieve significant infusion rates with a pressure bag or pump and are often included in trauma resuscitations when massive transfusion or fluids are needed. Intraosseous catheters provide ready vascular access in pediatric patients but are not preferred in the adult trauma patient due to limited flow rates, difficulty of placement, and potential complications.

14. **Answer D.** Flail chest occurs during blunt thoracic trauma when three or more ribs are each fractured in two places, causing a discrete chest wall segment that is unattached to the rest of the chest wall. Paradoxical motion of the flail segment is characteristic: The flail segment moves inward during inspiration and outward during expiration. Severity of the flail chest injury is due to the underlying pulmonary contusion that results from the blunt trauma. Diagnosis is made by physical examination and confirmed by either chest x-ray or CT. Management is directed at treating the underlying pulmonary contusion and should first involve administration of 100% oxygen to assess for the presence of severe pulmonary shunting. If the patient does not respond to noninvasive oxygen and is persistently hypoxemic, then endotracheal intubation should be performed. Hemothorax or pneumothorax may also be present and requires tube thoracostomy. Decubitus positioning is unlikely to be helpful in treating the flail chest and may exacerbate atelectasis in the contused lung region. A heavy weight placed on the flail segment is also likely to exacerbate the pulmonary contusion with little benefit.

15. **Answer B.** The recurrence rate after a single episode of uncomplicated diverticulitis is 20% to 30%. Furthermore, a high-fiber diet may help prevent further episodes. There is no evidence that avoiding nuts, corn kernels, popcorn, or seeds is associated with an increased rate of recurrence, despite the fact that patients are commonly advised against ingesting these substances. Young patients with diverticulitis are a special population because they tend to have more aggressive disease and the recurrence rate of diverticulitis is higher. Although resection of the disease segment remains elective, some authors recommend resection in all young patients due to their higher risk of recurrence. CT is the study of choice in the ED because it reliably visualizes the site of inflammation and is very useful for detecting various complications (e.g., abscesses, perforation, fistulas). Colonoscopy is useful to exclude colon cancer but

is deferred until the acute illness is treated. The mortality rate of hospitalized patients with diverticulitis is 1% to 6% for those requiring only medical management and 12% to 18% for those requiring surgery.

16. **Answer A.** Botulism occurs as a result of the toxin released by the anaerobic bacillus *Clostridium botulinum.* Botulinum toxin is considered the most potent poison known to humans, but it is not transmitted from person to person. Clinical botulism manifests as a descending paralysis, usually involving the cranial nerves. The mechanism is irreversible inhibition of presynaptic acetylcholine release. Antibiotics have little effect on treatment of botulism. Treatment involves supportive care, mechanical ventilation, and antitoxin therapy.

17. **Answer A.** Patients with testicular torsion will almost never exhibit a normal cremasteric reflex on the affected side. The sensitivity of this sign is extremely high (>95%). Prehn sign refers to relief of scrotal pain on elevation of the scrotum. Prehn sign was previously thought to distinguish epididymitis from testicular torsion but has been found to be inaccurate in this regard. Although urinalysis is usually normal, up to one-third of patients with torsion may have detectable urinary leukocytes. Fever is present in 20% and vomiting in 30% of cases, so absence of either should not be used to rule out the diagnosis.

18. **Answer B.** The patient's EKG appears to demonstrate an ectopic atrial rhythm with inverted P waves in lead II. However, the QRS axis is also flipped 180 degrees from normal. These findings indicate limb lead reversal. Specifically, the left leg and the right arm have been reversed. As a result, lead II becomes inverted, leads I and III become inverted *and* switch places, while leads aVR and aVF simply switch places. The only limb lead that is unaffected is aVL, which remains unchanged.

19. **Answer D.** The patient likely has Stevens–Johnson syndrome (SJS), most commonly caused by certain drug exposures. Sulfa drugs, allopurinol, carbamazepine, and phenytoin are usually implicated, though many other drugs have been known to cause SJS. SJS exists on the same spectrum as toxic epidermal necrolysis and can exhibit multiorgan involvement, though most cases are restricted to the skin and mucous membranes. Diagnosis is clinical, and treatment revolves around good supportive care, especially adequate IV hydration. Corticosteroid use is controversial. (Figure courtesy of Robert Hendrickson, MD. Reprinted from Hendrickson R. *Greenberg's Text-Atlas of Emergency Medicine.* Lippincott Williams & Wilkins; 2004:51, with permission.)

20. **Answer D.** Group A streptococci (GAS), *S. aureus,* and respiratory anaerobes are common causes of PTAs.

Thus, empiric antibiotics directed at these organisms are needed. In many communities, MRSA is prevalent and should be covered empirically. Thus, clindamycin is a common, effective agent for monotherapy. If MRSA resistance to clindamycin is significant, trimethoprim–sulfamethoxazole can be used to address MRSA, while clindamycin can be used to treat GAS and anaerobes. If they recur, 90% of recurrent PTAs develop within 1 year of the initial infection with the majority occurring very shortly after the initial infection. Therefore, many authors consider such recurrences an inadequately treated initial infection or simply a continuation of the same infection. Although tonsillectomy, whether it is performed emergently or after the initial infection has resolved, drastically reduces the rate of recurrence, PTAs have been known to occur after the tonsils have been removed. The treatment of PTAs is surgical with adjunctive antibiotic therapy. Needle aspiration is often the procedure of choice in select patients and is equally effective when performed correctly. Antibiotic therapy in the absence of surgical drainage is not effective. Finally, while CT scanning is not indicated in what otherwise appears to be an uncomplicated PTA, it is not possible to differentiate a PTA from peritonsillar cellulitis based on physical examination alone which sometimes leads to unnecessary surgical treatment.

21. **Answer C.** Coral snakes are part of the Elapidae family, whereas the remaining snakes listed are part of the Crotalidae family. Elapidae venom is neurotoxic, as several of the venom components block acetylcholine transmission. In contrast to victims of pit viper envenomation, victims of coral snake envenomation usually experience minimal pain and swelling at the bite site. However, signs of neurotoxicity may develop rapidly or be delayed for up to 12 hours. Ptosis is frequently the initial sign of neurotoxicity and may be followed by delirium, tremors, drowsiness, hypersalivation, and multiple cranial nerve abnormalities (dysarthria, diplopia, and dysphagia). In severe envenomations, respiratory muscle paralysis occurs, leading to respiratory failure and death.

22. **Answer B.** In a well newborn beyond the immediate neonatal period, without fever, hyponatremia is the most common cause of seizures. Water intoxication is the most common cause of hyponatremia during infancy. Infants are unable to adequately concentrate urine so parents who dilute formula or give their infants tap water put their infants at risk. Hypocalcemia is also a very common cause of seizures in the neonate, so serum calcium levels should be checked. In fact, all infants have a slight decline in serum calcium levels with a nadir at 24 to 48 hours. Symptomatic hypocalcemia is more common in infants of diabetic mothers, preterm infants, or infants with a history of anoxic encephalopathy. Hypomagnesemia is not as common as hypocalcemia, but

symptoms of hypomagnesemia mimic those of hypocalcemia and it is difficult to correct hypocalcemia if the serum magnesium is also low. Therefore, infants with seizures should have a comprehensive evaluation of their electrolytes. Hypokalemia is uncommon in infancy and does not typically cause seizures. Maple syrup urine disease is a rare disease resulting from the inability to catabolize branched chain amino acids. Infants typically present between 4 to 7 days of life with poor feeding, vomiting, or lethargy. Neurologic manifestations rapidly develop, such as alternating hypotonia and hypertonia, dystonia, seizures, and encephalopathy.

23. **Answer B.** Oral candidiasis is the most common form of candidal infection and *Candida* species colonize the oropharynx of 80% of healthy infants by 3 to 4 weeks of age. Oral candidiasis is also an AIDS-defining illness. Because *Candida* spp. are part of the normal flora of so many people, cultures are rarely useful. Instead, diagnosis is based on clinical examination and the finding of white, curd-like exudates on the buccal and gingival mucosa and less frequently on the tongue and soft palate. The exudates can be scraped away to reveal an erythematous, mildly eroded, and painful mucosa underneath. Although the infection is frequently self-limited, infants with thrush should be treated with oral nystatin suspension to hasten healing and primarily to prevent problems with feeding (due to pain). Tinea cruris is most commonly caused by *Trichophyton* spp., as with other dermatophyte infections. The hallmark of cutaneous candidiasis is the presence of satellite papules and pustules beyond the margins of a patch of macerated, sometimes weeping skin with scalloped borders. It typically occurs in intertriginous areas such as the groin, axilla, or underneath pendulous skin folds.

24. **Answer D.** The FAST examination has greater accuracy than any single element of the history or physical examination in blunt abdominal trauma. It is not as accurate for penetrating trauma as it is for blunt. Ultrasound cannot reliably distinguish between blood, urine, or other fluids (e.g., ascites). FAST has been associated with significant operational improvements, including time to surgery, CT utilization, and avoidable hospitalizations. Specificity tends to be higher than sensitivity, and blunt abdominal trauma patients who appear ill despite a negative FAST examination should have serial FAST examinations or CT imaging to fully evaluate the abdomen.

25. **Answer C.** The patient in this vignette has influenza, which tends to peak in winter. When it is started within the first 48 hours of illness, oseltamivir (Tamiflu) has been shown to reduce the duration of symptoms due to influenza by about half a day. However, patients taking it have more nausea and vomiting. In effect, using oseltamivir trades one category of symptoms for another. It

has not been shown to reduce complications or mortality from influenza, even among the elderly or chronically ill. Influenza vaccination does not hasten recovery in patients with active influenza.

26. **Answer C.** The patient has a ring-enhancing lesion seen in the left parietal area on contrast CT scan of the brain. In a patient with HIV, toxoplasmosis, due to the parasite *Toxoplasma gondii,* is the most likely cause. Treatment is with sulfadiazine, pyrimethamine, and adjunctive leucovorin. Corticosteroids may be used as adjunctive therapy in severe cases. Surgical excision is not indicated in toxoplasmosis. Mebendazole is an agent used to treat other parasitic infections. Clindamycin may be used to treat brain abscesses along with surgical drainage. (Figure reprinted with permission from Silverberg M. *Greenberg's Text-Atlas of Emergency Medicine.* Lippincott Williams & Wilkins; 2004:999.)

27. **Answer C.** Delayed sequence intubation (DSI) is a strategy to more safely secure a definitive airway in agitated, delirious patients whose agitation makes preoxygenation suboptimal or impossible. Historically, rapid sequence intubation (RSI) was emergently applied to all patients in need of a definitive airway. However, in hypoxic patients who resist preoxygenation efforts due to delirium or agitation, DSI offers an opportunity to safely preoxygenate patients prior to administering paralytics in preparation for intubation. To achieve this, serial doses of ketamine are used, typically starting at the low end of the scale, e.g., 1 mg/kg IV bolus followed by serial 0.5 mg/kg boluses until dissociation is achieved. Ketamine is an ideal agent because it doesn't depress airway reflexes or respiratory drive. Once the patient is dissociated and more compliant, preoxygenation can occur using a nonrebreather or a nasal cannula at 15 L/minute plus a noninvasive mask attached to a ventilator to provide CPAP at 5 to 15 mm Hg. As summarized by its creator, Scott Weingart, MD, another perspective is to think of DSI as procedural sedation, in which the procedure is effective preoxygenation. Once the patient is adequately preoxygenated, a paralytic agent can be given and intubation can proceed. Once dissociated, some patients experience such a profound improvement in their respiratory mechanics that DSI will obviate the need for intubation altogether.

28. **Answer D.** Intraoral lacerations are best repaired with absorbable sutures such as polyglactin 910 (Vicryl). Vicryl causes less tissue reactivity than silk and is preferred over nylon because it avoids the problem of a repeat visit for removal. Chromic gut is catgut that has been treated with chromium salts to improve longevity and is also appropriate for mucosal laceration repair. Large intraoral lacerations should be repaired primarily to prevent food particles from becoming entrapped and causing abscess formation and cellulitis. Small intraoral lacerations should be left to heal by secondary intention. Antibiotics (penicillin or clindamycin) may be given to patients who have through-and-through lacerations (through external skin and intraoral mucosa).

29. **Answer A.** Sepsis is the most common risk factor or condition, leading to the development of ARDS. ARDS is defined as the development of acute respiratory failure, with noncardiogenic pulmonary edema (established by the presence of bilateral infiltrates consistent with pulmonary edema on chest radiography and a pulmonary capillary wedge pressure ≤18 mm Hg indicating that the edema is noncardiogenic), and severe hypoxia such that the $Pao_2:Fio_2$ ratio ≤200. Identical findings in patients with a $Pao_2:Fio_2$ ratio ≤300 are diagnosed with acute lung injury (ALI), instead of ARDS, but the etiology of ALI is the same. Although sepsis is the most common cause of ARDS, severe trauma complicated by shock, multiple blood transfusions, and aspiration are all independent risk factors. Pancreatitis and near drowning may result in ARDS but are less common causes. Such causes also illustrate the idea that the ARDS may be due to direct lung injury (e.g., severe pneumonia with sepsis) or indirect lung injury (e.g., severe pancreatitis). The latter is presumably due to the widespread release of cytokines and other proinflammatory mediators.

30. **Answer E.** The initial intravenous resuscitation fluid of choice in pediatric patients is 0.9 normal saline. It is given in a 20 mL/kg bolus and may need to be repeated twice in patients with severe dehydration (up to 60 mL/kg). Dextrose-containing half-normal saline is adequate for maintenance, but the initial concern is volume repletion, so normal saline should be administered. When sufficient bolus hydration has been given, maintenance fluids according to the "4/2/1 rule" are instituted: 4 mL/kg/hour for the first 10 kg of body weight, 2 mL/kg/hour for the next 10 kg, and 1 mL/kg/hour for every 10 kg after that. The maintenance fluid composition varies by age and may be looked up in a reference.

31. **Answer C.** GERD is a very common cause of vomiting during infancy. Emesis is typically nonbilious and begins in early infancy, remaining fairly constant over time. It does not demonstrate the progressive pattern to projectile emesis that characterizes pyloric stenosis. Most infants respond to conservative measures. In the past, ranitidine (an H2 histamine receptor antagonist) or metoclopramide (which increases lower esophageal tone and gastric emptying) was used to help control symptoms. However, metoclopramide is not considered useful in infants <1 year of age with uncomplicated GERD and prokinetic agents such as metoclopramide, have considerable side effects. Proton pump inhibitors, such as omeprazole, have replaced histamine blockers,

such as ranitidine, when acid reduction is required. Most infants continue to gain weight normally and only rarely do infants demonstrate failure to thrive. For the most part, infant GERD peaks at 4 months and resolves by 12 months with nearly all cases resolved by 24 months of age (as the lower esophageal sphincter becomes more competent with age).

32. **Answer A.** The patient has avascular necrosis of the femoral head, or Legg–Calve–Perthes (LCP) disease. It is much more common in boys than girls and is usually unilateral (though 10% to 20% of patients have bilateral involvement). Pain may be referred to the groin or the knee. Young children are affected more commonly than young adolescents. Etiology is unknown. Obesity is a risk factor for slipped capital femoral epiphysis (SCFE), but not LCP disease. Management may be surgical, but this is considered on a case-by-case basis. Joint aspiration is useful to rule out septic arthritis as a cause for the symptoms, but radiography and MRI are the cornerstones of diagnosis of LCP disease. Emergency management consists of prompt orthopedic referral or consultation for consideration of surgical management. Leg-length discrepancy, deformity, and limitation of movement are important long-term sequelae. (Figure courtesy of James T Guille, MD. Reprinted with permission from Guille JT. *Greenberg's Text-Atlas of Emergency Medicine.* Lippincott Williams & Wilkins; 2004:601.)

33. **Answer C.** Patients with acute symptoms of stroke should be immediately evaluated for hypoglycemia. Hypoglycemia can mimic acute stroke and the management of this condition is radically different from acute ischemic or hemorrhagic stroke. Typically, blood glucose checking is performed by EMS, but patients who are brought in by other means do not have access to this. Obtaining an EKG is important, but it will not change the hyperacute management of potential stroke, even if it shows atrial fibrillation, which could be the etiology of the stroke. Temperature is certainly important as well, but should not delay checking of blood glucose in this particular patient as targeted treatment of an elevated temperature with focal neurologic findings cannot occur immediately. Prolactin levels were used for evaluation of seizure activity, but inadequate sensitivity and specificity have caused it to fall out of favor. Oral challenge should never be pursued in patients with possibility for acute stroke as they have a high risk of pharyngeal compromise and can aspirate.

34. **Answer C.** The optimal criteria used to determine which patients require an LP after a first febrile seizure are constantly evolving and remain unclear. However, the American Academy of Pediatrics (AAP) released new, less aggressive guidelines in 2011. According to its most recent guidelines, the AAP states that an LP should be considered for all infants aged 6 to 12 months who are inadequately vaccinated against *H. influenzae* or Streptococcus *pneumoniae* or in whom the vaccination status is not known. In addition, an LP should be considered for any infant receiving current antibiotic therapy since the use of antibiotics may mask meningeal signs and symptoms. Other higher risk groups include patients with focal or prolonged seizures, abnormal physical examinations, or toxic appearance. Regardless of vaccination status, older patients are able to participate in a complete physical examination to aid the physician in determining whether meningitis is a consideration. Most ordinary febrile seizures are treated symptomatically with antipyretics. Approximately one-third of patients with febrile seizures will have at least one more febrile seizure episode. Risk factors for this include young age at first seizure, lower temperature with the seizure episode, a first-degree relative with febrile seizure, and short duration between fever onset and seizure event. Patients with febrile seizures are twice as likely to develop epilepsy compared to the general population.

35. **Answer B.** Reduction of anterior shoulder dislocations may be accomplished through a variety of methods, none of which is clearly superior to the others. A high rate of complications is associated with use of the Kocher method (leverage, adduction, and internal rotation) and the Hippocratic method (axillary traction with the physician's foot). The most important factor in determining success of relocation is adequate muscle relaxation, which may be ensured by either procedural sedation or intra-articular anesthesia. Scapular manipulation may be performed with a patient sitting erect, but it should not be performed with pregnant patients in the third trimester in the prone position due to compression of the uterus.

36. **Answer D.** Sternoclavicular dislocations may occur in the anterior or posterior direction. Anterior dislocations are more common and occur because of a medially directed force to the shoulder. These injuries are unlikely to cause serious injury beyond the dislocation itself. Posterior dislocations result from a posteriorly directed force to the sternoclavicular joint and may cause great vessel, mediastinal, or airway injury. CT is more accurate than either plain films or ultrasound for the diagnosis of both anterior and posterior sternoclavicular dislocations.

37. **Answer D.** Patients with acute sigmoid diverticulitis usually have pain in the left lower quadrant as well as a change in bowel habits, either constipation or diarrhea. Vomiting, hematochezia, dysuria, and anorexia are seen in lower frequencies in acute diverticulitis. Anorexia is particularly sensitive for acute appendicitis if associated with right lower quadrant pain.

38. **Answer B.** Nitroprusside is a strong arterial and venous dilator only available as an IV drip. It is easily titrated and provides effective and predictable BP control. Extravasation of nitroprusside causes severe skin necrosis. Nitroprusside is metabolized to thiocyanate and excreted renally. Cyanide toxicity is not common, but thiocyanate toxicity can occur in renal failure, causing systemic symptoms. Nitroprusside may increase cerebral blood flow and ICP. Thiocyanate may cause damage to the fetal thyroid, and nitroprusside should be avoided during pregnancy. Nitroprusside is extremely fast acting, with a rapid onset and offset, making it ideal for rapid, predictable BP control.

39. **Answer E.** The potential space in this right upper quadrant view of the FAST scan is called Morison pouch. In trauma, free fluid (assumed to be blood) will accumulate preferentially in the right upper quadrant in a supine patient—this process will intensify with Trendelenburg positioning. The rectouterine pouch is known as the pouch of Douglas and it is the most posterior part of the peritoneal cavity. Morison pouch is part of the peritoneal cavity, not retroperitoneum (which cannot be adequately visualized with the FAST scan). The pericardial view should be the first view obtained in the FAST scan, as it addresses the most immediate life threat in trauma after the primary survey (pericardial tamponade). (Figure from Fleisher GR; Ludwig S. *Textbook of Pediatric Emergency Medicine.* 6th ed. Philadelphia, PA: Wolters Kluwer; 2010.)

40. **Answer B.** Hydralazine, isoniazid, and procainamide may all precipitate a lupus-like syndrome. SLE typically affects the hands, wrists, and knees and is most common in young women of childbearing age.

41. **Answer B.** Roux-en-Y bypass creates potential areas of herniation in the mesentery which are closed at the time of surgery. Despite closure, some patients experience intestinal herniation through mesenteric defects, resulting in abdominal pain. Herniation is often intermittent and difficult to diagnose by CT. While the classic "mesenteric swirl sign" may be present, the majority of patients may have a normal CT. Thus, patients with otherwise unexplained abdominal pain status post bypass surgery may need repeat exploration to exclude an internal hernia. Gastrogastric fistulas most often occur in patients with a stapled but undivided stomach (the fistula forms between the remaining stomach "pouch" and the undivided remnant), a procedure that was performed in early gastric bypass procedures. In contrast to common beliefs, gastroesophageal reflux is not a common complication of gastric bypass surgery. Cholelithiasis is a common complication of gastric bypass but the patient's history is not suggestive of biliary colic as his symptoms are not tied to eating.

42. **Answer C.** The abdominal radiograph demonstrates multiple, radiopaque packets consistent with body packing of recreational drugs. Because cocaine and other sympathomimetic agents are often packed, cardiac monitoring is indicated for these patients. Asymptomatic patients may not require any specific therapy, but symptomatic patients should be evaluated carefully for signs of systemic toxicity and treated with supportive care and antidotes as indicated. Patients may be given polyethylene glycol to induce whole bowel irrigation to promote more rapid transit of the packets through the GI tract. MRI is not indicated in patients with body packets, as it will not change management and adds little to the diagnosis. Surgical removal is indicated for signs of severe toxicity or bowel obstruction. NG aspiration is unlikely to provide any benefit and may instead cause retching and vomiting. Endotracheal intubation is not indicated in the absence of severe systemic toxicity. (Figure courtesy of Robert Hendrickson, MD. Reprinted with permission from Hendrickson R. *Greenberg's Text-Atlas of Emergency Medicine.* Lippincott Williams & Wilkins; 2004:805.)

43. **Answer B.** The OAR are a set of criteria that were devised to limit unnecessary ankle radiography in patients presenting with ankle pain. The criteria require ankle radiography in any patient with ankle pain who has the following:

1. Unable to ambulate four steps both at the time of injury and in the ED, or
2. Bony tenderness to palpation of the tip of either malleolus or tenderness of the distal 6 cm posterior to either malleolus.

The original paper, published in 1992, described a sensitivity of 100% and a specificity of 40%. Since then, however, several other studies have published a variety of other values, suggesting a wide variability for specificity and sensitivity somewhere >96%. However, even in the original paper (sensitivity of 100%), occasional patients had "insignificant" fractures such as chip fractures that would be managed in the same way as a sprain. The squeeze test involves squeezing the tibia and fibula approximately 5 cm proximal to the malleoli in an effort to provoke pain in the ankle. Increased ankle pain indicates disruption of the distal tibiofibular syndesmosis. The OAR have not been validated for pediatric use. Like other clinical decision rules, the OAR should not be used in unreliable patients such as patients with decreased mental status or intoxicated patients.

44. **Answer B.** This patient has dysfunctional uterine bleeding (DUB), which is defined as excessive, prolonged, or erratic uterine bleeding that is not related to an underlying anatomic uterine defect or systemic disease. Therefore, DUB is a diagnosis of exclusion.

However, anovulation is by far the most common cause of irregular vaginal bleeding in an adolescent. Although anovulatory menstrual cycles are most common in the first 2 to 3 years after menarche, it may take up to 6 years before most cycles become ovulatory. Oral contraceptive pills are very effective for the management of DUB. Nearly any regimen can be used, and the most common involves combination oral contraceptives (containing both estrogen and progesterone) with at least 30 to 35 mg of ethinyl estradiol. The pills are initially used four times daily in women with more extensive bleeding (and concomitantly low hemoglobin levels) and are gradually tapered by one pill every 3 days until only one pill is being used on a daily basis. Antiemetics may be needed due to the nausea that is a frequent side effect of high-dose estrogen therapy. In addition, iron supplementation should be used to boost red blood cell production.

45. **Answer D.** Sickle cell disease is a hemoglobinopathy causing sickling of red blood cells with any systemic stress, which results in diffuse microinfarctions. Sickle cell trait is present in approximately 10% of all African Americans, and sickle cell disease is primarily a disease of this population. Symptoms involve multiple organ systems and result in specific acute crises—vaso-occlusive, acute chest syndrome, splenic sequestration, and aplastic. Aplastic crises are characterized by the acute onset of worsening anemia combined with bone marrow failure. Laboratory abnormalities demonstrate a drop of hemoglobin of 2 g/dL from stable levels and an inadequate reticulocyte response (<2%) from the bone marrow to this sudden anemia. Aplastic crises are usually postinfectious and are responsible for 5% of all deaths in sickle cell patients.

46. **Answer E.** The patient is exhibiting signs of the Jarisch–Herxheimer reaction after treatment for secondary syphilis with penicillin G. The reaction occurs because massive death of spirochetes on exposure to the penicillin causes systemic symptoms in a serum sickness-like reaction. Treatment is symptomatic with acetaminophen or ibuprofen. An allergic reaction to the antibiotic that he was given is possible, but there were no urticaria demonstrated on physical examination and the rash that was present was already there before the antibiotic treatment. The patient should not be intubated or given epinephrine because of the lack of upper airway or pulmonary symptoms. Prednisone, diphenhydramine, and famotidine would be useful in an allergic reaction but have little role in the management of the Jarisch–Herxheimer reaction.

47. **Answer E.** ETEC is responsible for 45% to 50% of traveler's diarrhea. *Shigella* is the second most common cause of traveler's diarrhea, whereas viral causes and protozoa make up the remainder.

48. **Answer D.** Generalized seizures can result in a significant lactic acidosis due to anaerobic metabolism in the affected musculature as the muscles undergo repeated contractions. In generalized seizures, the amount of lactate produced can be significant resulting in a profound systemic acidosis. While the acidosis will eventually resolve without intervention provided the patient has normal renal function and stops seizing, intravenous bicarbonate should be given to normalize the acid–base status as soon as possible to address the patient's bradycardia. While dopamine and epinephrine have chronotropic effects due to their β1-agonist activity, neither medication will help resolve the patient's acidosis. Albuterol is an effective, though transient, treatment for severe hyperkalemia as it induces a potassium shift into cells.

49. **Answer D.** Gonococcus can cause either a migratory, polyarticular arthritis or monoarticular arthritis. Synovial fluid Gram stain is positive more often than culture. It is the most common cause of septic arthritis in the young, sexually active adult, and is much more common in women than men. The most common joints affected are the knees, wrists, and ankles. A clinical syndrome of arthritis, tenosynovitis, and dermatitis (discrete hemorrhagic pustules) may occur. Although urethral and cervical cultures are high-yield, patients rarely complain of associated symptoms. Treatment involves intravenous antibiotics (third-generation cephalosporin) and inpatient observation. Although orthopedic consultation is warranted, open drainage is rarely necessary.

50. **Answer C.** Initial treatment should focus on reducing the patient's blood pressure to a systolic blood pressure of 100 to 120 mm Hg or lower if the patient can tolerate it using parenteral beta-blockers (labetalol, esmolol, propranolol). Beta-blockers are the preferred agent because they also reduce heart rate and aortic wall stress by reducing the rate of systolic blood pressure rise. The nonselective calcium channel blockers (CCBs) (verapamil and diltiazem) are reasonable alternatives in patients who are unable to tolerate beta-blockers (e.g., due to bronchospasm). If the patient's blood pressure remains elevated above this range despite maximal beta-blocker therapy, or if the patient's blood pressure is at goal, with normal mentation, urine output, and renal function, then the blood pressure can be further reduced using nitroprusside. Nitroprusside is not considered a first-line agent because its use triggers reactive tachycardia and increased contractility. Thus, it is important to use it only in patients who have first achieved effective beta-blockade. As a direct arterial vasodilator, hydralazine should be avoided because its use results in reflex tachycardia and it has an unpredictable blood pressure response curve. Otherwise, each of the remaining agents may be used as a second-line agent after beta-blockade is initiated.

51. **Answer B.** The patient has a lytic lesion with fever in a subacute course consistent with osteomyelitis. The most common cause in all patients is *Salmonella*. Other gram-negative organisms such as *E. coli*, may also cause osteomyelitis in sickle cell patients. *S. aureus* is the primary cause of osteomyelitis in healthy hosts. Interestingly, though *Salmonella* is the most common cause of osteomyelitis in sickle cell patients, *S. aureus* remains the predominant cause of septic arthritis. *Aspergillus* is a rare cause of septic arthritis. Gonococcus is the most common cause of septic arthritis in the young, sexually active adult. *Pseudomonas* causes osteomyelitis in patients with puncture wounds to the feet and IV drug users.

52. **Answer E.** This patient has herpes zoster (shingles). Although shingles may be more likely to occur in patients with leukemia, Hodgkin lymphoma as well as other malignancies, most cases occur in otherwise healthy patients. (Figure reprinted with permission from Weber J. *Health Assessment in Nursing*. 2nd ed. Lippincott Williams & Wilkins; 2002.)

53. **Answer B.** D-dimer values increase naturally with age, and a recent review revealed that using an age-adjusted d-dimer cutoff value determined by multiplying the patient's age in years × 10 mcg/L reduces false positives without substantially increasing false negatives. As with the normal cutoff value, the patient should meet low-risk criteria prior to d-dimer testing. The PE rule-out criteria ("PERC" rule) applies only to patients <50 years old. A CT pulmonary angiogram would not likely be needed in patients with negative d-dimer tests. Patients who are low-risk by Wells criteria have <2% risk of venous thromboembolism. Thus, it may be reasonable to avoid further testing if an alternative diagnosis is made. However, given the morbidity and mortality associated with undiagnosed and untreated pulmonary embolism, further testing should be pursued in the absence of an alternative explanation for the patient's symptoms. Negative lower extremity Doppler imaging does not exclude a PE.

54. **Answer B.** *C. trachomatis* causes ocular trachoma in many third-world countries (considered the most common cause of preventable blindness worldwide) and is an important sexually transmitted disease in the United States. In the United States, *C. trachomatis* is a major cause of pelvic inflammatory disease (or cervicitis) as well as urethritis in men. A different serotype of the organism is also responsible for lymphogranuloma venereum (LGV), a more invasive sexually transmitted disease.

55. **Answer D.** Rh-negative patients with significant trauma should have RhIG administered to prevent isoimmunization. The dosage varies with gestational age—in gestational age <12 weeks, a 50-mcg dose is sufficient to prevent isoimmunization though there is some evidence that treatment at all may be unnecessary. Patients at gestational age >12 weeks should have the 300-mcg dose. Patients at risk for greater fetomaternal hemorrhage (possible when gestational age >16 weeks) should have the Kleihauer–Betke test performed to determine whether additional doses of RhIG are needed. Transfusions of blood products in pregnant trauma patients should be performed if clinical situations suggest hemodynamic compromise, ongoing bleeding, or coagulopathy.

56. **Answer A.** Acute spinal cord compression due to vertebral column metastasis occurs with many cancers, including lung, breast, and prostate. Patients present with typical findings of epidural compression, including pain, weakness, or bowel/bladder dysfunction. Any patient suspected of having metastatic epidural compression should have an emergent MRI of the spine to evaluate the symptoms. Rapid diagnosis and management is essential to prevent irreversible neurologic sequelae. Corticosteroids may be started in the ED to reduce edema of the spinal cord. Radiation and spinal surgery are the primary treatments of malignancy-related epidural cord compression. Other specialties need not be emergently consulted in these cases.

57. **Answer A.** The patient likely has a rib fracture or contusion given the focal pain and tenderness in her fifth rib. However, the true danger of a rib fracture is not the bony injury itself, but potential injury to the underlying structures, such as pleura, lung, liver, spleen, or kidney. The fifth rib is cephalad enough that an intra-abdominal injury would be less likely than thoracic injury. A chest x-ray is indicated to evaluate the lung parenchyma and the pleural lines. Rib x-rays are not routinely indicated in patients with thoracic trauma, except in cases where multiple fractures are suspected or elderly patients are involved, as significant intrathoracic or intra-abdominal injuries occur at higher frequency in these instances. Abdominal CT scan may be indicated with corroborative physical examination findings, but is never undertaken before routine x-rays of the chest or pelvis in the trauma patient. Brain CT scan and cervical spine radiographs are not indicated without loss of consciousness, altered mental status, focal neurologic deficit, headache, or neck pain/tenderness.

58. **Answer C.** DAI is an important traumatic cause of coma that is not due to a mass lesion or frank intracerebral hemorrhage. Initial CT scan is almost always normal in patients with DAI, but MRI may show diffuse white matter disruption due to axonal fiber injury. Because of the difficulty in gauging DAI on neuroimaging, the prognosis is based totally on clinical parameters. The duration of coma obviously correlates with severity of injury. Patients with DAI who awaken from coma within 24 hours may have few permanent disabilities.

Those in coma for longer than 24 hours tend to have much more grim outcomes, including persistent vegetative state or extreme cognitive dysfunction. Most types of acute intracranial hemorrhage severe enough to lead to coma would be evident on initial CT scan, including epidural or subdural hematomas, cerebral contusions, and intraparenchymal hematoma. An important exception is subarachnoid hemorrhage, which may not be visible on CT scan and is a common hemorrhagic cause of altered mental status after trauma.

59. **Answer A.** The vasculitic syndromes have multiple areas of overlap in their clinical manifestations and it is sometimes difficult for rheumatologists to apply a specific diagnosis. However, classically, PAN causes mononeuritis multiplex and mesenteric ischemia. Cutaneous findings are also common. Takayasu arteritis is very common in Japan and results in coronary ischemia. Wegener granulomatosis initially presents with symptoms of upper airway problems such as sinusitis, otitis, and nasal congestion while developing glomerulonephritis at a later stage. Behçet disease is characterized by recurrent oral and genital ulcerations and recurrent hypopyon (it is rarely seen, but pathognomonic finding). Churg–Strauss syndrome involves the lungs and most patients have symptoms of asthma in the 2 years preceding a diagnosis.

60. **Answer D.** Therapeutic hypothermia is primarily used to mitigate the neurologic devastation that occurs in the setting of cardiac arrest. While the initial trials were conducted in patients with cardiac arrest due to ventricular fibrillation or pulseless ventricular tachycardia, most published guidelines suggest that it can be used after any cardiac arrest thought due to cardiac origin (e.g., pulseless electrical activity [PEA] or asystole). Emergency physicians should strongly consider using therapeutic hypothermia in all patients with successful ROSC after cardiac arrest who are hemodynamically stable with a MAP >65, yet who are comatose with a GCS <8. While there are no evidence-based guidelines, most guidelines suggest that therapeutic hypothermia should be considered in all patients with ROSC <1 hour after the beginning of resuscitative efforts and should be started within 6 hours. Hypotensive patients in cardiogenic shock may be candidates for therapeutic hypothermia provided their MAP can be stably maintained >65 with the use of vasopressors. The patient described in this vignette (MAP = 53) would require vasopressors prior to the initiation of cooling. Ongoing hypotension is a contraindication for therapeutic hypothermia. Other contraindications to therapeutic hypothermia include patients with a core temperature <30°C (86°F) upon arrival, patients with poor baseline mental status, terminally ill patients, pregnancy (relative), traumatic arrest (relative), and patients with inherited clotting disorders. Shivering is an expected and common side effect of therapy but is not benign. Shivering leads to increased oxygen consumption, an elevated heart rate, increased work of breathing, and a generalized increase in the stress response. The heat generated from shivering can also impede cooling. Shivering should be managed with analgesia and sedation, with paralytics used if all other methodologies fail.

61. **Answer D.** The United States has the highest rate of homicide due to firearms in the industrialized world. The ready availability of firearms in the United States combined with complex socioeconomic inequalities put urban African-American youths at the highest risk for firearm-related death. The leading cause of death in this subset of the population is due to homicide from handguns.

62. **Answer C.** Pregnant women develop appendicitis at the same rate as not pregnant women. Due to nearby gynecologic structures, women with appendicitis are more frequently misdiagnosed. As many as 33% of women with appendicitis are initially misdiagnosed, and as many as 45% of women with symptoms of appendicitis are found to have a normal appendix during surgery. Although CMT is more common in gynecologic diseases, as many as one-fourth of women with appendicitis have CMT upon physical examination. Even in the third trimester, most pregnant women still have pain in the right lower quadrant. In pregnant women, appendicitis occurs slightly more often in the second trimester, although the reasons for this are not known. Fetal abortion complicates perforated maternal appendicitis in 20% of cases.

63. **Answer C.** The patient has an open-book pelvis fracture in association with hypotension, which may be rapidly fatal if not treated promptly. Temporizing management revolves around reducing the effective volume into which hemorrhage can occur by tightly securing the pelvis with a commercial device or simple bedsheet. Definitive management involves angiography with embolization to control hemorrhage and surgical fixation to repair the pelvis fracture. Foley catheterization may be performed in patients with pelvic fractures if there are no hard signs of urethral trauma (e.g., blood at the urethral meatus), but priority should be given to hemorrhage control rather than evaluation of urethral trauma. CT should never be performed on the hemodynamically unstable trauma patient. Thoracotomy is not indicated in patients with blunt traumatic mechanisms as survival rates are dismally low. Additional radiographs of the pelvis should be performed after hemodynamic compromise has been addressed. (Figure courtesy of Mark Silverberg, MD. Reprinted with permission from Silverberg M. *Greenberg Text-Atlas of Emergency Medicine.* Lippincott Williams & Wilkins; 2004:659.)

64. **Answer E.** There are several normal physiologic changes that occur with aging and that place elderly patients at greater risk of serious injury from trauma. Cerebral atrophy results in stretching of the dural bridging veins, increasing the risk of subdural hematoma formation after falls and relatively minor head trauma. Degenerative joint disease and osteoporosis result in an increased tendency to fracture bones after falls and blunt trauma. Due to these degenerative changes, the cervical spine is less mobile in elderly patients and is more commonly fractured. Type 2 odontoid fractures are the most common cervical spine fractures in the elderly. In addition, hyperextension injuries lead to central cord syndrome in which the ligamentum flavum is thought to buckle into the spinal cord, resulting in a contusion to the cord's central elements. This results in flaccid paralysis of the upper extremities but relatively unaffected lower extremities (although they may suffer from spastic paralysis in large cord lesions). The chest wall becomes more rigid and the lungs become less compliant in elderly patients. This places them at risk for flail chest, even from relatively minor injuries such as a simple fall. Elderly patients with even single rib fractures should be admitted in the setting of concomitant lung disease such as COPD.

65. **Answer C.** Ipratropium is primarily useful as a second-line adjunctive agent in the treatment of patients with acute asthma exacerbations. Multiple trials in the late 1990s as well as a few meta-analyses have demonstrated benefit in patients treated with a combination of albuterol and ipratropium versus albuterol alone. In pediatric populations, combination therapy decreases treatment time in the ED, albuterol dose requirements before discharge, as well as hospitalization rates. In adults, combination therapy has been shown to increase peak expiratory flow rate more than albuterol alone. However, there are conflicting data regarding ipratropium, and some studies have failed to demonstrate benefit. Owing to this conflicting data, ipratropium has been relegated to use as a second-line agent. As it appears to be safe and well tolerated, most experts advice using it as an adjunctive agent in severe asthma exacerbations. It is not recommended for use as a single agent primarily because of its slower onset of action and because it only alleviates cholinergically mediated bronchoconstriction. The main benefit of ipratropium over atropine is its superior side effect profile.

66. **Answer A.** IV drug uses (IVDUs) have bacteria that are transmitted through the skin to superficial veins, into the greater venous circulation, and eventually to the heart. These pathogens (*S. aureus* in more than three-fourths of cases) lodge most commonly in the tricuspid valve to cause right-heart endocarditis and may lead to septic pulmonary emboli.

67. **Answer C.** This patient has an aortoenteric fistula until proven otherwise. The classic presentation is abdominal pain and GI bleeding that resolves spontaneously (the so-called herald bleed) in a patient with a prior history of aortic graft. The initial bleeding is thought to stop when splanchnic pressure drops and allows adequate clot to form. However, the initial bleed is often followed by a massive and often fatal hemorrhage days or possibly weeks later. The fistula is caused by *S. aureus* or *Escherichia coli* infection of the prior graft and typically forms between the aorta and the distal duodenum. Therefore, all patients with a history of aortic graft and GI bleeding should undergo esophagogastroduodenoscopy to search for a fistula in the distal duodenum. Most of these patients, however, have an alternative, more common cause of GI bleeding.

68. **Answer D.** There are numerous risk factors for PE, which can be divided into inherited and acquired disorders. Inherited hypercoagulable disorders should be suspected in patients with a documented PE who are younger than 40 years old, or in similar patients who have a positive family history or who have recurrent PEs. Of the inherited disorders, factor V Leiden is the most common, and may be present in as many as 20% of patients with venous thromboembolic disease. In normal individuals, factor V is normally inactivated (along with factor VIII) by protein C, thereby disrupting the normal clotting cascade. Patients with factor V Leiden have a factor V protein that is resistant to inactivation by protein C, which allows the coagulation cascade to continue in an unregulated manner, resulting in a thrombophilic state. Plasminogen deficiency and protein S deficiency are also inherited disorders that increase the risk of thromboembolic disease, but they are far less common. Nephrotic syndrome is also associated with an increased risk of PE due to a relative deficiency of coagulation cascade regulatory proteins, which are lost in the urine. Cancer in any form is a well-described risk factor for PE.

69. **Answer B.** In adult blunt trauma patients, the indications to perform an evaluation for renal injury include gross hematuria, microscopic hematuria plus hypotension, or significant deceleration injury. In the absence of shock, microscopic hematuria is not an indication for CT in blunt trauma patients. However, microscopic hematuria may also be a marker of urethral or bladder injury and may warrant further investigation depending on the mechanism of injury and findings on physical examination. The presence of flank physical examination findings is not indicative of renal injury significant enough to warrant imaging. Penile involvement can certainly cause urethral damage, but it does not confer a higher risk of renal injury.

70. **Answer E.** This patient experienced scombroid fish poisoning. Although not an allergic reaction, the symptoms are due to excessive histamine levels in the fish and results in symptoms that are very similar to an allergic response. This patient's prior history of avid seafood intake also points against allergy. Histamine levels build up in inadequately refrigerated, or inadequately preserved dark-muscled fish due to the action of histidine decarboxylase by enteric bacteria in the fish. Symptoms usually occur within minutes of eating the fish and include severe throbbing headache, facial flushing and a sense of diffuse warmth, a burning sensation in the mouth and throat, palpitations, nausea, anorexia, vomiting, abdominal cramps, conjunctival injection, and pruritus. Symptoms are rapidly relieved after the injection of parenteral antihistamines such as diphenhydramine or cimetidine and most symptoms will have completely abated within 6 hours. The patient should not be told that he or she has an allergic reaction and they should not be prevented from eating fish in the future.

71. **Answer D.** Posterior shoulder dislocations occur much less commonly than anterior dislocations. Mechanisms include seizure (due to stronger internal rotator muscles compared with external rotator muscles), electrocution, and fall on an outstretched hand. Patients with posterior shoulder dislocation are almost never able to abduct or externally rotate their affected arms. Neurovascular injury is much less common than with anterior dislocations due to the anterior position of the neurovascular structures. Posterior shoulder dislocation is often confused with adhesive capsulitis and may simply present as stiffness and limited range of motion rather than frank pain. Recurrent injury does occur, but less commonly than in anterior shoulder dislocations. Management is with early reduction and orthopedic consultation.

72. **Answer C.** The capitate articulates directly with the lunate and dorsally dislocates when there is enough carpal instability due to fracture or ligamentous injury. On lateral radiographs, the lunate is in proper position relative to the radius, but the capitate falls posterior to the lunate and may even articulate with the distal radius. In lunate dislocation, the lunate dislocates volarly relative to the radius and the capitate is in line with radius. The median nerve is the most common peripheral nerve injured in cases of lunate or perilunate dislocation.

73. **Answer B.** Carditis complicates approximately 5% of untreated patients with Lyme disease, and more commonly affects men. Cardiac manifestations occur during the early phase of the illness, typically within a few weeks to a few months of infection. The most common manifestation is AV block of varying degrees. Patients with a PR interval >300 milliseconds are at highest risk for progressing to complete heart block. Occasionally, patients

require permanent or temporary pacemakers. However, most patients recover quickly without sequelae within 1 to a few weeks. Occasionally, patients have persistent first-degree heart block. Patients less commonly suffer from myopericarditis and symptoms of CHF. When present, myopericarditis is typically asymptomatic and not clinically relevant. Overall, the prognosis for patients with Lyme carditis is very good. The diagnosis is made when patients with appropriate findings give a history of tick exposure, or have positive antibody tests. While patients with early *localized* Lyme disease can have false-negative antibody, most patients with Lyme carditis are sero-positive.

74. **Answer C.** This patient presents with atrial fibrillation with a rapid ventricular response (AFib with RVR). Traditionally, electrical cardioversion has been a treatment option to restore normal sinus rhythm as long as the patient has been symptomatic for <48 hours. However, there are increasing data suggesting that the risk of a cardiac thrombus rises as early as 12 hours after onset. A transesophageal echocardiogram (TEE) should be performed to exclude a thrombus. Furthermore, evidence suggests that patients older than 65 have better outcomes when treatment focuses on rate control rather than rhythm control. Diltiazem or beta-blockers such as metoprolol are the treatment agents of choice. While digoxin may be useful, it has a narrower therapeutic window and more side effects of therapy. If electrical cardioversion is performed, it is unclear whether anterior–posterior (front and back) or anterior–lateral (right upper front and left lower front) pad placement is best. Anticoagulation is often necessary for patients who convert to normal sinus rhythm. The CHA_2DS_2–VASc is the current scoring system used to determine annual stroke risk and the need for anticoagulation. The scoring system is heavily tied to age, and females also earn an extra point for their gender. Given this patient's history of hypertension and diabetes, she will easily be considered high-risk and anticoagulation will be recommended.

75. **Answer E.** The patient has failed outpatient therapy for pyelonephritis. The possible reasons for this include antibiotic noncompliance, antibiotic resistance, a concomitant kidney stone, or a renal abscess. The patient has had 2 weeks of appropriate antibiotic therapy for pyelonephritis, which should be adequate for clinical cure unless a kidney stone or renal abscess is present. CT is recommended if such a complication is suspected. Initiating treatment with a more narrow-spectrum antibiotic such as TMP-SMX or metronidazole is not indicated, especially if no urine culture is performed beforehand. In this patient's case, the urine culture suggests that ciprofloxacin should normally be adequate therapy. However, given the resistance rates in many communities, the best empiric choice for outpatient treatment of

pyelonephritis is a third-generation oral cephalosporin such as cefixime. Extending the course of ciprofloxacin beyond 2 weeks is only indicated in cases of male prostatitis.

76. **Answer D.** Clinician judgment is extremely important in determining the disposition of patients with persistent abdominal tenderness after major trauma despite negative CT imaging. However, studies of this patient population reveal that, in general, it is safe to discharge them home with careful instructions to return for worrisome symptoms. Repeat CT imaging with oral contrast is neither necessary nor advisable since it increases radiation exposure without a significant improvement in diagnostic yield. Furthermore, isolated abdominal tenderness is not predictive for worrisome intraabdominal injury. However, disposition decisions should be individualized depending on clinician concern and degree of suspicion.

77. **Answer C.** The patient has evidence of acute testicular torsion, with scrotal pain, nausea, vomiting, and testicular tenderness. Pathophysiology involves twisting of the testis on the spermatic cord due to an anatomic abnormality or trauma. The most sensitive physical examination finding is the cremasteric reflex—presence of this reflex virtually rules out the diagnosis. Diagnosis can be made clinically in some cases, but confirmation is made with color Doppler ultrasonography, which has excellent sensitivity and specificity when performed by experienced operators. Prompt diagnosis is essential, as testicular survival is directly dependent on duration of symptoms—if surgical management is instituted within 6 hours of pain, approximately 100% of cases are salvageable. Advanced imaging techniques such as CT and MRI scans do not add to the diagnostic accuracy of testicular torsion and waste valuable time. Retrograde urethrogram is used to diagnose traumatic injuries to the urethra and is not indicated here. The bulbocavernosus reflex is used to evaluate spinal cord injuries in trauma patients and has no role in the evaluation of the acute scrotum.

78. **Answer A.** The patient has asymptomatic first-degree atrioventricular (AV) block with a prolonged PR interval but no dropped beats. This is commonly seen in healthy individuals, has no prognostic significance, and requires no further evaluation or management.

79. **Answer B.** SIDS is defined as the sudden, inexplicable death of any infant whose cause cannot even be diagnosed by autopsy. The peak age for SIDS is 2 to 4 months. Risk factors include maternal smoking, young maternal age, preterm age, among others. Apnea and hypoventilation are the most likely explanations, but dysrhythmias, airway obstruction, and trauma are all proposed as possible contributors. Infants should be placed on their backs to sleep to help reduce the incidence of SIDS.

80. **Answer B.** The patient has clear clinical evidence of meningitis. Given the time course, it is unclear whether the etiology is viral or bacterial, so a cautious approach should be taken. Ideally, the patient should have a lumbar puncture as soon as possible, but antibiotics should not be delayed in such cases as they do not appear to significantly affect culture results in the first 4 hours of therapy. Corticosteroids are now part of the standard of care for treatment of suspected bacterial meningitis as they improve functional outcomes. The indications for CT scan before lumbar puncture are altered mental status, focal neurologic deficit, suspected brain mass lesion, and signs of increased intracranial pressure. MRI of the brain has little role in the emergent evaluation of meningitis.

81. **Answer D.** Due to the anterior communicating artery, lesions of the anterior cerebral artery proximal to the communicating artery are generally well tolerated. Lesions distal to this anastomosis result predominantly in leg weakness and sensory loss as well as a variety of personality and behavioral changes. These changes include abulia, which is the inability of patients to make decisions. The upper extremities may be involved but are typically only mildly affected. Furthermore, the deficits are usually most marked distally. The tongue and the face are generally spared.

82. **Answer C.** The patient has a large central corneal abrasion as demonstrated by the irregular patch of fluorescein uptake from 3 o'clock to 6 o'clock. Treatment of corneal abrasions involves pain control with topical or oral analgesics, short-acting cycloplegics, and topical antibiotics to prevent secondary infection. Topical antivirals would be indicated in patients with herpes simplex or zoster keratitis, which are signaled by the presence of dendrites or pseudodendrites, respectively. Topical steroids should never be given by the emergency physician (EP) without ophthalmologic consultation beforehand, as consequences may be devastating in patients with herpetic keratitis. Acetazolamide is used to increase aqueous humor excretion as part of noninvasive temporizing therapies for acute glaucoma attacks. Emergent ophthalmologic consultation is not indicated in patients with corneal abrasions, even in patients with abrasions associated with contact lenses. If there is suspicion of corneal ulcer (which would appear as a yellowish spot on the cornea), then consultation should be obtained emergently. (Figure from Rapuano CJ. Wills Eye Institute – Cornea. 2nd edition. Philadelphia: Wolters Kluwer, 2011.)

83. **Answer E.** Modern, multidetector CT scanners, which are ubiquitous in the United States, are nearly 100% sensitive in detecting clinically significant cervical spine injuries. Flexion and extension views don't add

additional information. While MRI is more sensitive for detecting ligamentous injuries, those injuries are almost never clinically relevant in patients without neurologic complaints or findings. Symptomatic patients most commonly have stable traumatic cervical disk herniations and symptoms and findings can guide management. Patients with persistent tenderness without neurologic complaints or findings may be discharged home with outpatient follow-up. Some guidelines suggest discharging patients in a rigid collar (such as a Miami-J, Aspen, or Philadelphia collar) with short-term follow-up, ideally in consultation with the trauma or neurosurgical team.

84. **Answer E.** Multiple sclerosis (MS) is the most common autoimmune inflammatory demyelinating disease of the central nervous system. In patients with symptoms and findings of an acute episode of demyelination, steroids remain the mainstay of treatment. While a 5-day course of 1,000 mg IV methylprednisolone is the most common therapy given, oral prednisone regimens are equally effective, except in patients with optic neuritis. One trial demonstrated higher relapse rates in patients with optic neuritis who were given an oral prednisone regimen versus the group given IV methylprednisolone. Plasma exchange is reserved for patients who don't respond to steroids. Finally, since this patient has known MS, and since her symptoms and findings are suggestive of MS, there is no indication for neuroimaging.

85. **Answer B.** The patient has conjunctival injection around the limbus (the junction of the clear cornea and white sclera), also known as perilimbic injection or ciliary flush. This is usually due to iritis or anterior uveitis. Corneal abrasion can occur concomitantly with an iritis, but without a history of trauma, this would be atypical. Acute angle closure glaucoma would not be likely in a 37-year-old male without any prior history. Furthermore, the pupil would likely be fixed, mid-dilated, or cloudy with significant loss of vision. Pinguecula and pterygium are both chronic, benign growths in the conjunctiva of little clinical significance except cosmesis. Pterygia can invade the line of vision and needs to be corrected in those cases. (Figure courtesy of Gary N Foulks and Joseph A Halabis, OD, In: Allingham RR, Damji KF, Freedman SF, et al. *Shields Textbook of Glaucoma.* 6th ed. Philadelphia, PA: Wolters Kluwer; 2010.)

86. **Answer B.** Although handlebar injuries are simply a form of blunt abdominal trauma, which therefore put patients at risk for liver and spleen injuries, there is an increased risk of pancreatic and small bowel injuries. Classically, pancreatic or duodenal injuries are associated with pediatric handlebar injuries. Patients with pancreatic injury often develop delayed symptoms and

may have a relatively benign presentation initially. Eventually, they develop abdominal pain, nausea, and vomiting and have evidence of pancreatic injury by elevated enzymes on laboratory analysis. Acute closed-loop small bowel obstruction and rupture may also occur with handlebar injuries. Owing to the lack of significant blood loss, patients may again be relatively asymptomatic. Since the small bowel contains relatively little air, up to 85% of cases will have a normal upright abdominal film (i.e., no free air) and 50% will have no signs of peritonitis on examination. Therefore, physicians must maintain a high suspicion for injury in cases of pediatric handlebar trauma.

87. **Answer D.** In neonates, the heart rate is the most sensitive indicator of adequate cardiopulmonary status. In addition to inadequate respiratory effort, infants with bradycardia, specifically when the heart rate falls below 100, need positive pressure ventilation (PPV). PPV is delivered with bag–mask ventilation (BMV) at a rate of 40 to 60 times per minute for 30 seconds, after which the heart rate is assessed to determine the effectiveness of the resuscitation. Tracheal intubation is ultimately required if the infant's heart rate doesn't improve despite these efforts.

88. **Answer C.** Antiviral therapy has been shown to hasten recovery from the shingles rash as well as the acute neuritis that accompanies it. However, neither steroids, nor antivirals, nor a combination of the two has been shown to decrease postherpetic neuralgia. Steroids are not recommended for patients with shingles. Antiviral therapy is only recommended for patients presenting within 72 hours of onset. There is no role for the shingles vaccine in patients with active shingles.

89. **Answer C.** The thoracic outlet syndrome comprises a group of pathologic conditions associated with compression of the structures at the junction of the upper extremity and trunk. The findings are neurologic (95%), venous (4%), and arterial (1%). The most commonly affected structure is the ulnar nerve.

90. **Answer D.** Nausea and vomiting are common in patients with SAH, occurring in about three-quarters of all cases. Unfortunately, many other headache syndromes will also cause nausea and vomiting, so they are not specific for SAH. About half of all patients with SAH have alteration of mental status, which is the next most common associated sign/symptom. Focal neurologic deficit, preceding exertional activity, seizure, and intraocular hemorrhage each are present in less than a quarter of all cases. Preceding exertional activity does confer a roughly threefold increased likelihood that the headache is due to SAH, but sensitivity of this finding is low.

91. **Answer B.** Patients with an upper extremity DVT tend to be younger and leaner than their lower extremity DVT counterparts. They less commonly have an inherited or acquired hypercoagulable state but more commonly have an underlying diagnosis of cancer. In fact, most upper extremity DVTs are associated with an indwelling catheter (often used for chemotherapy or long-term antibiotics). Though patients with an upper extremity DVT experience complications less often than patients with lower extremity DVTs, approximately 6% of patients still develop a PE (versus as many as one-third of patients with a lower extremity DVT), so patients require long-term anticoagulation, typically for 3 to 6 months after diagnosis.

92. **Answer C.** Postintubation hypotension is a common problem in asthmatics, occurring in as many as 20% of intubated patients. The presence of severe airflow obstruction can cause air trapping even in the setting of normal minute ventilation. Air trapping causes elevated intrathoracic pressures, which decreases venous return and subsequently cardiac output and BP. These problems are exacerbated in patients who are relatively hypovolemic, and for this reason, some experts recommend bolusing asthmatics with 1 L of crystalloid before intubation. In the setting of the "crashing" patient, excessive or overzealous "bagging" is often mistakenly applied in an attempt to resuscitate the patient. This creates the perfect setup for postintubation hypotension by insufflating the chest with a large volume of air. Because connecting the ventilator was the trigger for this patient's hypotension, the most prudent step is to immediately disconnect the ventilator and allow the patient to exhale for 30 seconds (the apnea test). Immediate recovery suggests the hypotension was caused by auto-positive end-expiratory pressure (PEEP) and lung hyperinflation. Persistent hypotension suggests a tension pneumothorax and should prompt an immediate needle thoracostomy once the pneumothorax is located. Pneumothorax should be suspected anytime there is a sudden clinical deterioration. Needle thoracostomy may be required in the setting of severe hypotension with or without concomitant tracheal deviation.

93. **Answer D.** Thyroid storm treatment requires sequential inhibition of the following: hormone synthesis, hormone release, and peripheral conversion from T_4 to T_3. Thionamides, including propylthiouracil and methimazole, prevent the synthesis of new thyroid hormone. Potassium iodide serves as a source of inorganic iodide, which prevents release of preformed hormone from the thyroid gland. In the acute setting potassium iodide can actually promote new hormone synthesis and should, therefore, always be given *after* thionamide therapy in thyroid storm. Propranolol is used next to treat cardiovascular effects of thyrotoxicosis as well as to block peripheral conversion of T_4 to the more metabolically active T_3. Glucocorticoids are used to treat any underlying adrenal insufficiency and may have some effect in preventing peripheral conversion.

94. **Answer A.** Between 30% and 80% of alcoholics have magnesium deficiency. Patients with hypomagnesemia are frequently asymptomatic or manifest only nonspecific symptoms. The most prominent symptoms in the ED are neuromuscular and cardiovascular, and magnesium deficiency tends to mimic calcium deficiency. The mechanism of hypomagnesemia in alcoholism is thought to be a combination of malnutrition, increased renal excretion, and GI losses from vomiting and diarrhea. Diuretic therapy is also a very prevalent cause of hypomagnesemia, although the subsequent volume loss increases magnesium reabsorption in the proximal tubule. Therefore, magnesium depletion in the setting of diuretic therapy tends to be modest. Hypomagnesemia is the most common electrolyte abnormality in ambulatory diabetic patients and is also common in DKA. In these patients, magnesium is lost through the urine due to glycosuria.

95. **Answer C.** Sulfonylureas fall into the "one pill can kill" category of toxic ingestions among pediatric patients. Glyburide is a commonly used second-generation sulfonylurea with a long half-life (10 hours) as well as active metabolites. Insulin release is increased within 1 hour after ingestion, and hypoglycemia rapidly follows. As with several other sulfonylureas, the peak effect does not occur for 2 to 6 hours, and because of the drug's prolonged half-life, persistent or delayed effects both occur. Many pediatric patients are asymptomatic with euglycemia at presentation. However, most experts recommend admission to the hospital for prolonged observation, even among such patients. Patients with symptoms at presentation, such as the patient in this question, should be admitted. In contrast to adults, children should receive more dilute preparations of dextrose to manage hypoglycemia. D25W can be given to young children while D10W is preferred for neonates and infants, though it can also be given to older children. While the exact dextrose dose can deviate from this rule, the easiest way to remember the amount of dextrose to deliver in acutely hypoglycemic, symptomatic neonates is to follow the "rule of 50." The basic formula is % dextrose × mL/kg volume = 50. So:

D5 × 10 mL/kg = 5 × 10 = 50. For a 5 kg child, bolus 10 mL/kg or 50 mL of D5

D10 × 5 mL/kg = 10 × 5 = 50. For a 5 kg child, bolus 5 mL/kg or 25 mL of D10 (as in this patient)

D25 × 2 mL/kg = 25 × 2 = 50. For a 5 kg child, bolus 2 mL/kg or 10 mL of D25.

While some experts recommend octreotide therapy to all symptomatic patients receiving dextrose, others recommend octreotide only in settings of refractory hypoglycemia. Octreotide works by decreasing calcium influx in pancreatic beta islet cells, which results in decreased calcium-mediated insulin release.

96. **Answer A.** Dysuria in all patients is most commonly due to bacterial UTI. Gram-negative enteric rods are the number one causative group, with *E. coli* as the single most likely etiologic agent. Urethritis due to *Chlamydia* and *gonococcus* is also extremely common, as are candidal vaginitis and bacterial vaginosis. Viral and parasitic infections are uncommon causes of dysuria. Allergic urethritis may be responsible in patients who have long-term foreign bodies (such as Foley catheters) in place.

97. **Answer A.** Due to their significant airflow obstruction, mechanically ventilated asthmatics are at risk for lung hyperinflation and concomitantly elevated airway pressures. To avoid these problems, the most commonly used ventilatory strategy is "permissive hypercapnia." In this strategy, the patient is ventilated at settings that ensure adequate time for exhalation, which limits air trapping and subsequent auto-PEEP and lung hyperinflation (with elevated plateau pressures). Expiratory time can be maximized by limiting the time spent during inspiration (by setting high inspiratory flow rates and by using a square-wave form), as well as by decreasing minute ventilation (by decreasing *either* V_T or RR). The byproduct of these changes is hypercapnia. Previous approaches aimed to normalize alveolar CO_2 by using higher respiratory rates and tidal volumes but resulted in increased morbidity and mortality from airway barotrauma. Peak pressure reflects the pressure applied to the large- and medium-sized airways as air is pushed into the lungs by the ventilator. It strongly reflects airway resistance and tends to be very high in asthmatics due to their significant airway obstruction. Plateau pressure reflects the pressure applied to the small airways and alveoli after the air settles in the lungs. It is extremely important to monitor plateau pressure and ensure that it remains <35 cm H_2O to avoid alveolar overdistension and barotrauma. When plateau pressure is normal and intrinsic PEEP is <15 cm H_2O, peak pressure elevations are immaterial. Therefore, while high inspiratory flow rates elevate the peak pressure, it is unnecessary to reduce flow rates to decrease peak pressure. In fact, it is most often necessary to *increase* the inspiratory flow rate in order to decrease inspiratory time, which also results in *increased* peak pressure. Peak pressure is determined by the rate of airflow, not the absolute volume of air nor the respiratory rate.

98. **Answer E.** Although the patient has an obvious leg fracture, her hypotension suggests that there may be another, more significant injury present. In general, only a few sites of injury in adults can cause enough hemorrhage

to result in hypotension. These include thorax, intraperitoneum, retroperitoneum, pelvis, and bilateral femurs. Tibial fractures by themselves do not usually result in hypotension due to hemorrhage. Appropriate adjuncts to the primary survey include radiographs of the chest and pelvis and focused assessment of sonography in trauma (FAST) scan. These tests should be done *before* any management of the open tibial fracture. Specific management of the open tibial fracture can occur only if there are extra care providers to perform this concomitantly with the adjuncts to the primary survey. Tetanus immunization can be carried out at any time within 72 hours of the injury and need not be an emergency procedure.

99. **Answer E.** The patient has herpes zoster ophthalmicus. Though the illness is focal, most patients have a systemic prodrome of headache, fever, and generalized malaise. Hutchinson sign describes a vesicular eruption over the nose which occurs due to varicella zoster virus (VZV) involvement of the nasociliary branch of the trigeminal nerve. Since this same branch innervates the globe, such patients are at increased risk for ocular involvement, and should receive treatment as for patients who have clear evidence of ocular involvement. Treatment involves systemic oral antivirals and topical steroids. Topical antivirals can be used as adjunctive therapy and topical antibiotics can also be used as optional adjunctive therapy if the diagnosis is in doubt. Urgent ophthalmologic consultation is generally pursued. Corneal hypoesthesia is common and over three-fourths of patients recover completely. The ophthalmic division of cranial nerve V is involved. Anterior uveitis occurs often in herpes zoster ophthalmicus and the frequency is independent of severity of corneal involvement.

100. **Answer C.** Spontaneous remission is the rule in trigeminal neuralgia as >50% of patients will experience a remission for 6 months. Antiviral medications directed at herpes and corticosteroids should be used for patients with postherpetic neuralgia. This is a separate entity from trigeminal neuralgia and patients should not be placed on antivirals unless they have a history of herpes zoster (shingles) involving the face. All patients with trigeminal neuralgia should be referred to a neurologist for further evaluation. Up to 2% to 4% of patients with trigeminal neuralgia also have multiple sclerosis and up to 10% of patients have intracranial lesion. Therefore, all such patients should receive an MRI on an outpatient basis. Unfortunately, roughly 30% of patients will fail medical therapy and require surgical ablation. Phenytoin is not indicated for trigeminal neuralgia. Carbamazepine is the standard front-line agent and is started at 100 to 200 mg b.i.d. Although carbamazepine is sometimes poorly tolerated, it produces a significant positive response in most patients with classic trigeminal neuralgia.

TEST 2

1. Which of the following is the preferred imaging modality to diagnose a parapharyngeal abscess in the ED?
   - A. Lateral neck x-ray
   - B. Anterior–posterior neck x-ray
   - C. CT scan of the neck
   - D. Magnetic resonance imaging (MRI) of the neck
   - E. Ultrasonography of the neck

2. Which of the following is true regarding falls from buildings?
   - A. Mortality is unrelated to height of the fall.
   - B. Feet-first falls cause retroperitoneal bleeding more often than intraperitoneal bleeding.
   - C. Renal injury is uncommon in falls onto supine position.
   - D. Calcaneal fracture is the most common cause of death from all falls.
   - E. Falls onto prone position almost never result in death.

3. A 45-year-old male presents in a coma after being exposed to smoke from a building fire. The patient is immediately intubated. An arterial blood gas (ABG) demonstrates metabolic acidosis and an extremely elevated lactate level. Which of the following is the most important medication to administer?
   - A. Amyl nitrite
   - B. Sodium nitrite
   - C. Sodium thiosulfate
   - D. Methylene blue
   - E. Dexamethasone

4. A 44-year-old male presents after a motor vehicle crash (MVC) with scrotal pain. Blood was noticed initially at the urethral meatus, but a 16-Fr Foley catheter was mistakenly placed with return of yellow urine. Which of the following is the most appropriate next step in management?
   - A. Remove the 16-Fr catheter and place a 12-Fr Foley catheter
   - B. Remove the 16-Fr catheter and place a 12-Fr Coude catheter
   - C. Remove the 16-Fr catheter and perform retrograde urethrogram
   - D. Remove the 16-Fr catheter and perform retrograde cystogram
   - E. Leave the catheter in place and obtain urologic consultation

5. A 19-year-old male presents with acute onset of right testicular pain and nausea for 5 hours. Physical examination reveals a markedly swollen and tender testis in a horizontal lie with an absent right cremasteric reflex. Which of the following is the most appropriate definitive management?
   - A. Antibiotics
   - B. Analgesia
   - C. Manual detorsion
   - D. Operative orchidopexy
   - E. Extracorporeal shockwave lithotripsy

6. Which of the following physiologic changes is expected in hypothermic patients?
   - A. Hemoconcentration
   - B. Hypoglycemia
   - C. Metabolic alkalosis
   - D. Oliguria
   - E. Seizures

7. Which of the following is true regarding troponin I in acute myocardial infarction (MI)?
   - A. Starts elevating 12 hours after MI
   - B. Peaks at 36 hours after MI
   - C. Returns to baseline within 72 hours
   - D. Sensitivity at 6 hours after MI is 95%
   - E. Specificity at 6 hours after MI is 95%

8. Which of the following is true regarding lung abscesses?

   A. The most common pathogen is *Streptococcus pneumococcus*.

   B. Patients with anaerobic lung abscesses typically present with acute-onset chest pain, cough, and fever.

   C. Lung abscess occurs most commonly in patients with poor oral hygiene.

   D. Thoracotomy with abscess excision is the cornerstone of therapy.

   E. Lung abscesses most commonly develop as a complication of pediatric pneumonia.

9. A 45-year-old female is referred to the ED from an optometrist with a diagnosis of bilateral papilledema and "rule out pseudotumor cerebri." Which of the following is true about pseudotumor cerebri (also known as *idiopathic intracranial hypertension*)?

   A. Brain stem compression is the most feared complication.

   B. CT scanning will demonstrate hydrocephalus in 80% of cases.

   C. Oculomotor nerve palsy is the most common associated cranial nerve palsy.

   D. Men outnumber women 4:1.

   E. Headaches are the most common presenting symptom.

10. A previously healthy 35-year-old male is brought to the ED with a chief complaint of fever and altered mental status. The patient had been well until 1 day prior to admission, when he developed a fever and general malaise. He was too ill to work on the day of evaluation, and when his wife returned from work, she found him hot, sweaty, and "out of it." The patient presents with a temperature of 102.1 F, P 103, RR 18, BP 125/75, SaO$_2$ 97% RA. He is awake, but somnolent and confused. A lumbar puncture is performed which reveals gram-positive cocci in pairs. His wife asks about receiving prophylactic therapy. Which of the following is most appropriate?

   A. Doxycycline 100 mg PO BID × 3 days

   B. Ciprofloxacin 500 mg PO × 1 dose

   C. Rocephin 250 mg IM × 1 dose

   D. Rifampin 600 mg PO × 2 days

   E. No prophylaxis is indicated.

11. Which of the following is true regarding toxic alcohols?

   A. Alcohol dehydrogenase has greater affinity for methanol than for ethanol.

   B. Alcohol dehydrogenase has greater affinity for ethylene glycol than for ethanol.

   C. Alcohol dehydrogenase has greater affinity for ethylene glycol than for methanol.

   D. As little as one tablespoon of 40% methanol may be lethal in adults.

   E. Gastrointestinal (GI) absorption of both methanol and ethylene glycol takes 4 to 5 hours.

12. A 33-year-old female presents with a chief complaint of dysphagia. She feels a sensation of foods, particularly solids, getting "stuck" in her chest and she sometimes needs to raise her arms above her head or straighten her back after eating to help things pass. She also complains of intermittent substernal burning chest pain. Her doctor has been treating her for gastroesophageal reflux disease (GERD) for the last 9 months but she seems to be getting worse. What is the likely cause of her symptoms?

   A. Nutcracker esophagus

   B. Diffuse esophageal spasm

   C. Schatzki ring

   D. Achalasia

   E. Zenker diverticulum

13. A 38-year-old female who has a history of "infertility" presents to the ED with low abdominal pain. She recently became pregnant after using in vitro fertilization. Her physical examination reveals mild low abdominal tenderness, no adnexal mass, and a closed cervical os with a normal bimanual examination. An ultrasonography demonstrates a live intrauterine gestation appropriately sized for dates but also reveals a slightly enlarged left ovary. Which of the following is the approximate risk of a heterotopic pregnancy in this patient?

   A. 0.25%

   B. 1%

   C. 10%

   D. 25%

   E. 50%

14. Which of the following is true about fungal pulmonary disease?

   A. Most cases of primary pulmonary infection with *Histoplasma capsulatum* are undetected and resolve without treatment.

   B. *Cryptococcus neoformans, Blastomyces dermatiditis, H. capsulatum*, and *Coccidioides imitis* all have a specific geographic distribution.

   C. Patients with fungal pneumonia are generally contagious to other patients.

   D. Fungal pneumonias generally cause acute, self-limiting illness in healthy patients.

   E. *C. imitis* pulmonary infection most commonly results in disseminated disease.

15. A 5-year-old male is brought for evaluation of penile erythema. He is uncircumcised and has erythema, edema, and a semisolid discharge around the glans without accompanying phimosis or paraphimosis. He has had several similar episodes in the past with identification of yeast. Which of the following is the most appropriate diagnostic test?

A. Liver function tests
B. Postvoid residual
C. Intravenous pyelogram
D. Serum glucose
E. Retrograde urethrogram

16. A 44-year-old alcoholic man presents with shortness of breath, fever, and productive cough. Chest x-ray demonstrates a left lower lobe infiltrate. The diagnosis of pneumonia is made. Which of the following is the most likely cause?

A. *Staphylococcus aureus*
B. *Streptococcus pneumoniae*
C. *Klebsiella pneumoniae*
D. *Mycobacterium tuberculosis*
E. *Mycoplasma pneumoniae*

17. Which of the following is true regarding transient ischemic attack (TIA)?

A. Neurologic findings in patients with TIAs are more commonly "positive" (tingling or involuntary movements) than "negative" (aphasia, weakness, numbness).
B. A "march" of symptoms affecting various body parts in succession is common in TIAs.
C. TIA was recently redefined as transient neurologic dysfunction that resolves within 1 hour.
D. Confusion and generalized weakness are common in patients with a TIA.
E. The most common mimic of symptoms caused by a TIA is a complicated migraine.

18. A 52-year-old male with a history of alcoholism presents with nausea and vomiting. He has been drinking more excessively than usual over the last few days after his wife left him. He has mild, epigastric abdominal pain. Vital signs are 98.5°F, 104, 22, 165/93, 100% RA. His physical examination is normal except for mild regular tachycardia and dry mucous membranes. His labs are shown below.

WBC: 6.5
Hb: 12.2
Plt: 125K
Na: 132
K: 4.4
Cl: 90
HCO$_3$: 12
BUN: 36
Cr: 1.4
Glu: 106

Which of the following is the most appropriate next step in management?

A. Insulin 10 units IV
B. Sodium bicarbonate 1 amp IV
C. Metoprolol 5 mg IV
D. D5 0.9 NS 1 L
E. Hydralazine 20 mg IV

19. Which of the following oral medications is most likely to cause serious damage to the esophageal mucosa when swallowed?

A. Amoxicillin
B. Potassium chloride
C. Metoprolol
D. Lovastatin
E. Hydrochlorothiazide

20. A 36-year-old pregnant female at 27 weeks of gestation presents to your community ED after a motor vehicle accident. The patient was a restrained passenger (three-point restraints) in a vehicle traveling approximately 30 mph when it collided with a stationary vehicle. Air bags deployed, but the patient self-extricated and was found sitting next to the car at the scene. She has not had any vaginal bleeding or leakage, but she is complaining of painful contractions. Which of the following is true?

A. Uterine rupture has occurred.
B. The patient most likely has placental abruption.
C. Uterine contractions usually resolve spontaneously.
D. The patient should be started on a terbutaline infusion and immediately transferred to a tertiary care facility.
E. Digital examination should be performed to determine whether there is cervical dilation and the patient is in active labor.

21. A 23-year-old female with a history of sickle cell disease presents with fever, chills, cough, and dyspnea. A chest x-ray demonstrates a focal infiltrate in the right lower lobe. Which of the following is the most appropriate management at this time?

A. Heparin, intravenous fluids, and antibiotics
B. Tissue plasminogen activator to treat pulmonary veno-occlusion
C. Intravenous fluids and oxygen
D. Intravenous fluids, albuterol, prednisone, and antibiotics
E. Intravenous fluids and antibiotics alone

22. Which of the following is the most common cardiac rhythm in patients with pulmonary embolism (PE)?

A. Normal sinus rhythm
B. Atrial fibrillation
C. Atrial flutter
D. Ventricular tachycardia
E. Sinus tachycardia

23. A 9-year-old male presents with progressively worsening right eyelid swelling, pain, and redness, for 3 days. He denies blurry vision. Which of the following is more characteristic of orbital cellulitis than periorbital cellulitis?

A. Fever

B. Periorbital edema

C. Eye tenderness

D. *S. aureus* as the etiologic agent

E. Restricted eye movement

24. A 48-year-old female with a history of a pulmonary embolism on warfarin is brought in by EMS with an intracerebral hemorrhage. Which of the following is an advantage of prothrombin complex concentrates (PCCs) over fresh frozen plasma (FFP)?

A. PCC can be infused faster than FFP

B. PCC causes a greater increase in clotting factors

C. PCC has a smaller volume than FFP

D. PCC does not require thawing or blood-type matching

E. All of the above

25. A 67-year-old female with a history of hypertension and hyperlipidemia is brought in to the ED after a syncopal episode. The patient reports eating lunch with a friend when she began to feel dizzy. She can't recall anything else. No seizure activity or chest pain was noted. Her EKG is shown. Which of the following is true? (Fig. 2-1)

A. Since the patient's rhythm is normal, there is no increased risk of a serious cardiac outcome

B. The patient has a right bundle branch block, which is not associated with an increased risk of a serious cardiac outcome

C. The patient is at increased risk for a serious cardiac outcome

D. T inversions in leads I and aVL combined with <1 mm ST depression in V6 are concerning for ischemia

E. The patient is likely symptomatic from her low heart rate as a result of beta blocker therapy

26. A 52-year-old male is brought to the ED after a high-speed motor vehicle crash. His primary survey is as follows:

Airway: Intact
Breathing: Intact breath sounds bilaterally
Circulation: Normal pulses throughout
Disability: Moves and feels all extremities
Exposure: Ecchymosis to left upper chest

His vital signs are 99.0, 90, 22, 155/85, 92% RA. Chest x-ray is shown in Figure 2-2. Which of the following is the next best step in management?

A. Left needle thoracostomy

B. Left tube thoracostomy

C. Right needle thoracostomy

D. Right tube thoracostomy

E. Supplemental oxygen

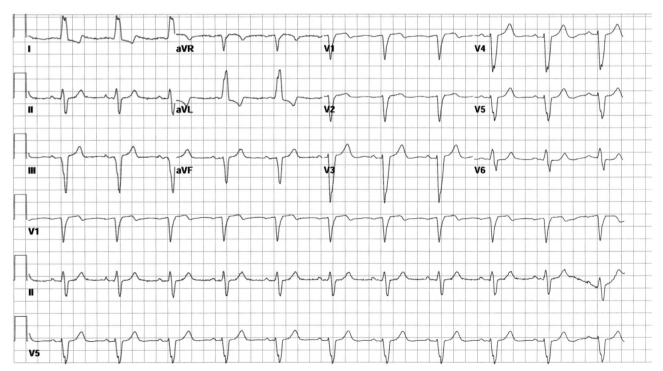

Figure 2-1

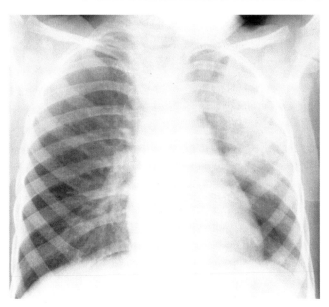

Figure 2-2

27. Which of the following therapies has the fastest onset of action in reducing serum potassium levels in cases of hyperkalemia?

   A. Intravenous calcium
   B. Nebulized albuterol
   C. Intravenous insulin and glucose
   D. Oral sodium polystyrene sulfonate (Kayexalate)
   E. Intravenous sodium bicarbonate

28. A 1-week-old term male infant who was delivered at home is brought to the ED by his parents with abdominal distension, difficulty passing stools, failure to thrive, and bilious vomiting. Digital rectal examination reveals an empty rectal vault but stimulates significant stool and gas production once the finger is removed. Which of the following is the most likely cause of these symptoms?

   A. Intussusception
   B. Pyloric stenosis
   C. Gastroesophageal reflux disease (GERD)
   D. Hirschsprung disease
   E. Incarcerated hernia

29. The earliest indicator of acute radiation syndrome is:

   A. Thrombocytopenia
   B. Eosinophilia
   C. Decrease in absolute lymphocyte count
   D. Aplastic anemia
   E. Increase in the number of atypical lymphocytes

30. Cholelithiasis is an uncommon disease entity in children. Which of the following is most commonly associated with biliary colic in children?

   A. Cystic fibrosis (CF)
   B. Hemolytic anemia

   C. Obesity
   D. Diabetes
   E. Cerebral palsy

31. A first-time mother brings in her 4-day-old male infant to the ED with a chief complaint of abdominal pain and sudden yellowish-green vomiting. She notes that he had been "fussy" all day but became ill only a few hours earlier. On examination, he appears ill and has a mildly distended abdomen. An abdominal film is shown in Figure 2-3. Which of the following is the next best step in management?

   A. Barium enema
   B. Emergent surgical consultation
   C. Broad spectrum antibiotics for presumed necrotizing enterocolitis
   D. Obtain an ultrasound to rule out pyloric stenosis
   E. Recommend smaller, thickened feedings, frequent burping, and discharge home

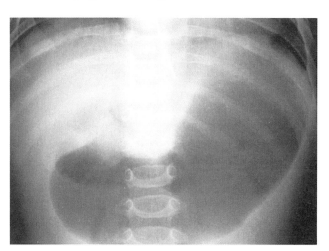

Figure 2-3

32. Which of the following is true regarding viral hepatitis?

   A. Adult patients infected with acute hepatitis B are more likely to become chronic carriers than patients infected with acute hepatitis C.
   B. Hepatitis C is most commonly acquired through sexual intercourse with an infected person.
   C. Hepatitis C is the most common viral cause of fulminant hepatic failure.
   D. Both direct and indirect bilirubin are typically elevated in roughly equal amounts.
   E. Leukocytosis is a harbinger of fulminant hepatic failure.

33. A 55-year-old male presents with a seizure. He has never had a seizure before and developed tonic–clonic movements for 1 minute followed by a postictal confusional state lasting about 10 minutes. Physical examination is normal, and the patient is amnestic to the event. Blood glucose is normal. Which of the following is the most appropriate next step in management?

A. MRI brain
B. CT brain
C. Phenobarbital loading dose
D. Lumbar puncture
E. Prolactin level

34. Which of the following is associated with a normal anion gap in overdose?

A. Salicylates
B. Methanol
C. Isopropanol
D. Ethylene glycol
E. Isoniazid

35. A 24-year-old male presents with headache, stiff neck, fever, and rash shown (Fig. 2-4). Which of the following is the next best step in management?

A. CT brain without contrast
B. CT brain with contrast
C. Lumbar puncture
D. Ceftriaxone
E. Vancomycin

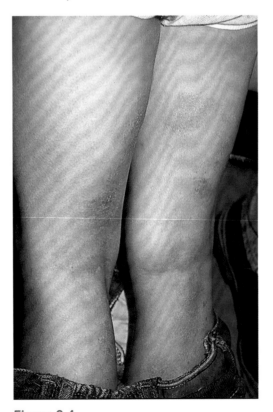

Figure 2-4

36. Which of the following is the most common cause of acute food poisoning in the United States?

A. *Clostridium perfringens*
B. *S. aureus*
C. *Escherichia coli*
D. *Bacillus cereus*
E. *Vibrio parahaemolyticus*

37. A 27-year-old male is brought to the ED after an accident riding an all terrain vehicle (ATV). He was riding in an open field with a helmet and body armor when he ran into a wire fence that struck him in the neck, knocked him off the bike and knocked him out. He now complains of a mild headache and neck and back soreness but is otherwise without complaints. His examination reveals left-sided ptosis and anisocoria with a smaller left pupil. Which of the following is most likely to reveal significant injury?

A. CT head without contrast
B. CT angiography
C. Laryngoscopy
D. Cervical spine series
E. Chest x-ray

38. A 7-year-old female presents with syncope without a prodrome. EKG shows QT prolongation. Family history is most likely to reveal which of the following?

A. Cystic fibrosis
B. Hirschsprung disease
C. Juvenile rheumatoid arthritis
D. Deafness
E. Short stature

39. A 22-year-old female presents to the ED with symptoms of extreme panic. She tells you that she just used lysergic acid diethylamine (LSD) for the first time. Which of the following is true regarding this patient?

A. Lorazepam may be used to reduce agitation.
B. The patient is likely to get addicted to LSD.
C. LSD is structurally and functionally similar to γ-aminobutyric acid (GABA).
D. The lethal dose of LSD is very close to the typical dose taken to induce a "trip."
E. The patient is unlikely to develop tolerance with repeated uses of LSD.

40. Which of the following is the most effective treatment for fibromyalgia syndrome?

A. Prednisone
B. IV immunoglobulin (IVIG)
C. Aerobic exercise
D. Acupuncture
E. Physical therapy

41. Which of the following is true regarding EKGs in posterior wall MI?

   A. Abnormalities are most commonly seen in V3.
   B. ST elevations in precordial leads are diagnostic.
   C. Tall R waves are the earliest findings.
   D. T-wave inversions are common in V1–V3.
   E. Posteriorly placed leads are more accurate than anterior leads.

42. The most common associated finding in pharyngitis caused by adenovirus is which of the following?

   A. Pneumonia
   B. Encephalitis
   C. Peritonsillar abscess
   D. Scarlatiniform rash
   E. Conjunctivitis

43. A 53-year-old female presents 3 days after extraction of a premolar tooth with exquisite pain and tenderness in the area unrelieved by ibuprofen. Halitosis is present. Which of the following is true regarding this patient?

   A. Trismus is likely present.
   B. Irrigation and packing are generally of no benefit.
   C. Pathophysiology involves premature loss of clot from the socket.
   D. Treatment involves inducing mild bleeding to form a clot.
   E. Antibiotics and nonsteroidal anti-inflammatory drugs (NSAIDs) play no role in management.

44. Which of the following is a potential complication of *Bordetella pertussis* infection?

   A. Pneumonia
   B. Subconjunctival hemorrhage
   C. Pneumothorax
   D. Otitis media
   E. All of the above

45. Which of the following is indicated as supplemental treatment for patients with ethylene glycol poisoning?

   A. Folate and niacin
   B. Thiamine and pyridoxine
   C. Vitamin D and vitamin K
   D. Cobalamin and vitamin A
   E. Potassium and selenium

46. An 82-year-old male with a history of osteoporosis presents for evaluation of back pain after a fall. The patient reports he slipped in his kitchen and fell to his buttocks.

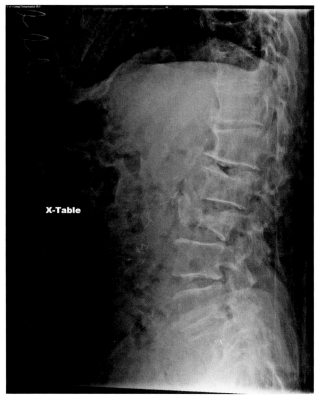

X-Table

Figure 2-5

He presents for evaluation of lumbar back pain. His x-ray is shown. Which of the following is the best next step in management? (Fig. 2-5)

   A. Admission for kyphoplasty
   B. MRI to assess retropulsion
   C. Consult spine surgery
   D. TLSO bracing
   E. Ambulatory walking trial, pain medicine

47. Which of the following toxins is most commonly associated with seizures?

   A. Cocaine
   B. Alcohol
   C. Opiates
   D. Ecstasy
   E. Ephedra

48. A 42-year-old male presents with left ear and posterior periauricular pain for 3 days. The ear is shown in Figure 2-6. Which of the following is the most important next step in diagnosis?

   A. X-rays
   B. Computed tomography (CT)
   C. MRI
   D. Tympanocentesis
   E. Lumbar puncture

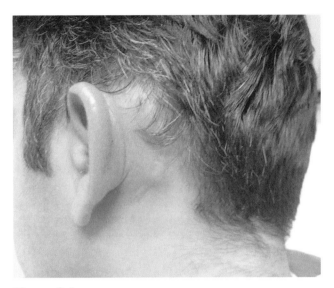

Figure 2-6

49. Applying a magnet to the chest of a patient with a pacemaker:

   A. Turns the pacing function off
   B. Turns the sensing function off
   C. Changes the pacemaker response to sensing from inhibition of impulse generation
   D. Completely deactivates all functions of the pacemaker
   E. Converts a dual chamber pacemaker into a single chamber pacemaker

50. You are consulting the thoracic surgery service after having recently placed a chest tube in a 22-year-old male for a 25% spontaneous pneumothorax. The consultant asks you whether there is still an "air leak" present. Assuming the patient's lung re-expanded appropriately, what is the most likely significance of an air leak?

   A. All patients will have an air leak after chest tube insertion.
   B. The chest tube was inserted into a branch of the patient's tracheobronchial tree.
   C. The suction holes on the chest tube are not completely inserted into the chest cavity.
   D. The water seal chamber does not have enough water in it.
   E. There is still an unhealed defect in the patient's bronchial tree.

51. Which of the following constitutes definitive treatment for ethylene glycol poisoning?

   A. Ethanol drip
   B. Fomepizole
   C. Pyridoxine
   D. Thiamine
   E. Dialysis

52. A 27-year-old male is brought to the ED after a motor vehicle accident complaining of right arm pain. His arm is swollen and shortened compared with the unaffected side. His x-ray reveals the image shown in Figure 2-7. Which of the following associated findings is most likely to be present upon physical examination?

   A. Inability to extend the wrist
   B. Loss of two-point discrimination at the volar tip of the index finger
   C. Absence of a radial pulse
   D. Inability to oppose the thumb
   E. Hypoesthesia of the palmar aspect of the little and ring fingers

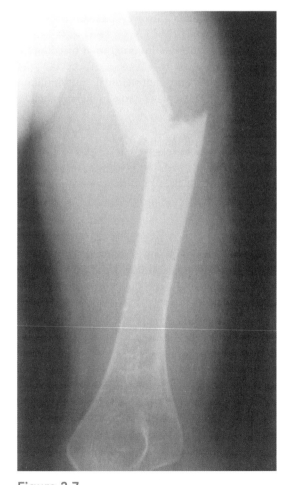

Figure 2-7

53. A 57-year-old female with hypertension who has not seen a doctor in 30 years presents with weakness and

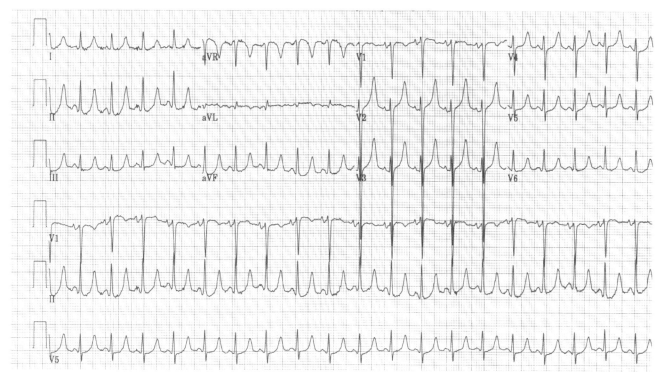

Figure 2-8

fatigue. The EKG is shown in Figure 2-8. After appropriate further evaluation, which of the following is most likely the appropriate next step in management?

A. Defibrillation at 200 J
B. Cardioversion at 50 J
C. Lidocaine 150 mg IV
D. Calcium gluconate 100 mg/kg IV
E. No acute management, follow-up with primary care

54. Which of the following is the most common cause of encephalitis?

A. Herpes virus
B. Mumps virus
C. Enteroviruses
D. Neurocysticercosis
E. Adenovirus

55. A 45-year-old female presents with intermittent epigastric pain and nausea for several weeks. She denies fever, diarrhea, cough, and chest pain. She does not take medications, drink alcohol, or smoke. She has had an extensive workup including CT scan of the abdomen and pelvis, gall bladder ultrasound, and cardiac stress testing, all of which were normal. You suspect gastritis. Which of the following is the most likely cause?

A. *Helicobacter pylori* infection
B. NSAID use
C. Alcohol use
D. Peppermint gum chewing
E. Radon exposure

56. A 22-year-old male is dropped off by his friends at the ED who stated he was shot with a gun in the middle of his abdomen. The most likely structure to be injured is the:

A. Liver
B. Small intestine
C. Spleen
D. Colon
E. Diaphragm

57. In patients receiving a normal 12-lead EKG, which of the following is true regarding reciprocal ST depressions seen in acute MI?

A. They have little prognostic significance.
B. They are more commonly seen in inferior MIs than anterior MIs.
C. They have poor specificity for acute MI.
D. They are more commonly seen in acute pericarditis than acute MI.
E. They are usually upsloping when seen in the setting of acute MI.

58. When compared to burns of other depths, deep partial-thickness burns:

A. Will impair joint function after healing if they involve a joint
B. Invariably heal with hypertrophic scarring
C. Are often difficult to differentiate clinically from full-thickness burns
D. Are typically painful only when direct pressure is applied
E. All of the above

59. Which of the following patients has the highest statistical chance of completed suicide?

    A. 75-year-old black man
    B. 75-year-old white man
    C. 18-year-old black woman
    D. 35-year-old pregnant woman
    E. 50-year-old married white man

60. EMS arrives with a 32-year-old female in active labor who spontaneously delivers her infant while she is still on the EMS stretcher. Upon initial evaluation, the infant is lying on its side on the stretcher, between the mother's legs, appearing cyanotic, breathing spontaneously but not crying. What is the next step?

    A. Deliver respirations with a bag-valve mask to improve oxygenation
    B. Suction the mouth and nose with a suction bulb
    C. Double clamp and cut the umbilical cord
    D. Dry the baby with a towel
    E. Deliver the placenta

61. A 63-year-old female with a history of "kidney problems" presents with a chief complaint of dizziness and lightheadedness. An EKG reveals profound bradycardia with a rate of 30 that fails to improve after atropine or transcutaneous pacing. Which of the following may be useful?

    A. Calcium
    B. Epinephrine
    C. Defibrillation
    D. Dopamine
    E. Norepinephrine

62. A 52-year-old male with a longstanding history of diabetes and hypertension presents for evaluation of vertigo. A head thrust maneuver (head impulse test) is abnormal when his head is turned to the right. There is no direction-changing nystagmus. There is no skew deviation. Which of the following is true?

    A. The patient likely has a vestibular lesion on the right
    B. The etiology is likely a viral infection
    C. The patient's symptoms are consistent with central vertigo
    D. The patient likely has ipsilateral facial muscle weakness
    E. The patient likely has a right-sided cerebellar stroke

63. A 44-year-old alcoholic man presents with hematemesis. Which of the following is the most likely cause?

    A. Peptic ulcer disease
    B. Gastric varices

    C. Esophageal varices
    D. Boerhaave syndrome
    E. Arteriovenous malformation

64. A 64-year-old female presents with a 3-week history of a constant, moderately intense, dull right-sided fronto-temporal headache. She also complains of occasional jaw pain as well as muscle aches and weakness in her shoulders. She denies any visual complaints, fever, or vomiting. She has a normal eye and neurologic examination. A noncontrast CT brain is normal. Which of the following is the most appropriate next step?

    A. Obtain MRI brain
    B. Perform lumbar puncture
    C. Check C-reactive protein (CRP)
    D. Prescribe carbamazepine
    E. Order migraine vasodilation stimulation test

65. A 43-year-old female presents with acute onset of upper abdominal pain. She has right upper quadrant tenderness, but lacks rebound tenderness or a Murphy sign. She has no fever and normal labs and her pain has resolved. Her abdominal ultrasound is shown Fig. 2-9. Which of the following is the next best step in management?

    A. Intravenous antibiotics
    B. Endoscopic retrograde cholangiopancreatography (ERCP)
    C. Percutaneous biliary drain
    D. Cholescintigraphy with 99mTc-hepatic iminodiacetic acid (HIDA scan)
    E. Close outpatient follow-up with surgery

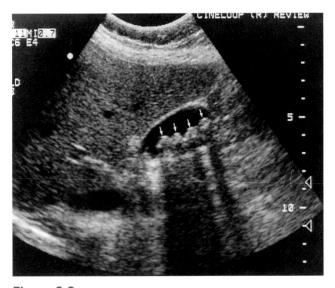

Figure 2-9

66. A 55-year-old female presents with a progressively worsening, painful, swollen, and discolored left leg shown in Figure 2-10. Which of the following is the most likely pathophysiologic mechanism?

    A. Thrombosis

    B. Embolus

    C. Infection

    D. Autoimmune

    E. Allergy

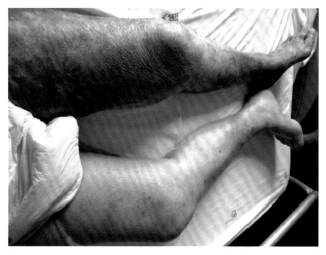

Figure 2-10

67. Which of the following is the most common finding in propanolol overdoses in adults?

    A. Ventricular tachycardia

    B. Hypoglycemia

    C. Hyperkalemia

    D. Seizure

    E. Renal failure

68. Which of the following is true about extrapulmonary tuberculosis (TB) infection?

    A. Pericarditis is a potential manifestation.

    B. Painful lymphadenopathy is common.

    C. The central nervous system (CNS) is typically spared.

    D. Skeletal TB most commonly involves the pelvis.

    E. Adrenal TB is typically unilateral.

69. A 7-year-old male is brought in for evaluation of elbow pain after a fall on an outstretched hand. His x-ray is shown. Which of the following is the most likely diagnosis? (Fig. 2-11)

    A. Radial head fracture

    B. Olecranon fracture

    C. Sprain of the radial annular ligament

    D. Radial head dislocation

    E. Supracondylar humerus fracture

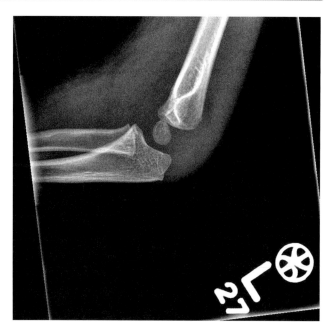

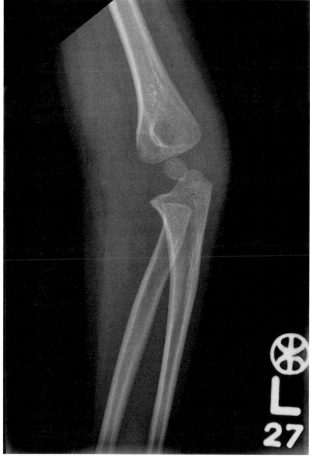

Figure 2-11

70. An 18-year-old primigravida at 35 weeks of gestation presents with abdominal pain, vaginal discharge, and a low-grade fever. She states that she was well until two days ago when, after coughing, she experienced a small stream of fluid running down her leg which she thought was urine. Her temperature is 102°F and her pulse is 108. Her examination reveals a yellowish discharge in the vaginal vault with a tender uterus. What is the most likely cause of her symptoms?

    A. Abruptio placentae
    B. Pelvic inflammatory disease
    C. Bacterial vaginitis
    D. Pyelonephritis
    E. Chorioamnionitis

71. A 26-year-old G_2P_2 presents to the ED 3 days after spontaneous vaginal delivery of a healthy male infant with a chief complaint of crampy low abdominal pain and a foul smelling vaginal discharge. On examination, she has a fever of 102°F and a tender uterus on bimanual pelvic examination. Which of the following is true?

    A. This condition is more common after vaginal delivery than cesarean section.
    B. She has postpartum pelvic inflammatory disease.
    C. *Chlamydia* and *Mycoplasma* are the most common etiologic agents.
    D. Premature rupture of membranes (PROM) is a risk factor for her condition.
    E. All of the above.

72. A 58-year-old female presents to the ED with a chief complaint of acute-onset painless flashes and floaters in her left eye. She denies any other changes to her vision and states she can read normally. However, on confrontation visual field testing, there is a visual field deficit in the upper temporal quadrant of her right eye. Which of the following is likely present?

    A. Vitreous hemorrhage
    B. Posterior vitreous detachment (PVD)
    C. Diabetic proliferative retinopathy
    D. Retinal detachment
    E. Posterior uveitis

73. In patients older than 85 years, which of the following is the most common symptom during MI?

    A. Chest pain
    B. Dyspnea
    C. Syncope
    D. Altered mental status
    E. Fever

74. A 3-day-old male infant is brought into the ED by his parents with a rash consistent with erythema toxicum neonatorum. Which of the following is true?

    A. He was likely born at least 5 weeks premature
    B. He probably has lesions on his palms and soles
    C. He should be treated with ketoconazole cream
    D. The rash will look like macules and pustules on an erythematous base
    E. All of the above

75. A 47-year-old female presents with a severe occipital headache and a general feeling of malaise. Her neurologic examination is normal. A stat head CT is shown in the image (see Fig. 2-12). Which of the following is true about this patient?

    A. The development of hydrocephalus requires urgent neurosurgical intervention.
    B. The patient should be given stat IV corticosteroids and loaded with an anticonvulsant.
    C. Such patients often succumb to uncal herniation.
    D. A Cushing response should be suspected if there is a drop in blood pressure.
    E. All of the above.

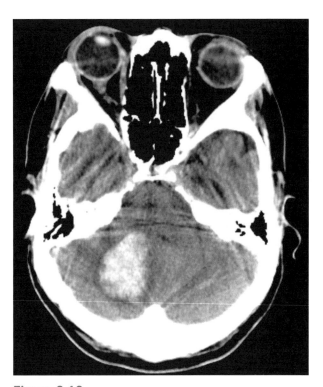

Figure 2-12

76. A 62-year-old female with a history of hypertension, diabetes mellitus, and emphysema presents with a 3-week history of dyspnea on exertion, three-pillow orthopnea, and bilateral lower extremity edema. She denies fevers, cough, or chest pain. A chest x-ray is shown in Figure 2-13A,B. The patient's electrocardiogram (EKG) does not show any ischemic changes. Her vitals are: Respiratory rate 22 per minute, pulse 108, BP 154/88, pulse oximetry 88% on room air. What is the next best step in management?

    A. Perform an immediate therapeutic thoracentesis
    B. Perform a diagnostic thoracentesis to rule out empyema
    C. Administer oxygen, nitrates, and furosemide
    D. Perform rapid sequence intubation
    E. Order a B-type natriuretic (BNP) level in order to determine the best management.

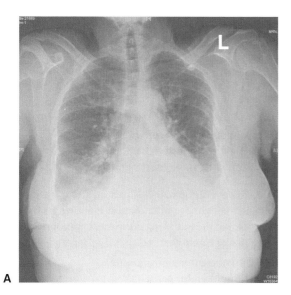

A

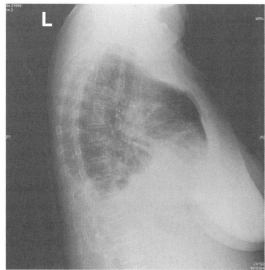

B

Figure 2-13

77. Which of the following is an ingredient in sitz baths?

    A. Baking soda
    B. Salicylate
    C. Corticosteroids
    D. Insoluble fiber
    E. None of the above

78. Which of the following is usually the earliest symptom to occur in patients with aortic stenosis (AS)?

    A. Lower extremity edema
    B. Angina
    C. Syncope
    D. Orthopnea
    E. Paroxysmal nocturnal dyspnea

79. A 3-day-old female neonate is brought to the ED with a chief complaint of rectal bleeding. A guaiac test of the stool is positive. Which of the following tests can help to determine whether the blood in the stool is of fetal origin?

    A. Kleihauer–Betke test (KBT)
    B. Meckel scan
    C. Rosette test
    D. Apt test
    E. All of the above

80. Which of the following is true regarding perimortem cesarean section?

    A. The fetus should be delivered within 5 minutes of maternal cardiac arrest.
    B. Family consent should be obtained before the procedure.
    C. It should only be performed if the fetal age is determined to be >20 weeks of gestation.
    D. A low horizontal abdominal incision affords the best opportunity for fetal recovery.
    E. A lateral approach is best in cases of a suspected anterior placenta.

81. A 12-year-old male is brought in by his parents for evaluation of three episodes of bloody diarrhea. There has been a recent outbreak of *E. coli* 0157:H7 traced to a petting zoo. The patient appears fatigued but nontoxic with a benign abdominal exam and vitals T 100.1°F, P 98, R 18, BP 110/77, and SaO$_2$ 97% on RA. His blood tests reveal a white blood cell count of 16,100/mm^3, hemoglobin 12.6 g/dL, platelets 142,000/mm^3, HCO$_3$ of 17 mEq/L, BUN 28 mg/dL and creatinine 1.1 mg/dL. Which of the following is true?

    A. Antibiotics will hasten recovery and reduce complications
    B. The patient has hemolytic uremic syndrome
    C. Treatment is generally supportive
    D. Diphenoxylate–atropine (Lomotil) is a useful adjunct in these patients
    E. Hemolytic uremic syndrome occurs in 85% of kids with hemorrhagic diarrhea

82. A 19-year-old female is brought to the ED after an accidental submersion. She was drinking with friends at a dock when she accidentally fell into the water. She was submerged in the water for approximately 1 minute before her friends pulled her out. She was gagging and coughing when they pulled her from the water but she did not require cardiopulmonary resuscitation. Her blood alcohol level is 120 mg/dL and her pulse oximetry reveals an oxygen saturation of 94% on room air. An initial chest x-ray is normal. Assuming the remainder of her examination is normal and she has no signs of trauma, what is the best course of management?

    A. Admission to the hospital for overnight observation.
    B. Observation for 4 hours, then discharge if she is asymptomatic with SaO$_2$ >94% on room air.
    C. Repeat chest x-ray in 8 hours, then discharge if she is asymptomatic with SaO$_2$ >94% on room air.
    D. Observe for 6 hours, administer oral steroids, prescribe a short pulse of steroids to limit aspiration pneumonitis and discharge home if SaO$_2$ >94% on room air.
    E. Administer oral antibiotics and oral steroids, prescribe a course of both medicines, and discharge home without observation.

83. A 26-year-old female presents for evaluation of an eye injury. There is significant periorbital soft tissue swelling and the globe can't be visualized at the bedside. Bedside ultrasound can be used to help diagnose which of the following?

    A. Retinal detachment
    B. Vitreous hemorrhage
    C. Lens dislocation
    D. Retrobulbar hemorrhage
    E. All of the above

84. A 44-year-old female presents after a motor vehicle collision with a complaint of neck pain. Neurologic examination reveals that bilateral upper extremity strength is 1/5 and bilateral lower extremity strength is 4/5. Which of the following is the most likely pathophysiologic process?

    A. Anterior cord syndrome
    B. Central cord syndrome
    C. Brown–Séquard syndrome
    D. Cauda equina syndrome
    E. Complete cord injury

85. What is the clinical factor that best differentiates heat stroke from heat exhaustion?

    A. Core temperature >102°F
    B. The presence of anhidrosis
    C. Elevation of hepatic transaminases
    D. Central nervous system (CNS) dysfunction
    E. History of exertion in a hot environment

86. Which of the following is true about primary spontaneous pneumothorax?

    A. Most patients develop primary pneumothorax during vigorous exercise.
    B. Expiratory chest x-rays are critical to make a diagnosis.
    C. It is typically a less dangerous finding than primary spontaneous pneumomediastinum.
    D. Hamman crunch is pathognomonic for the diagnosis.
    E. Smoking is the most significant risk factor.

87. A 23-year-old female is struck in the eye with a soccer ball. Penlight eye examination is shown in Figure 2-14. Which of the following is the most appropriate next step in management?

    A. Trendelenburg positioning
    B. Ibuprofen for pain
    C. Activated factor VII
    D. Eye shielding
    E. IV antibiotics

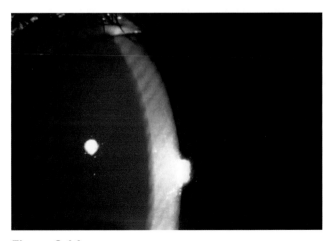

Figure 2-14

88. A 64-year-old male with a history of well-controlled, mild hypertension presents to the ED with a chief complaint of an abrupt episode of "flashes of light" and floaters in his right eye. He states that he was watching television when he experienced a brief episode in which many "glittery lights" flashed in his right eye. The episode resolved, but he has subsequently noted a couple of gray spots floating in his vision. He denies decreased visual acuity. Direct ophthalmoscopy is unrevealing. Which of the following is the most likely cause of his symptoms?

   A. Retinal detachment
   B. Ocular migraine
   C. Occipital lobe ischemia
   D. Vitreous detachment
   E. Optic neuritis

89. What is the approximate sensitivity and specificity of the monospot test for infectious mononucleosis due to Epstein Barr virus (EBV)?

   A. 50%, 50%
   B. 80%, 80%
   C. 95%, 80%
   D. 80%, 95%
   E. 95%, 95%

90. Which of the following is true regarding patients with a primary spontaneous pneumothorax?

   A. Pleuritic chest pain and dyspnea are the most common symptoms.
   B. Hemoptysis is present in most patients.
   C. It occurs most frequently in women aged 20 to 40 years.
   D. Without treatment, symptoms tend to intensify within 24 to 48 hours.
   E. Atrial fibrillation is the most common cardiac rhythm in the acute setting of a spontaneous pneumothorax.

91. A 4-year-old previously healthy girl presents to the ED with a 2-day history of cough productive of yellow sputum, fevers up to 102.4°F, pleuritic chest pain, and dyspnea. On examination, she is tachypneic and mildly toxic appearing. Her chest x-ray reveals a right middle lobe infiltrate. Which of the following organisms is the most likely cause of this problem?

   A. *Klebsiella pneumoniae*
   B. *Mycoplasma pneumoniae*
   C. *Chlamydia trachomatis*
   D. *Respiratory syncytial virus* (RSV)
   E. *Streptococcus pneumoniae*

92. Among patients presenting with an NSTEMI, which of the following describes the appropriate use of antiplatelet therapy?

   A. Aspirin alone, given in doses of 162 to 325 mg, is the standard of care.
   B. Aspirin plus a GPIIbIIIa inhibitor should be given in all cases.
   C. Either clopidogrel or a GPIIbIIIa inhibitor should be used in addition to aspirin.
   D. Patients should only receive clopidogrel in addition to aspirin if no percutaneous intervention (PCI) is planned.
   E. Clopidogrel is only indicated for patients who are intolerant of aspirin.

93. Which of the following is true regarding urine analysis?

   A. Urine dipstick is 99% sensitive for microscopic hematuria.
   B. Red blood cell (RBC) casts indicate interstitial cystitis.
   C. White blood cell casts indicate renal parenchymal inflammation.
   D. Transitional cells indicate bladder cancer.
   E. Normal urinary pH is 9 to 11.

94. Which of the following is the most specific finding in diagnosing necrotizing enterocolitis (NEC)?

   A. Abdominal radiograph demonstrating multiple dilated loops of small bowel
   B. Abdominal radiograph with a "double bubble" sign
   C. Abdominal radiograph with pneumatosis intestinalis
   D. The presence of abdominal distension, bilious emesis, and guaiac positive stools
   E. The presence of portal vein thrombosis upon US examination

95. A 56-year-old male with a history of a prosthetic aortic valve presents for evaluation of fever and chills for 1 week. Echocardiogram reveals vegetations on the prosthetic valve. Which of the following is the most likely etiologic organism?

   A. Coagulase-negative *Staphylococcus*
   B. *Streptococcus viridans*
   C. *Haemophilus influenzae*
   D. *Pseudomonas aeruginosa*
   E. *Klebsiella pneumoniae*

96. Which of the following is a risk factor for development of kidney stones?

   A. Female gender
   B. Hypoparathyroidism
   C. Crohn disease
   D. Hyperthyroidism
   E. Diabetes mellitus

97. A 26-year-old male with no significant past medical history is brought to the emergency room by his father and wife. The patient's boss called his wife, asking why the patient had not shown up for work over the past 2 days. The patient's wife was unaware the patient had not been going to work, since he had been leaving the house on a daily basis, though he had been "saying strange things" for several months. His vital signs are normal. A urine drug screen is negative. He is not known to abuse alcohol and has an undetectable blood alcohol level. Upon evaluating the patient, it is clear that he is experiencing auditory hallucinations as he is having a conversation with someone who is not physically present. When you introduce yourself, he says that "the CEO of your company is getting together with the CEO of my company to cut down all the trees." Which of the following is most likely true of his underlying condition?

A. He has mania complicated by psychotic features.
B. He abuses LSD, which is not commonly tested on drug screens.
C. His risk of suicide is highest in the early stage of his illness.
D. Visual hallucinations are the most common form of hallucinations.
E. Hallucinations are more common than delusions.

98. Which of the following is the most common sign or symptom in patients with normal pressure hydrocephalus (NPH)?

A. Ataxia
B. Dementia
C. Papilledema
D. Urinary incontinence
E. Headache

99. What is the duration of action of naloxone?

A. 30 minutes
B. 1 hour
C. 5 hours
D. 10 hours
E. 20 hours

100. Which of the following is the most appropriate initial antihypertensive medication for hypertensive crises in pregnant patients?

A. Nitroprusside
B. Nitroglycerin
C. Clonidine
D. Labetalol
E. Hydrochlorothiazide

ANSWERS AND EXPLANATIONS

1. **Answer C.** As with other deep space infections of the neck, CT is the most valuable diagnostic tool. Although lateral neck x-rays are the preferred *initial* imaging modality for suspected retropharyngeal space infections, they do not typically provide useful information in patients with suspected parapharyngeal infections. Furthermore, CT is better able to localize the specific site of infection in patients with retropharyngeal abscesses. Anterior–posterior plain films of the neck are occasionally used to support a diagnosis of croup (steeple sign), but have no role in the diagnosis of parapharyngeal space infections. Both MRI and ultrasonography are capable of providing useful information, but MRI is limited by time and access constraints and ultrasonography provides much less detail and is less able to accurately localize the site of the problem.

2. **Answer B.** Falls from buildings are an important mechanism of multisystem blunt trauma. Feet-first falls tend to cause lower extremity, spinous, and pelvic injuries, the last of which results in retroperitoneal bleeding. Mortality is related to the height of the fall—half the number of patients who fall from four stories die. Falls onto the back commonly cause spinous and retroperitoneal injuries, including serious trauma to the kidneys. Calcaneal fracture often occurs in patients with feet-first falls but rarely by itself causes mortality. Instead, it is a sign of other potential injury, including spinous or pelvic fracture. Falls onto prone position can cause serious abdominal and thoracic injuries and may easily result in death.

3. **Answer C.** Patients with smoke inhalation from building fires are exposed to two major toxins, carbon monoxide and hydrogen cyanide. A metabolic acidosis with elevated lactate level in these patients is highly suggestive of dual toxicity. Carbon monoxide binds to hemoglobin with more than 200 times greater affinity than oxygen, and prevents hemoglobin from carrying oxygen. Cyanide poisons complex IV of the mitochondrial electron transport chain. Treatment of carbon monoxide alone is 100% oxygen and hyperbaric oxygen is severe cases. Treatment of hydrogen cyanide alone involves two major steps: Induction of methemoglobinemia with nitrites, which pulls the cyanide molecule off the electron transport chain, and detoxification of cyanide with thiosulfate. When there is poisoning with both cyanide and carbon monoxide, induction of methemoglobinemia by nitrites should be avoided, as it would further prevent hemoglobin from carrying oxygen. The treatment of choice in this case would be sodium thiosulfate.

Methylene blue is the treatment for severe methemoglobinemia. Dexamethasone has no role in the management of carbon monoxide or cyanide poisonings.

4. **Answer E.** Urethral injury occurs most commonly in men due to the length of the male urethra. The injury is suspected on physical examination by a variety of findings—blood at the urethral meatus, scrotal/penile hematoma, severe pelvic fracture, or high-riding or mobile prostate. Evaluation of suspected urethral injury generally involves retrograde urethrogram to assess for extravasation of contrast. However, once a Foley catheter is successfully placed and the bladder is drained of urine, it should not be removed until urologic consultation is obtained. The key to managing urethral injuries is to prevent urine from leaking out of the bladder into the retroperitoneum, pelvis, or abdomen. If the Foley has already successfully decompressed the bladder, the urethral injury may be evaluated later in the operating room (OR) or with a modified bedside urethrogram around the Foley, if needed. Removal of the Foley can convert a partial urethral disruption into a complete one and should be avoided.

5. **Answer D.** Testicular torsion is the most likely diagnosis because of the acute testicular pain, nausea, and absence of ipsilateral cremasteric reflex. Pathophysiology involves twisting of the testis on the spermatic cord due to an anatomic abnormality or trauma. In unclear cases, color Doppler ultrasonography is the diagnostic test of choice, but in textbook cases such as this, emergent urologic consultation is indicated. Prompt diagnosis is essential, as testicular survival is directly dependent on duration of symptoms—if surgical management is instituted within 6 hours of pain, approximately 100% of cases are salvageable. Definitive surgical management involves bilateral orchidopexy. Antibiotics are used to treat epididymitis, a common condition in the differential diagnosis of the acute scrotum. Analgesics and antiemetics should be considered conjunctive therapy in patients with testicular torsion but do not affect the disease process itself. Manual detorsion may be used as a temporizing measure, but should never be considered definitive therapy. Lithotripsy is used to treat kidney stones, and has no role in the management of testicular torsion.

6. **Answer A.** Due to decreased plasma volume, the hematocrit increases approximately 2% for every 1°C decrease in the core temperature. This is thought to be due to increased vascular permeability and third spacing of fluids as well as cold-induced diuresis and free water

loss. In acute hypothermia in otherwise healthy individuals, hyperglycemia occurs because of the circulating catecholamines and cold-related inhibition of insulin secretion. There is a tendency toward metabolic acidosis in hypothermic patients although limited experimental data suggest that patients may present either acidotic or alkalotic. Patients experience respiratory depression with decreasing temperature, in part due to the decrease in metabolism that occurs as the body cools. This raises the Pco_2 and decreases the pH. Other factors that contribute to the acidotic state include lactate production from shivering and decreased tissue perfusion and impaired hepatic function. These effects are blunted somewhat because of the fact that as blood cools, it becomes more alkalotic. A progressive diuresis, not oliguria, occurs as the temperature cools. The most common neurologic finding in hypothermic patients is a decreased level of consciousness. EEGs in hypothermic patients demonstrate generalized slowing and decreased amplitude. In addition, pupillary responses and deep tendon reflexes are decreased and patients tend to have increased muscle tone.

7. **Answer E.** Troponin I is highly specific for cardiac muscle. It starts rising between 3 and 6 hours after infarction, peaks at 12 to 24 hours, and returns to normal within 7 days. The specificity of troponin I is excellent at 6 hours postinfarction, but the sensitivity does not approach 100% until 12 hours.

8. **Answer C.** The development of a lung abscess is most commonly a consequence of aspiration in patients with poor oral hygiene. Less commonly, it may occur as a result of necrotizing pneumonia. Classically it has been thought that anaerobic bacteria are responsible for the great majority of lung abscesses. However, recent studies have revealed that the microbiology may differ between immunocompetent and immunocompromised patients. Although anaerobes are predominant in immunocompetent patients, patients with depressed immune systems are more frequently infected with aerobic bacteria such as *S. aureus, Pseudomonas aeruginosa, Klebsiella pneumoniae,* and *H. influenzae*. Frequently, however, infections are polymicrobial. Nonbacterial organisms such as fungi and parasites may also cause lung abscesses. *S. pneumococcus* is not a common cause. Patients with anaerobic or fungal lung abscesses typically experience an indolent course of fever, productive cough, night sweats, anorexia, and weight loss. The sputum is classically malodorous, which should be a clue to the diagnosis. Immunocompromised patients presenting with a lung abscess as a result of aerobic necrotizing pneumonia present with acute symptoms of pneumonia and may be quite ill. Chest radiography typically reveals a cavitary lesion with an air–fluid level. Antibiotics remain the cornerstone of therapy although surgical

management may ultimately be necessary. Typical surgical indications are medical treatment failure, suspected cancer, or congenital lung malformation. Lung abscesses very rarely develop in the setting of pediatric community acquired pneumonia and only occur typically in patients who are immunocompromised because of acquired immune deficiencies, malignancy or chemotherapy, and in patients who are predisposed to aspiration (children with neurologic disorders, decreased mental status, impaired cough, or swallowing dysfunction).

9. **Answer E.** Pseudotumor cerebri, also known as *idiopathic intracranial hypertension,* is a syndrome of increased ICP without an identifiable cause. To satisfy the diagnostic criteria for the disease, there can be no evidence of a mass or a structural or vascular lesion on neuroimaging. Furthermore, the composition of the cerebrospinal fluid must be normal, and any symptoms resulting from the disease must be completely attributable to papilledema or generalized elevated intracranial pressure (ICP). The most common presenting symptom is headache, which tends to be worse in the recumbent position and in the morning (after prolonged recumbency overnight). The most common serious complication is permanent vision loss. CT scan never reveals hydrocephalus. Abducens nerve palsy is the only cranial nerve palsy that commonly occurs and typically presents as intermittent or constant lateral binocular diplopia. Women are more commonly affected, with a 19 times increased incidence in obese women of childbearing age.

10. **Answer E.** The gram stain reveals gram-positive cocci most consistent with *Streptococcus pneumonia*. Chemoprophylaxis is only necessary for meningitis caused by *N. meningitidis* or *Haemophilus influenzae* (principally caused by *type B,* which is now quite rare in the United States due to the Hib vaccine), which are both gram-negative organisms (*Neisseria* are *diplococci* and *Haemophilus* are *bacilli*). The classic regimen in exposed adults is Ciprofloxacin 500 mg orally × 1 dose. Children should be treated with either Rocephin IM × 1 (125 mg IM × 1 in children <15 years of age) or oral Rifampin (age-based dosing twice daily for 2 days). There is some evidence of Ciprofloxacin resistance in certain parts of Minnesota and North Dakota, where Ciprofloxacin becomes a second-line agent. Therefore, Rocephin and Rifampin are also reasonable alternatives in adult patients who have had close contact with an affected individual. Azithromycin is another alternative if local isolates demonstrate resistance to Ciprofloxacin.

11. **Answer D.** Ingestion of even small quantities of methanol is extremely lethal without appropriate therapy. One tablespoon of 40% methanol can kill an adult, and less than one teaspoon is enough to cause blindness. Methanol is metabolized to formaldehyde by alcohol

dehydrogenase, and formaldehyde is converted to formic acid by aldehyde dehydrogenase. Ethylene glycol is metabolized to glycolaldehyde by alcohol dehydrogenase, and glycolaldehyde is converted to glycolic acid by aldehyde dehydrogenase. Alcohol dehydrogenase has greatest affinity for ethanol, then methanol, then ethylene glycol. GI absorption is very rapid for both ethylene glycol and methanol, usually occurring within 1 hour.

12. **Answer D.** Achalasia is an esophageal motility disorder due to failure of the lower esophageal sphincter to relax and a complete absence of esophageal peristalsis. It affects men and women equally and presents between the third and fifth decade. Dysphagia is the most common symptom. All patients have difficulty with solid foods but two-thirds of patients describe dysphagia with liquids as well. Patients may stand after eating, raise their arms above their head, or straighten their back to increase esophageal pressure and help esophageal emptying. Patients with achalasia have symptoms for an average of 2 years before diagnosis and they are often treated for GERD due to the presence of burning chest pain. Diffuse esophageal spasm and nutcracker esophagus are hypermotility disorders, resulting in exceedingly strong esophageal peristaltic contractions. The most common complaint is chest pain, although the presence of dysphagia is less common and more variable. Schatzki ring is a fibrous band-like stricture in the distal esophagus that is present in up to 15% of the normal population. Patients who develop symptoms typically present with acute esophageal obstruction.

13. **Answer B.** The baseline risk of a heterotopic pregnancy is reported to be 1 in 4,000 pregnancies or 0.25%. However, in vitro fertilization and other assisted reproductive technologies (ART) dramatically increase the risk of heterotopic pregnancy. The risk of a heterotopic pregnancy in the setting of in vitro fertilization is approximately 1%, whereas the risk in the setting of some ART therapies may be as high as 4.5%. The key aspect to recognize is that ART is the primary risk factor for heterotopic pregnancy, and the resulting risk of heterotopic pregnancy is approximately the same as the risk for ectopic pregnancy in the general population.

14. **Answer A.** *H. capsulatum* is the most common pulmonary fungal infection worldwide. It may infect immunocompetent as well as immunocompromised individuals, but primary infection is almost always asymptomatic and very few cases are ever brought to the attention of a physician. In endemic regions, at least 80% to 90% of the population has positive skin testing by the age of 20. *Histoplasma* and *Blastomyces* are endemic to the Mississippi and Ohio River valleys in the United States, whereas *Coccidioides* is found in the arid southwest. In contrast, *Cryptococcus* is ubiquitous throughout the world, without a specific distribution. It generally causes disease in immunocompromised hosts, and is the most common cause of life-threatening fungal infection in patients with human immunodeficiency virus (HIV). Except in a few rare cases, patients with fungal pulmonary infection are not capable of transmitting disease to others. Of the fungi that cause systemic mycoses, *Blastomyces* most commonly causes disseminated disease.

15. **Answer D.** The patient has evidence of fungal balanoposthitis, or infection of the foreskin and glans. Recurrent such infections may be due to an immune-compromised state, most commonly diabetes. Balanoposthitis most often occurs in patients who are uncircumcised and is usually due to infection from typical skin flora. Urinalysis may be indicated to evaluate for sexually transmitted infection. Treatment is with penile hygiene and antibiotics directed at the most likely organisms. Liver function tests would not be helpful in evaluation of penile infection. Postvoid residual volume and intravenous pyelogram evaluate for urinary obstruction. Retrograde urethrogram is used in patients with pelvic trauma and suspected urethral injury.

16. **Answer B.** Although the incidence of *K. pneumonia* is higher in alcoholics than nonalcoholics, the overall most common cause of CAP in the alcoholic patient is still pneumococcus. Alcoholic patients tend to have a higher incidence of aspiration pneumonia and tuberculous disease compared with the general population. Alcohol itself is immunosuppressive and predisposes patients to a higher incidence of bacterial infections. Treatment of CAP in the alcoholic patient is similar to that of the general population—third-generation cephalosporin plus a macrolide or a fluoroquinolone. Anaerobic coverage may be added for patients who are at particular risk for aspiration pneumonia.

17. **Answer C.** In 2002, the Transient Ischemic Attack Working Group redefined TIA as "a brief episode of neurologic dysfunction caused by focal brain or retinal ischemia, with clinical symptoms typically lasting less than 1 hour, and without evidence of acute infarction." In 2009, the American Heart Association and American Stroke Association endorsed similar guidelines that emphasized that the diagnosis can only be considered in patients without evidence of central nervous system infarction. Positive findings such as tingling or involuntary movements are the exception in patients with a TIA. In addition, symptoms affecting multiple different body parts usually occur simultaneously. "Marching" symptoms are more common in patients with migraines or seizures. Nonfocal symptoms such as generalized weakness, dizziness, lightheadedness, and confusion are not commonly due to a TIA. Finally, the most common mimic of symptoms attributable to a TIA is hypoglycemia.

18. **Answer D.** The patient has a significant anion-gap acidosis ($132 - 90 - 12 = 30$) with a history of alcohol abuse and no history of diabetes. Alcoholic ketoacidosis (AKA) is the most likely cause, resulting from the lack of nutrition other than alcohol, which causes the formation of ketone bodies. A common mistake in treatment of AKA is to give only saline fluids (without glucose). Treatment requires glucose (dextrose), either with food or IV fluids, to halt the formation of ketone bodies from ethanol metabolism. It is important to note that urine dipstick tests can be negative for ketones despite the severity of AKA. This is because dipstick tests only assess for the presence of acetoacetate, not beta-hydroxybutyrate. AKA has an even higher ratio of beta-hydroxybutyrate to acetoacetate compared to diabetic ketoacidosis (DKA). Insulin is contraindicated in patients with AKA, as it can precipitously drop glucose levels in an already glycogen-depleted state. Bicarbonate is not generally recommended in the management of anion-gap acidosis; treatment instead should focus on the underlying cause. For the same reason, metoprolol is not indicated in what is likely sinus tachycardia. Giving IV hydralazine to treat a moderately elevated blood pressure without signs of end-organ dysfunction is not recommended.

19. **Answer B.** Certain oral medications cause severe esophageal irritation when swallowed—doxycycline, tetracycline, aspirin, and potassium chloride. Of these, potassium chloride is the most caustic, sometimes leading to esophageal perforation and penetration into the mediastinal great vessels.

20. **Answer C.** The development of uterine contractions is the most common consequence of maternal trauma. This is due to stimulatory prostaglandins that are released upon contusion to the maternal uterus. Ninety percent of contractions stop spontaneously, and tocolytics are generally not used. However, all pregnant patients with a viable fetus should undergo continuous cardiotocographic monitoring. In patients with abdominal pain and overt contractions, most authors recommend admission for 24 hours of monitoring. Though placental abruption is the most common cause of fetal loss related to trauma, the presence of uterine contractions is not enough to make this diagnosis. Fetal distress and persistent uterine irritability upon cardiotocographic monitoring is the most sensitive indicator of placental abruption. Uterine rupture is rare and most commonly occurs in women who have a history of prior cesarean delivery. It may be difficult to diagnose and is associated with a very high fetal mortality. Digital examination should never be performed after the first trimester because ED physicians could trigger catastrophic bleeding in patients with undiagnosed placenta previa. Such examinations are best left for the obstetrician after US has verified placental position and fetal viability.

21. **Answer E.** The patient has acute chest syndrome, as indicated by the presence of fever, cough, dyspnea, and new infiltrate on chest x-ray in the setting of sickle cell disease. The diagnosis is based on the presence of a new infiltrate plus at least one of the following: chest pain, a temperature >38.5°C, or respiratory distress manifest by increased work of breathing or cough, wheezing, tachypnea, or hypoxemia (or a combination). It is a very common cause of death in patients with sickle cell disease. The most common cause of acute chest syndrome is infection (pneumonia), while pulmonary infarction and fat embolism are the next most common causes. Overall, however, the etiology cannot be determined in more than one-third of cases. Treatment involves fluids, analgesics, oxygen, and antibiotics. Heparin is used to manage pulmonary thromboembolism but is not indicated in patients with undifferentiated acute chest syndrome. It may be indicated in patients with acute chest syndrome due to pulmonary thromboembolism, but this is evaluated on a case-by-case basis in close consultation with a hematologist. Tissue plasminogen activator may be indicated for acute stroke, MI, or severe pulmonary thromboembolism. Angioplasty is indicated for acute STEMI but has no role in the management of acute chest syndrome. Albuterol and prednisone are used to treat bronchospastic lung disease, which is not part of the pathophysiologic process of acute chest syndrome though reactive airway disease may also be present since it is such a common entity.

22. **Answer A.** Although sinus tachycardia is the most common *arrhythmia* in patients with PE, normal sinus rhythm remains the most common cardiac rhythm. A recent study demonstrated that roughly two-third of patients with PE have normal sinus rhythm (there was no significant difference from control patients). That doesn't suggest, however, that most patients with PE have normal EKGs, as rhythm is only one aspect of EKG analysis. In fact, most patients with PEs have been found to have abnormal EKGs, but no single abnormality has been shown to have sufficient sensitivity or specificity to aid in the diagnosis. Therefore, the role of EKG in the evaluation of PE is to rule out the presence of alternative diagnoses, such as cardiac ischemia or pericarditis.

23. **Answer E.** Patients with periorbital (preseptal) cellulitis may have fever, periorbital edema, and eye tenderness, but ophthalmoplegia is characteristic of orbital cellulitis. Gram-positive cocci are common causes of both conditions, but *S. aureus* is more commonly implicated in periorbital cellulitis. Orbital cellulitis is usually caused by *S. pneumoniae, H. influenzae, M. catarrhalis, S. pyogenes,* and polymicrobial infections. Diagnosis can be definitively made by CT scan of the brain and orbits. Orbital cellulitis mandates hospital admission with IV antibiotics, whereas uncomplicated

cases of periorbital cellulitis may be managed on an outpatient basis.

24. **Answer E.** Prothrombin complex concentrates (PCCs) are pooled plasma products that contain vitamin-K–dependent coagulation factors as well as therapeutic levels of protein C and S, which inhibit clot formation. Commercially available PCCs contain factors II, IX, and X but are categorized further as three-factor (3F-PCC) or four-factor (4F-PCC) PCCs depending on whether they also contain clinically useful amounts of factor VII. While PCCs are plasma products, they exist in a dried, concentrated powder form, are stored at room temperature so they do not need to be thawed, are purified so they do not need ABO typing, can be prepared within minutes and are delivered in much smaller volumes with much shorter infusion times than plasma. Recent studies have also demonstrated that PCCs are far more effective than fresh frozen plasma at correcting the coagulopathy and elevated INR associated with vitamin K antagonists like warfarin.

25. **Answer C.** The patient's EKG reveals a left bundle branch block (LBBB) which is associated with a greater than three times risk of a serious cardiac cause. Any left bundle conduction abnormality, including an anterior or posterior hemiblock is associated with a serious cardiac outcome. Also predictive of serious cardiac outcomes though not quite as strongly is any nonsinus rhythm either on EKG or on cardiac monitoring. Right bundle blocks, Q waves, and nonspecific ST segment changes are not predictive of more serious cardiac outcomes.

26. **Answer E.** The patient has a large left upper lobe consolidation, which in the clinical setting of blunt trauma is likely pulmonary contusion. No definite pneumothorax is seen on either side. Hemothorax is on the differential diagnosis but would either appear as diffuse haziness of the lung fields on a supine radiograph or inferior layering (like a pleural effusion) on an upright radiograph. Pulmonary contusions can cause inadequate oxygenation and lead to pneumonia. Treatment is largely supportive, with optimal hydration and supplemental oxygenation. Needle thoracostomy should be reserved for cases of hemodynamically unstable traumatic pneumothorax. (Figure courtesy of John H Harris, William H Harris. *Radiology of Emergency Medicine.* 4th ed. Philadelphia, PA: Lippincott Williams & Wilkins; 1999, with permission.)

27. **Answer B.** Hyperkalemia predisposes patients to serious dysrhythmias. The management of hyperkalemia involves all of the answer choices given in the preceding text. Catecholamines, such as albuterol, activate Na^+–K^+ ATPase pumps via the β2 receptor, which lowers potassium by shifting it into cells. The effects of nebulized albuterol are essentially immediate, although peak effects may not occur until 60 to 90 minutes after administra-

tion. Sodium bicarbonate has been part of the traditional treatment regimen for hyperkalemia, but its role is increasingly questioned as some studies have shown no change in potassium levels after its use. Although calcium salts are a critical part of hyperkalemia therapy and are effective within 5 minutes, they do not reduce potassium levels but rather function to stabilize the cardiac myocyte membrane to prevent the deleterious effects of hyperkalemia. Insulin and glucose begin to work in 30 minutes, and Kayexalate starts to exchange sodium for potassium in 1 hour. Hemodialysis is the management of choice in cases of hyperkalemia that are refractory to the medical management given in the preceding text.

28. **Answer D.** Hirschsprung disease accounts for roughly 20% of cases of partial intestinal obstruction in early infancy. Although intussusception is the most common cause of intestinal obstruction in children younger than 2 years, the typical presentation is one of acute-onset, severe abdominal pain which may be associated with vomiting and bloody stools. Patients with pyloric stenosis present with progressive nonbilious projectile emesis. Patients with GERD do not develop signs of obstruction and most commonly have nonbilious emesis. Hirschsprung disease is usually diagnosed in the newborn nursery due to failure of newborns to pass meconium. Ninety-nine percent of full-term infants pass meconium within 48 hours of birth. However, because there is a spectrum of disease, some infants may present in a delayed manner and may have a subtle presentation. Since this infant was delivered at home, he was not observed in the newborn nursery, where stool production is monitored. The absence of stool in the rectal vault followed by copious stool and gas production following digital examination indicates a likely distal colonic obstruction (created by the narrowed, aganglionic segment of bowel) which is transiently relieved by digital examination. These findings in concert with the patient's symptoms of obstruction should bring about the consideration of Hirschsprung disease. Diagnosis is first confirmed through an abnormal "string sign" on barium enema. This is followed by rectal biopsy revealing the aganglionic segment of bowel responsible for the disease.

29. **Answer C.** The absolute lymphocyte count is not only the earliest indicator of the acute radiation syndrome but it also provides prognostic information. Patients with an absolute lymphocyte count <500 have a very poor prognosis with very high lethality when the absolute lymphocyte count is <100. In contrast, patients with an absolute lymphocyte count >1,000 have significant, but usually nonlethal injuries.

30. **Answer B.** Patients with hemolytic disorders, such as sickle cell anemia or hereditary spherocytosis, represent the largest group of pediatric patients with symptomatic

cholelithiasis. Hemolysis puts these patients at risk for the formation of pigmented gallstones. CF and obesity also put children at risk for cholelithiasis. In CF, patients experience inspissated biliary secretions, leading to stone formation. Diabetes and cerebral palsy are unrelated diseases. Neonates often have multiple factors predisposing to gallstones, but these patients are usually diagnosed in the neonatal intensive care unit (ICU), before discharge and presentation in the ED. Examples of neonatal risk factors include prematurity, parenteral nutrition, surgery, blood transfusion, sepsis, and diuretic administration.

31. **Answer B.** The abdominal film demonstrates gastric and duodenal dilation. Malrotation with midgut volvulus must be a leading consideration in any toxic-appearing infant with a history of sudden-onset bilious emesis. Malrotation occurs in approximately 1 in 500 live births, or about half as often as pyloric stenosis. Of all infants with malrotation, 75% will develop volvulus and 75% of these infants will present in the first month (most in the first week). Most infants present with acute-onset bilious emesis and obstruction. Plain films are usually nonspecific and may be normal, but they may also reveal the "double bubble" sign which reflects the dilated stomach and proximal duodenum (the intervening pylorus separates the two "bubbles," not shown in Fig. 2-3). This may also be seen with duodenal atresia but that is an illness that presents in the newborn nursery. Malrotation with midgut volvulus is a life-threatening illness that requires emergent surgical intervention to reduce the volvulus and relieve the ischemia caused by constriction of the bowel's mesenteric blood supply. Necrosis of the bowel may occur in as little as 3 hours. (Figure reprinted with permission from Fleisher GR. *Atlas of Pediatric Emergency Medicine.* Philadelphia, PA: Lippincott Williams & Wilkins; 2003.)

32. **Answer D.** Adult patients infected with hepatitis B develop chronic hepatitis B <5% of the time. In contrast, patients with acute hepatitis C infection become chronic carriers 80% to 90% of the time. Hepatitis C is most commonly acquired by intravenous drug use (IVDU) or blood transfusions. In the United States, both blood donors and the donated blood are screened for hepatitis C, so the risk of infection through this route is quite low and IVDU predominates. However, worldwide, <40% of the blood supply is tested for hepatitis C. Hepatitis C is the least common viral cause of fulminant hepatic failure. Coinfection with hepatitis B and D is the most common. The white blood cell count has almost no utility in the setting of hepatitis infection.

33. **Answer B.** Patients presenting to the ED with a first-time generalized seizure should receive a CT brain to evaluate for intracranial hemorrhage or mass lesion. MRI should be reserved for those patients who do exhibit a mass lesion on CT that requires further characterization. Starting antiepileptic therapy in patients with first-time seizures is established on a case-by-case basis with neurology consultation. Regardless, phenobarbital is almost never the initial therapy. Lumbar puncture may be pursued if an infectious source is suspected, but should always be preceded by a CT to exclude mass lesion in the setting of seizure. Prolactin levels were initially touted as a way to definitively diagnose a generalized seizure, but later research has shown an inability to distinguish accurately between seizure and syncope.

34. **Answer C.** Isopropanol classically does not cause elevated anion gap when ingested. The osmolar gap, however, is elevated and should be calculated and measured when there is suspicion of toxic alcohol overdose. Elevation of the anion gap due to lactic acidosis can occur in cases of severe isopropanol poisoning if there is associated coma, gastrointestinal hemorrhage, or hypotension. Choices A, B, D, and E all cause an elevation in the anion gap at some point during their metabolism.

35. **Answer D.** The purpura and clinical history are both consistent with meningococcemia and meningitis due to *N. meningiditis.* This causes a fulminant, overwhelming septic picture which can lead quickly to death if not treated immediately. As a gram-negative organism, meningococcus should be treated with ceftriaxone. Although formal diagnosis of bacterial meningitis involves CT brain in most cases before a lumbar puncture to obtain cerebrospinal fluid (CSF), in cases where critical illness is evident, antibiotics and steroids should be given before confirmatory diagnostic maneuvers. Vancomycin is certainly an important antibiotic to give in most cases of meningitis (as it kills gram-positive organisms such as pneumococcus), but it should not precede ceftriaxone in cases where meningococcus is likely. (From Goodheart HP. *Goodheart's Photoguide of Common Skin Disorders.* 2nd ed. Philadelphia, PA: Wolters Kluwer; 2003.)

36. **Answer A.** Although *C. perfringens* is probably the most common cause of acute food poisoning in the United States, all of the above bacteria may cause foodborne illness. Their classic associations are given below.

- *C. perfringens:* Toxin-mediated, predominantly diarrheal illness that occurs 6 to 12 hours after ingestion and is common in meats, poultry, and gravies. Requires ingestion of live organisms because the toxin is produced in vivo. The illness resolves in 24 hours with supportive care.
- *S. aureus:* Toxin-mediated emetogenic illness that occurs 1 to 6 hours after ingestion. Common in high-protein foods such as ham, eggs, poultry, custard-based pastries as well as potato or egg salads. Symptoms typically resolve within 8 hours without specific treatment.

- *B. cereus:* Causes two distinct illnesses. First is toxin-mediated illness that results in acute food poisoning, predominantly characterized by vomiting. Very similar to the syndrome caused by *S. aureus* except it almost always occurs after ingestion of fried rice. Second illness is a diarrheal illness almost indistinguishable from the illness caused by *C. perfringens.* As with *C. perfringens,* it is a toxin-mediated event but requires ingestion of live organisms as the toxin is produced in vivo.
- *V. parahaemolyticus* is increasingly a cause of food-borne illness in raw or undercooked fish or shellfish. It causes disease through direct intestinal invasion as well as enterotoxin production and is almost always characterized by explosive watery diarrhea and crampy abdominal pain. Vomiting and bloody stools may occur but are less common.

37. **Answer B.** This patient has Horner syndrome caused by disruption to the sympathetic fibers that encircle the carotid artery. Division of the sympathetics results in ptosis, miosis, and anhidrosis on the side of the injury and can occur after either blunt or penetrating trauma. Though the presence of Horner syndrome is not a life-threatening emergency, it may represent a life-threatening vascular emergency due to the proximity of the sympathetic chain to the carotid artery. Therefore, all patients with Horner syndrome should have a definitive evaluation of the carotid artery to exclude intimal injury (e.g., carotid angiography or helical CT angiography, which has largely replaced dedicated angiography in most centers). Interestingly, delayed presentation of neurologic deficits is typical of vascular injuries to the neck due to blunt trauma. In the absence of Horner syndrome, most patients experience stroke symptoms between 1 and 24 hours after injury due to carotid or vertebral artery dissection or thrombosis. Vascular injury should be suspected in all patients with neurologic findings that are incongruent with head CT findings.

38. **Answer D.** Prolongation of the QT interval may be due to congenital or acquired causes. Congenital long QT syndromes may be associated with deafness (Jervell–Lange–Nielsen syndrome) or without deafness (Romano–Ward syndrome). Acquired causes can be from electrolyte abnormalities, environmental conditions, or medication effects. Excessive prolongation can result in potentially fatal ventricular dysrhythmias, such as ventricular fibrillation and *torsades de pointes.* Treatment is usually with magnesium and standard advanced cardiac life support (ACLS) protocols. Prevention of ventricular dysrhythmias is with chronic β-blocker therapy and sometimes pacemakers/defibrillators.

39. **Answer A.** LSD is part of a class of substances known as *psychedelics,* which produces hallucinations, generally without confusion or disorientation. Users are usually aware that they are experiencing drug-induced hallucinations. Panic and agitation are the most common unintended effects of these substances—benzodiazepines are indicated as first-line therapy, along with placement in a low-stimulation atmosphere (dark, quiet room). Addiction to LSD is rare, but tolerance occurs with repeated use. LSD is structurally and functionally similar to serotonin. The lethal dose of LSD far exceeds the typical hallucinogenic dose, and lethal overdoses are rare and are usually due to contaminants, such as phencyclidine or cocaine.

40. **Answer C.** Aerobic exercise is the most effective therapy for treatment of fibromyalgia syndrome at this time. Resistance exercise may also be effective and is currently being studied. Fibromyalgia syndrome is a noninflammatory condition of chronic hypersensitivity of muscles in response to painful stimuli. Patients with fibromyalgia syndrome experience pain at lower thresholds of somatic stimuli. Over 90% of patients with fibromyalgia exhibit fatigue and over 50% carry a concomitant diagnosis of mood disorder. Sleep is frequently affected as well. Prednisone and IVIG do not improve fibromyalgia syndrome, as there is no inflammatory component to target. Acupuncture and physical therapy have been shown to be ineffective in the majority of patients.

41. **Answer E.** Posterior wall MIs occur with infarction of the right coronary artery or left circumflex artery, depending on the anatomic dominance of the patient. Standard EKG electrodes are anteriorly placed and may not exhibit infarction patterns of ST elevation—posterior electrodes are more accurate at diagnosing posterior wall MIs. Infarction patterns in posterior wall MIs are opposite of those in anterior wall MIs—posterior MIs will show ST depression instead of ST elevation, R waves instead of Q waves, and upright T waves instead of T-wave inversions. Leads V1 and V2 are the most specific anterior leads for posterior wall infarction. Tall R waves, like Q waves, are the latest findings in posterior MIs.

42. **Answer E.** Approximately 30% to 50% of patients with adenovirus pharyngitis have an associated conjunctivitis, which is typically a unilateral, follicular conjunctivitis. Patients presenting with conjunctivitis, pharyngitis, and fever are said to have pharyngoconjunctival fever, which is diagnostic for adenovirus infection. No further testing is required. Outbreaks of community-acquired pharyngoconjunctival fever due to adenovirus have been attributed to exposure to water from contaminated swimming pools as well as fomites from shared pool towels. The EP should keep this in mind when treating young children with pharyngitis and conjunctivitis in the summer. In the absence of conjunctivitis, it is not possible to differentiate adenovirus-induced pharyngitis from group A β-hemolytic

streptococcal pharyngitis as both organisms may cause an intense exudative pharyngitis.

43. **Answer C.** The patient has dry socket, or acute alveolar osteitis. It occurs in 5% to 20% of all tooth extractions, and the posterior mandibular teeth are at highest risk. Age, smoking, and poor dental hygiene are strong risk factors. Dry socket is distinguished from normal postextraction pain by the severity, delayed onset, and lack of relief with NSAIDs. Halitosis is almost always present in patients with dry socket. Trismus is not present. Direct anesthesia, irrigation, and gentle packing are indicated. Treatment may also include NSAIDs and narcotics for pain and penicillin. Recreating a clot is associated with a higher incidence of osteomyelitis.

44. **Answer E.** There are numerous potential complications of *B. pertussis* infection and complications are not uncommon. They can be divided into mechanical complications as a result of severe cough and infectious complications. Mechanical complications include subconjunctival hemorrhage, Mallory–Weiss tears, pneumothorax and pneumomediastinum, atelectasis, urinary incontinence (increases with age), syncope, rib fractures, facial and truncal petechiae, abdominal and inguinal hernias, and back pain. Infectious complications include pneumonia (up to 20% in children, versus only 2% to 4% in adults), sinusitis, and otitis media (most common infectious complication). The most serious complication in young infants is apnea, leading to hypoxia, cyanosis, and possibly death. It is because of this complication, that all infants with *B. pertussis* infection should be admitted to an intensive care unit (ICU) setting for appropriate monitoring. This complication most commonly occurs in infants just a few weeks old. Pneumonia may be primarily caused by *B. pertussis* in young infants, whereas the pneumonia that occurs in adolescents and adults is usually caused by a secondary infection. Other rare complications include seizures (0.3% to 0.6%), encephalopathy (0.1%), and even carotid artery dissection.

45. **Answer B.** During the metabolism of ethylene glycol, glyoxylic acid is produced. Glyoxylic acid may be metabolized in three ways—two pathways form nontoxic compounds and the third forms the toxic oxalic acid, which predisposes to calcium oxalate crystals. Pyridoxine and thiamine are each cofactors in the two pathways that form nontoxic compounds and are recommended as supplemental therapy in addition to the standard treatment of ethylene glycol poisoning (bicarbonate, competitive alcohol dehydrogenase inhibitors such as alcohol or 4-methylpyrazole [Fomepizole], dialysis).

46. **Answer E.** The x-ray demonstrates a significant vertebral compression deformity. Fortunately, vertebral compression fractures are stable fractures with few neurologic complications. While retropulsed fragments can impact the spinal cord or cause cauda equine syndrome, this patient has no neurologic symptoms that would mandate an MRI. CT scans are sometimes performed to determine stability in patients with wedge fractures but this patient's injury is clearly a compression deformity which is a stable injury. A thoracolumbosacral orthosis (TLSO) is a very large brace intended to immobilize the spine typically after spinal surgery. While smaller lumbar braces can be used (e.g. "chair back" braces), they can't be used while sitting, limit mobility which can lead to other problems, and aren't clearly efficacious. Kyphoplasty, a form of vertebral augmentation meant to reduce the fracture is reserved for patients with persistent pain who fail conservative management. Most patients with these injuries remain able to ambulate and can be discharged from the hospital with pain control and follow-up.

47. **Answer B.** Alcohol is the toxin most commonly associated with seizures. Most alcohol-related seizures are due to alcohol withdrawal and typically occur between 6 and 48 hours after discontinuation of drinking. However, alcohol withdrawal seizures have been known to occur as long as 7 days after discontinuation of drinking, particularly in cases of polysubstance abuse with benzodiazepines and barbiturates. Interestingly, acute alcohol intoxication can also provoke seizures, and there is some electroencephalographic evidence to suggest a lowered seizure threshold in this setting.

48. **Answer B.** The patient has acute mastoiditis. There is erythema behind the auricle in the setting of otic pain. Mastoiditis is usually seen as a complication of otitis media and occurs when the mastoid air cells are blocked by infectious debris. Streptococci are the most common cause. The infection can spread to cause a generalized skull osteomyelitis with associated cranial neuropathies and meningitis. Diagnosis is primarily made clinically, but CT scan of the mastoid area can provide important information for the consulting ENT doctor. Plain radiographs are too insensitive for the diagnosis. MRI is not necessary in the acute setting. Tympanocentesis is unlikely to change management. Lumbar puncture is indicated only in the setting of signs and symptoms of associated meningitis, but a CT scan should be performed first to assess for the possibility of mass effect from localized infection. (Figure courtesy of Mark Silverberg, MD. Reprinted with permission from Greenberg MI, Hendrickson RG, Silverberg M, et al. *Greenberg's Text-Atlas of Emergency Medicine.* Philadelphia, PA: Lippincott Williams & Wilkins; 2004:135.)

49. **Answer B.** Applying a magnet to the pulse generator causes the pacemaker to default to asynchronous pacing

function by turning off (or bypassing) the sense amplifier. In other words, a magnet "turns the sensing function off." The pacemaker will deliver impulses (pacer spikes) at its predefined default rate (sometimes called the "magnet rate") regardless of the heart's intrinsic electrical activity. The result is an irregular heart rate, since the pacemaker ignores the patient's intrinsic rhythm and is therefore not synchronized to the patient's intrinsic rhythm.

50. **Answer E.** Tube thoracostomy is the most common procedure performed in the setting of thoracic trauma. It is also the primary means by which a primary or secondary spontaneous pneumothorax is treated (a small pneumothorax may be observed without intervention). The presence of a pneumothorax must have been caused by a defect in the patient's bronchial tree resulting in communication between the bronchioles and the pleural space. The chest tube is placed within the pleural space such that when suction is applied to the chest tube the accumulated pleural air will be removed allowing the lung to expand. However, because the original lesion does not heal instantaneously, the application of suction to the pleural space may also remove air directly from the bronchial system through the original defect that caused the pneumothorax. The expectation is that the rate of air accumulation in the pleural space through the defect is slower than the rate of air removal, thereby allowing the lung to expand. The vacuum is maintained until there is no longer any evidence of a leak (therefore signifying that the defect has healed). The easiest way to test for the presence of a leak is to ask the patient to cough and then examine the water seal chamber for air bubbling up through the column of water. Coughing increases intrathoracic pressure which forces air through the defect, if one is still present. In the case of a very small defect, there may not be a detectable leak after correct tube placement. Leaks can also be due to inadequate insertion of the chest tube such that some of the suction holes lie outside the pleural cavity. Alternatively, there may simply be a leak in the vacuum tubing or connectors. In these cases, however, the lungs will frequently fail to expand as the suction capacity is "wasted" by continuously removing air from the limitless ambient environment instead of the pleural space. This will be evident by virtue of a constant bubbling in the water seal chamber. The amount of water in the water seal chamber has no effect on the amount of air escaping from the system.

51. **Answer E.** Only dialysis can definitively remove ethylene glycol from the body. Ethanol and fomepizole are temporizing measures to inhibit alcohol dehydrogenase from catalyzing the conversion of toxic alcohols into their toxic metabolites. Pyridoxine and thiamine are cofactors in the conversion of glyoxylic acid, a toxic metabolite of ethylene glycol, to nontoxic compounds.

They are useful as adjunctive therapies for ethylene glycol poisoning but do not constitute definitive therapy.

52. **Answer A.** The radial nerve may be injured in as many as 20% of humeral shaft fractures because of its close proximity to the humerus as it travels posteriorly in the spiral groove. Most of these injuries are transient neurapraxias and will improve without intervention. Therefore, such injuries should be well documented and followed by close outpatient observation. Injuries to the radial nerve in this area result primarily in wrist drop along with weakness of finger extension and hypoesthesia and decreased two-point discrimination in the distribution of the radial nerve. The radial nerve also innervates the supinators of the wrist, resulting in difficulty with supination. Because the radial nerve sends branches to the triceps before its entrance into the spiral groove, elbow extension is unaffected (although it may be weak due to pain resulting from the fracture). (Figure from Reece RM, Ludwig S. *Child Abuse: Medical Diagnosis and Management.* 2nd ed. Philadelphia, PA: Lippincott Williams & Wilkins; 2001:150, with permission.)

53. **Answer D.** The EKG demonstrates diffuse tall T waves consistent with hyperkalemia. The history of absence of medical care, untreated hypertension, weakness, and fatigue suggests the possibility of renal failure as the underlying cause of hyperkalemia. Potassium levels should obviously be confirmed on laboratory tests, but cardioprotective agents such as calcium chloride or calcium gluconate should be ordered early. Defibrillation should never be performed in awake patients. Cardioversion should only be performed with a clear history of hemodynamic instability. Lidocaine is used for wide-complex tachycardias but has generally been supplanted by amiodarone for acute use.

54. **Answer C.** Enteroviruses, such as coxsackievirus, account for more than half of all the cases of encephalitis. Herpes virus is the most common cause of severe encephalitis in the United States. Typically, in frank infections of the brain parenchyma (encephalitis), there is some degree of concomitant infection and inflammation of the meninges. Therefore, *meningoencephalitis* is a more accurate term describing most of these infections. When the infection is limited to the meninges, it is termed *meningitis,* reflecting meningitis in the absence of a pyogenic organism. Mumps is another important cause of aseptic meningitis, especially in the setting of outbreaks of the virus such as in Iowa in early 2006. Meningoencephalitis is the most common complication of childhood mumps and frequently occurs at the same time as parotitis. Neurocysticercosis is a rare cause typically found in immigrants from areas where undercooked pork harboring the parasite *Taenia solium* may be eaten. Adenovirus is an uncommon cause.

55. **Answer A.** *Helicobacter pylori* infection is the most common cause of gastritis and peptic ulcer disease. *H. pylori* is a gram-negative bacillus that causes gastric and duodenal mucosal inflammation. It is implicated in over half of all cases of gastritis and peptic ulcer disease. Treatment is with combinations of proton pump inhibitors and antibiotics (e.g., lansoprazole + amoxicillin + clarithromycin). The next most common cause of gastritis and peptic ulcer disease is NSAID use. Although the patient denies history of medication use, NSAIDs should be specifically queried about as patients frequently forget over-the-counter medications that they are taking. Alcohol can cause gastritis but usually in moderate to large quantities and regular use. Peppermint puts patients at risk for GERD exacerbations but does not usually cause frank gastritis. Radon gas exposure is likely the number one source of background ionizing radiation and puts patients at risk for lung cancer but does not usually directly cause gastritis.

56. **Answer B.** In order of decreasing frequency, the small intestine, liver, and colon are the most commonly injured abdominal organs in the setting of penetrating abdominal trauma.

57. **Answer B.** Reciprocal ST depressions associated with ST elevations have high specificity for acute MI (reported to be >90%) and are not usually present in nonischemic conditions. Their presence confers a higher risk of poor outcomes. Reciprocal ST depressions are usually downsloping. Most inferior wall MIs exhibit reciprocal ST depressions, whereas most anterior wall MIs do not.

58. **Answer E.** The traditional scheme for categorizing burn injuries has been replaced by a surgical model which describes burns as superficial (first degree), superficial partial-thickness (superficial second degree), deep partial-thickness (often requiring surgery), and full-thickness (third degree). The term "fourth degree" is still used to describe burns that injure subcutaneous tissues, including muscle, tendons, and bone. One significant problem with initial burn wound evaluation is that the character of the wound may change over time in a process known as "wound conversion." Superficial wounds may become deeper over time depending on the adequacy of blood flow and healing, as well as the patient's underlying medical problems. In addition, the depth of injury is often variable throughout the wound such that both deep and superficial components may be present. Deep partial-thickness wounds invariably heal with significant, hypertrophic scarring that impedes joint function. Such burns are not painful unless palpated, and they do not blanch when pressure is applied. Clinically, they are often difficult to differentiate from full-thickness burns. Furthermore, deep partial-thickness burns leave very few viable epithelial cells remaining, so wound healing (via re-epithelialization) is extremely slow and often requires skin grafting.

59. **Answer B.** Elderly white men have the highest rate of completed suicide, representing more than three-fourths of all suicide deaths, and women have the highest rate of suicide attempts. White patients are more likely to commit suicide than blacks or Hispanics, and non-pregnant women of childbearing age are more likely than pregnant women to do so. Divorced patients have higher rates than unmarried patients, who, in turn, have higher rates than married patients. Most successful suicide attempts involve firearms and most unsuccessful attempts involve drug ingestions. The presence of a firearm in the house is an independent risk factor for completed suicide, and the patient should be directly asked about this on history. Substance abuse, especially alcohol and cocaine, is extremely common in patients who complete suicide. Patients who present to the ED with attempted suicide must be evaluated for medical illness that may masquerade as mood disorder or thought disorder leading to the suicide attempt. Roughly 20% of patients with major depression and 10% of patients with schizophrenia commit suicide.

60. **Answer B.** Cyanosis is normal after birth and acrocyanosis can persist for as long as 10 minutes in many infants. Thus, cyanosis alone is not a good indicator of neonatal respiratory distress. If the neonate appears to have consistent, spontaneous respirations with a good effort, then the neonate should first be suctioned in the mouth and nose. This clears oropharyngeal and nasopharyngeal secretions that may be impeding airflow. It also stimulates the baby helping to provide an indicator of neonatal wellness and responsiveness. In routine deliveries, in which the neonate's respiratory effort is clearly strong, suctioning with a bulb syringe is unnecessary and oral and nasal secretions can be wiped away with a clean towel. However, in cases in which there is a question about neonatal respiratory effort, suctioning is the first step before moving forward to positive pressure ventilation.

61. **Answer A.** In the setting of renal disease, hyperkalemia is the likely culprit of the patient's bradycardia. Calcium and bicarbonate should be used to help reverse the patient's bradycardia. Many patients with acute renal failure or an acute exacerbation of chronic kidney disease are acidotic and it is this acidosis that prevents the heart from responding to typical treatments for bradycardia such as atropine and transcutaneous pacing. While bicarbonate targets the root issue, calcium opposes potassium's effects on the myocardium, restoring the cardiac resting membrane potential, allowing cardiac myocytes to conduct electricity normally. None of the other treatments listed are helpful in patients with hyperkalemia.

62. **Answer A.** The combination of the head impulse test (head thrust maneuver), evaluation of direction-changing nystagmus, and evaluation of eye skew devia-

tion comprise the HINTS (head impulse–nystagmus–test of skew) test to determine whether vertigo is due to a central or peripheral lesion. Of specific concern is differentiating peripheral vertigo from a cerebellar stroke. In the head impulse test, the patient fixates his gaze on a distant object while the physician rotates the patient's head from side to side before randomly "thrusting it" rapidly back to the midline. In an abnormal test, the patient is unable to maintain fixation during the thrust and the eyes slowly march back to the midline in a saccadic fashion as they re-fixate on the object. A positive test indicates a problem in the vestibuloocular reflex (VOR) and a peripheral lesion. In patients with peripheral lesions, the fast phase of nystagmus will always occur in the same direction regardless of whether the patient is looking left or right. It is easier to detect if the patient does not fixate on an object. In central lesions the direction of nystagmus may (or may not) change depending on the direction of gaze. In testing for skew deviation, the physician asks the patient to fixate on an object while covering and then uncovering and eye while examining the eye for vertical movement, which is abnormal, after it is uncovered. A normal head impulse test, or the presence of direction-changing nystagmus or skew deviation all make a brainstem or cerebellar lesion more likely and MRI imaging should be pursued.

63. **Answer A.** The most common cause of upper GI bleeding in both the general population and alcoholics is peptic ulcer disease. When combined with NSAIDs and other ulcerogenic drugs, alcohol can contribute to the loss of protective gastric mucosal lining. Treatment in alcoholics is the same as for nonalcoholics, with special attention to electrolyte management, prevention of alcohol withdrawal, and attention to seizure precautions. Gastric and esophageal varices occur at a higher rate in those alcoholics who have a history of portal hypertension from cirrhosis. Boerhaave syndrome refers to rupture of the esophagus from forceful vomiting. It usually occurs in alcoholics, and presents more often as sepsis and hypovolemia due to mediastinitis rather than GI bleed. Arteriovenous malformation is a more common cause of lower GI bleed than upper GI bleed.

64. **Answer C.** There is strong clinical evidence of temporal arteritis, with the unilateral frontotemporal headache and jaw claudication in a late middle-aged patient. The shoulder muscle pain and weakness are symptoms of polymyalgia rheumatica, which occurs concomitantly in as many as half of all cases of temporal arteritis. Diagnosis is suspected with elevated ESR or CRP. CRP is more sensitive than erythrocyte sedimentation rate (ESR) (97% vs. 86%) and does not increase with normal aging like ESR does. Confirmation can be made with temporal artery biopsy. The major dangerous com-

plication of temporal arteritis is blindness from ophthalmic artery inflammation. Treatment for known or suspected cases of temporal arteritis is with parenteral steroids. MRI for evaluation of subacute headache with a normal head CT does not generally yield an emergent diagnosis. Lumbar puncture is a reasonable choice here but does not account for the more emergent diagnosis, which is temporal arteritis. Carbamazepine is first-line treatment for trigeminal neuralgia, which is on the differential diagnosis of unilateral headache and jaw pain. However, the pain from trigeminal neuralgia tends to be episodic, lancinating pain rather than constant, dull pain. To this author's knowledge (and moderate consternation), there is no such thing as the migraine vasodilation stimulation test.

65. **Answer E.** The patient's gall bladder ultrasound shows multiple gallstones with shadowing. Given the absence of fever, leukocytosis, or Murphy sign, there is no strong clinical evidence to suggest acute cholecystitis. There is also no pericholecystic fluid and no mention is made of a sonographic Murphy sign, both of which would be signs of acute cholecystitis. In a patient with symptomatic gallstones, surgical evaluation can be undertaken to assess for need for cholecystectomy—this does not need to be emergent (though urgent outpatient referral is preferred to reduce repeated visits for biliary colic). Intravenous antibiotics are used for acute cholecystitis. ERCP is preferred in cases of gallstone pancreatitis, when the lipase is elevated in the presence of gallstones. Percutaneous biliary drains are not used often in the emergency setting. HIDA scan is only used when ultrasound is equivocal for biliary pathology in cases with strong clinical suspicion. (From Daffner RH. *Clinical Radiology: The Essentials.* 2nd ed. Philadelphia, PA: Lippincott Williams & Wilkins; 1999.)

66. **Answer A.** The patient has phlegmasia cerulea dolens, which is diagnosed by the clinical triad of cyanosis, pain, and edema due to massive lower extremity venous thrombosis. The cyanosis is due to a combination of increased venous backflow and compromised arterial flow. Phlegmasia alba dolens is similar but lacks cyanosis and instead appears as a blanched extremity. Treatment involves admission, intravenous anticoagulation, and possibly surgical thrombectomy and fasciotomy. (Figure From Mumoli N, Invernizzi C, Luschi R, et al. Phlegmasia cerulea dolens. *Circulation.* 2012;125(8):1056–1057.)

67. **Answer D.** Propanolol is the most dangerous β-blocker in overdose. It is highly lipophilic and readily enters the CNS, causing seizures and coma. β-Blocker overdoses commonly cause bradycardia, AV block, and hypotension, and less often lead to tachydysrhythmias. Hypoglycemia is much more common in children than in adults, and glucose should be part of the cocktail of

atropine, glucagon, and insulin therapy for patients with β-blocker overdose. Hyperkalemia and renal failure may also occur, but much less often than seizure.

68. **Answer A.** *Mycobacterium tuberculosis* can affect nearly any organ system in the body. The most common extrapulmonary manifestation is *painless* lymphadenopathy, usually in the cervical region. Although classically described as a disease of childhood, the peak incidence is between 20 and 40 years of age. Although the nodes are initially discrete, they may form a firm, matted, nontender mass over time. Pericarditis may result from direct extension of TB from mediastinal lymph nodes, or the spine, lungs, or sternum. The onset may be insidious or acute and may result in a restrictive pericarditis. The CNS is not spared in extrapulmonary TB, and tuberculous meningitis is the most common presentation of neurologic TB disease. In such cases, the CSF usually reveals very high protein levels, ranging from 100 to 500 mg/dL, although levels as high as 2 to 6 g/dL have been reported. In contrast, CSF glucose concentration usually is <45 mg/dL. Skeletal TB most commonly involves the spine (Pott disease), with most lesions in the thoracic pine. Vertebral destruction usually begins at the anteroinferior portion of the vertebral body, eventually resulting in an anterior wedge defect and a palpable bony prominence posteriorly (termed *Gibbus*). *M. tuberculosis* typically spreads to the bilateral adrenal glands, causing bilateral adrenal enlargement and subsequent destruction which ultimately causes adrenal insufficiency.

69. **Answer E.** Supracondylar fractures are the most common pediatric elbow fractures. They frequently occur after a fall on an outstretched hand with the elbow "locked" in extension or hyperextension. The supracondylar region of bone is thin and weak making it prone to fracture. This patient's x-ray reveals an anterior and posterior fat pad sign as well as a very subtle fracture of the anterior and posterior cortex (Fig. 2-15). Even without these latter findings, a supracondylar fracture should be suspected and the patient should be placed into a long arm posterior splint. Volkmann ischemic contracture is the classic complication of brachial artery injury that can occur in posteriorly displaced supracondylar fractures.

70. **Answer E.** This patient experienced preterm PPROM 2 days before presentation, which dramatically increased her risk for developing chorioamnionitis. Chorioamnionitis is an intra-amniotic infection that is most commonly due to vaginal flora that has gained entry to the amniotic cavity. Risk factors include young age, low socioeconomic status, nulliparity, extended duration of labor and ruptured membranes, multiple vaginal examinations, and pre-existing infections of the lower genital tract. The typical causative organisms are group B *streptococci* and *E. coli* and the most widely used antibiotic regimen is a combination of ampicillin and gentamicin.

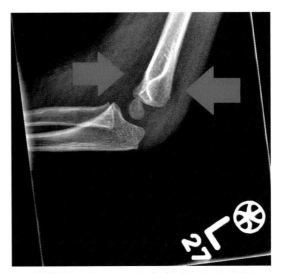

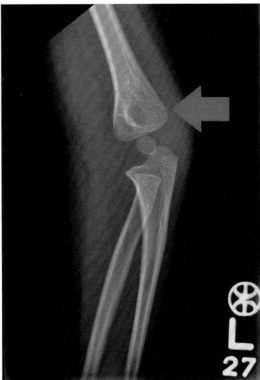

Figure 2-15

Ampicillin may be replaced with vancomycin, erythromycin, or clindamycin in penicillin-allergic patients.

71. **Answer D.** This patient has endometritis, which is the most common puerperal infection. The primary risk factor for endometritis is cesarean section, although young age, low socioeconomic status, prolonged stage 2 of labor, prolonged ruptured membranes, and multiple vaginal examinations are also risk factors. Patients typically present 2 to 3 days after delivery with fever, abdominal pain, and foul smelling lochia. Infections are polymicrobial and are most commonly caused by gram-negative enteric pathogens as well as *Bacteroides* and

Prevotella species. *Chlamydia* is rarely responsible and may cause late-onset puerperal infection.

72. **Answer D.** Patients presenting with the triad of flashes, floaters, and field deficits should be emergently referred to an ophthalmologist for presumed retinal detachment. Patients may not recognize small peripheral detachments that do not affect visual acuity. Many patients, however, complain of progressive partial vision loss in the affected field. PVD causes both flashes and floaters but does not cause a field deficit. Vitreous hemorrhage most commonly results from diabetic proliferative retinopathy, PVD, and trauma. If the degree of hemorrhage is significant, overall visual acuity will be decreased. Furthermore, the presence of vitreous hemorrhage significantly increases the likelihood of retinal detachment. In addition to vitreous hemorrhage, the presence of retinal pigment within the vitreous (called vitreous pigment or "tobacco dust") strongly increases the likelihood of retinal detachment (LR+ = 44). Posterior uveitis is an umbrella term referring to inflammation of the posterior portions of the middle layer of the eye (e.g., choroiditis). It is characterized by painless floaters that often cause blurred vision.

73. **Answer B.** Elderly, diabetic, and female patients frequently have atypical anginal symptoms. The extreme elderly (>85 years) experience shortness of breath as the most common symptom during an MI. Nausea, typical chest pain, syncope, and fatigue may also be present. The emergency physician (EP) can never clinically rule out the diagnosis of acute coronary syndrome in elderly patients just because they lack frank chest pain. Choices D and E occur more frequently in dehydration and infection than in MI.

74. **Answer D.** Erythema toxicum neonatorum is a very common, benign rash which is most common in full-term infants (incidence declines with decreasing gestational age) (see Fig. 2-16). It is thought to be due to a

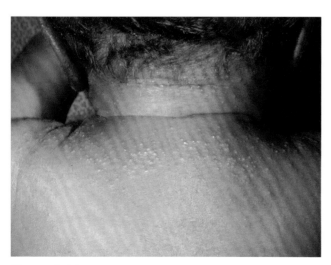

Figure 2-16

problem with sebaceous glands within hair follicles called pilosebaceous follicles. It is most common on the trunk and proximal extremities and spares the palms and soles. As it resolves spontaneously it requires no treatment. (From Lugo-Somolinos A, McKinley-Grant L, Goldsmith LA, et al., eds. *VisualDx: Essential Dermatology in Pigmented Skin.* Philadelphia, PA: Wolters Kluwer; 2011.)

75. **Answer A.** The patient's head CT demonstrates an acute cerebellar hemorrhage. Surgical intervention has been the mainstay of management of cerebellar hemorrhage. However, in awake patients with relatively small infarcts (<3 cm), patients may be candidates for observation in an intensive care setting. All patients with cerebellar hemorrhage, however, may deteriorate rapidly due to hydrocephalus or progressive brainstem compression. Due to the local mass effect, the fourth ventricle may become compressed, resulting in an obstructive hydrocephalus. This requires emergent ventricular drainage. Due to the possibility of rapid deterioration, all patients with cerebellar infarction should be admitted to an intensive care setting. Corticosteroids and anticonvulsants have no role in the management of cerebellar hemorrhage. Corticosteroids help to reduce the vasogenic edema associated with tumors, but not the cytotoxic edema associated with infarction. Prophylactic anticonvulsants have not proved to be useful, and because seizures are initiated in the cortex, cerebellar lesions should not trigger epileptic events. Herniation may occur in these patients, but results in upward transtentorial herniation, not uncal herniation. Finally, the Cushing response may occur, but results in very high BPs, with systolic pressures in the neighborhood of 200 mm Hg. This degree of hypertension usually portends a bad outcome. (Figure courtesy of Mark Silverberg, MD. Reprinted in Silverberg M. *Greenberg's Text-Atlas of Emergency Medicine.* Philadelphia, PA: Lippincott Williams & Wilkins; 2004:46, with permission.)

76. **Answer C.** This patient has an exacerbation of congestive heart failure (CHF). Although she has no prior diagnosis of CHF, her clinical history is consistent with the diagnosis. Pleural effusions are common in CHF and thoracentesis generally has no role in their management because they typically resolve with diuretics. This patient also lacks infectious symptoms, which would suggest the presence of pneumonia or a parapneumonic effusion. In patients with severe respiratory compromise as a result of large pleural effusions in the setting of CHF, a secure airway through rapid sequence intubation would be the first step. Although this patient is hypoxic, she has not yet been given supplemental oxygen, so it is premature to intubate this patient at this point. Furthermore, non-invasive ventilation might be attempted before establishing a secure airway in patients with only mild to moderate respiratory distress. BNP levels may be helpful in determining the etiology of respiratory distress in

patients who have mixed cardiopulmonary disease without a clear clinical picture. This patient's clinical picture clearly points toward a diagnosis of CHF, so a BNP level would not provide any additional information.

77. **Answer E.** Sitz is a word that comes from the German word, *sitzen,* meaning "to sit." A *sitz bath* refers to any device that allows a patient to immerse only the perineum and buttocks in water while draping the rest of their body outside the tub. While patients may add various medications to the water, it is not recommended and there is no evidence that such additives help. Sitz baths are thought to help a variety of perianal complaints, such as hemorrhoids, because anal canal pressure decreases significantly in warm water (40°C) and blood flow improves.

78. **Answer B.** AS usually occurs due to congenital bicuspid structure, calcific degeneration, or rheumatic heart disease. The classic murmur is a systolic crescendo–decrescendo murmur at the right upper sternal border or cardiac base. The natural history of AS usually follows a sequence of findings, starting with angina, followed by syncope, and then heart failure. As each subsequent finding occurs, the mortality increases significantly. Valve replacement is the only definitive treatment once symptoms appear.

79. **Answer D.** Swallowed maternal blood is a common cause of factitious GI bleeding in young neonates. The apt test involves the application of alkali to a small sample of bloody stool. Owing to its different composition from adult hemoglobin, fetal hemoglobin (which is composed of two α and two γ subunits instead of two α and two β subunits as in adult hemoglobin) is resistant to denaturation by this application. After the application of alkali, fetal hemoglobin will remain pinkish red upon microscopic examination whereas adult hemoglobin will appear brownish. Both the Rosette test and the KBT are used to detect the presence of fetal maternal hemorrhage.

80. **Answer A.** Perimortem cesarean section should be performed in all pregnant patients suffering traumatic cardiac arrest with a fetus >24 weeks of gestational age. Maternal resuscitation always takes precedence over the fetus, but once cardiac arrest has occurred, an immediate decision to undergo perimortem cesarean section must be made. Seventy percent of fetuses will survive if delivered within 5 minutes of maternal arrest. None will survive after 25 minutes. Consent is unnecessary and should not be sought before the procedure. If the fetal gestational age is unknown, cesarean delivery should be performed if the fundal height exceeds the umbilicus. To perform the procedure, a large midline vertical incision ("classic" midline incision) is made from the subxiphoid process to the symphysis pubis. If an anterior placenta is encountered upon entering the uterus, it should be incised to reach the fetus, as bleeding can be addressed after the procedure. Ideally, verification of fetal viability through fetal heart tones would be documented before the procedure, but absence of this information is not a contraindication and no time should be wasted attempting to document fetal viability.

81. **Answer C.** Enterohemorrhagic *E. coli* (EHEC) is a common cause of pediatric bloody diarrhea. The bacterium produces a Shiga-like toxin which is responsible for hemolytic uremic syndrome (HUS). Though EHEC is the most common cause of HUS, HUS occurs in fewer than 10% of patients with EHEC infections. HUS develops 5 to 10 days after the onset of diarrhea and classically comprises hemolytic anemia, thrombocytopenia, and acute kidney injury with as many as 50% of patients requiring dialysis. The patient in this vignette doesn't have any of these symptoms. In well patients like him with symptoms only of hemorrhagic colitis, treatment is supportive, consisting of rehydration, and electrolyte management. Antibiotics may increase the rate of HUS because their use can induce expression and release of Shiga toxin. Antidiarrheals can also worsen systemic symptoms and should be avoided.

82. **Answer B.** Neither antibiotics nor corticosteroids have any role in prophylactic therapy of potential aspiration. Corticosteroids may be of use in patients with a history of reactive airway disease, who have active symptoms upon presentation to the ED. Otherwise, asymptomatic patients should be observed for a minimum of 4 hours in the ED. Repeat x-rays are not required. If the patient remains asymptomatic and maintains an oxygen saturation >94% without supplemental oxygen, she may be safely discharged.

83. **Answer E.** Bedside ultrasound of the orbit is one of the easiest and also the most effective uses of ultrasound. Since the eyelids represent the only tissue between the ultrasound probe and the eye, resolution is excellent. Using the high frequency, flat probe (7.5 to 10 MHz linear transducer), the eye can be scanned in both the long and short axes in 1 minute. In addition to retinal detachment (thick band lying anterior to the retina in the posterior globe), vitreous hemorrhage (echogenic material within the usually clear black vitreous), lens dislocation (lens located in a different place than is seen on the normal contralateral eye), and retrobulbar hemorrhage (hypoechoic fluid collection posterior to the eye not seen on the contralateral eye), it can be used to diagnose vitreous detachment (thin membrane just anterior to retina), globe rupture (decreased globe volume with distorted shape), and intraocular foreign body. As noted above, ultrasound can be used in patients with globe rupture, but a lot of gel should be used and excessive pressure should not be applied to the eye.

84. **Answer B.** The classic neurologic deficit seen in central cord syndrome is upper extremity weakness greater

than lower extremity weakness. This is because of the cervical motor axons being closer to the midline than the lumbar motor axons. Large central cord injuries can initially be clinically indistinguishable from complete cord syndromes. Anterior cord syndrome results in deficits of bilateral motor function and pain/temperature sensation with sparing of vibration/position sensation. Brown–Séquard syndrome, or cord hemisection, results in deficits in ipsilateral motor function and vibration/position sensation and contralateral pain/temperature sensation. Cauda equina syndrome, usually due to disk herniation, preferentially affects the lower extremities and bowel/bladder function. Complete cord injury affects all neurologic functions below the level of injury.

85. **Answer D.** Neurologic dysfunction is the hallmark of heatstroke. Patients with heat *exhaustion* present with intact mental status, although they may present with generalized malaise, fatigue, headache, impaired judgment, vertigo, as well as nausea and vomiting. Patients with heat exhaustion also typically present with persistent and profuse sweating, with a core temperature that may be only mildly elevated and which is always <104°F. Patients with heat stroke usually have a core temperature >105°F, resulting in multiorgan failure. Patients may be anhidrotic and have elevated hepatic transaminases, although these findings are not required for the diagnosis. In addition, patients with heat exhaustion may also develop elevated hepatic transaminases although the increase is less severe. Most significantly, patients with heat stroke have an altered sensorium (delirium) and may develop coma or seizures.

86. **Answer E.** Although it may be counterintuitive, most patients develop primary spontaneous pneumothorax while at rest. Traditionally, expiratory chest x-rays were thought to aid in the diagnosis of pneumothorax. Because the relative size of the chest cavity is thought to decrease during expiration, and since the size of the pneumothorax is theoretically constant, the pneumothorax should occupy a greater fraction of the chest cavity and, therefore, be easier to detect upon expiration. Clinically, however, expiratory films have not demonstrated much utility. Pneumomediastinum is a less common but generally benign finding, and is frequently self-limited. It is usually due to persistent elevations in intrathoracic pressure such as that caused by repetitive severe coughing, asthma exacerbations, or seizures. In contrast, secondary pneumomediastinum is a morbid diagnosis that results from significant underlying disease such as Boerhaave syndrome. Hamman sign or crunch is a physical examination finding in the setting of pneumomediastinum. It describes the crunch-like sound heard upon cardiac auscultation as the heart expands against the mediastinal air. The most frequent physical examination finding in pneumomediastinum

is SQ emphysema, frequently in the neck. Male smokers have more than a 20-fold increased risk of developing a spontaneous pneumothorax, whereas woman smokers have a more than 10-fold increased risk. Other risk factors include tall height and cold weather. There is an increased incidence in the fall and winter.

87. **Answer D.** The patient has a total (or "eight-ball") hyphema. The pupil is almost completely obscured by blood in the anterior chamber due to the ocular trauma. ED management is with ophthalmologic consultation, topical steroids (under the direction of the ophthalmologist only), head elevation, eye shielding, and tetanus booster. The eye is shielded to prevent secondary injury and further bleeding. Trendelenburg positioning and NSAIDs will likely worsen the bleed and are contraindicated. Although factor VII has important procoagulant activities, it has currently not been approved for use in patients with hyphemas. IV antibiotics are not indicated except in patients with evidence of globe rupture. (From Rhee D, ed. *Color Atlas and Synopsis of Clinical Ophthalmology: Wills Eye Institute – Glaucoma.* Philadelphia, PA: Wolters Kluwer; 2012.)

88. **Answer D.** PVD is an extremely common problem, and in otherwise healthy adults, it is a normal occurrence with aging. Over time, pockets of fluid called premacular bursa develop within the normally gelatinous vitreous. Their presence destabilizes the vitreous which contracts, eventually pulling away from its posterior attachment to the retina. The detachment stimulates retinal photoreceptors, resulting in "flashes" of light. The posterior edge of the vitreous subsequently hangs in front of the remaining retina and is seen as floaters in the visual field. PVD is occasionally associated with vitreous hemorrhage, which typically resolves without treatment. Patients with diabetes may experience vitreous hemorrhage independent of PVD, which reflects underlying proliferative retinopathy requiring ophthalmologic referral. Rarely, PVD is associated with retinal tears and subsequent retinal detachment. Retinal detachment is typically visible on direct ophthalmoscopy, particularly when the pupil is first dilated. Retinal detachment is associated with decreased vision in the area of the defect. Thus, patients who present with complaints of flashes, floaters, *and* visual field loss ("the three Fs") require emergent referral for repair to prevent extension of the defect to the fovea. Patients with normal acuity should be referred just as emergently, since their prognosis with repair is better as normal acuity suggests that the fovea is not involved in the detachment.

89. **Answer D.** The heterophile antibody test, or monospot, is a rapid assay for the diagnosis of infectious mononucleosis due to EBV. It has lower sensitivity early in the illness (<70% in the first week) but steadily improves in the next few weeks. Specificity is excellent and reported

to be near 100%. It is important to tell patients suspected of having infectious mononucleosis with a negative monospot test that either the illness is early in its course or a non-EBV cause is possible. Infectious mononucleosis is subacute to chronic multisystem syndrome of pharyngitis, lymphadenopathy, splenomegaly, hepatitis, and fatigue. Splenomegaly is perhaps the most important clinical feature for the emergency physician as demonstration of this finding requires strict avoidance of contact sports and aggressive physical activity to prevent splenic rupture. Treatment is supportive. Almost one-third of all patients with infectious mononucleosis carries group A *Streptococcus* (GAS), which confounds the diagnosis of a patient with febrile pharyngitis and leads to inappropriate antibiotic use.

90. **Answer A.** Ipsilateral pleuritic chest pain and dyspnea are the most common symptoms of a primary spontaneous pneumothorax. Hemoptysis is uncommon in spontaneous pneumothorax and would signify a specific etiology for the pneumothorax such as tumor. Patients may occasionally be asymptomatic or have nonspecific complaints. Many patients delay treatment for up to 1 week, and symptoms tend to resolve without treatment in 24 to 48 hours. Primary spontaneous pneumothorax is three times more common in men than in women and typically occurs in tall, healthy young men. Other factors associated with spontaneous pneumothorax are smoking, changes in atmospheric pressure, mitral valve prolapse, and Marfan syndrome. The most common arrhythmia is a mild sinus tachycardia.

91. **Answer E.** *S. Pneumoniae* (also known as *Pneumococcus*) is the most common *bacterial* cause of pneumonia in preschool-aged children (6 months to 5 years). Overall, viruses are the most common pathogens causing pneumonia in this age group, with RSV being the most common, followed by parainfluenza and influenza viruses, as well as adenovirus and rhinovirus. However, this patient did not present with a viral prodrome and is mildly toxic upon examination. It is critical, therefore, to treat this patient with antibiotics that target *S. Pneumoniae*. Because of increasing resistance among *S. Pneumoniae* isolates, high-dose amoxicillin is the drug of choice, although patients who are hospitalized may require ampicillin, cefuroxime, or cefotaxime delivered intravenously. *K. pneumoniae* is an uncommon cause of pneumonia in children though it can cause severe infections in immunocompromised hosts. Community-acquired *Klebsiella* is primarily a disease of debilitated older men with a history of alcoholism. *M. pneumoniae* is the most common pathogen causing pneumonia in children aged 5 to 15 years. *C. trachomatis* may cause pneumonia in infants aged 3 weeks to 3 months, typically causing an afebrile, subacute interstitial pneumonia. RSV bronchiolitis and pneumonia are the primary causes for hospitalization during the first year of life.

92. **Answer C.** Dual antiplatelet therapy is the recommended approach in patients with NSTEMI. Upon arrival to the ED, all patients should be given between 162 and 325 mg of uncoated aspirin to be chewed immediately. Uncoated aspirin is preferred over enteric coated aspirin because of its more rapid absorption. At these doses, aspirin nearly immediately, completely, and permanently (until a new platelet is made) inhibits thromboxane A2 production which is critical for platelet aggregation. In addition to aspirin, patients should receive either clopidogrel (a thienopyridine, along with ticlopidine and prasugrel) or a GPIIbIIIa inhibitor, such as abciximab, eptifibatide, or tirofiban. Most guidelines recommend clopidogrel as the first-line agent in patients being managed without PCI while clopidogrel or a GPI-IbIIIa inhibitor can be used in patients subjected to an invasive strategy. While some studies have suggested that higher loading doses should be used, the recommended loading dose of clopidogrel in the setting of NSTEMI remains 300 mg *unless* immediate catheterization is going to be performed (in which case the recommended dose is 600 mg).

93. **Answer C.** Urinalysis is a crucial diagnostic tool for the evaluation of all urinary system conditions. The presence of casts in the urine indicates a renal source—RBC casts are associated with glomerulonephritis and white blood cell casts with parenchymal inflammation, such as pyelonephritis. Urine dipstick is a rapid screening tool to detect the presence of glucose, leukocytes, protein, and blood. Unfortunately, sensitivity for most of these parameters is only on the order of 75% to 85% and negative dipstick should not be used to rule out their presence. Transitional cells are from a bladder source but are usually a normal finding and do not necessarily indicate a malignant process. Normal urinary pH is from 5 to 8 and usually mirrors serum pH except in certain disease states, such as renal tubular acidosis or urinary tract infection.

94. **Answer C.** NEC is the most common GI emergency affecting neonates. However, because premature infants are predominantly affected, it is a disease that is most commonly diagnosed in the neonatal intensive care unit (NICU) and only rarely seen in the ED. Interestingly, however, the age at onset of NEC is inversely related to the gestational age and birth weight. Therefore, low–birth-weight infants who initially look well in the NICU may be discharged home before the development of NEC. Initial findings in NEC are nonspecific and include ileus (multiple dilated loops of small bowel) or an asymmetric bowel gas pattern. With the progression of the disease, however, air spreads through ulcerated GI mucosal epithelium resulting in pneumatosis intestinalis or air within the biliary tract (portal venous). Pneumatosis intestinalis occurs in 75% of infants with NEC and is the most specific finding.

95. Answer A. The patient has endocarditis of a prosthetic valve, which is most commonly due to coagulase-negative staphylococci. *S. viridans* is the most common cause of native valve endocarditis. Choices C, D, and E are uncommon causes of native valve endocarditis.

96. Answer C. Kidney stones most commonly occur in middle-aged patients, usually men. Risk factors include age, male gender, family history, and conditions which increase serum and urinary calcium levels. Kidney stones are divided into four main categories—calcium, magnesium ammonium phosphate, uric acid, and cystine. Calcium stones represent approximately two-third of all stones and occur more often in patients with common precipitants of hypercalcemia, including hyperparathyroidism, milk–alkali syndrome, laxative abuse, and sarcoidosis. Inflammatory bowel disease also leads to the formation of calcium oxalate stones, due to hyperoxaliuria. Magnesium ammonium phosphate (struvite) stones account for one-fifth of all calculi and occur in patients with UTIs due to *Proteus, Klebsiella,* and *Pseudomonas.* Uric acid stones occur in patients with hyperuricemia, often due to gout. They are usually radiolucent and missed on plain radiographs. Cystine stones are the least common and are due to hypercystinuria, an inborn error of metabolism usually diagnosed at birth.

97. Answer C. The patient most likely has schizophrenia, a chronic, debilitating psychiatric condition, characterized by a combination of psychosis (delusions, hallucinations, and disorganized thoughts), negative symptoms (e.g., flat affect, social withdrawal, and decreased verbal expression), cognitive impairment (affecting attention, language, memory, and executive function), and a mood disorder. The presentation can be highly variable, and none of these findings is pathognomonic for the diagnosis. However, this patient's chronic course ("saying strange things" for months) leading to an acute "psychotic break" involving auditory hallucinations (auditory hallucinations, usually in the form of hearing voices, are more common than other hallucinations) is typical of schizophrenia. Psychosis related to drug abuse and withdrawal is common but develops acutely and in the setting of a history of abuse or findings that support abuse (e.g., a positive drug screen). Two-thirds of patients with schizophrenia have delusions, which are the most common "positive symptom" (positive symptoms are synonymous with "psychosis"). Suicide is reported in as many as 10% of patients with the diagnosis and is most common early in the course of the illness at the beginning of treatment or shortly after the resolution of an acute psychotic episode. It also occurs *more* commonly among patients with *mild* impairment, which is thought to reflect the higher executive functioning and better insight among such patients. Improved self-recognition may lead to more severe depression, while intact executive functioning allows such patients to act on suicidal thoughts.

98. Answer A. NPH was initially described in 1965 as a triad of difficulties of gait (ataxia), altered mentation (dementia), and urinary sphincter dysfunction (incontinence) in concert with enlarged ventricles (hydrocephalus) but apparently normal cerebrospinal fluid (CSF) pressure upon LP. Recent research has shown that while the CSF pressure may be normal during a single LP, patients with NPH experience transient increases in CSF pressure which can now be appreciated in centers capable of performing CSF monitoring. Therefore, many authors have advocated changing the name of this illness to "chronic hydrocephalus." Though there is no "classic" gait, walking difficulties are the most consistent and prominent feature of NPH. Furthermore, ataxia is most likely to improve after CSF shunting. Alterations in cognition and mentation may be so mild that they are not noticed by either the patient or the patient's family and the term *dementia* is overly broad generalization. Urinary incontinence is present only in the later stages although a sensation of urinary urgency is almost always present. Papilledema is a sign of increased intracranial pressure. Headache is not a typical feature of patients with NPH.

99. Answer B. Naloxone is a pure opioid antagonist with an extremely rapid onset of action, duration of 1 to 2 hours, and the ability to be delivered by a variety of routes (IM, IV, subcutaneous [SC], endotracheal [ET]). The duration is of prime importance, as patients with opiate overdose who are given a one-time naloxone dose in the ambulance often become acutely intoxicated again once the naloxone wears off. All opiates have longer durations of action than naloxone, even heroin, which can last as long as 2 to 3 hours if used by the SC route. For this reason, all patients with severe opiate overdose should be monitored carefully in the ED at least as long as the expected peak effect of the particular opiate.

100. Answer D. Intravenous medications are most appropriate for rapid control of BP. Labetalol is safe and effective during pregnancy and produces predictable control of BP during hypertensive crises such as eclampsia. Hydralazine is an antihypertensive medicine that is also commonly used. Nitroprusside also provides excellent BP control but has not been proven safe during pregnancy. Nitroglycerin causes preload reduction but has little effect on afterload reduction, which is the more important intended mechanism of action for antihypertensive agents during crises. Clonidine and hydrochlorothiazide are oral medications that have a limited role in acute management of BP during hypertensive crises due to unreliable absorption and efficacy.

QUESTIONS

1. A 34-year-old female with a history of seizure disorder presents with a generalized tonic–clonic seizure. She is on phenytoin for her seizures. Her postictal state has elapsed and she is alert and oriented now. Vital signs are 99°F, 85, 155/80, 99% RA. Physical examination is normal. Which of the following is the most likely cause for her seizure?

   A. Alcohol use
   B. Febrile seizure
   C. Medication noncompliance
   D. Central nervous system (CNS) infection
   E. Mass lesion

2. A 26-year-old female presents to the ED with ankle pain. She was playing tag with her kids in the yard when her foot got caught in an open pipe, snapping it outward as she fell to the ground. Her x-ray is shown in Figure 3-1. Which of the following is true?

   A. This is a stable injury.
   B. The deltoid ligament is probably intact.
   C. The syndesmosis is probably intact.
   D. This is a Maisonneuve fracture.
   E. None of the above.

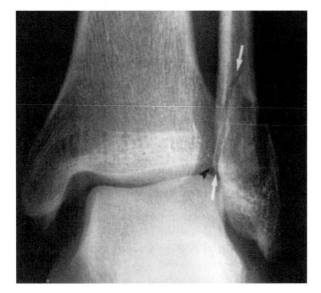

Figure 3-1

3. A 33-year-old male with a history of type I diabetes presents with nausea, vomiting, and altered mental status. His wife states that he did not take his insulin for the past few days. His chemistry panel is below:

   Na: 125
   K: 3.8
   Cl: 90
   HCO$_3$: 10
   BUN: 30
   Cr: 1.4
   Glu: 727

   In addition to insulin and IV fluids, which of the following is the most important step in management?

   A. Sodium bicarbonate
   B. Potassium
   C. Fomepizole
   D. Glucagon
   E. Ceftriaxone plus azithromycin

4. A 66-year-old female who recently completed chemotherapy for colon cancer through a right chest Port-a-Cath presents with a chief complaint of right arm pain, swelling, and weakness. The right hand is warm, and well perfused. The radial pulse is equal to the contralateral side. There is no evidence of cellulitis. An upper extremity deep venous thrombosis (DVT) is suspected. Which of the following is the next best test?

   A. Magnetic resonance angiography (MRA)
   B. Direct venography by interventional radiology
   C. D-dimer
   D. Compression Doppler ultrasound
   E. CT angiography

5. A 48-year-old female presents with chronic intermittent abdominal pain and diarrhea for 1 year. She reports having episodes of moderate abdominal cramping four to five times per week. She has normal vital signs and an unremarkable abdominal examination. The patient has had multiple negative diagnostic studies, including gall bladder ultrasound, CT abdomen/pelvis, MRI abdomen/pelvis, stool studies, and colonoscopy. You suspect irritable

bowel syndrome. Which of the following is the best next step in management until she sees her primary care physician?

A. Ondansetron 4 mg po qd
B. Polyethylene glycol po bid
C. Prednisone 20 mg po qd
D. Ciprofloxacin 500 mg po bid
E. Psyllium fiber therapy

6. A 35-year-old male presents with severe head trauma. Funduscopic examination demonstrates papilledema and increased intracranial pressure (ICP) and impending herniation is suspected. Mannitol is given and a decision is made to hyperventilate the patient as a last-ditch effort while waiting for neurosurgical evaluation. Which of the following is an appropriate target level of PCO_2 for therapeutic hyperventilation?

A. 22 mm Hg
B. 27 mm Hg
C. 32 mm Hg
D. 37 mm Hg
E. 42 mm Hg

7. A previously healthy 5-year-old male presents with painless rectal bleeding. The bleeding seems to have resolved but his mother states that he had four or five large, brick-colored stools earlier in the day. His stool guaiac test is positive. Which of the following is the most likely cause of his symptoms?

A. Duodenal ulcer
B. Meckel diverticulum
C. Esophagitis
D. Anal fissure
E. Inflammatory bowel disease

8. Which of the following is seen in almost all patients with Guillain–Barre syndrome within the first week of illness?

A. Albuminocytologic dissociation
B. Muscle weakness
C. Sensory deficits
D. Areflexia
E. Diarrhea

9. A significantly elevated lactate dehydrogenase level (LDH) in a patient with a left ventricular assistance device (LVAD) likely indicates which of the following?

A. Fluid overload
B. Right heart failure
C. Worsening native cardiac function
D. Opportunistic infection
E. Thrombosis within the pump

10. A 24-year-old male ingests liquid drain cleaner and immediately presents to the ED. Which of the following is the most appropriate treatment?

A. Ingestion of a small cup of water
B. Calcium gluconate
C. Dexamethasone
D. Ampicillin
E. Neutralization therapy with hydrochloric acid

11. Which of the following is the most commonly ingested alcohol after ethanol?

A. Methanol
B. Ethylene glycol
C. Isopropanol
D. Propylene glycol
E. Acetone

12. A 51-year-old female presented for evaluation of left wrist pain after a fall on an outstretched hand. Her x-ray is shown. In the course of her evaluation, it is clear that she has a neurologic deficit due to an injury to a nerve. Which of the following findings is most likely? (Fig. 3-2)

A. Weakness of thumb and index finger flexion
B. Numbness of the dorsum of the hand
C. Weakness of ring and pinky finger extension
D. Weakness of wrist extension
E. Numbness of the volar ring and pinky finger

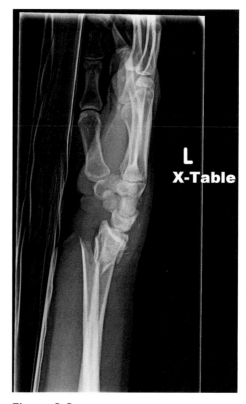

Figure 3-2

13. Which of the following is true regarding brown recluse spiders?

    A. Most bites require no treatment and resolve without complications.
    B. Hemorrhagic lesions require urgent dermatologic consultation for excision.
    C. Dapsone is used to prevent secondary bacterial infection of brown recluse bites.
    D. Topical steroids decrease the severity of the tissue reaction.
    E. Aspirin should be used to decrease platelet aggregation and thrombosis.

14. A 40-year-old male presents with delirium, polyuria, and a serum calcium level of 15 mg/dL. Which of the following is true?

    A. Nifedipine is the agent of choice for initial treatment.
    B. Thiazide diuretics are more helpful than loop diuretics in promoting urine calcium excretion.
    C. Calcitonin can be used as monotherapy in the treatment of hypercalcemia.
    D. Sodium bicarbonate infusion will increase the amount of ionized calcium.
    E. Glucocorticoids may be helpful if the patient has an underlying hematologic malignancy or granulomatous disease.

15. Which of the following tick-borne illnesses characteristically exhibits a centripetal rash?

    A. Lyme disease
    B. Babesiosis
    C. Rocky Mountain spotted fever
    D. Ehrlichiosis
    E. Tularemia

16. Which of the following is classically contraindicated in patients with presumed acute digoxin toxicity?

    A. Transvenous pacing
    B. Electrical cardioversion
    C. Calcium gluconate infusion
    D. Transthoracic pacing
    E. All of the above

17. A 27-year-old male is hammering nails at a construction site without eye protection and feels something strike his right eye. After washing out the eye, he still complains of pain and presents to the ED. Which of the following is the safest and most accurate modality for locating the potential foreign body?

    A. X-ray
    B. Ultrasonography
    C. MRI
    D. CT scan
    E. Nuclear medicine scan

18. Which of the following is true about gastric volvulus?

    A. It is usually associated with a large umbilical hernia.
    B. It most commonly results from twisting about its short axis.
    C. It most commonly occurs in infants younger than 1 year.
    D. In most cases, a nasogastric tube cannot be passed into the stomach.
    E. Gastric infarction and death occur in 80% of patients if not rapidly diagnosed and treated.

19. A 34-year-old male with schizophrenia is brought to the ED by his family because he "keeps ignoring" them. They report that for the last few hours, when they argue with him about taking his risperidone, he stares off into the space and does not acknowledge them in any way. This lasts for a few minutes and gradually improves until the next conversation. They want to speak with the psychiatrist about putting him on a new antipsychotic medication. His vital signs are normal and physical examination is unremarkable except that when you question him about his medication, he becomes visibly angry and his eyes look up to the ceiling. After he calms down in a few minutes, he resumes normal eye contact and conversation. Which of the following is the most appropriate action at this time?

    A. Discharge home with outpatient psychiatry follow-up
    B. Consult psychiatry for alprazolam prescription
    C. Haloperidol 5 mg IM
    D. Lorazepam 2 mg IM
    E. Benztropine 1 mg IM

20. A 42-year-old male presents with a swollen, erythematous, and tender left knee. He is in a long-term monogamous relationship. A concomitant history of recurrent renal stones in this man suggests a diagnosis of:

    A. Reactive arthritis
    B. Systemic lupus erythematosus
    C. Rheumatoid arthritis
    D. Gout
    E. Nongonococcal septic arthritis

21. A 3-week-old term neonate is brought by his parents with a fever of 102.0°F. He appears active and nontoxic, but his right tympanic membrane (TM) is red, and moderately swollen. The rest of the physical examination is completely unremarkable. Which of the following is the most appropriate next step in management?

    A. Discharge home with high-dose amoxicillin and routine follow-up.
    B. Discharge home with high-dose amoxicillin–clavulanic acid and next-day follow-up.
    C. Administer a single dose of IM ceftriaxone and discharge home with next-day follow-up.
    D. Admit for observation with prophylactic antibiotics.
    E. Admit for observation with prophylactic antibiotics and blood, urine, and cerebrospinal fluid (CSF) cultures.

22. Of the following, which is the strongest risk factor for an ectopic pregnancy?

   A. Prior ectopic pregnancy
   B. History of pelvic inflammatory disease (PID)
   C. Current use of an intrauterine device (IUD)
   D. Prior C-section
   E. Oral contraceptives

23. A 34-year-old female who takes phenelzine for depression presents with agitation, severe hypertension, mydriasis, and hyperthermia. Which of the following foods did she most likely eat before presentation?

   A. Oranges
   B. Apples
   C. Graham crackers
   D. Cheese
   E. Ice cream

24. Which of the following most commonly complicates normal labor and delivery?

   A. Face presentation
   B. Breech presentation
   C. Shoulder dystocia
   D. Brow presentation
   E. Abnormal fetal lie

25. Which of the following is the most common cause of death among nursing home residents?

   A. Congestive heart failure
   B. Pneumonia
   C. Urosepsis
   D. Massive stroke
   E. Myocardial infarction

26. Which of the following spinal injuries is most likely to be stable?

   A. Flexion teardrop fracture
   B. Bilateral facet dislocation
   C. Transverse process fracture
   D. Hangman fracture
   E. Jefferson fracture

27. A 27-year-old female, G_2P_1, at 5 weeks by dates, presents with abdominal pain. She has had minor "spotting" but no frank vaginal bleeding, her internal cervical os is closed, and her serum β-hCG is 750 mIU/mL. Which of the following is true?

   A. She should be diagnosed with a threatened abortion and asked to return in 2 days for a repeat quantitative β-hCG level.
   B. She has a missed abortion.
   C. She should receive an ultrasound to assess uterine contents and the adnexa.

   D. She should be diagnosed with an early pregnancy versus an ectopic pregnancy and told to return in 2 days for a repeat quantitative β-hCG level and an ultrasound.
   E. She has an inevitable abortion.

28. A 19-month-old female toddler is brought to the ED by her parents with a limp. She has not been fussy and her parents can't recall when her limp started. Her mother states that she appeared to "walk a little strangely" in the morning for the last week but it "seemed to go away." The limp has since become more persistent, and her parents have noted some swelling in her left knee. She has not had a recent infectious illness, and the patient has no hip pain. Her examination reveals a mildly swollen knee with minimal warmth, no erythema, and good range of motion. X-rays of the knee are normal. Which of the following is true?

   A. Morbidity is primarily related to the development of uveitis.
   B. Fever, rash, and irritability are common in association with the disorder.
   C. Her symptoms are due to toxic synovitis.
   D. She likely has septic arthritis.
   E. Plain films will likely reveal Legg–Calvé–Perthes disease.

29. A 47-year-old female without any past medical history presents with several days of progressively worsening left eye pain, blurry vision, and redness. Visual acuity in the left eye is slightly reduced. The patient notes that exposure of the right eye to light causes increased pain in her left eye. Her left pupil is constricted and minimally reactive to light with perilimbic conjunctival injection. There is no discharge. Which of the following is the most appropriate treatment?

   A. Topical antibiotics
   B. Hypertonic eye drops
   C. IV mannitol
   D. Ocular massage
   E. Topical cycloplegic mydriatics

30. Which of the following patients should be placed in respiratory isolation?

   A. A 72-year-old female nursing home resident being treated for a chronic obstructive pulmonary disease exacerbation.
   B. A 46-year-old male with community-acquired pneumonia.
   C. A 23-year-old male who thinks he was exposed to anthrax.
   D. A 3-month-old female ex-premature infant being admitted with bronchiolitis.
   E. A 28-year-old asymptomatic medical student who recently had a positive pressure differential (PPD) test.

TEST 3

31. A 38-year-old mildly obese primigravida at 34 weeks' gestation presents with a chief complaint of "swollen legs" and abdominal pain. Her blood pressure is 170/100 and she has 3+ protein on urine dipstick. After giving her magnesium for prophylaxis of her seizures and hydralazine for blood pressure control, the nurse tells you that her urine output seems a bit low, and asks you what you want to do about her significant edema. The next best step in management is:

    A. Furosemide 40 mg IV push
    B. Maintenance intravenous fluids
    C. Hydrochlorothiazide 25 mg orally
    D. Mannitol 0.5 mg/kg IV push
    E. 25% albumin given intravenously at 1 g/kg

32. Which of the following is true for patients with suspected globe rupture?

    A. Succinylcholine is the paralytic of choice for rapid-sequence intubation.
    B. Tonometry is indicated to assess for concomitant glaucoma.
    C. Eye shielding should be avoided due to infectious complications.
    D. Intravenous antibiotics should be given.
    E. Tetanus immunization is contraindicated.

33. A 44-year-old previously healthy male presents for evaluation of a headache after falling backward 8 feet from a ladder. The patient's neurologic examination is unrevealing and his Glasgow Coma Scale (GCS) is 15. CT reveals an occipital epidural hemorrhage. Which of the following is true?

    A. The patient should be admitted to an ICU for close monitoring
    B. The patient should undergo an emergent suboccipital craniectomy to evacuate the blood
    C. Hypertonic saline infusions help to reduce the increased intracranial pressure associated with these injuries
    D. The lack of pupillary findings suggests this lesion is probably benign
    E. Most patients suffer cortical blindness as a result of the injury

34. A 45-year-old obese woman presents with right upper quadrant abdominal pain for several weeks. Her pain is worse after she eats. Which of the following clinical features supports the diagnosis of biliary colic?

    A. Worsened pain on eating protein
    B. Colicky spasms of abdominal pain lasting 15 minutes
    C. Radiation of pain to right shoulder
    D. Fever >101.5°F
    E. Antecedent use of nonsteroidal anti-inflammatory drugs (NSAIDs)

35. Which of the following is true regarding the diagnosis of kidney stones?

    A. Normal urinalysis essentially rules out the diagnosis.
    B. KUB radiograph has >90% specificity.
    C. Most kidney stones are radiolucent.
    D. Ultrasonography has >90% sensitivity.
    E. CT scan has roughly 90% sensitivity and specificity.

36. A 28-year-old female presents with a painful left index finger after it was inadvertently caught in a car door. X-rays are negative for a fracture, but there is a 50% subungual hematoma. The volar finger pad and paronychial tissues appear intact. Which of the following is true?

    A. The nail should be removed to find and repair any nailbed laceration.
    B. Trephination should be done to relieve pressure before the nail is removed.
    C. Trephination alone results in similar cosmetic and functional outcomes as nail removal.
    D. 2-Octyl cyanoacrylate glue cannot be used to repair nailbed lacerations.
    E. Prophylactic antibiotics have been shown to decrease complications and improve outcome.

37. In a patient with refractory hypotension after blunt abdominal trauma, the pictured finding on FAST examination, as shown in Figure 3-3:

    A. Is an indication for exploratory laparotomy.
    B. Indicates that at least 2.5 L of blood is present in the peritoneum.
    C. Indicates a liver laceration is present.
    D. Should be followed by a CT scan to elucidate the injury.
    E. Shows all of the above are true.

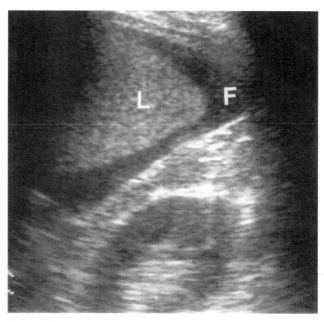

Figure 3-3

38. Diagnosis of which of the following findings is the primary utility of the focused assessment with sonography in trauma (FAST) scan?

    A. Pelvic fracture
    B. Renal injury
    C. Diaphragmatic rupture
    D. Hemoperitoneum
    E. Aortic injury

39. A 32-year-old G_3P_2 at 39 weeks' gestation presented to your community ED after spontaneous rupture of membranes and with regular uterine contractions roughly 3 minutes apart. Although the fetal head delivers without difficulty, the shoulders appear to be trapped and you suspect shoulder dystocia. The next best step in management should be:

    A. Midline episiotomy
    B. McRoberts maneuver
    C. Increased traction
    D. Rubin maneuver
    E. Wood corkscrew maneuver

40. A 23-year-old female presents for right ear pain and drainage after being struck on the side of the head with a basketball. Her distal external auditory canal and tympanic membrane are shown in Figure 3-4. Which of the following is the most appropriate next step in management?

    A. Prednisone 40 mg PO q.d. × 4 days
    B. Doxycycline 100 mg PO b.i.d. × 10 days
    C. Gentamicin 100 mg IV t.i.d. × 7 days
    D. Copious ear irrigation with saline and peroxide
    E. No specific therapy

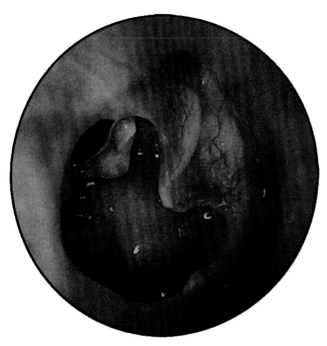

Figure 3-4

41. A 24-year-old female presents with bilateral eye redness and pain on waking. She states that her eyes are extremely watery and irritated but denies purulent discharge. She states her roommate had the same symptoms a few days ago. She does not wear contact lenses. Her visual acuities are normal. Physical examination demonstrates bilateral conjunctival infection without discharge. Slit lamp examination is unremarkable. Which of the following is the most likely etiology?

    A. HSV-1
    B. Varicella zoster virus (VZV)
    C. Adenovirus
    D. *S. pneumoniae*
    E. *Pseudomonas aeruginosa*

42. A 14-year-old male is brought to the ED by his mother concerned about Lyme disease. The patient has a 2-cm circular, erythematous rash on his leg. Which of the following is true?

    A. Serologic testing should only be performed in patients with a rash
    B. The patient should not be treated unless they recall a tick bite
    C. Positive serologic tests indicate active Lyme disease
    D. If the rash is uniformly red without central clearing, Lyme is unlikely
    E. The patient should be given a course of doxycycline

43. Which of the following is a reasonable indication to perform tube thoracostomy in a patient with a parapneumonic pleural effusion?

    A. Pleural fluid:serum LDH ratio <0.6
    B. Serum–pleural fluid albumin gradient >1.1
    C. Pleural fluid pH <7.0
    D. Pleural fluid glucose >100 mg/dL
    E. Fever >101.5°F after first dose of appropriate antibiotics

44. Which of the following is the most common error leading to malpractice claims?

    A. Failure to diagnose
    B. Improper performance of a procedure
    C. Delay in treatment
    D. Delay in diagnosis
    E. Improper medical management

45. A 47-year-old female on rivaroxaban for a DVT is brought to the emergency department with a scalp abrasion after falling on an icy sidewalk. Head CT is negative. Which is the best next step?

    A. Administer oral vitamin K and discharge with close follow-up
    B. Administer a prothrombin complex concentrate and admit for observation
    C. Discharge home with a family member and close follow-up
    D. Admit for observation and repeat CT
    E. Observe in the ED with repeat CT in 6 hours

46. Appropriate initial therapy in an adult patient with epiglottitis includes which of the following?

    A. Nebulized racemic epinephrine, IV levofloxacin
    B. Humidified oxygen, IV ceftriaxone
    C. Nebulized racemic epinephrine, IV dexamethasone, IV ampicillin
    D. Humidified oxygen, IV levofloxacin
    E. IV dexamethasone, IM penicillin G benzathine

47. A 54-year-old female presents with acute onset of dizziness, vertigo, and nausea. You note nystagmus on her examination. Which of the following characteristic of nystagmus is most likely to be associated with a central cause?

    A. Horizontal
    B. Fatigable
    C. Direction-changing
    D. Intensity-changing
    E. All of the above

48. A 22-year-old Latino male who recently emigrated from Mexico presents to the ED with fever, chills, abdominal pain, and intermittent nausea and vomiting. A CT scan of his abdomen is shown in Figure 3-5. Which of the following is true?

    A. This condition requires immediate surgical drainage.
    B. Transmission is typically fecal–oral.
    C. Infections are usually polymicrobial.
    D. Hyperbilirubinemia is the most commonly abnormal laboratory finding.
    E. All of the above.

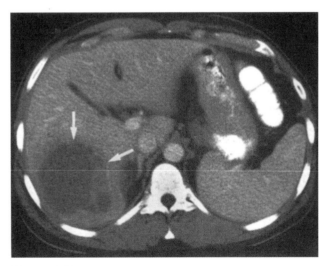

Figure 3-5

49. A 22-year-old male presents to the ED after being struck by lightning. He feels fine now but has a rash on his back in a feather or fern pattern. Which of the following is the best step in management of this complication?

    A. Doxycycline 100 mg PO BID × 10 days
    B. Hydrocortisone 2% ointment × 7 days
    C. Terbinafine 1% cream × 4 weeks
    D. Polymyxin B-neomycin-bacitracin antibiotic ointment
    E. No specific therapy

50. A 56-year-old female with longstanding hypertension, renal failure on dialysis, and a seizure disorder presents to the emergency department after a generalized seizure. Though the patient returned to her neurologic baseline, she has a persistently bleeding tongue wound over the margin of the tongue. Lab tests are significant for moderate anemia with a hemoglobin of 9.1 g/dL, a platelet count of 162,000 per uL, and severe uremia with a BUN of 108 mg/dL. Which of the following is the best approach to this patient's bleeding?

    A. Platelet transfusion
    B. Emergent hemodialysis
    C. IV desmopressin (dDAVP)
    D. Suture repair of the tongue wound
    E. IV estrogen

51. A 22-year-old female presents with a chief complaint of a painful vaginal lump and vulvar pain while walking (Fig. 3-6). She denies any vaginal discharge, fevers, or abdominal pain. Her urine human chronic gonadotropin (β-hCG) is negative. Which of the following is true?

    A. *N. gonorrhoeae* and *Chlamydia trachomatis* cause most infections.
    B. Antibiotics should be given to cover typical polymicrobial vaginal flora.
    C. When not infected, this gland is palpable at the 5 o'clock and 7 o'clock positions around the vaginal introitus.
    D. A Word catheter should be placed after incision and drainage and left in place for 6 to 8 weeks.
    E. If left untreated, ascending cystitis, pyelonephritis, and sepsis occur in 35% of patients.

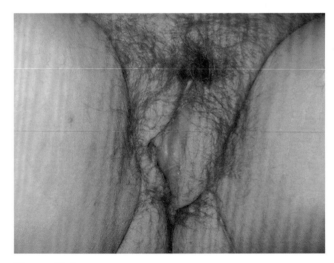

Figure 3-6

52. A 27-year-old female with pneumonia requires tracheal intubation. Which of the following is the best position to maximize the duration of safe apnea during intubation?

    A. Trendelenburg
    B. Reverse Trendelenburg
    C. Sitting up, chin to chest
    D. Supine
    E. Semi-upright, head forward

53. A 47-year-old male with a history of alcoholism presents with a chief complaint of jaundice, right upper quadrant pain, and a low-grade fever. He had his last drink earlier in the day. Which of the following is true?

    A. His AST and ALT levels will be more than 10 times normal.
    B. He should be transferred for immediate liver transplantation.
    C. The patient's fever suggests an infectious cause of his symptoms is most likely.
    D. Reactive leukopenia is the most common cellular laboratory abnormality.
    E. Hepatomegaly is the most common physical examination finding.

54. A 5-year-old male is brought to the ED by his parents for diarrhea. He has had multiple, loose bowel movements mixed with blood for 2 days, associated with shaking chills. The patient has not traveled or been exposed to antibiotics. He appears dehydrated and ill. Which of the following is the most likely cause?

    A. *Clostridium difficile*
    B. *Campylobacter*
    C. Adenovirus
    D. Enterotoxigenic *Escherichia coli* (ETEC)
    E. *Giardia*

55. A 28-year-old female complaining of bilateral left-sided visual field problems most likely has:

    A. Bilateral optic neuritis
    B. A lesion in the right occipital lobe
    C. A pituitary tumor
    D. Multiple sclerosis
    E. A lesion affecting the left optic nerve

56. A 34-year-old female presents with several weeks of bilateral hand numbness and tingling. She notes that it is most prominent in the mornings and improves over the course of the day. You strongly suspect carpal tunnel syndrome. Which of the following is the most sensitive diagnostic test for this diagnosis?

    A. Tinel test
    B. Phalen test
    C. Allen test
    D. Hoffman sign
    E. Eichoff test

57. The treatment of choice for scabies (*Sarcoptes scabiei*) is:

    A. Permethrin 5% cream
    B. Lindane 1% lotion
    C. Malathion 0.5% lotion
    D. Fluconazole 150 mg PO
    E. Ivermectin 200 mg/kg PO

58. A 44-year-old male presents with a 1-week history of painful, swollen, bleeding gums as well as malaise and intermittent fever. He smokes, takes no medicines, and denies weight loss, night sweats, or family history of hematologic malignancy. Examination reveals poor dental hygiene, inflamed gingival tissue, and mild regional lymphadenopathy. Which of the following is true regarding this patient?

    A. Analgesics alone are sufficient for therapy.
    B. Spirochetes and fusobacteria are commonly present in gingival creases.
    C. Follow-up with a dentist is generally not necessary.
    D. Vincent angina, a common complication, involves extension to the buccal mucosa.
    E. The disease is communicable by direct contact with secretions.

59. Patients with thoracic outlet syndrome most commonly present with:

    A. Neurologic symptoms
    B. Ischemic symptoms
    C. Infectious symptoms
    D. Pain
    E. All of the above

60. A 15-year-old male is brought to the ED after being submerged in a lake for "a minute or two." He had been water skiing when he lost control and "wiped out" and then was lying face down in the water without moving. He was not breathing when his friends pulled him out of the water, but he regained spontaneous respirations after they performed cardiopulmonary resuscitation. In the ED, he is awake, but somnolent, breathing spontaneously with a pulse oximetry of 95% on room air and making purposeful movements and following commands. The next most important step in management is:

    A. IV antibiotics
    B. Rapid sequence intubation
    C. IV dexamethasone
    D. Cervical spine imaging
    E. ED thoracotomy

61. A 25-year-old previously healthy black woman presents to the ED complaining of a facial rash over her nose, mild fever, and achy wrists. She just returned from an annual weekend trip to the Florida beaches with a bunch of girlfriends. Which of the following is the most sensitive test to aid in her diagnosis?

    A. Rheumatoid factor (RF)
    B. Anti-Smith antibody (anti-Sm)
    C. Antidouble stranded deoxyribonucleic acid antibody (anti-dsDNA)
    D. Antisingle strand deoxyribonucleic acid antibody (anti-ssDNA)
    E. Antinuclear antibody (ANA)

62. A 44-year-old male presents with acute onset of severe abdominal pain. His abdomen is tender throughout and he exhibits rebound tenderness. His x-ray is shown in Figure 3-7. Which of the following is the next best step in management?

    A. Heparin
    B. Azithromycin
    C. Octreotide
    D. Paracentesis
    E. Surgical consultation

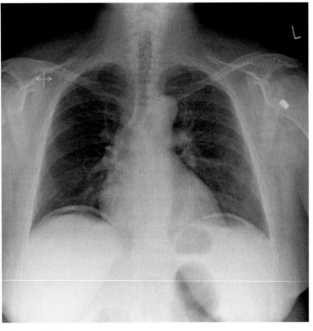

Figure 3-7

63. Which of the following joints is most commonly affected in septic arthritis?

    A. Hip
    B. Knee
    C. Ankle
    D. Wrist
    E. Shoulder

64. A 4-year-old male presents with a 1-day history of generalized abdominal pain and multiple episodes of bloody diarrhea. His mother says he had a hamburger at a local fast-food restaurant 5 days ago but that "they eat there all the time." His symptoms began with watery diarrhea and mild abdominal pain but have progressed to more severe pain with bloody diarrhea. He has no fever. Which of the following statements is true?

    A. TMP-SMX is the treatment of choice
    B. Up to 25% of children may develop hemolytic–uremic syndrome (HUS)
    C. Most affected children have a very high fever
    D. Thrombotic thrombocytopenic purpura (TTP) is the most common systemic complication
    E. The hamburger is likely unrelated to this patient's diarrheal illness as the incubation period is more commonly 12 to 24 hours

65. A 41-year-old male with diabetes and hypertension presents with acute left facial weakness, the inability to close his left eye, and a loudness sensation in his left ear. He has no weakness or numbness in his left arm or leg. His symptoms started yesterday and he is concerned that he has had a stroke. Which of the following is true?

    A. A CT scan of his brain should be performed to rule out the possibility of stroke.
    B. A vesicular rash over the ear indicates a better prognosis.
    C. The patient should be given a prescription for prednisone and acyclovir.
    D. The patient's diabetes and hypertension do not affect the outcome of his illness.
    E. After recovery, he has a 50% chance of having another episode in his lifetime.

66. A 25-year-old male presents with bright red blood after having a bowel movement. He reports some itching and pain in his rectum. Examination reveals a nonthrombosed external hemorrhoid. Which of the following is the most appropriate, long-term management option?

    A. Hydrocodone–acetaminophen
    B. Topical corticosteroids
    C. Warm water, stool softeners, high-fiber diet
    D. Topical nitroglycerin
    E. Topical nifedipine

67. A 54-year-old diabetic woman presents with perineal pain, fever, and lethargy. Her perineal examination is shown in Figure 3-8. Which of the following is the most appropriate next step in management?

    A. Corticosteroids
    B. Oral antibiotics
    C. Intravenous antibiotics
    D. Intravenous antibiotics and surgical debridement
    E. MRI of pelvis

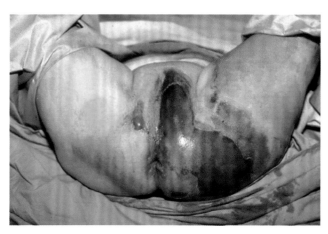

Figure 3-8

68. Which of the following has the highest resistance to electricity?

   A. Nerve
   B. Blood
   C. Muscle
   D. Fat
   E. Mucous membrane

69. A 44-year-old male without past medical history presents with fever and cough. His vital signs are: 100.2, 89, 18, 122/72, 99% RA. His chest x-ray is shown (Fig. 3-9). Which of the following is the most appropriate therapy for this patient?

   A. Supportive care
   B. Oseltamivir
   C. Doxycycline
   D. Piperacillin–tazobactam
   E. Vancomycin and cefepime

70. After toxic acetaminophen ingestion, what is the maximum amount of time after which N-acetylcysteine (NAC) administration still results in 100% prevention of hepatic injury?

   A. 2 hours
   B. 4 hours
   C. 8 hours
   D. 12 hours
   E. 24 hours

71. A 9-year-old male presents with fever, sore throat, and refusal to eat or drink because of severe odynophagia. His oropharyngeal examination is shown in Figure 3-10. Which of the following is the most likely etiology?

   A. Aphthous stomatitis
   B. *Streptococcus pyogenes*
   C. *Corynebacterium diphtheriae*
   D. Coxsackievirus
   E. Herpes simplex virus

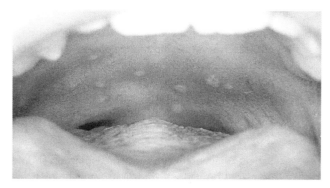

Figure 3-10

72. Which of the following is the most specific EKG finding in acute pericarditis?

   A. Concave ST elevations
   B. Convex ST elevations
   C. PR depressions
   D. Hyperacute T waves
   E. Primary atrioventricular (AV) block

73. Urine containing crystals suggests ingestion of which of the following substances?

   A. Ethylene glycol
   B. Methanol
   C. Isopropanol
   D. Salicylates
   E. Acetaminophen

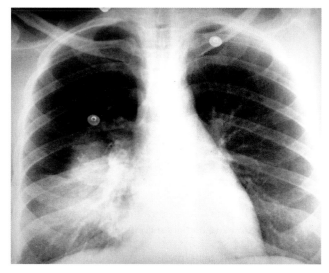

Figure 3-9

74. Which of the following is true regarding adrenal insufficiency?

    A. Patients with secondary adrenal insufficiency frequently have hyperpigmentation.
    B. Hypernatremia is the most common electrolyte abnormality.
    C. Hyperkalemia is a common side effect of prednisone or hydrocortisone therapy.
    D. Nausea and vomiting are present in >50% of patients.
    E. All of the above.

75. Which of the following is the treatment of choice for acute cluster headache?

    A. 100% oxygen
    B. Sumatriptan
    C. Morphine
    D. Lorazepam
    E. Dexamethasone

76. Which of the following is true regarding spontaneous abortion?

    A. Patients diagnosed with threatened abortion should not receive anti-D immunoglobulin (RhoGAM) because the antibody may provoke an immune response to the live fetus.
    B. When a fetal heartbeat is seen on ultrasonograph, patients diagnosed with threatened abortion will experience a spontaneous miscarriage 50% of the time.
    C. Patients diagnosed with threatened abortion should be placed on bedrest restrictions until the bleeding resolves.
    D. All patients who present to the ED with fetal or placental tissue and resolution of vaginal bleeding can be diagnosed with a complete abortion and discharged.
    E. Up to 80% of women with first-trimester spontaneous abortion complete the abortion without intervention.

77. A 52-year-old previously healthy American-born male presents 2 months after having a purified protein derivative (PPD) placed on his left forearm. He had been in Central America approximately 6 months ago with the Peace Corps. He states that the injection site became quite large, red, and firm, but he never followed up with a doctor. He now wants to know what to do. He denies cough, weight loss, drenching night sweats, or fever. His chest x-ray is unrevealing. Which of the following is most likely true?

    A. He has active TB and requires isolation and a multidrug treatment regimen.
    B. He is not infected with TB as he has no symptoms of TB.
    C. He has latent TB infection and he may infect other persons.

    D. He has latent TB infection and requires prolonged treatment with INH and B6.
    E. He must be admitted for acid-fast bacilli sputum cultures to determine if he has been infected with TB.

78. A 64-year-old male presents to the ED with several weeks of heel pain. He used to have pain only with heavy exercise, but gradually it has started limiting walking as well. It even occurs in the morning when he wakes up and walks for the first time. He decided not to inform his primary care doctor about this pain and came to the ED for evaluation. He has mild tenderness to palpation on the proximal plantar heel but an otherwise unremarkable physical examination. Radiographs are normal. Which of the following is the most appropriate next step in management?

    A. Discharge with stirrup ankle brace
    B. Discharge with Achilles tendon stretching exercises
    C. Admit for magnetic resonance imaging (MRI) of his foot
    D. Admit for orthopedic surgery consultation
    E. Admit for vascular surgery consultation

79. A 5-year-old male presents with right hip pain. There is no history of trauma. Which of the following is the most likely cause?

    A. Femoral neck fracture
    B. Osteogenesis imperfecta
    C. Transient synovitis
    D. Slipped capital femoral epiphysis (SCFE)
    E. Legg–Calve–Perthes disease

80. Which of the following are common findings in patients diagnosed with *Pneumocystis carinii* pneumonia (PCP)?

    A. Elevated transaminases (aspartate aminotransferase, alanine transaminase)
    B. Respiratory acidosis due to CO_2 retention
    C. Pleural effusions
    D. Elevated arterial lactate levels
    E. Elevated lactate dehydrogenase (LDH) levels

81. Which of the following deficits below the level of injury is consistent with an anterior cord syndrome?

    A. Loss of total sensation and motor function.
    B. Bladder and bowel incontinence and loss of motor function.
    C. Loss of motor function only.
    D. Loss of vibration and position sensation and motor function.
    E. Loss of pain and temperature sensation and motor function and bladder incontinence.

82. A 38-year-old male presents with right-sided thoracic pain after tripping and falling against a counter. His vital signs are: 98.6, 80, 16, 122/72, and 100% on RA. He has tenderness along the mid axillary line at the level of

the nipple. He has no abdominal pain or tenderness. PA and lateral chest x-rays are negative for pneumothorax or hemothorax. He is very anxious about a rib injury. What is the most important next step in management?

A. Order a full rib x-ray series
B. Order a CT chest without contrast
C. Order a CT chest with contrast
D. Have hospital security escort him outside to compose himself
E. Provide pain control, education, and reassurance

83. Which of the following associations is true?

A. Mallet finger: Disruption of the flexor digitorum profundus (FDP) tendon.
B. Bennett fracture: Extra-articular fracture of the base of the thumb metacarpal.
C. Trigger finger: Volar plate entrapment.
D. Jersey finger: Primary involvement of the ring finger.
E. Gamekeeper thumb: Radial collateral ligament injury.

84. Which of the following is true of domestic violence?

A. Domestic violence often begins or worsens during pregnancy.
B. Most states mandate reporting of domestic violence against competent adult women.
C. Noncompliance is uncommon among abused women.
D. Domestic violence is less common among gay couples.
E. All of the above

85. A 56-year-old male presents with generalized fatigue, weakness, and vomiting. He tells you that he has taken an overdose of his doxepin medication. His BP is 155/95, and his EKG demonstrates a regular, wide-complex tachycardia. Which of the following is the most appropriate next step in management?

A. Cardioversion at 50 J
B. Lidocaine
C. Procainamide
D. Sodium bicarbonate
E. Propafenone

86. A patient presents with findings concerning for endocarditis. Which of the following findings is most sensitive in endocarditis?

A. Signs of embolic stroke
B. Painful subcutaneous nodules on finger pads
C. Heart murmur
D. Splenomegaly
E. Petechiae

87. Which of the following is true regarding diabetic keto-acidosis (DKA) and hyperosmolar hyperglycemic syndrome or state (HHS)?

A. Fluid depletion is larger in DKA.
B. Seizures are the most common fatal manifestation in HHS.
C. All patients with HHS have potassium deficiency.
D. Thromboembolic events are more common in DKA.
E. All of the above.

88. Which of the following is the most common complication of Epstein–Barr virus (EBV) pharyngitis?

A. Asymptomatic elevated transaminases
B. Airway obstruction
C. Splenic rupture
D. Hemolytic anemia
E. Meningoencephalitis

89. A 78-year-old female presents with acute onset of right-sided arm and leg weakness 1 hour prior to arrival. You suspect stroke and immediately order a noncontrast CT brain. The CT of brain is unremarkable. Which of the following is the most appropriate conclusion to draw from this CT result?

A. There is no stroke.
B. There is no ischemic stroke.
C. There is no meningitis.
D. There is no intracranial hemorrhage.
E. There is no cervical artery dissection.

90. A 22-year-old male presents with a swollen area on his scrotum shown in Figure 3-11. The area is firm and non-tender to palpation and does not transilluminate. Which of the following is the most appropriate next step in management?

A. Emergent surgery
B. Azithromycin PO
C. Outpatient urology referral
D. Scrotal elevation
E. Corticosteroids

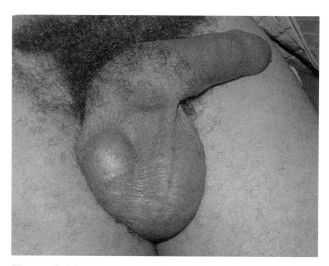

Figure 3-11

91. Which is the most appropriate management for a patient with suspected smallpox lesions?

    A. Acyclovir
    B. Vaccination
    C. Ganciclovir
    D. Rifampin
    E. Isolation

92. A 74-year-old male with a history of hyperlipidemia is brought in by emergency medical services (EMS) with an acute ischemic right hemispheric stroke. Soon after returning from CT, he has a generalized seizure which terminates without treatment after 1 minute. Which of the following is true about this patient?

    A. The patient should have been treated with prophylactic phenytoin as soon as the diagnosis of ischemic stroke was made.
    B. The patient should be given a loading dose of phenytoin after his seizure.
    C. Status epilepticus occurs more commonly in the setting of ischemic strokes than in other stroke syndromes.
    D. Phenytoin is contraindicated in patients with ischemic stroke due to its potential for causing ataxia.
    E. Although isolated seizures are common in patients with ischemic strokes, treatment with antiepileptic drugs is unnecessary because recurrence is uncommon.

93. A 42-year-old male with a history of alcohol abuse presents with acute epigastric abdominal pain. His workup reveals acute pancreatitis and he denies any prior history of pancreatitis. A CT scan that was ordered as part of his workup is shown in Figure 3-12. Which of the following is true?

    A. The CT is indicative of chronic pancreatitis.
    B. An urgent surgical consult is required for drainage.
    C. The patient should be given broad-spectrum antibiotic therapy.

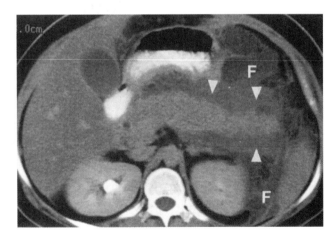

Figure 3-12

D. This finding increases his mortality 10-fold.
E. This finding is common and normally resolves without intervention.

94. A pregnant patient is receiving a magnesium infusion for pre-eclampsia. Which of the following findings is the earliest indicator of significant toxicity?

    A. Diaphoresis
    B. Loss of deep tendon reflexes
    C. Slowed respiratory rate
    D. Sinus tachycardia
    E. Visual floaters

95. Which of the following is true regarding retropharyngeal abscesses (RPAs)?

    A. RPAs are usually preceded by foreign body aspiration in children.
    B. Patients with RPAs generally prefer to lie supine.
    C. Prevertebral soft tissue swelling in excess of 22 mm at the level of C2 is diagnostic for RPA in children and adults.
    D. *Mycobacterium* spp. are the most common cause of RPAs.
    E. Atlantoaxial separation is the most common fatal complication of RPAs.

96. A 32-year-old female presents with recurrent episodes of headaches, palpitations, and profuse diaphoresis. Her primary care doctor diagnosed her with an anxiety disorder after her thyroid function "came back normal" but various selective serotonin reuptake inhibitors have been ineffective. In the ED, her vital signs include a temperature of 99.0°F, a pulse of 90, and a blood pressure of 175/100. Which of the following is the best agent to treat her hypertension?

    A. Metoprolol
    B. Hydrochlorothiazide
    C. Phenoxybenzamine
    D. Nifedipine
    E. Enalapril

97. A 53-year-old female with a high-grade non-Hodgkin lymphoma develops tumor lysis syndrome (TLS) after undergoing induction chemotherapy. Which of the following substances will have a *lower* concentration than normal upon laboratory testing?

    A. Calcium
    B. Uric acid
    C. Phosphate
    D. Iron
    E. Lactate dehydrogenase

98. A 25-year-old male is punched in the face at a bar and presents to you with dental pain. On examination, his right lower first premolar has a fracture exposing a yellowish surface. No blood is seen on the tooth. Which of the following is the correct type of fracture and what is the proper management?

    A. Ellis I; follow-up in dental clinic in 1 week
    B. Ellis I; follow-up in dental clinic next day
    C. Ellis II; follow-up in dental clinic in 1 week
    D. Ellis II; follow-up in dental clinic next day
    E. Ellis III; immediate dental consultation

99. Erosion into the carotid artery is most commonly a complication of which of the following?

    A. Ludwig angina
    B. Parapharyngeal abscesses
    C. Peritonsillar abscesses
    D. Retropharyngeal abscesses
    E. Epiglottitis

100. Which of the following is true regarding malaria?

    A. The causative organism is a parasite.
    B. The vector is the male *Anopheles* mosquito.
    C. Human-to-human transmission may occur through saliva.
    D. *Vivax* malaria is the most severe variety.
    E. Blackwater fever is usually caused by *ovale* malaria.

ANSWERS AND EXPLANATIONS

1. **Answer C.** The number one cause of seizures in patients with a history of seizure disorder is medication noncompliance. Other important causes include alcohol use, alcohol withdrawal, and sleep deprivation. Febrile seizures are extremely rare in adults. Central nervous system infection would be unlikely in a patient without fever, abnormal physical examination, or suggestive historical findings. Mass lesion is often diagnosed during first-time seizures, but patients with a history of a seizure disorder often already have had adequate neuroimaging to evaluate this.

2. **Answer E.** This woman has an oblique fracture of the distal fibula at the level of the mortise as well as rupture of the deltoid ligament. It is clear that the deltoid ligament is disrupted because of the widened medial joint space on the mortise view. Such an injury would be classified as a Weber class B (supination external rotation) fracture. It is the most common fibular fracture and results in an oblique injury at the tibio-fibular syndesmosis which is usually disrupted. On the lateral view, a "spike" seen on the posterior apex of the distal fragment is diagnostic. Since this patient has widening of the deltoid ligament, her injury is unstable and requires operative repair. The Maisonneuve fracture is also an eversion injury resulting in a medial malleolar fracture or rupture of the deltoid ligament in concert with an oblique fracture of the proximal fibula. Any patient with a medial malleolar fracture or deltoid ligament rupture (medial joint space widening) as well as lateral displacement of the fibula without a fracture of the distal fibula should be suspected of having a Maisonneuve fracture and the examination should include palpation of the proximal fibula. (Figure reprinted with permission from Harris JH. *The Radiology of Emergency Medicine.* 4th ed. Lippincott Williams & Wilkins; 1999:856.)

3. **Answer B.** The patient has an anion-gap acidosis (125 − 90 − 10 = 25) in the presence of elevated blood sugar, which is DKA until proven otherwise. The most common cause of DKA is medication noncompliance, followed by infection, myocardial ischemia, and other body stressors. Treatment with insulin and IV fluids should be supplemented with aggressive potassium management. The presence of significant acidosis causes the body to shunt hydrogen ion into cells and exchange them for potassium ions, which are moved into the bloodstream. This results in a false elevation of potassium levels. When insulin is given, this level can drop precipitously as the acidosis is corrected, allowing potassium to move back out of the blood stream and into cells. In DKA,

potassium levels above normal should be left alone (unless there are significant EKG signs of hyperkalemia). Potassium levels in the normal range should be gently supplemented, and potassium levels below normal should be aggressively supplemented. Bicarbonate is not routinely indicated in most cases of anion-gap acidosis and likely has no positive effect on outcomes. Fomepizole is an alcohol dehydrogenase inhibitor used to prevent formation of metabolites in toxic alcohol ingestion. Glucagon has opposite effects to insulin and would likely exacerbate the problem of severe insulin deficiency seen in this DKA example. Although infection is a common trigger of DKA, and aggressive efforts to seek a source should be pursued, empiric antibiotics are not indicated, especially in the setting of known decreased insulin compliance.

4. **Answer D.** Doppler ultrasonography is the standard test for evaluating the presence of both lower and upper extremity DVT. While MRA has excellent specificity, it is only 80% sensitive for the diagnosis of upper extremity DVT. CT angiography has not been evaluated extensively, and its test characteristics are not yet known. Direct venography is a highly accurate method of diagnosing upper extremity DVT, but it is invasive and time consuming, so it should only be used in cases in which ultrasound is nondiagnostic though suspicion remains high. Finally, while negative D-dimers can be used in low-risk patients to exclude the presence of a lower extremity DVT, no validated criteria exist for proper risk stratification among patients with a possible upper extremity DVT. Therefore, the D-dimer cannot be used to exclude upper extremity DVT.

5. **Answer A.** The diagnosis of irritable bowel syndrome (IBS) is made when patients have at least 3 days of abdominal pain per month over 3 months along with changes in stool frequency and appearance. The patient likely has diarrhea-type IBS (IBS-D), as opposed to constipation-type (IBS-C) or mixed-type (IBS-M). Ondansetron, a serotonin-3 receptor blocker that reduces intestinal fluid secretion, is a reasonable starting treatment for IBS-D. Polyethylene glycol and psyllium fiber therapies are reasonable treatments for IBS-C, but may worsen IBS-D, as they promote stool production. Most patients with IBS do not have a significant inflammatory or acute infectious component, so prednisone and ciprofloxacin are not indicated.

6. **Answer C.** In the past, patients with signs of intracranial hypertension after head trauma were hyperventilated to PCO_2 <25 mm Hg in order to cause reflex

cerebral vasoconstriction and reduced cerebral blood volume. However, more recent research suggests that reducing the PCO_2 levels to below 30 mm Hg may cause cerebral hypoxia in many areas of the brain, potentially worsening the chances for neurologic recovery. The appropriate PCO_2 range for hyperventilation appears to be between 30 and 35 mm Hg—this will result in modest cerebral vasoconstriction without hypoxia. An arterial catheter is useful for measuring rapid, serial blood gases to maintain the PCO_2 in this range.

7. **Answer B.** Meckel diverticulum is the most common cause of substantial GI bleeding in children. The diverticulum is a remnant of the omphalomesenteric (or vitelline duct), which is frequently lined with gastric mucosa or other heterotopic tissues. It follows the "rule of 2s." It is present in 2% of the population, and only 2% of patients will ever develop symptoms or complications. It contains two types of tissue (it includes gastric tissue which produces acid occasionally causing bleeding ulcers). It is located within 2 feet proximal to the ileocecal valve, is 2 cm long and 2 cm wide. Half of all patients develop symptoms by the age of 2. Bleeding is usually painless and often resolves spontaneously due to splanchnic vasoconstriction. Meckel scan which is performed with technetium Tc 99 m pertechnetate is the diagnostic test of choice.

8. **Answer B.** Patients with Guillain–Barre syndrome (GBS) almost always have muscle weakness that begins early in the course of illness (within the first week). Usually, this is extremity muscle weakness but the Miller Fisher variant of GBS has oculomotor weakness. Hyporeflexia is also commonly seen early, but true areflexia is not as common. Sensory deficits are also often seen, but several variants of GBS lack sensory findings completely (i.e., acute motor axonal neuropathy, Miller Fisher). Diarrhea as part of antecedent *Campylobacter* infection may be reported before neurologic symptoms occur, but this is seen in less than half of cases.

9. **Answer E.** Pump thrombosis is one of the most common, serious complications of left ventricular assist devices (LVADs). All patients with LVADs are anticoagulated to reduce this risk. Thrombosis within the pump leads to hemolysis which releases lactate dehydrogenase (LDH), a common intracellular enzyme. LDH levels >1,000 are strongly suggestive of pump thrombosis. In addition, patients with pump thrombosis may have a seemingly paradoxically increased palpable pulse on examination as blood is no longer routed through the pump, as well as symptoms and findings of worsening heart failure. Right ventricular heart failure is a possible complication of LVAD most often because of the increased workload placed on the right ventricle as the LVAD increases overall cardiac output. However, LVAD patients are also susceptible to malignant dysrhythmias like ventricular tachycardia and ventricular fibrillation as well as pulmonary embolism which can also present with right ventricular failure. Since circulation in patients with LVADs is dependent on a mechanical device, these patients may not be aware when they experience a malignant rhythm such as ventricular fibrillation or ventricular tachycardia.

10. **Answer A.** Liquid drain cleaner usually contains a strong base, such as sodium or potassium hydroxide. The treatment of caustic ingestions is generally supportive and involves diagnosis of severe esophageal burns with endoscopy. Small amounts of water or milk may be taken immediately after the ingestion to wash away the excess caustic material. Large amounts of fluids should never be taken, as this may precipitate vomiting, which will dramatically worsen esophageal injury. Calcium gluconate is indicated in patients with hydrofluoric acid exposure to replete the calcium, which is bound by the extremely electronegative fluoride ion. Steroids have not been proved to be beneficial in patients with most caustic injuries, although it may offer some benefit in patients with moderate esophageal injuries. Antibiotics should not be given unless that patient has received steroids or unless there are clear signs of perforation. Neutralization therapy with acid or base should never be pursued, as this will lead to further injury.

11. **Answer C.** Isopropanol is the second most commonly ingested alcohol after ethanol. Choices A, B, and D are less commonly ingested. Choice E, acetone, is not an alcohol because it lacks a hydroxyl group.

12. **Answer A.** This patient has an angulated, displaced, comminuted distal radius fracture. These injuries are associated with median nerve injuries, the most important of which is muscle weakness in the thumb and index finger. While sensory abnormalities may be present, they are usually due to a nerve compression and resolve uneventfully. Answers B, C, and D all result from a radial nerve injury while answer E results from an ulnar nerve injury. Neither of these nerves is commonly injured in patients with a distal radius fracture.

13. **Answer A.** As with other spider or insect bites, a diagnosis of a brown recluse spider bite cannot be reliably made without the spider. Furthermore, there remains no evidence for any of the variety of therapies for brown recluse spider bites, including early surgical excision, dapsone, electric shock, steroids, hyperbaric oxygen, colchicine, antihistamines, anticoagulants, or prophylactic antibiotics. Despite this, many of these therapies are still used. Dapsone, in particular, has been advocated as a means of limiting the toxic effects of the venom. It is not used as an antibiotic. Most bites result in burning

pain, mild erythema, pruritus, and minimal swelling. Occasionally, hemorrhagic vesicles develop along with central necrosis in the days following the bite. Even in the case of these more severe bites, supportive therapy is all that is required.

14. **Answer E.** This patient has hypercalcemic crisis (generally defined as any patient with a serum calcium >14 mg/dL), which is typically characterized by altered mental status, polyuria, and dehydration. The initial goals are to restore intravascular volume with intravenous saline and to rapidly lower the serum calcium level by enhancing urinary excretion and reducing bone resorption (primarily through osteoclast inhibitors such as pamidronate or other bisphosphonates). Calcium channel blockers (CCBs) such as nifedipine, play no role in the treatment of hypercalcemia. Loop diuretics are the most effective drugs in enhancing urinary calcium elimination. In contrast, thiazides increase calcium reabsorption in the distal tubule resulting in a further increase in serum calcium levels. Calcitonin is the fastest acting, but weakest agent in reducing serum calcium and cannot be used for monotherapy. Bicarbonate is not useful in hypercalcemia. However, in the setting of a true alkalosis, more free calcium will be bound to albumin, thereby decreasing the amount of free ionized calcium. Glucocorticoids are useful in patients with hypercalcemia caused by an underlying hematologic malignancy or granulomatous disease due to their effects on vitamin D metabolism and cytokine release. Glucocorticoids do not exert their effect for 1 to 2 days after initiation of treatment.

15. **Answer C.** Rocky Mountain spotted fever (RMSF), caused by *Rickettsia rickettsii* transmitted by the *Dermacentor* tick, causes a centripetal rash, spreading from the wrists and ankles toward the trunk. Despite its name, cases are seen most commonly in the southeastern states, but nearly all states have reported cases. The characteristic symptoms are fever, constitutional symptoms, abdominal pain, along with the centripetal rash. Antibiotic therapy (specifically with doxycycline) has steadily improved the mortality to about 1%. Doxycycline can even be given to children for optimal treatment of RMSF, as no other antibiotic improves outcomes as well. The other tick-borne diseases mentioned are rarely associated with a centripetal rash. Syphilis, dengue, Kaposi sarcoma, and coxsackievirus can also cause centripetal rashes.

16. **Answer E.** There are several "classic" contraindications in the setting of digoxin toxicity. The most commonly cited is to avoid using calcium to treat hyperkalemia that frequently accompanies digoxin toxicity (since digoxin inhibits the Na^+/K^+ ATPase). Interestingly, while hyperkalemia is a reliable marker of digoxin toxicity, hyperkalemia is not the cause of death in severely poisoned

patients (death is caused by fatal arrhythmias induced by digoxin's direct effects on cardiac automaticity and excessive vagal tone) and treatment of hyperkalemia has not been shown to decrease the risk of death. While there is almost no evidence to support the idea that "stone heart" (tetany of the myocardium) will result from calcium administration in the setting of hyperkalemia-associated digoxin toxicity, elevated levels of *intracellular* calcium are already present, and hyperkalemia is not the chief problem (but rather reflects the degree of toxicity). Therefore, intravenous calcium should not be used to treat hyperkalemia in digoxin toxicity. In addition, patients with digoxin toxicity have an exceptionally excitable myocardium, so transvenous and transthoracic pacing as well as electrical cardioversion are all classically contraindicated. Atropine can be used as a temporizing measure in patients with severe bradycardia, but Fab fragments should be given as soon as possible after the diagnosis of a digoxin-associated arrhythmia is made. While there remains scant evidence, there is a theoretical increased risk of developing more malignant arrhythmias in response to pacing and cardioversion (e.g., ventricular fibrillation and pulseless ventricular tachycardia).

17. **Answer D.** MRI is the most sensitive test to detect ocular foreign body, but should never be used when a metallic ocular foreign body is suspected. Plain radiographs are useful but are not as sensitive as CT scan. Ultrasonography is highly operator dependent. Nuclear medicine scans have no role in ocular foreign body detection.

18. **Answer D.** Gastric volvulus is a rare disorder that chiefly occurs in older people and results from twisting of the stomach about its long axis (organoaxial volvulus). Twenty percent of cases occur in infants younger than 1 year due to congenital diaphragmatic defects. In older people, it is frequently associated with large paraesophageal hiatal hernias. The classic triad is known as *Borchardt triad*, and consists of severe epigastric pain and abdominal distension, vomiting, and the inability to pass a nasogastric tube. If the diagnosis is suspected, the ED physicians should attempt to pass a nasogastric tube because this occasionally reduces the volvulus. Due to its redundant blood supply, gastric infarction is uncommon, even in delayed cases, occurring in as many as 25% of cases.

19. **Answer E.** The patient appears to have evidence of a specific dystonic reaction known as the *oculogyric crisis*, where both the patient's eyes stare upward and do not come back to the neutral position. Symptoms can fluctuate based on emotional state. Dystonic reactions are usually due to an excess of cholinergic activity due to overblockade of dopaminergic receptors by antipsychotic medications. The normally inhibitory effect of

dopamine on the cholinergic neurons is reduced with the use of antipsychotic agents. Treatment for acute dystonic reactions is with an anticholinergic agent, either benztropine or diphenhydramine. Discharging the patient home neither treats the patient nor adequately manages the social situation. Psychiatric consultation for a new psychotropic medication prescription is not appropriate until the primary cause of the complaint has been evaluated and addressed. Haloperidol would further worsen the oculogyric crisis. Lorazepam might sedate the patient but would probably not improve the dystonia.

20. **Answer D.** Ten percent to 25% of patients with gout have renal stones, and the rate correlates with the degree of hyperuricemia. For example, >50% of patients with a serum uric acid level >13 mg/dL have stones. Reactive arthritis is the name, which is now given to arthritis, urethritis, and conjunctivitis that occurs after an infection (thus, "reactive") and which was formerly called Reiter syndrome.

21. **Answer E.** The approach to the neonate with fever is constantly evolving. However, all neonates less than 28 days old still require a full "septic workup" with blood, urine, and CSF cultures, as well as prophylactic antibiotics and admission for observation. In this age-group, serious bacterial infection is common and often completely undetectable by physical examination or routine blood tests. Current guidelines enable the emergency physician (EP) to use considerable discretion in the evaluation of older (>28 days) febrile neonates. It is extremely important to obtain a thorough vaccination status of young infants, since the standard vaccine schedule aggressively immunizes infants in the first year of life. Although there is no perfect algorithm for evaluating older neonates, clinicians can use a CBC to help stratify well-appearing infants >28 days old into high- and low-risk categories for further evaluation. In addition, urinary tract infections are a common cause of occult fever among female infants as well as uncircumcised male infants. Catheterized urinalysis and culture should be sought in all febrile female infants <24 months as well as in all uncircumcised, febrile male infants <12 months in whom there is no alternative source of infection. The potential presence of otitis media should never result in outpatient management of the febrile neonate. Antibiotic administration without appropriate culture and laboratory analysis results in the inability to diagnose serious bacterial infection.

22. **Answer A.** History of prior ectopic pregnancy is the *strongest* risk factor for current ectopic pregnancy. The *most common* risk factor is PID. The sequelae of PID account for approximately half of all cases of ectopic pregnancy. Although IUD use increases the relative risk of ectopic versus intrauterine pregnancy, it decreases the *overall* risk of all pregnancy significantly. C-section increases the risk of placenta previa, but not of ectopic pregnancy. Oral contraceptive use may reduce the symptoms of PID (thus predisposing to more untreated PID), but overall pregnancy rate (including ectopic) is reduced.

23. **Answer D.** The patient has the characteristic "wine-and-cheese" reaction due to ingestion of a tyramine-containing food with pharmacologic MAOI activity. Tyramine is normally converted to endogenous stimulatory amines, and monoamine oxidase (MAO) functions to break these down. Use of monoamine oxidase inhibitors (MAOIs) inhibits this degradation function and excess dietary tyramine in this setting causes a disorder similar to serotonin syndrome or a sympathomimetic crisis. Tyramine is present in high quantities in cheese, alcohol, dried meats and fruits, and soy.

24. **Answer B.** Breech presentation occurs in approximately 4% of births or roughly 1 per 25 live births. Shoulder dystocia and abnormal fetal lie each occurs in roughly 1 per 300 live births. Face presentation occurs when the fetus is in longitudinal lie and there is full extension of the fetal head, with the occiput against the upper back. It is associated with an increased risk of perinatal mortality (2% to 3%) and fetal anomalies (e.g., anencephaly) and it occurs in roughly 1 per 550 live births. Brow presentation occurs when the fetal head is inadequately flexed in a longitudinal lie, taking an intermediate position between flexion and extension. Further extension results in face presentation. Brow presentation is also associated with an increased perinatal mortality rate of 1% to 8% and occurs in approximately 1 per 1,400 live births.

25. **Answer B.** Pneumonia is the most common cause of death among residents of long-term care facilities. It is also the most common reason for transfer to such a facility. As with many other diseases, the clinical presentation of pneumonia in the elderly may be very vague or atypical. Frequently, elderly patients may lack fever, cough, chest pain, headache, and myalgias. They may also not be strong enough or oriented enough to vocalize complaints about dyspnea. Studies have revealed that in general, elderly persons manifest fewer overall symptoms than do their younger cohort in the setting of pneumonia. *S. pneumoniae* remains the most common pathogen in both community-acquired pneumonia (CAP) and in pneumonia acquired in a nursing home setting. Although the etiology of nursing home-acquired pneumonia is often undetermined, the microbiology more closely resembles CAP than nosocomial pneumonia. Interestingly, the risk of *invasive* pneumococcal disease is fourfold higher in the nursing home population than in elderly persons living in the community.

Although its efficacy has not been 100% validated, most authors agree that all patients of long-term care facilities should be vaccinated against both influenza and *Streptococcus pneumoniae*.

26. **Answer C.** Spinal injuries are classified by the mechanism of injury and mechanical stability in reference to their potential to cause neurologic damage. Unstable injuries are considered likely to cause spinal cord damage and usually require surgical stabilization. Stable spinal injuries are more common than unstable ones and are easier to remember because there are only a few types—wedge fracture, spinous and transverse process fractures, unilateral facet dislocation, and vertebral burst fracture (with the exception of a Jefferson fracture, which is a burst fracture of C1). All other spinal injuries are considered potentially or definitely unstable. A flexion teardrop fracture occurs when the anterior portion of the vertebral body shears off from a flexion force, causing ligamentous disruption. Bilateral facet dislocation is an extremely unstable injury resulting from significant flexion, causing the superior facets of the inferior vertebra to lose their articulation with the inferior facets of the vertebra immediately superior to it. Spinal cord injury is common due to the significant displacement of the vertebrae. Solitary transverse process fracture is usually of no clinical significance as it is far removed from the articular surfaces of the vertebrae and spinal cord. A Hangman fracture occurs from extreme extensor forces, causing bilateral fractures of the pedicles of C2 and dislocation of C2 from C1. Unlike the past where hanging gave this fracture its name, the common mechanism now is motor vehicle collision. The Jefferson fracture results from vertical compression forces causing the anterior and posterior portions of the ring of C1 to break and putting the spinal cord at extreme risk for severe injury.

27. **Answer C.** Although this patient may have an early normal pregnancy and a threatened abortion, she is at risk for an ectopic pregnancy. Because the patient's serum β-hCG level is below the discriminatory threshold (the level at which a normal pregnancy can be detected by ultrasonography), the main reason for obtaining an ultrasonograph is to search for an ectopic pregnancy. Approximately 50% of women with an ectopic pregnancy have a β-hCG level <3,000 mIU/mL and symptomatic patients with a β-hCG level <1,000 mIU/mL are four times more likely to have an ectopic pregnancy than those patients with higher β-hCG levels. If the ultrasonograph is nondiagnostic and the patient is otherwise stable, she can be discharged with instructions to follow-up with her OB in 2 days for a serial β-hCG level. In that case, her diagnosis remains unclear, so she could be given a diagnosis of "possible ectopic pregnancy versus threatened abortion." Once her β-hCG level has risen

beyond the discriminatory zone, her ultrasonogram should be repeated to evaluate for the presence of a normal pregnancy.

28. **Answer A.** This patient's presentation is most consistent with pauciarticular (also called oligoarticular) juvenile arthritis, which is the most common type of juvenile arthritis. When systemic symptoms are present in the setting of arthritis, patients are diagnosed with systemic onset juvenile arthritis (previously known as Still disease). Pauciarticular juvenile arthritis affects females more than males, typically begins in the second year of life, and is rare in children older than 10. The hip joint is almost never affected, but the other large joints, such as the knees, ankles, elbows, and wrists, are commonly affected. This patient's presentation of a painless morning limp that improves throughout the day is common. The course of the illness is frequently benign, as 50% of patients will experience complete resolution within 6 months. The disease is most often nonsteroidal anti-inflammatory drug-responsive and rarely requires more powerful therapies. The development of uveitis is the only extra-articular complication common to the disease. Permanent injury typically precedes symptom onset with respect to uveitis, so referral to an ophthalmologist is critical. Toxic synovitis is an aseptic inflammatory disorder of the hip, which is typically postinfectious. Patients with septic arthritis have erythema, pain, and limited range of motion on examination. Legg–Calvé–Perthes disease is idiopathic avascular necrosis of the hip.

29. **Answer E.** The patient has iritis, which is treated primarily with topical steroids and mydriatics. Ophthalmologic consultation is generally pursued before the initiation of steroids. The history of consensual photophobia and physical examination demonstrating perilimbic conjunctival injection (ciliary flush) is characteristic. Topical antibiotics are used to prevent bacterial superinfection in corneal abrasions or viral conjunctivitis. Hypertonic eye drops are used for corneal hydrops (extreme corneal edema). Mannitol therapy for lowering intraocular pressure is indicated for patients with glaucoma. Ocular massage is indicated for patients with central retinal artery occlusion to try to dislodge embolus or thrombus and cause it to migrate to a more distal site in the circulation.

30. **Answer D.** Respiratory syncytial virus (RSV) is the most common cause of bronchiolitis, followed by parainfluenza, influenza, adenovirus, and rhinovirus. To avoid infecting other uninfected patients and health care workers (who then transmit infections to yet more patients), patients with RSV bronchiolitis should be placed in respiratory isolation on droplet precautions. If multiple patients with RSV bronchiolitis are admitted,

then the group could be isolated as a cohort until discharge. Bacillus anthracis is not transmitted from person to person. Patients with COPD exacerbations and CAP also do not require isolation. Finally, the medical student with a PPD but no symptoms of active TB has latent TB infection and is not contagious to other people.

31. **Answer B.** Pre-eclampsia is associated with vasospasm, reduced renal blood flow and glomerular filtration rate, and increased total body water resulting in edema. However, hypovolemia results in decreased uteroplacental blood flow and possible fetal injury. Diuretics and hyperosmotic agents should, therefore, never be used in the setting of pre-eclampsia. Although volume expanders such as albumin may sound like a good idea, they do not reverse vasospasm or improve uteroplacental blood flow. Instead, maintenance fluids should be given although recommendations between authors vary. Due to the risk of pulmonary edema and the inability of intravenous fluids to reverse vasospasm, however, aggressive large fluid boluses should also be avoided. One author recommends 5% dextrose in lactated Ringers solution with close monitoring of urine output, which is maintained at approximately 30 mL/hour. Excessive urine output may indicate fluid overload, placing patients at risk for pulmonary edema.

32. **Answer D.** Globe rupture is a true ophthalmologic emergency, usually requiring operative care. Antibiotics and tetanus boosters should be given to all patients with suspected globe rupture to prevent infectious complications. Succinylcholine without pretreatment with nondepolarizing paralytics can increase intraocular pressure. Tonometry is contraindicated as this will also increase intraocular pressure. Eye shielding is mandatory to prevent further damage to the injured eye and to restrict eye movement.

33. **Answer A.** Traumatic epidural hemorrhage in the posterior fossa is less common than other locations. However, even patients who are initially well appearing with a normal examination can rapidly deteriorate due to sudden brainstem compression. Thus, such patients are best observed in a highly monitored setting such as an ICU. Suboccipital craniectomy is the appropriate procedure to evacuate occipital epidural hematomas but the procedure isn't usually necessary in patients without neurologic complaints or findings. Hypertonic saline is not an accepted adjunct to treatment of these patients. While visual field cuts may occur after an occipital lobe injury, complete cortical blindness is uncommon because it requires an injury affecting the bilateral occipital lobes.

34. **Answer C.** Biliary colic, also known as symptomatic cholelithiasis, refers to upper abdominal pain caused by gallstones. The name "colic" is actually a misnomer—

biliary colic usually causes constant, steady pain occurring from 2 to 6 hours, often starting 1 to 2 hours after eating. "Colicky," spasmodic pain is rare. Radiation of pain to the right scapula or shoulder increases the likelihood of biliary disease but is not at all sensitive. Biliary colic is no worse on eating protein, but may be worse after eating fatty foods. Fever is more characteristic of acute cholecystitis or other intra-abdominal inflammation rather than simple biliary colic. Antecedent use of NSAIDs supports a diagnosis of gastritis, peptic ulcer disease, or viscous perforation rather than biliary colic. Gallstone formation *is*, however, increased by fibrates, octreotide, oral contraceptive agents, and total parenteral nutrition.

35. **Answer E.** CT has become the test of choice for diagnosis of kidney stones, replacing the intravenous pyelogram in this regard. It has excellent sensitivity and specificity and is helpful in evaluating other conditions in the differential diagnosis of flank pain. Twenty percent of kidney stones have normal urinalyses, without microscopic hematuria, so a normal urinalysis in highly suspicious cases by no means rules out the diagnosis of kidney stone. Radiographs have <75% specificity for the diagnosis, and false positives from phleboliths, calcified lymph nodes, and bone shadowing are common. Most kidney stones are radiopaque—uric acid stones, representing approximately 10% of all stones, are radiolucent. Ultrasonography, although possessing good sensitivity and excellent specificity for hydronephrosis, has relatively poor sensitivity for ruling out the diagnosis of kidney stone.

36. **Answer C.** Historically, nail removal with subsequent primary repair of any nailbed laceration was the standard approach to patients with subungual hematomas. However, patients with intact nail folds and an intact volar pad do not require nail removal. In such patients, trephination alone results in identical cosmetic and functional outcomes. Studies to date suggest that the outcome is the same regardless of the size of the hematoma, which has sometimes been used to determine which patients require nail removal. Leaving the nail in place provides a splinting effect that likely maintains apposition of the underlying nailbed while small lacerations heal. Patients with a clear nail deformity, or a laceration of the nail should have the nail removed to explore the nailbed. If a laceration is present, 6-0 absorbable sutures or 2-octyl cyanoacrylate glue can be used to achieve closure. Patients with simple subungual hematomas do not require prophylactic antibiotic treatment. Distal phalanx fractures associated with subungual hematomas are considered "open" fractures. However, even among such patients, antibiotic prophylaxis has not improved outcome or decreased the infection rate in otherwise healthy patients. Admittedly, usage of the language

"open fracture" will continue to encourage antibiotic use in the setting of a distal phalanx fracture, regardless of whether this practice improves outcomes.

37. **Answer A.** The image demonstrates hemoperitoneum with blood in Morison pouch (right upper quadrant). In an unstable patient, this is an indication for immediate laparotomy. In unmistakably stable patients, a CT scan of the abdomen should be performed to better delineate the injury and the potential need for surgery. The sensitivity of FAST for the detection of 100 to 500 mL of blood is as high as 95%. Therefore, while at least 500 mL of blood is present, it is not possible to state unequivocally that 2.5 L is present. Furthermore, 2.5 L of blood loss would place the average adult male in class IV hemorrhagic shock which typically presents with a systolic blood pressure <70 mm Hg and a heart rate >140. After confirming the presence of hemoperitoneum by ultrasonography, CT scanning should only be performed in undoubtedly stable patients if a clear reason for laparotomy does not already exist. (Figure reprinted with permission from Harris JH. *The Radiology of Emergency Medicine.* 4th ed. Lippincott Williams & Wilkins; 1999:694.)

38. **Answer D.** The FAST scan consists of a series of ultrasonographic images designed to assess for the presence of hemoperitoneum. Ultrasonography of the right upper quadrant, left upper quadrant, and suprapubic regions aids in this determination. A fourth view in the subxiphoid region focuses on the pericardium to assess for effusion or tamponade. The FAST scan is ideally performed in the patient with blunt trauma just after the primary survey is complete and in conjunction with plain radiographs of the chest and pelvis. Pelvic fracture is assessed by the initial radiograph of the pelvis. The kidneys and abdominal aorta are retroperitoneal structures which cannot be diagnosed with the use of FAST scan. Diaphragmatic injury is notoriously difficult to diagnose with noninvasive studies (including CT, FAST, and diagnostic peritoneal lavage [DPL]) and may require thoracoscopy or laparoscopy for definitive diagnosis.

39. **Answer B.** Shoulder dystocia occurs when further progression of fetal delivery is halted by impaction of the fetal shoulders within the maternal pelvis. Although it is more common in diabetic mothers with infants weighing >4,000 g, more than half the cases involve infants <4,000 g and without other risk factors. Rapid recognition and treatment is critical because of an increased risk of fetal hypoxia and irreversible neurologic damage. Other injuries that complicate shoulder dystocia include brachial plexus injuries and humerus and clavicular fractures. With the exception of increased traction, all of the maneuvers listed may be used to help relieve shoulder dystocia. Most experts advocate using the least invasive maneuvers first. The best first step is the McRoberts maneuver in concert with suprapubic pressure. The McRoberts maneuver involves hyperflexion of the maternal hips (placing the maternal knees up to the chest), which moves the symphysis pubis over the fetal anterior shoulder. This is done in conjunction with moderate suprapubic pressure to push the fetal anterior shoulder below the symphysis. If this fails, more invasive maneuvers can be used such as the Rubin or Wood corkscrew maneuvers. The Rubin involves pushing the posterior fetal shoulder toward the fetal chest by placing a hand inside the vagina. The Wood corkscrew maneuver involves rotating the fetus 180 degrees (preferably clockwise) in an attempt to free the shoulders. In general, a liberal median episiotomy creates more space to allow the posterior shoulder to pass but does not, by itself, relieve dystocia, and it increases maternal morbidity. If all of these efforts fail, the posterior arm can be grasped, placed on the fetal chest, and swept over the face and out of the vagina. This maneuver (Barnum maneuver) may result in fractures or brachial plexus injury.

40. **Answer E.** The figure demonstrates a TM perforation in the setting of head trauma. Treatment of traumatic TM perforations in a dry environment is purely supportive with close ENT follow-up. Perforations in a wet environment require prophylaxis with antipseudomonal antibiotics. Perforations associated with preceding symptoms of otitis media also require standard antibiotic therapy with an aminopenicillin. All patients should be instructed to keep the ear canal dry. Healing of TM perforations occurs over several weeks to months. (Figure Courtesy of Handler SD. In: Chung EK, Atkinson-McEvoy LR, Lai NL, Michelle Terry M, eds. *Visual Diagnosis and Treatment in Pediatrics.* 3rd ed. Philadelphia: Wolters Kluwer, 2014.)

41. **Answer C.** The patient likely has uncomplicated viral conjunctivitis, which is most commonly caused by adenovirus, given the lack of dendrites (HSV), pseudo-dendrites or facial rash (VZV), or purulence on physical examination (bacterial). Viral conjunctivitis is extremely contagious and a sick contact is usually identified. Bacterial conjunctivitis may be difficult to distinguish early in the course from viral but is much less common. Contact lens use is the major risk factor for pseudomonal conjunctivitis.

42. **Answer E.** While erythema migrans is classically associated with central clearing, it is more commonly uniformly erythematous and sometimes has increased central erythema. Furthermore, a minority of patients recall a tick bite (this varies, but probably about 25%). Serologic testing should be avoided in the emergency department as it's often falsely negative in early Lyme,

and positive tests do not indicate active Lyme, particularly in patients who live in an endemic area. Alternative tests are being developed. Doxycycline remains the treatment of choice for Lyme even in children. Concerns about dental staining in children <8 years old given a course of doxycycline are unfounded and not supported by recent published evidence. In children with allergies, amoxicillin and cefuroxime are alternatives.

43. **Answer C.** Parapneumonic effusions can be uncomplicated, complicated, or frankly empyematous. Pleural fluid analysis can help guide optimal therapy. Patients with uncomplicated parapneumonic effusions usually improve with antibiotics alone. Patients with complicated parapneumonic effusions and frank empyema benefit from adjunctive tube thoracostomy drainage. Much like other body cavities which normally contain sterile, transudative fluid (such as the intraperitoneal space, CSF, and synovial capsules), the presence of increased WBCs, increased neutrophils, increased protein, reduced glucose, and lowered pH all indicate the presence of inflammation and likely significant infection. Pleural fluid pH <7 is the only one of the choices that adheres to these principles. A pleural fluid:serum LDH ratio of less than 0.6 and a serum:pleural fluid albumin gradient of greater than 1.1 actually point to a transudative cause (i.e., *less* protein in the pleural fluid). A high pleural fluid glucose indicates that there are not inflammatory cells or bacteria present to lower the glucose in any appreciable fashion. Lack of immediate response of fever to initial antibiotic therapy is not an indication to perform tube thoracostomy.

44. **Answer A.** Failure to make the correct diagnosis accounts for two-third of malpractice claims. Delay in diagnosis and improper medical management account for most of the remainder. Procedural errors and delay in treatment are less commonly cited reasons for malpractice claims.

45. **Answer C.** Anticoagulated patients with negative head CTs after head trauma rarely develop clinically relevant delayed bleeding. There is no evidence that repeat head CT is helpful or required. Furthermore, in the absence of bleeding, no reversal agents are needed. Admission for observation or ED observation without repeat imaging is a reasonable strategy. However, it is reasonable to discharge patients home with a reliable family member who can monitor them for signs of clinical decompensation. Better guidelines about how to manage these patients will slowly be developed as their use proliferates. Data thus far appear to demonstrate lower or similar risks of bleeding complications compared to warfarin.

46. **Answer B.** Despite their widespread use, neither intravenous corticosteroids nor racemic epinephrine has been shown to be beneficial in the management of adult epiglottitis. The foundation of effective management is the early administration of appropriate antibiotics and airway management, which may include early intubation or observation in a monitored setting. While *H. influenzae* type B remains an important cause of this disease in adults (the *H. influenzae* type b [Hib] vaccine has drastically reduced this entity in children), it is found in as few as 17% of cases. Other important bacterial causes include *Streptococcus,* and numerous gram-negative organisms. Although ampicillin was a drug of choice in the past, *H. influenzae* and other pathogens are increasingly resistant to this therapy due to the presence of β-lactamase. Therefore, second- and third-generation cephalosporins are the drugs of choice (e.g., ceftriaxone, cefotaxime, and ceftizoxime). Humidified oxygen is another component of epiglottitis therapy that has no proven benefit. However, because there is little potential harm in humidifying delivered oxygen; it remains a part of recommended treatment.

47. **Answer C.** Patients with nystagmus that changes direction based on the gaze direction (i.e., looking right causes fast-phase of nystagmus to the right, looking left causes fast-phase of nystagmus to the left) are at high risk for central cause of their nystagmus. Vertical nystagmus also predicts a central cause. Horizontal, fatiguable, and intensity-changing (beating faster, but not changing the direction of the fast component, in response to head movements) nystagmus are all commonly associated with peripheral causes.

48. **Answer B.** Amebiasis occurs in 10% of the world's population and amebic liver abscess is the most common extraintestinal manifestation of the disease. Patients with amebic liver abscesses more commonly have an acute presentation than patients with pyogenic liver abscesses. Transmission occurs through the fecal–oral route and is usually due to contaminated water or food products. Infections are always caused by *Entamoeba histolytica* and bacterial superinfections are uncommon. Alkaline phosphatase is elevated in 75% of patients and aminotransferases are increased in 50%. Elevated bilirubin levels are uncommon and reflect biliary obstruction. In contrast to pyogenic liver abscesses, the treatment is nonsurgical, and involves metronidazole 750 mg t.i.d. for 7 days. Following metronidazole, some authorities recommend an additional course of a luminal amebicide such as iodoquinol, diloxanide furoate, or paromomycin. (Figure reprinted with permission from Harris JH. *The Radiology of Emergency Medicine.* 4th ed. Lippincott Williams & Wilkins; 1999:613.)

49. **Answer E.** The patient has a feathering rash caused by lightning. It is not an actual burn injury, but rather a local irritation to electron showering that can occur

during a lightning strike. The rash is temporary and requires no specific management. Antibiotic, steroid, and antifungal therapy is not indicated. Preventive therapy with a triple antibiotic ointment is not useful (as there is no actual burn present) and may put patients at risk for neomycin-induced contact dermatitis.

50. **Answer C.** While hemodialysis and intravenous estrogen can positively impact platelet dysfunction in uremic patients and reduce bleeding, desmopressin is the least complicated, fastest approach to address this patient's ongoing bleeding. Desmopressin is thought to work by promoting the release of large factor VIII:von Willebrand factor multimers from endothelial cells. Therefore, it tends to reach maximal effectiveness after two doses as its use depletes existing multimer stores. Hemodialysis is the most definitive means of correcting uremic bleeding, but it's a slow process, and won't help to gain control of bleeding within the emergency department. Estrogens can also be used to help control uremic bleeding but they are slow in onset and aren't useful for urgent applications. This patient has an adequate number of platelets so a transfusion won't be beneficial and suture repair is traumatic and may induce additional bleeding.

51. **Answer D.** This patient has a Bartholin gland abscess, which is an infection of fluid that has accumulated in the gland. Healthy Bartholin glands are located at 5 o'clock and 7 o'clock positions around the vaginal introitus and are not palpable. Nonspecific inflammation or trauma may obstruct the glandular duct, however, resulting in accumulation of glandular fluid inside the gland and a Bartholin gland cyst. Asymptomatic cysts in young women do not require treatment. Older women should have the cyst excised by a specialist in order to search for glandular adenocarcinoma. All patients with an abscess should have incision and drainage followed by the placement of a Word catheter. The catheter is left in place for 6 to 8 weeks to allow formation of a fistulous tract, which enables ongoing drainage and prevents recurrence. Bartholin gland abscesses are almost always caused by polymicrobial vaginal flora. Antibiotics are unnecessary unless there is an associated cellulitis or unless sexually transmitted organisms are suspected. Cultures of the abscess can be obtained if there is concern about the etiology. (Figure from Sherman SC, Ross C, Nordquist E, Wang E, Cico S, (eds). *Atlas of Clinical Emergency Medicine.* 1st ed. Philadelphia: Wolters Kluwer, 2015.)

52. **Answer E.** Multiple studies after demonstrated a longer time to desaturation in patients placed in a head upright (head of bed elevated ≥20 to 30 degrees) and chin forward position (external auditory meatus aligned with the sternal notch). In immobilized patients who

can't bend the spine can be placed into reverse Trendelenburg, in which the head of the bed is elevated at least 30 degrees higher than the foot of the bed.

53. **Answer E.** This patient has acute alcoholic hepatitis. Although most cases of alcoholic hepatitis are subclinical or asymptomatic, it may be life threatening. Patients presenting for treatment are characterized by fever, right upper quadrant pain, jaundice, anorexia, and occasionally nausea and vomiting. Physical examination most commonly reveals hepatomegaly (as opposed to the shriveled, firm liver in patients with cirrhosis), jaundice, ascites, splenomegaly, and signs of alcohol withdrawal. AST and ALT levels are only modestly elevated, typically remaining below 300 U/L, and the ratio of AST:ALT is usually greater than 2:1. Bilirubin levels are elevated but are variable depending on the severity of the disease. Leukocytosis is common, with a mean WBC count of 12,400 per mm^3, whereas counts up to 20,000 are not uncommon. Fever is a common finding but concomitant infection is uncommon. Bilirubin levels and the prothrombin time (PT) have been classically used to stratify patients into low- or high-risk categories by calculating the Maddrey discriminant function.

$$\text{Discriminant function} = 4.6 \times (\text{PT in seconds} - \text{control in seconds}) + \text{bilirubin (mg/dL)}.$$

Levels over 32 correspond with severe disease and a 1-month mortality >50%.

54. **Answer B.** The patient has evidence of gastroenteritis with bloody, loose bowel movements, also known as dysentery. Dysentery is more likely to be due to a bacterial source than viral or parasitic. Although viruses cause the majority of cases of gastroenteritis, *Campylobacter* is one of the most common causes of bacterial gastroenteritis and dysentery. *C. difficile* should be suspected in any patient with a history of exposure to antibiotics. Adenovirus is a common cause of pediatric viral gastroenteritis but is usually associated with watery rather than bloody diarrhea. ETEC is the most common cause of traveler's diarrhea, but rarely causes dysentery especially when there is no history of foreign travel. *Giardia* causes a subacute, watery diarrhea, often with a history of camping.

55. **Answer B.** Patients with visual field complaints affecting both eyes must have lesions affecting either the optic chiasm or retrochiasmal pathways (posterior to or "before" the optic chiasm) including the optic tracts, lateral geniculate body, the optic radiations, and the occipital cortex. This patient complains of a homonymous hemianopia meaning that she is experiencing trouble with her vision in the same visual field of both eyes. The most common reason for this problem is a stroke, but in a young person, a tumor is more likely. While pituitary

tumors are common, such tumors affect the optic chiasm and classically produce a bitemporal anopia, which causes difficulty with vision in the outer half of each eye's visual field. This is because the central portion of the optic chiasm contains the fibers from the nasal portion of both retinas which in turn detect light from the temporal visual fields.

56. **Answer B.** Phalen test (holding hands dorsum-to-dorsum with the wrists flexed at 90 degrees) is probably the most sensitive physical examination maneuver for evaluation of carpal tunnel syndrome, though sensitivity is reported to be as low as 51%. Tinel test (tapping the volar wrist for elicitation of numbness or tingling) has been shown to be useless in the evaluation of carpal tunnel syndrome and should be eliminated from routine physical examination. Allen test (compression of radial and ulnar arteries to assess blood flow before a radial arterial cannulation) has no relationship to carpal tunnel syndrome and is another test of dubious utility. Hoffman sign (flicking the distal phalanx of the middle finger and looking for movement of the thumb and index fingers) aims to evaluate cervical spinal cord compression. Recent rigorous testing of this physical examination finding has also found poor sensitivity and specificity. The Eichoff test (tucking the thumb into the palm and ulnarly deviating the wrist causes pain in the radial wrist) is used to evaluate deQuervain tendonitis—the Eichoff test is commonly mislabeled as the Finkelstein test. Importantly, the Eichoff test is not particularly accurate at evaluating deQuervain tendonitis.

57. **Answer A.** Permethrin has become the treatment of choice for scabies because it is equally efficacious to lindane, yet it is not appreciably absorbed through the skin making systemic side effects less likely. Malathion shampoo can be used for pediculosis capitis (head lice), although permethrin is still preferred because of its more pleasant odor and more rapid administration (malathion requires 8 to 10 hours of administration in cases of head lice while permethrin requires only 10 minutes).

58. **Answer B.** The patient has acute necrotizing ulcerative gingivitis, commonly known as *trench mouth*. The gingiva is painful and friable, unlike ordinary gingivitis. Treatment involves oral antibiotics and good oral hygiene. Spirochetes and fusobacteria predominate in what is likely a bacterial overgrowth process. Vincent angina refers to extension of acute necrotizing ulcerative gingivitis (ANUG) to the tonsils, and cancrum oris refers to extension to the lips and buccal mucosa. Direct contact with secretions does not confer increased risk.

59. **Answer A.** The thoracic outlet syndrome comprises a group of pathologic conditions associated with compression of the structures at the junction of the upper extremity and trunk. The findings are neurologic (95%), venous (4%), and arterial (1%). The elevated arm stress test is the best physical examination tool to determine the presence of thoracic outlet syndrome. The test involves abducting the shoulders to 90 degrees with the elbows flexed at 90 while opening and closing the fists for 3 minutes. A positive result is indicated by arm fatigue and pain, and the inability to keep it abducted.

60. **Answer D.** Trauma in the setting of submersion injuries is usually because of motor vehicle accidents (in which the vehicle crashes into water) or accidents involving diving, boating, or falls from a height into water. Although antibiotics are of use in patients who were submerged in grossly contaminated fluid (e.g., sewage), they have no role in routine fresh or saltwater submersion. Corticosteroids also have no role in drowning patients unless patients have a history of reactive airway disease and have evidence of bronchospasm on physical examination. Since the patient is breathing spontaneously and appears to be able to protect his airway, intubation is not indicated. However, because this patient was involved in a high-speed crash, trauma-related injury should be the next most important issue after ensuring an adequate airway, breathing, and circulation.

61. **Answer E.** This patient has features of systemic lupus erythematosus (SLE). Black women of childbearing age are most at risk for developing SLE. This patient is presenting with the classic malar rash after sun exposure in concert with fever and arthralgias. As in rheumatoid arthritis, arthralgias in SLE are typically symmetric and most commonly involve in the fingers, hands, wrists, and knees. Fevers are very common in patients with SLE, and nearly all patients will develop a fever at some point in their course, although greater than one-third will present with a fever. Patients with SLE have numerous autoantibodies. However, testing for ANA is most sensitive as 99% of patients with SLE have a positive ANA. The positive predictive value of ANA testing suffers because 5% to 7% of healthy individuals will also test positive for ANA. Anti-Sm is the most specific antibody, with a specificity of 99% and a positive predictive value of 97%. However, its sensitivity is only 25% so it is not a good screening test.

62. **Answer E.** The patient's x-ray shows evidence of free air, indicating a likely viscus perforation. Broad-spectrum antibiotics, NPO status, and surgical consultation are mandatory. Anticoagulation would be contraindicated in someone who is likely going to the operating room for bowel surgery. Azithromycin would not be adequate treatment for bowel surgery as it would miss important gram-negative and anaerobic pathogens. Octreotide is used for cirrhotic patients with acute variceal bleeding

and does not have a role in the management of viscus perforation. Paracentesis should be used as a diagnostic maneuver to evaluate spontaneous bacterial peritonitis in patients with cirrhosis. (From Smith WL. *Radiology 101*. 4th ed. Philadelphia, PA: Wolters Kluwer; 2013.)

63. **Answer B.** The most commonly affected joints in septic arthritis are knee (40% to 50%), hip (13% to 20%), shoulder (10% to 15%), ankle (6% to 8%), wrist (5% to 8%), and elbow (3% to 7%).

64. **Answer B.** *E. coli* O157:H7 (also known as enterohemorrhagic *E. coli* or enterohemorrhagic *E. coli* [EHEC]) is the most important strain of *E. coli* that commonly causes diarrhea in the United States. It is most frequently associated with eating undercooked ground beef. However, outbreaks from contamination of apple cider, raw milk, and most recently, spinach, have also been reported. Antibiotics are contraindicated in all cases because they may induce the expression and release of toxins (Shiga toxins), which may worsen the disease and increase the risk of developing HUS. HUS is a syndrome characterized by microangiopathic hemolytic anemia, thrombocytopenia, and renal failure and occurs in as many as 25% of cases (most of which occur in children). HUS is the most common cause of renal failure in children. TTP is a less frequent complication of EHEC infection and more commonly occurs in the elderly or immunocompromised. Infection with EHEC results in a hemorrhagic colitis after an incubation period, which ranges from 3 to 8 days. Fever is atypical and a different pathogen should be considered if fever is present.

65. **Answer C.** This patient has Bell palsy. Bell palsy is defined as paresis or paralysis of the facial nerve (seventh cranial nerve), which is usually unilateral. The first step in the diagnosis is to determine that the paresis or paralysis is due to a peripheral instead of a CNS lesion. In patients with CNS lesions, furrowing of the eyebrows and closure of the eye is unaffected. This is due to the fact that the neurons of the facial nucleus that innervate the upper face receive input from both cerebral hemispheres (whereas the neurons of the facial nucleus that innervate the lower face receive input primarily from the contralateral cerebral hemisphere). A CT scan would only be necessary in patients with evidence of a CNS lesion upon physical examination. The presence of a vesicular rash over the ear indicates Ramsay–Hunt syndrome. Ramsay–Hunt syndrome, also known as *herpes zoster oticus*, results from reactivation of varicella zoster virus in the geniculate ganglion of the facial nerve. It is much less common and carries a more severe prognosis for recovery than Bell palsy of unknown cause or Bell palsy due to reactivation of HSV. More than 75% of patients will recover without treatment. Therefore, medical treatment is aimed at the remaining population. Because it

is not possible to identify which patients will recover fully without treatment, all patients are generally treated upon making the diagnosis. The treatment for Bell palsy includes corticosteroids, antiviral agents directed against herpes viruses (acyclovir, valacyclovir, and famciclovir), and artificial tears and eye ointment to prevent corneal drying. There is disagreement over the best regimen (e.g., some experts recommend antivirals only in cases of a severe palsy) and the timing of presentation. However, it is generally felt that earlier treatment yields better results and that corticosteroids are of limited utility if a patient presents after 7 days of symptoms. Patients with diabetes and hypertension have a more severe course and less complete recovery. Recurrence of Bell palsy rarely occurs. In cases of recurrence, consideration should be given to alternative diagnoses.

66. **Answer C.** External hemorrhoids are best treated with nonpharmacologic therapies. The WASH regimen (warm water, analgesia, stool softeners, and high-fiber diet) is probably the most effective regimen and also the least likely to cause unacceptable side effects. Opioid pain relief without accompanying stool softeners is not recommended as they will further exacerbate constipation and straining. Topical corticosteroids can be used acutely (though little data exist for true benefit), but long-term use can cause skin atrophy. Topical nitroglycerin is used in patients with anal fissures but is not recommended in patients with nonthrombosed external hemorrhoids. Topical nifedipine may be used in anal fissures and thrombosed external hemorrhoids but is not recommended for nonthrombosed external hemorrhoids.

67. **Answer D.** The patient has evidence of necrotizing fasciitis of the perineal area, commonly referred to as *Fournier gangrene*. Fournier gangrene is a systemic, life-threatening, polymicrobial infection, which requires intravenous antibiotics and surgical debridement. Intravenous immunoglobulin and hyperbaric oxygen therapy may be helpful in certain cases. Corticosteroids are not indicated except in cases of concomitant adrenal insufficiency. Antibiotics without surgical debridement are not sufficient for management. The diagnosis is usually made clinically—in unclear cases, CT or MRI may aid the diagnosis but neither is 100% sensitive or specific. (Figure courtesy of Paul J Kovalcik, MD, In: Sherman SC, Ross C, Nordquist E, et al., eds. *Atlas of Clinical Emergency Medicine*. 1st ed. Philadelphia, PA: Wolters Kluwer; 2015.)

68. **Answer D.** Electrical resistance refers to the ability of the substance to resistant passage (conductance) of electricity. High-resistance tissues convert electrical energy to heat energy, damaging the tissue itself but putting other structures at less risk for damage. Low-resistance tissues

allow electricity to pass, which can cause potentially serious organ damage at sites away from the initial entry point. Fat, tendon, and bone have the highest electrical resistance. The other answer choices represent the least resistant tissues. Dry, undamaged skin is of intermediate resistance; calloused skin has high resistance, but wet skin has very low resistance.

69. **Answer C.** The chest x-ray shows a consolidation consistent with community-acquired pneumonia. A 44-year-old patient without comorbidities or abnormal vital signs would be a good candidate for outpatient therapy, including doxycycline or azithromycin. Fluoroquinolone therapy could also be pursued, but would carry the risk of musculoskeletal side effects without appreciable improvement in bacterial coverage in this previously healthy patient. Supportive care is not sufficient for patients with presumed bacterial pneumonia. Oseltamivir is not effective for patients without influenza. Piperacillin–tazobactam or vancomycin plus cefepime would be regimens used for severely ill patients with high risk for *Pseudomonas* infection (those with comorbidities, recent exposure to antibiotics, or recent hospital stays). (Figure from Daffner RH, Hartman MS. *Clinical Radiology.* 4th ed. Baltimore, MD: Lippincott Williams & Wilkins; 2014.)

70. **Answer C.** NAC promotes the metabolism of acetaminophen into a nontoxic compound by sulfation, through replenishment of glutathione. Prevention of hepatic injury is complete when the first dose of NAC is given within 8 hours of acute ingestion. Beneficial effects still occur as far out as 48 hours after ingestion, but efficacy in preventing hepatic injury decreases progressively starting at the 8-hour mark.

71. **Answer D.** The vesicular lesions on the soft palate are most characteristic of herpangina, which is usually caused by coxsackie viruses A and B. The clinical syndrome usually starts with fever, myalgias, dysphagia, and sometimes headache and stiff neck. Oral lesions of herpangina usually spare the gingiva and hard palate, unlike herpes simplex virus gingivostomatitis. Management of herpangina is completely supportive and ulcers will recede in 10 days. Attention to appropriate hydration is integral, as many patients will be unable to even drink liquids because of pain for the first few days of illness. Aphthous ulcers are classically present on the tongue, buccal mucosa, and soft palate, but they are rarely associated with systemic symptoms of infection. Group A *streptococci* may cause pharyngeal and tonsillar ulcers but not usually more proximal ulcers. Diphtheria classically causes a grayish tonsillar pseudomembrane without ulcerations. (Figure courtesy of Mark Silverberg, MD, In: Greenberg MI, Hendrickson RG, Silverberg M, et al., eds. *Greenberg's Text-Atlas of Emergency Medicine.*

Lippincott Williams & Wilkins; 2004:156, reprinted with permission.)

72. **Answer C.** The EKG changes over time in patients with pericarditis. Acutely, concave ST elevation and PR depression with tall T waves are seen. Depression of the PR segment is the most specific EKG finding for acute pericarditis. Concave ST elevation is also common, but can be seen in a variety of other conditions, including benign early repolarization and left ventricular hypertrophy. An ST-segment to T-wave ratio of >0.25 argues in favor of acute pericarditis. Convex ST elevations are more likely to be due to myocardial infarction than pericarditis. Hyperacute T waves are seen more often in hyperkalemia and infarction than in pericarditis. AV blocks are rarely seen in acute pericarditis. Chronic EKG changes associated with pericarditis include return of ST segments to baseline, T-wave flattening, T-wave inversion, and then complete normalization after a few weeks to months.

73. **Answer A.** The metabolism of ethylene glycol is ethylene glycol → glycoaldehyde → glycolic acid → → → oxalic acid. Oxalic acid forms calcium oxalate crystals which can deposit in the renal tubules and cause renal insufficiency, and the other metabolites of ethylene glycol are directly nephrotoxic as well. Approximately one-fourth of ethylene glycol is directly excreted in the kidneys, but hepatic metabolism with alcohol dehydrogenase catalyzes the formation of the toxic metabolites. The goals of therapy in patients with ethylene glycol toxicity are to block the availability of alcohol dehydrogenase with either fomepizole or ethanol and to hemodialyze the unmetabolized ethylene glycol. Methanol toxicity results in the formation of formic acid, which accumulates in the brain and causes blindness and death. Isopropanol causes generalized CNS depression similar to ethanol intoxication. Salicylate overdose results in direct nephrotoxicity, metabolic acidosis, electrolyte abnormalities, and pulmonary and cerebral edema. Acetaminophen overdose causes fulminant hepatic failure.

74. **Answer D.** Patients with primary adrenal insufficiency develop hyperpigmentation due to increased levels of corticotropin releasing hormone, which stimulates the synthesis of adrenocorticotropic hormone (ACTH) and of melanocyte stimulating hormone (MSH), which is cleaved from the same pre-peptide as ACTH. Adrenal insufficiency secondary to pituitary insufficiency results in low ACTH levels, so hyperpigmentation is not seen. Hyponatremia, hyperkalemia, and hypoglycemia are common electrolyte abnormalities as a result of adrenal insufficiency (specifically mineralocorticoid insufficiency). Therefore, hypokalemia may occur as a result of replacement therapy with prednisone or hydrocortisone

(but not with dexamethasone, which does not have mineralocorticoid activity). Nausea and vomiting are common GI manifestations of adrenal insufficiency.

75. **Answer A.** Oxygen is the standard of care for cluster headache. Seventy-five percent of patients with cluster headache given 100% oxygen through face mask will experience complete or near-complete relief within 15 minutes. Because attacks of cluster headaches are self-limited and typically last no longer than 90 minutes, patients may not have pain by the time they reach the ED. Therefore, oxygen is an inconvenient therapy. Sumatriptan is the most effective self-administered medication. It is administered as a nasal spray and is effective in more than 50% of patients within 15 minutes of use. However, its use is not recommended in patients who are having more than two attacks per day because this would result in an overdose of the medication. Dihydroergotamine and zolmitriptan are also effective treatments. Narcotics, benzodiazepines, and corticosteroids have no role in acute cluster headache management.

76. **Answer E.** All Rh-negative pregnant patients with first-trimester vaginal bleeding should be given RhoGAM. The dose in the first trimester is 50 μg, whereas the dose after the first trimester is 300 μg. RhoGAM has not been shown to cause fetal harm. The classic teaching is that 50% of patients diagnosed with a threatened abortion progress to spontaneous miscarriage. However, once a fetal heartbeat is identified on ultrasonograph, only 15% of such women will progress to spontaneous miscarriage whereas the remainder will carry the pregnancy normally to term. Patients with threatened abortion should be advised to carry out their normal activities although patients are often advised to avoid tampons, intercourse, and douching to prevent infection. Patients frequently confuse blood clots with tissue and even in the presence of laboratory confirmation of products of conception, a diagnosis of complete abortion is ill-advised. Only if a complete gestational sac or fetus is present should a diagnosis of complete abortion be considered. Otherwise, an ultrasound should be performed to determine if retained products of conception are present. Finally, approximately 80% of patients with first-trimester spontaneous abortion will complete the abortion without intervention. The classic teaching is that all patients diagnosed with an anembryonic pregnancy (or blighted ovum), intrauterine fetal demise, missed abortion, or incomplete abortion require surgical evacuation. However, current research demonstrates that the volume of intrauterine contents is the best predictor of the need for surgical evacuation and most women do not require intervention.

77. **Answer D.** The Mantoux test is the most common test used to screen for TB exposure and infection. It consists of an intradermal injection of 10 units (0.1 mL) of standardized PPD from *M. tuberculosis*. Positivity is determined by the amount of *induration*, not erythema, in response to the injection and is typically measured between 48 and 72 hours. Induration <5 mm in diameter is negative and induration >15 mm is positive. Induration between 5 and 15 mm may be positive, depending on other factors, such as prior immunization with Bacille Calmette–Guérin (BCG) or the presence of immunosuppression as in patients with HIV. As the BCG vaccine is not used in this country and because this patient is American-born, BCG is an unlikely cause of his positive test result. In this country, patients with HIV are considered to have a positive PPD if the amount of induration exceeds 5 mm, as are patients who have had close contact with active TB and patients who have a fibrotic chest x-ray. Patients in any other high-risk group are considered positive when the amount of induration exceeds 10 mm in diameter. Regardless of the group to which a patient belongs, a positive PPD means that a patient has been exposed to and infected with *M. tuberculosis* and that the organism remains in their body. Because this patient does not have symptoms of active disease (e.g., fever, cough, hemoptysis, night sweats, anorexia, and weight loss) and does not have any findings on his chest x-ray, he has latent, not active, disease. Patients with latent TB infection are not contagious, but they require treatment with INH to dramatically reduce their lifetime risk of developing active TB.

78. **Answer B.** The patient likely has plantar fasciitis, which is inflammation of the plantar surface of the foot, just distal to the calcaneus. Patients complain of moderate–severe heel pain on walking. Pain can be worse in the morning, when feet are allowed to remain in plantar flexion while sleeping. Treatment involves physical therapy exercises to stretch the Achilles tendon with dorsiflexion splints. Nonsteroidal anti-inflammatory drugs (NSAIDs) can also be employed for pain control. Corticosteroid injections are generally not recommended. Stirrup ankle braces are more useful for patients with ankle sprains to prevent inversion and eversion and do not help treat a pathologic process that involves plantarflexion and dorsiflexion. Admission for MRI or surgical consultation in this otherwise healthy patient with no signs of acute emergency requiring operative evaluation is not advisable. Optimal management in this case also involves encouragement for outpatient follow-up.

79. **Answer C.** Transient synovitis is the most common cause of atraumatic hip pain in children. It usually occurs in children <6 years old, and the cause is unknown. Referred pain to the knee may be the only complaint, so careful inspection of the hip is mandatory in all patients with isolated knee pain. Diagnosis is made by excluding other more serious causes of

hip pain, namely septic arthritis, fracture, SCFE, and Legg–Calve–Perthes disease. Patients with transient synovitis are less likely than those with septic arthritis to have fever, elevated erythrocyte sedimentation rate (ESR), and tenderness of the hip. Management of transient synovitis is purely supportive with rest and NSAIDs. Hip fracture in the pediatric patient is suggested by high-force trauma and severe tenderness is common. Osteogenesis imperfecta is a rare disease that causes problems in bone synthesis due to collagen defects. Frequent fractures are common and physical examination may demonstrate blue sclerae, deafness, and ligamentous laxity. Subclinical cases may be more common than previously recognized. SCFE occurs when the femoral epiphysis slips off the metaphysis, usually in adolescents. Legg–Calve–Perthes disease is avascular necrosis of the femoral head due to unknown reasons. It occurs from childhood to adolescence but is less common than transient synovitis.

80. **Answer E.** Because PCP cannot be cultured, and the gold standard in making the diagnosis remains invasive (bronchoscopy and subsequent staining), there has been much interest in trying to find surrogate serum markers to indicate the presence of *P. jirovecii*. Most of this interest has focused on LDH. Unfortunately, although it is true that LDH levels are elevated in the setting of PCP, this finding is not specific for PCP. However, the level of LDH appears to correlate with the degree of radiographic severity. This supports the idea that elevated LDH levels are more a reflection of generalized lung inflammation than a marker of any particular organism. Lactate levels and liver transaminases have no role in the diagnosis of PCP. Most patients with PCP and hypoxia have a respiratory alkalosis, as their respiratory rate (and depth) increases with the severity of their hypoxia. Finally, patients with CD4 counts <200 are most susceptible to PCP, and it is this population who should be on chemical prophylaxis. Pleural effusions are not common in PCP.

81. **Answer E.** In trauma patients, anterior cord syndrome most commonly occurs in hyper*flexion* injuries in which herniated vertebral discs or vertebral body fragments compress the anterior aspect of the spinal cord or the anterior spinal artery. The anterior spinal artery provides blood supply to the anterior two-thirds of the spinal cord. The primary structures affected in the spinal cord are the spinothalamic tract, which is responsible for the transmission of pain and temperature sensory input, and the corticospinal tract, which carries descending voluntary motor signals. In addition, anterior cord syndrome affects the descending autonomic tracts for bladder control, resulting in incontinence or variable degrees of bladder dysfunction. The dorsal or posterior columns, which are responsible for proprioception and vibration sensation, are unaffected so those functions are preserved.

82. **Answer E.** The patient may have a clinical rib fracture, which will require pain control and possibly incentive spirometry. However, most rib fractures do not need to be diagnosed radiographically, as management will not change irrespective of the rib x-ray result. Educating the patient that the rib may be fractured and that the important function of the ribs was fulfilled (i.e., protection of the lungs and pleura) is the best management. CT chest without contrast would be indicated if the patient were suspected of having an occult pneumothorax or hemothorax. CT chest with IV contrast is not typically indicated with this trauma mechanism and should be reserved for patients suspected of aortic injury. Hospital security action should be reserved for patients who represent physical danger to themselves or others.

83. **Answer D.** Mallet finger is the disruption of the extensor tendon at the level of distal interphalangeal (DIP) joint with or without an associated avulsion fracture of the dorsal base of the distal phalanx. It is caused by a flexion force on the volar tip with an extended DIP joint. Conversely, jersey finger results from avulsion of the FDP tendon at the level of the DIP joint. It most commonly occurs when an extension force is applied to a flexed DIP such as that occurs during tackling another player in football by grabbing his jersey. The ring finger is involved in 75% of cases. In contrast to the mallet finger, surgical repair is the treatment of choice in nearly all cases. A Bennett fracture is an intra-articular fracture of the base of the thumb metacarpal (at the carpometacarpal joint) with lateral displacement and retraction of the distal segment due to the abductor pollicis longus. Such fractures require thumb spica splinting and frequently need operative fixation. Trigger finger refers to a stenosing flexor tenosynovitis typically due to overuse. It results in the formation of a nodule in the flexor tendon sheath, which prevents extension of the digit at the level of the metacarpophalangeal (MCP) joint. It most commonly occurs in the ring and long fingers, and local corticosteroid injection usually results in significant improvement. Patients should then be splinted in extension and referred to a hand specialist for further evaluation. Gamekeeper thumb is an avulsion injury of the ulnar collateral ligament (UCL) at the thumb–MCP joint. It most commonly occurs during a skiing accident in which the patient's thumb is trapped in the loop of the pole, resulting in forced abduction and extension of the thumb. An avulsion fracture may also occur at the site of the UCL insertion. Patients should be placed in a thumb spica splint and referred to a hand surgeon for further evaluation. Volar plate entrapment may occur with dorsal proximal interphalangeal (PIP) dislocations preventing ED reduction.

84. **Answer A.** Domestic violence against women may occur in as many as 20% of pregnancies. If abuse is already present in a relationship, it often worsens during

pregnancy. Females (regardless of pregnancy) presenting for ED care are at increased risk for abuse relative to females presenting for primary care or nonurgent care. Specifically, women with chronic headaches, chronic abdominal pain, and trauma victims are all at increased risk for abuse. Noncompliance is also common among abused patients. With respect to abuse in general, while the majority of victims are women, up to 40% of abused patients may be men. Like abused females, these patients confront significant barriers against reporting abuse. There are myriad organizations who issue various and sometimes conflicting advice about the appropriate manner to screen for abused patients. The Massachusetts Medical Society Committee on Violence suggests asking the following single question: "At any time has a partner hit, kicked or otherwise hurt or threatened you?" Interestingly, the incidence of domestic violence is the same in gay couples as it is among straight couples. However, studies show that gay couples are infrequently screened for domestic violence.

85. **Answer D.** The treatment of choice for QRS prolongation and wide-complex tachycardias in patients with tricyclic antidepressant overdose is sodium bicarbonate. Tricyclics inhibit fast sodium channel conductance, and the sodium bicarbonate counteracts this effect. Stable dysrhythmias do not require immediate cardioversion. Lidocaine has no proven efficacy in patients with wide-complex tachycardia due to tricyclic overdose. Procainamide (IA antidysrhythmic) and propafenone (IC antidysrhythmic) further exacerbate the inhibition of sodium channel conductance and are contraindicated.

86. **Answer C.** Fever is the most common symptom in infective endocarditis but is nonspecific. Audible heart murmur or fever is present in almost 90% of patients with endocarditis. Murmurs are less common and fever is more common in IV drug users. Choices A, B, D, and E occur in less than half the number of patients with endocarditis. Some type of vasculitic skin lesion will occur in most patients, but a specific type such as Osler nodes, Janeway lesions, petechiae, or splinter hemorrhages each occur in less than one-fourth of patients. Splenomegaly is present in roughly one-third.

87. **Answer C.** Patients with HHS have a larger fluid deficit and more significant potassium deficiency than patients with DKA. Although seizures may occur in HHS, the most common immediate life threat is hypovolemic shock. Hypokalemia is the next most serious immediate risk to patients with HHS. Thromboembolic events may occur in either DKA or HHS but more commonly complicate HHS. Thromboembolic events occur as a result of severe dehydration and resulting hyperviscosity.

88. **Answer A.** In practice, probably the most common complication is the ampicillin- or amoxicillin-associated

rash that occurs when patients with EBV pharyngitis are mistakenly treated for a bacterial pharyngitis. Such a rash may occur in up to 95% of patients with EBV pharyngitis who are treated with one of these two medications. The rash occurs less commonly when patients are treated with other β-lactam antibiotics. Elevations of the hepatic enzymes AST and ALT commonly occur (up to 80%) to approximately four times the upper limit of normal and peak during the second to fourth week of illness. However, levels well over 1,000 may occur. Jaundice may also be seen (5%), but coagulopathy is not typical. Spontaneous recovery is the rule, and supportive care is the only required treatment. Airway obstruction is probably the most important complication for the emergency medicine physician. It is due to tonsillar hypertrophy and occurs more commonly in young children because of their prominent lymphoid tissue. Overall, however, this complication occurs in <5% of patients and can usually be managed conservatively by elevating the head of the bed, giving intravenous fluids and corticosteroids and using humidified air. Splenic rupture receives a lot of attention but occurs in <0.5% of adults with EBV infection. The rate in children is thought to be much lower. It most commonly occurs in the second and third week of illness and is rarely fatal when it does occur. Patients present with left upper quadrant abdominal pain, with or without radiation to the left shoulder (Kehr sign), and splenic rupture should be considered especially in the setting of shock. Numerous hematologic complications are associated with EBV infection, including autoimmune hemolytic anemia (3%), mild thrombocytopenia (25% to 50%), and mild transient neutropenia (50% to 80%). Headache is the most common neurologic manifestation of EBV infection (50%), although meningoencephalitis is the most common severe neurologic complication (1% to 5%).

89. **Answer D.** The role of noncontrast CT brain in the evaluation of an acute-onset, focal neurologic deficit is to establish the lack of hemorrhage or large space-occupying lesion in the brain. Noncontrast CT brain has poor sensitivity for ischemic stroke; because ischemic strokes represent over three-quarters of all strokes, the negative predictive value of noncontrast CT brain for stroke in general is also poor. Noncontrast CT brain is used to rule out intracranial hemorrhage to permit consideration for IV tissue plasminogen activator (TPA), which is the only effective treatment for acute ischemic stroke but is absolutely contraindicated in hemorrhagic stroke. Meningitis can only be definitively diagnosed using CSF analysis with lumbar puncture. Cervical artery dissection is best evaluated with either CT angiogram or MR angiogram of the head and neck.

90. **Answer C.** The patient likely has a testicular tumor, usually of germ-cell type in this age-group. Evaluation

may include screening for metastases with a chest x-ray and a CT scan of the abdomen and pelvis, although this may occur on an urgent outpatient (rather than emergent inpatient) basis. Emergent surgery is not indicated in patients with testicular tumors except in certain patients who have evidence of testicular torsion. Azithromycin may be used to treat chlamydial epididymitis but has no role in the management of testicular tumors. Scrotal elevation is often used as a diagnostic maneuver to distinguish between epididymitis and testicular torsion (relief is called *Prehn sign*), but it is an unreliable finding for this purpose. Corticosteroids may be used in patients with testicular tumors as part of certain chemotherapeutic regimens but has no role in the acute management. (Figure courtesy of Mark Silverberg, MD, In: Greenberg MI, Hendrickson RG, Silverberg M, et al., eds. *Greenberg's Text-Atlas of Emergency Medicine.* Lippincott Williams & Wilkins; 2004:330, reprinted with permission.)

91. **Answer E.** Smallpox is due to *Variola major*, a member of the poxvirus family. It was eradicated in the 1970s and now exists only in laboratories. Mortality of smallpox is almost 30% and contagiousness is extremely high. The only effective strategies for management are prevention, vaccination, and isolation. Vaccination is only effective if given before or within a few days of exposure. No antivirals or antibiotic are effective in management.

92. **Answer B.** The incidence of seizures after ischemic stroke is uncertain but is cited to be as high as 13%. Typically, patients with seizures after stroke are divided into patients who have seizures within 7 days (early seizures) and those who develop seizures after 7 days (late seizures). Prophylactic use of anticonvulsants in patients with ischemic stroke has not been shown to reduce either early or late seizures although there are limited data on this topic. Therefore, the prophylactic use of anticonvulsants in such patients is not recommended. When seizures do occur, their management is the same as "conventional" seizure management, and status epilepticus is rare. Current guidelines recommend that patients with an ischemic stroke in the ED who develop seizures warrant standard treatment (if necessary) to terminate the seizure followed by treatment with an anticonvulsant to prevent recurrence. There are no special contraindications to antiepileptic use in stroke patients.

93. **Answer E.** The CT scan reveals a hypodense fluid collection surrounding an inflamed pancreas. Acute fluid collection is associated with acute pancreatitis in 30% to 50% of patients. These fluid collections resolve spontaneously in most patients. A pseudocyst is a fluid collection that persists for 4 to 6 weeks and becomes encapsulated by a wall of fibrous or granulation tissue. Unless pancreatitis is *due* to an infectious agent, acute infection of fluid collections or of necrotic pancreatic

tissue is uncommon. Infection usually occurs within the first 2 weeks although abscess formation may not occur until 1 month after the acute infection. If an abscess does occur, urgent drainage is required. (Figure reprinted with permission from Harris JH. *The Radiology of Emergency Medicine.* 4th ed. Lippincott Williams & Wilkins; 1999:618.)

94. **Answer B.** Magnesium therapy is the cornerstone of seizure prophylaxis in patients with pre-eclampsia. The loss of deep tendon reflexes is the first reliable sign of impending, serious toxicity. This is followed by a slowed respiratory rate, respiratory arrest and finally, cardiac arrest. In the setting of lost deep tendon reflexes, the infusion should be stopped immediately. Calcium gluconate can be used as an adjunct to oppose magnesium's effects but is usually reserved for patients with respiratory depression. While nausea and vomiting, diaphoresis, flushing and warmth, headaches, paresthesias, visual changes, and palpitations may occur as side effects of therapy, they are not reliable indicators of significant toxicity.

95. **Answer B.** Patients with RPAs generally prefer to lie supine to prevent the abscess and posterior wall edema from infringing upon their airway. Such patients should never be forced to sit upright. Although aggressive treatment of pediatric pharyngitis with early antibiotics has reduced the incidence of subsequent RPAs, children remain the most commonly affected group. This is due to the presence of large retropharyngeal lymph nodes in children younger than 4 years, which may become infected and subsequently develop into RPAs. Adults frequently present with a history of antecedent trauma, such as ingestion of a fish bone or caustic agents as well as vertebral fractures. Since the retropharyngeal lymph nodes rapidly involute after the ages of 4 to 6, adults usually require some insult to the intact retropharyngeal mucosa in order to develop a subsequent infection. An RPA should be suspected if the prevertebral soft tissue from the anteroinferior aspect of C2 to the border of the tracheal air column is >7mm in children and adults or the same space at the level of C6 is >14 mm in children and 22 mm in adults. Although *M. tuberculosis* may cause an RPA, the most common cause is *Staphylococcus*. Finally, the most common fatal complication is airway obstruction. Atlantoaxial separation may occur due to damage of the transverse ligament of the atlas by the abscess. Such patients present with neurologic symptoms and an enlarged predental space. All patients diagnosed with an RPA require immediate ENT consultation, admission to the ICU for airway monitoring, and broad-spectrum antibiotic coverage.

96. **Answer C.** This patient has a pheochromocytoma. Pheochromocytomas are catecholamine producing tumors

that account for <1% of cases of hypertension. They are most commonly found in the adrenal medulla although 10% are extra-adrenal (the rule of "10s" in pheochromocytoma: 10% bilateral, 10% malignant, 10% extra-adrenal, 10% associated with familial disorders, e.g., multiple endocrine neoplasia). The diagnosis is based on detection of urinary metanephrines and vanillylmandelic acid (VMA) and has a diagnostic sensitivity of 98% for detecting pheochromocytoma. Assays for plasma metanephrines may also be performed. Finally, CT or MRI is used for tumor localization. Hypertension has traditionally been treated with phenoxybenzamine, an α-blocker, whereas β-blockers should be avoided (β-blockers lead to unopposed α stimulation, which may result in a worsening of hypertension). Due to associated peripheral edema and orthostatic hypotension, other α-blockers have also been used such as terazosin or doxazosin.

97. **Answer A.** TLS describes the constellation of problems that arises from massive cell death that occurs in the setting of chemotherapy of rapidly growing, highly chemosensitive malignancies. Hyperuricemia, hyperkalemia, hyperphosphatemia, and hypocalcemia are the most common problems. The laboratory diagnosis of TLS is made when two of these four abnormalities are present simultaneously or whenever symptomatic hypocalcemia is present. Clinical TLS occurs when the laboratory findings are accompanied by renal failure, seizures, cardiac arrhythmias, or death. Though elevated levels of lactate dehydrogenase are not required to make a diagnosis of TLS, they will typically be significantly elevated in the setting of massive cellular death. Hyperkalemia is the most immediate life threat, while hypocalcemia can be symptomatic (tetany) or life threatening. Hyperuricemia results in significant calcium urate precipitation (which causes hypocalcemia) and subsequent calcium urate deposition in the kidneys which leads to renal failure. Aggressive IV hydration is the cornerstone of management of TLS. In addition, it is critical to reduce the level of uric acid to decrease the likelihood of renal injury. Traditionally, this has been achieved with allopurinol, which blocks the metabolism of hypoxanthine and xanthine to uric acid by inhibiting xanthine oxidase. Since allopurinol does not affect existing uric acid concentrations, rasburicase (a recombinant *uric acid oxidase* given parenterally) is used for those with pre-existing hyperuricemia and will likely supplant allopurinol as the standard of care.

98. **Answer D.** Tooth fractures are classified by the Ellis system—type I is through the enamel and the tooth appears white; type II is through the dentin and the tooth appears yellow; and type III is through the pulp and the tooth has a spot of blood which reappears when wiped away. Tooth fractures should all be followed up by a dentist—the time of follow-up varies by type. Type I requires only routine follow-up within 1 week, and types II and III require either immediate dental consultation or next day follow-up. Calcium hydroxide paste may be placed on type II and III fractures to cover the exposed dentin and pulp.

99. **Answer B.** Posterior parapharyngeal space infections are more dangerous than anterior infections as they may encroach on the cervical sympathetic chain as well as the carotid artery and jugular vein. Patients with such infections may develop an ipsilateral Horner syndrome or cranial neuropathies of cranial nerves IX, X, XI, and XII. Jugular vein thrombosis may also occur along with erosion of the carotid artery, resulting in life-threatening hemorrhage or aneurysm formation. Involvement of the jugular vein may result in septic thrombophlebitis and a subsequent Lemierre syndrome, which is also known as postanginal septicemia. Patients with this problem present with symptoms of severe sepsis after their symptoms of pharyngitis have resolved. All deep space neck infections have the capability of causing such severe complications by virtue of their ability to extend to adjacent spaces resulting in a posterior parapharyngeal space infection. However, as the posterior pharyngeal space lies alongside the carotid sheath, infections in this area most commonly erode into the adjacent vasculature.

100. **Answer A.** Malaria is caused by the *Plasmodium* parasite, which is transmitted to humans through bites from the female *Anopheles* mosquito. *Plasmodium falciparum* has the capacity to cause severe systemic malaria, cerebral malaria, and blackwater fever, a syndrome of hemoglobinuria associated with chronic infection. Human-to-human transmission is rare and generally occurs only with blood transfusion or organ transplantation. Malaria is suspected in patients who travel to an endemic area and develop symptoms of fever, chills, headache, abdominal pain, nausea, and myalgias. Episodic fevers at a regular frequency is classic for malaria. Diagnosis involves thick blood smears to identify *Plasmodium* and thin smears to identify the specific organism. Treatment is with oral quinine plus doxycycline or intravenous quinidine.

TEST 4

QUESTIONS

1. A rash that starts on the wrists and ankles is typical in cases of:

   A. Meningococcemia
   B. Rubella (German measles)
   C. Rubeola (measles)
   D. Henoch–Schönlein purpura (HSP)
   E. Pityriasis rosea

2. What is the most common cause of immediate post-partum hemorrhage?

   A. Retained products of conception
   B. Vaginal or vulvar tears
   C. Uterine atony
   D. Placenta accrete
   E. Uterine rupture

3. A 1-week-old infant is brought to the emergency department (ED) with fast breathing, irritability, and poor feeding. Room air pulse oximetry is 88% and the patient appears to have decreased activity. His temperature is 99.8°F. Chest x-ray reveals a slightly enlarged heart with increased pulmonary consolidation. Lung examination reveals mild wheezes with good air exchange. Albuterol and oxygen are initiated. Which of the following medications is indicated?

   A. Prostaglandin
   B. Indomethacin
   C. Ribavirin
   D. Cefotaxime
   E. Propanolol

4. A 38-year-old pregnant woman presents to the ED with vaginal bleeding and abdominal pain radiating to the back. She is 25 weeks by dates and has had an uncomplicated pregnancy with routine prenatal care. She admits to smoking one pack of cigarettes per day and otherwise has no significant history. Her uterus is firm and tender on examination and there is bright red blood oozing from the cervical os. The most likely diagnosis is:

   A. Appendicitis
   B. Placenta previa
   C. Vasa previa
   D. Fibroid degeneration
   E. Abruptio placentae

5. A 7-year-old is diagnosed with appendicitis after returning to the ED a day after first presenting with abdominal pain. Missed cases of appendicitis are most often initially diagnosed as:

   A. Mesenteric adenitis
   B. Intussusception
   C. Gastroenteritis
   D. Inflammatory bowel disease
   E. Pancreatitis

6. A 24-year-old female presents to the ED with left facial pain. She had been diagnosed with right-sided trigeminal neuralgia 1 year ago and was started on carbamazepine. Although her symptoms resolved over several weeks, she is now complaining of similar symptoms on the left side of her face. In addition, she notes a history of mild right arm weakness and numbness several months ago that seems to have resolved without any intervention. Which of the following should be considered in this patient?

   A. Lyme disease
   B. Multiple sclerosis (MS)
   C. Guillain–Barre syndrome
   D. Myasthenia gravis (MG)
   E. Cerebellopontine angle tumor

7. A 59-year-old female with a history of sick sinus syndrome status post pacemaker placement presents to the ED with a chief complaint of dizziness and shortness of breath. Her vital signs are T 98.6, P 42, BP 96/48, and SaO_2 97% on RA. Her initial EKG demonstrates sinus bradycardia, with occasional ventricular escape beats. No pacer spikes are observed. After a magnet is applied to the patient's pacemaker, a repeat EKG demonstrates a paced rhythm at a rate of 70 beats per minute. Which of the following is the most likely cause of the patient's pacemaker dysfunction?

   A. Oversensing
   B. Impulse generation failure (failure to pace)
   C. Battery depletion
   D. Failure to sense
   E. Failure to capture

8. A 34-year-old male presents with chronic intermittent abdominal pain and constipation. His primary care physician and gastroenterologist gave him the diagnosis of irritable bowel syndrome. Which of the following is true regarding irritable bowel syndrome?

   A. It is associated with cancer of the jejunum
   B. Treatment often involves partial colectomy
   C. It is considered a mild subtype of schizophrenia
   D. Affirmation of the diagnosis and reassurance are effective
   E. Weight loss is a frequent finding

9. A 15-year-old previously healthy female is brought to the ED by her parents with a chief complaint of shortness of breath (SOB), palpitations, lightheadedness, and severe fatigue. The patient had been diagnosed with "a viral infection" by her pediatrician 5 days before presenting to the ED. While she initially seemed to improve, she complains of feeling SOB with a sense that her heart is "beating out of her chest" for the past day. Her parents noted she was breathing fast, and she appeared to be "winded" even when sitting down. Upon arrival, she is pale and ill-appearing, with vitals of T 98.6, P 143, RR 28, BP 105/70, and SaO_2 of 92% on RA. A chest x-ray demonstrates fluffy bilateral infiltrates. Her lung examination reveals tachypnea with increased work of breathing, and rales without wheezes. Which of the following is true of the patient's likely underlying problem?

   A. The patient's EKG will most likely reveal supraventricular tachycardia.

   B. An elevated MB isoenzyme of creatine kinase (CK-MB) helps to confirm the patient's diagnosis and direct therapy.
   C. Loop diuretics and inotropes may be helpful in her management.
   D. Two sets of blood cultures should be drawn and IV antibiotics, and aggressive IV fluids should be administered to treat a likely superimposed bacterial infection.
   E. Echocardiography will likely reveal previously undiagnosed congenital heart disease.

10. A 26-year-old previously healthy man is brought to the ED after being found unconscious outside a bar after having vomited on himself. He is drunk and afebrile, and his pulse oximetry reveals a saturation of 96%. His chest x-ray reveals a minimal right-sided streaky infiltrate (Fig. 4-1). Which of the following is true?

    A. The patient likely has a developing bacterial pneumonia and requires broad-spectrum antibiotics.
    B. The patient likely has a chemical pneumonitis caused by the aspiration of acidic gastric contents, which may later develop into pneumonia.
    C. Antibiotics should be started early in chemical pneumonitis to prevent the subsequent development of bacterial superinfection.
    D. Corticosteroids have been proven to be beneficial in patients such as these.
    E. This patient is probably suffering from a combination of chemical pneumonitis and bacterial infection.

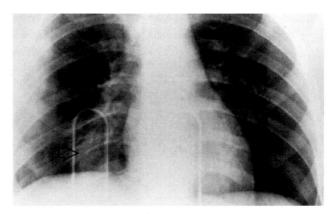

Figure 4-1

11. A 50-year-old male without past medical history presents with acute onset of cough, shortness of breath, and fever for 2 days. He has crackles in his left middle lung field and chest x-ray is shown in Figure 4-2. Which of the following is the most likely etiologic cause?

   A. *Streptococcus pneumoniae*
   B. *Haemophilus influenza*
   C. *Staphylococcus aureus*
   D. *Mycoplasma pneumoniae*
   E. *Klebsiella pneumoniae*

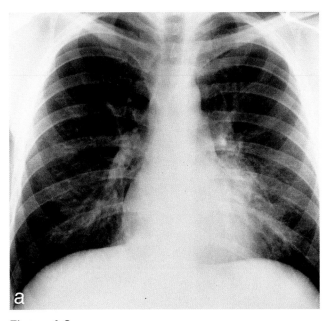

Figure 4-2

12. A 23-year-old female presents with fever, myalgias, and headache for 3 days. She then developed a rash, which started on her wrists and ankles and has now spread all over her body. The nonblanching rash is shown in Figure 4-3. Which of the following is the most likely etiology?

   A. *Rickettsia rickettsii*
   B. *Borrelia burgdorferi*
   C. Coxsackievirus
   D. *N. gonorrhoeae*
   E. *N. meningitidis*

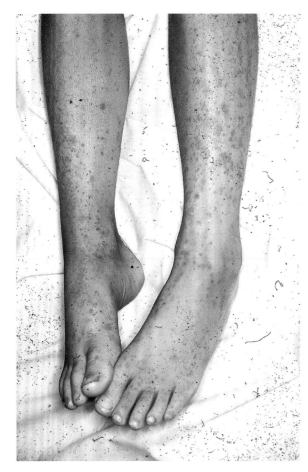

Figure 4-3

13. Physical examination of a patient with reactive arthritis (formerly known as Reiter syndrome) may be expected to reveal:

   A. Waxy plaques on the palms and soles
   B. Sausage-like swelling of the fingers
   C. Painful, shallow ulcers in the mouth
   D. Conjunctival injection
   E. All of the above

14. Which of the following x-ray findings is diagnostic for pulmonary embolism (PE)?

   A. Atelectasis
   B. Hampton hump (pleural wedge density)
   C. Elevated hemidiaphragm
   D. Westermark sign (oligemia)
   E. None of the above

15. Which of the following is the correct diagnosis of the injury shown in Figure 4-4?

A. Trigger finger

B. Mallet finger

C. Bennett fracture

D. Jersey finger

E. None of the above

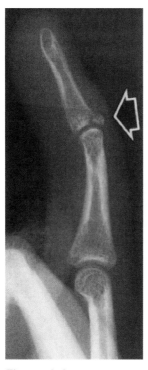

Figure 4-4

16. A 22-year-old female presents with a 3-day history of a severe sore throat and painful swallowing. She has a muffled voice, but no respiratory distress. Examination reveals "two-finger" trismus, an erythematous pharynx, swelling of the left anterior pillar, and uvular deviation to her right. Which of the following is true?

A. *Fusobacterium* species are the most commonly isolated organisms.

B. This patient requires urgent tonsillectomy.

C. Trismus is an uncommon finding that indicates extension of the infection to the deeper neck tissues.

D. Most of these infections are polymicrobial.

E. Absence of pus upon aspiration rules out the presence of an abscess.

17. The daughter of an 82-year-old female brings her mother in with a chief complaint of a "foreign body" in her vagina (see Fig. 4-5). The patient had reported the uncomfortable sensation of sitting on a ball and of something "falling out" of her vagina. Which of the following is the next best step in management?

A. Consultation with obstetrics and gynecology (OB-GYN) for immediate hysterectomy.

B. Discharge the patient with a prescription for metronidazole and an appointment with OB-GYN in 2 days.

C. Manually reduce the mass.

D. Incision and drainage of the mass.

E. None of the above.

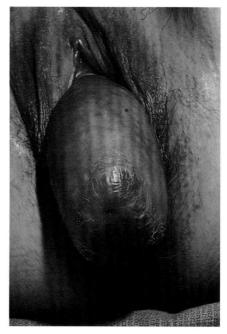

Figure 4-5

18. A 38-year-old female presents to the ED complaining of throat irritation and a 3-week history of an episodic spastic cough. The cough is worse at night and is occasionally so forceful that she vomits after she coughs. She is accompanied by her teenage son who has had a similar illness for 6 weeks without abating. She is a nonsmoker. What is the most likely cause of her illness?

A. *Corynebacterium diphtheriae*

B. *Legionella pneumophila*

C. *Bordetella pertussis*

D. *M. pneumoniae*

E. *S. pneumoniae*

19. Which of the following is true regarding prosthetic heart valves?

A. Bioprosthetic (porcine) valves require anticoagulation therapy with Coumadin.

B. Prophylactic anticoagulation should be maintained at international normalized ratios (INRs) between 1 and 2.

C. Chronic hemolysis occurs in most patients.

D. In patients with mechanical valves, auscultation of a metallic closure sound indicates serious valvular dysfunction.

E. Endocarditis develops in most patients.

20. A 11-year-old male presents after a motor vehicle collision. Primary survey is intact and vital signs are normal. Genitourinary examination is shown in Figure 4-6. Which of the following is the most appropriate next step in management?

A. Foley catheter placement
B. Retrograde urethrogram
C. Retrograde cystogram
D. Urinalysis
E. Aspiration of the corpora cavernosa

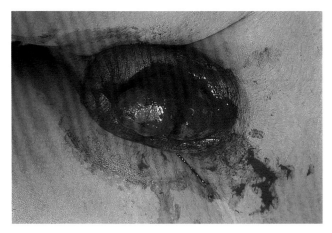

Figure 4-6

21. Which of the following is true regarding transverse myelitis?

A. Older adults represent the majority of cases
B. Cerebrospinal fluid (CSF) glucose is usually elevated
C. Albuminocytologic dissociation is usually present
D. Bilateral clinical findings are common
E. Cord compressive lesion is evident

22. Which of the following is the average duration of a typical generalized tonic–clonic seizure?

A. 15 seconds
B. 30 seconds
C. 1 minute
D. 2 minutes
E. 3 minutes

23. Which of the following routes of administration causes the fastest onset of action of cocaine?

A. Intranasal
B. Sublingual
C. Oral
D. Inhalation
E. Transdermal

24. While working in the ED, a paramedic calls from emergency medical services (EMS) to provide a mass casualty alert from a local stadium. Many fans watching a basketball game in a small arena became suddenly ill, and several slumped to the ground and either lost consciousness or seemed to be "convulsing." The building was rapidly evacuated. Ambulatory evacuees complained of severe headache, diaphoresis, excessive "spit" and runny nose, as well as shortness of breath with a frothy cough, nausea, vomiting, and muscle aches. Though several survivors noted a "mist" coming from some of the vents inside the building, there was no significant odor noted. In addition to high-flow oxygen, which of the following is the best course of treatment among survivors?

A. Pralidoxime (PM) and atropine
B. Amyl nitrite
C. Sodium thiosulfate and sodium nitrite
D. Diazepam and atropine
E. Succinylcholine and etomidate for rapid sequence intubation

25. In which of the following hematologic malignancies is a hyperviscosity syndrome (leukostasis) due to elevated numbers of WBCs most likely to occur?

A. Acute lymphoblastic leukemia (ALL)
B. Chronic myelogenous leukemia (CML)
C. Non-Hodgkin lymphoma
D. Acute myelogenous leukemia (AML)
E. Chronic lymphocytic leukemia (CLL)

26. Which of the following is true regarding interpersonal violence and intimate partner abuse (IPA)?

A. Most violence against women is perpetrated by strangers.
B. Most of the violence against men is perpetrated by intimate partners.
C. Less than 1% of all men report an incident of IPA.
D. Victim substance abuse contributes to IPA.
E. Most patients will not report IPA unless directly asked.

27. A 42-year-old male presented for evaluation of posterior shoulder pain after a fall backward from a ladder. X-rays reveal a scapular fracture. Which of the following is true?

A. Associated thoracic injury is usually more serious than the fracture itself.
B. Operative repair is usually required.
C. Avascular necrosis of the humeral head is a common complication.
D. The arm is usually held in full abduction at presentation.
E. Associated contralateral scapular fracture is common.

28. Among close contacts of a patient diagnosed with meningitis caused by *Neisseria meningitidis,* what is the approximate likelihood of transmission *without* prophylactic antibiotic therapy?

    A. <1%
    B. 5%
    C. 25%
    D. 50%
    E. 90%

29. When evaluating and managing patients with unstable pelvic fractures, pelvic binders:

    A. Should never be used
    B. Should be applied over the bilateral greater trochanters extending above the umbilicus
    C. Help to control arterial bleeding
    D. Are as effective as external fixation in controlling bleeding
    E. Have more complications than military antishock trousers

30. Which of the following is the most characteristic finding on funduscopic examination for central retinal artery occlusion?

    A. Pale gray retina with cherry red fovea
    B. Cloudy cornea with mid-dilated pupil
    C. Disc edema with tortuous veins
    D. Reddish haze with black reflex
    E. Grayish-green subretinal membrane

31. Which of the following is true regarding isopropanol poisoning?

    A. Blood urea nitrogen (BUN) may be falsely elevated.
    B. Ketosis without acidosis is the characteristic lab abnormality.
    C. Elevated anion gap is seen in most patients.
    D. Ocular accumulation causing blindness is the typical pathophysiologic finding.
    E. Fomepizole should be administered empirically in patients with high suspicion of isopropanol poisoning.

32. A 28-year-old male presents with an acute, progressively worsening headache and fever for 1 day. Physical examination reveals a toxic-appearing, slightly confused patient with fever and meningismus. Which of the following is the most appropriate next step in management?

    A. CT brain without contrast
    B. CT brain with contrast
    C. Lumbar puncture
    D. Ceftriaxone and vancomycin
    E. Ceftriaxone, vancomycin, and dexamethasone

33. Which of the following is true regarding control of hypertension and stroke?

    A. Patients with both ischemic and hemorrhagic strokes should have their BP reduced to an SBP of 140 to 160 mm Hg or prestroke levels.
    B. BP should not be controlled in any stroke patient unless the patient is a candidate for tissue plasminogen activator (tPA).
    C. Only patients with ischemic infarcts should have their BP reduced to a target SBP of 140 to 160 mm Hg or prestroke levels.
    D. Only patients with intracerebral hemorrhage should have their BP reduced to a target SBP of 140 to 160 mm Hg or prestroke levels.
    E. All stroke patients who experience clinical deterioration in the ED should have emergent BP control to a target SBP of 140 to 160 mm Hg or prestroke levels.

34. A 34-year-old male with AIDS presents with cough, malaise, and exertional dyspnea for 8 days. He stopped his highly active antiretroviral therapy several weeks prior due to side effects. His vital signs are 100.4°F, 95, 22, 165/85, 95% RA. Chest radiography shows an interstitial pneumonia pattern. Which of the following is the most appropriate treatment?

    A. Clindamycin
    B. Trimethoprim–sulfamethoxazole
    C. Doxycycline
    D. Piperacillin–tazobactam
    E. Primaquine

35. Upon starting your shift, you receive sign-out on a 46-year-old male diabetic patient who is being treated with an intravenous insulin drip for diabetic ketoacidosis (DKA). Two hours later, a repeat chemistry panel reveals the following: Na^+ 141 mEq/L, Cl^- 112 mEq/L, HCO_3^- 17 mEq/L, blood urea nitrogen (BUN) 16 mg/dL, creatinine 0.9 mg/dL, glucose 278 mg/dL. Which of the following is true?

    A. The patient has a mixed high anion gap (AG) ketoacidosis and nonanion gap hyperchloremic metabolic acidosis (HCMA).
    B. He should be given subcutaneous insulin and his insulin infusion can be discontinued after 30 to 60 minutes.
    C. His DKA is not yet resolved and he requires an ongoing intravenous insulin infusion.
    D. The patient should be given bicarbonate replacement therapy.
    E. A repeat arterial blood gas (ABG) should be performed to guide further therapy.

36. A 4-year-old male presents with progressive periorbital edema, weight gain, anorexia, and nausea for several weeks. Hypertension is noted on physical examination. Urinalysis demonstrates 4+ protein. Which of the following is most likely to be present in this patient?

    A. Hyperalbuminemia
    B. Thrombophilia
    C. Hypotriglyceridemia
    D. Urinary bacteria
    E. Gross hematuria

37. A 12-year-old female is brought in by EMS after a gunshot wound. The patient was injured incidentally when her older brother was "showing off" his gun to his friends. She presents with two soft-tissue wounds to her right leg, with significant swelling about the right knee. An x-ray demonstrates a small amount of shrapnel, and a small fracture to the distal cortex of her femur. Clinically, there is expanding, nonpulsatile, swelling in the area of the knee. Which of the following is the next best step?

    A. Take her to the operating room (OR) for vascular repair
    B. CT angiography of the leg
    C. Take her to the OR for open reduction and internal fixation of her femur
    D. Ultrasound of the leg
    E. Angiography of the leg

38. A 22-year-old female presents after a drug overdose in a suicide attempt. She states she took 60 of her fluoxetine tablets 2 hours before presentation. She is asymptomatic, awake, and alert, and vital signs and physical examination are normal. Which of the following is true regarding this patient?

    A. Death from dysrhythmia is the most likely outcome.
    B. Ipecac is indicated to prevent gastric absorption.
    C. Cyproheptadine has not been proven to improve outcomes.
    D. Sodium bicarbonate should be used for ventricular dysrhythmias.
    E. Hemodialysis may be helpful in massive overdose.

39. What is the primary risk factor for uterine rupture among pregnant women?

    A. Vaginal delivery after a prior cesarean-section
    B. Diabetes
    C. Large for gestational age fetus
    D. Prolonged use of oxytocin
    E. Maternal collagen vascular disease

40. A 75-year-old male with a history of atrial fibrillation presents with fatigue, nausea, and halos in his vision. He states that he has been depressed lately and took some pills in an effort to commit suicide. The serum digoxin level is elevated. Which of the following is an indication to administer digitalis antibody (Fab) fragments?

    A. Atrial fibrillation with ventricular rate of 120
    B. Potassium level of 6 mEq/L
    C. Digoxin level of 3 ng/mL
    D. Total digoxin ingestion of 3 mg
    E. Magnesium level of 3 mEq/L

41. A 5-year-old male presents with bloody diarrhea for several days, associated with fatigue, pallor, and malaise. Several kids at school have similar complaints. Blood tests at his pediatrician's office demonstrate severe anemia, thrombocytopenia, and renal insufficiency. Which of the following is the most likely cause?

    A. *Shigella*
    B. *Salmonella*
    C. *Escherichia coli*
    D. Rotavirus
    E. Child abuse

42. A 52-year-old male presents with acute, right-sided flank pain. He has a history of kidney stones and states that he feels this is the same kind of pain. You confirm the diagnosis of a 3-mm, distal ureteral stone with CT imaging. His vital signs, physical examination, urinalysis, and creatinine are all normal. His pain is under control after parenteral analgesics. Which of the following is the most important next step in management?

    A. Discharge home with instructions to drink 10 L of water per day to "flush out" the stone
    B. Discharge home with instructions to take ibuprofen 600 mg every 6 hours as needed for pain
    C. Discharge home with instructions to take clonidine 0.1 mg three times a day
    D. Consult urologist in ED for consideration of lithotripsy
    E. Admit to the hospital for next-day urologic consultation

TEST 4

43. An 18-year old male presents with the rash shown (see Fig. 4-7). Which of the following substances is the likely trigger?

    A. Arsenic
    B. Brass
    C. Nickel
    D. Dermatium
    E. *Rhus* species

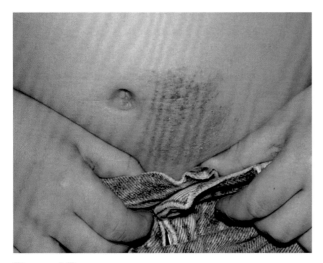

Figure 4-7

44. The amount of time after which a limb exposed to ischemia at room temperature ("warm ischemia") begins to develop irreversible damage is:

    A. 1 hour
    B. 3 hours
    C. 6 hours
    D. 12 hours
    E. 24 hours

45. A 62-year-old male is being transported to the hospital by EMS with a chief complaint of chest pain and shortness of breath. After placing the patient on oxygen and giving aspirin and sublingual nitroglycerin, the EMS providers transmit the initial 12-lead EKG, which is shown in Figure 4-8. Which of the following is the most appropriate next step upon EMS arrival?

    A. Prepare the catheterization laboratory's ST-elevation myocardial infarction (STEMI) team for immediate cardiac catheterization.
    B. Start a nitroglycerin drip to be titrated until the patient is pain-free, and give a loading dose of low–molecular-weight heparin.
    C. Start a nitroglycerin drip, and give a loading dose of clopidogrel, and a loading dose of low–molecular-weight heparin.
    D. Start a nitroglycerin drip, and give 25 mg of oral metoprolol, and a loading dose of low–molecular-weight heparin.
    E. Place nitroglycerin paste on the patient's chest, and give a loading dose of clopidogrel, oral metoprolol, and a loading dose of low–molecular-weight heparin.

46. In patients with a peritonsillar abscess (PTA), the area of greatest fluctuance is most commonly:

    A. Superior to the tonsil
    B. Lateral to the tonsil
    C. Inferior to the tonsil
    D. Within the tonsil itself
    E. None of the above

47. Which of the following is the most common complication of mitral stenosis (MS)?

    A. Atrial fibrillation
    B. Endocarditis
    C. Congestive heart failure
    D. Myocardial infarction (MI)
    E. Pneumonia

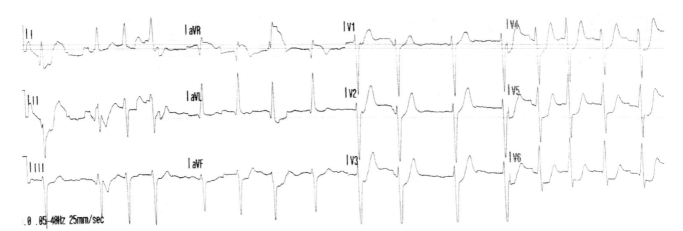

Figure 4-8

48. A 65-year-old female presents with the rash shown (Fig. 4-9). Which of the following is the best treatment plan?

   A. Supportive care
   B. Trimethoprim–sulfamethoxazole plus cephalexin
   C. Valacyclovir
   D. Acyclovir plus prednisone
   E. Acyclovir plus amitriptyline

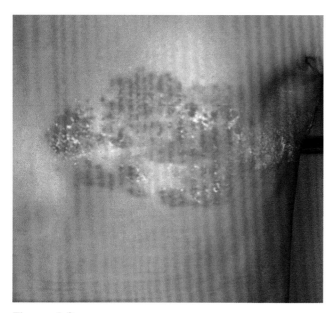

Figure 4-9

49. A patient presents with new-onset psychosis. Which of the following suggests a medical, rather than a psychiatric, cause for the symptoms?

   A. Auditory hallucinations
   B. Age <35
   C. Gradual onset
   D. Aphasia
   E. Flat affect

50. Which of the following describes the appropriate means of examining the pelvis in a trauma patient?

   A. Anterior–posterior compression over the symphysis pubis
   B. Superior and posterior force applied to the bilateral anterior–superior iliac spine (ASIS) to "rock" the pelvis back and forth
   C. Lateral compression of the iliac wings
   D. Palpate the bilateral ASIS and "open" the pelvis like a book
   E. All of the above

51. A 25-year-old female presents to the ED with worsening left-sided pelvic pain and vaginal discharge. She states that she was seen in the office by her primary care doctor 3 days ago for similar problems, received an injection of an antibiotic, and was given a prescription that she has not had a chance to fill. In the ED, she has a fever, purulent vaginal discharge, cervical motion tenderness, and a palpable, tender left-sided adnexal mass. Which of the following is true?

   A. She has Fitz–Hugh–Curtis syndrome.
   B. Aspiration and culture of the mass is likely to reveal *Neisseria gonorrhoeae.*
   C. If untreated, rupture of the mass and secondary peritonitis may occur.
   D. The patient should be kept NPO for emergent surgery.
   E. The patient most likely has a hemorrhagic ovarian cyst.

52. Which of the following is the most appropriate medication to induce rapid, measured reduction of blood pressure in hypertensive crises?

   A. Nifedipine
   B. Isoproterenol
   C. Phenoxybenzamine
   D. Nitroprusside
   E. Hydrochlorothiazide

53. An 8-year-old male restrained back-seat passenger is brought to the ED after a car accident. He was wearing a lap belt only when the car in which he was riding was struck in a front-end collision with another vehicle at high speed. The restraint puts him at increased risk for which of the following injuries?

   A. Jejunal perforation
   B. Chance fracture of the lumbar spine
   C. Abdominal wall contusion
   D. Pancreas hematoma
   E. All of the above

54. The most common cause of acute mesenteric ischemia is:

   A. Thrombosis in the superior mesenteric artery (SMA).
   B. Mesenteric vein thrombosis.
   C. Nonocclusive mesenteric vascular disease.
   D. SMA embolism.
   E. Abdominal aortic aneurysm involving the SMA.

55. A 44-year-old female presents with the rash shown (see Fig. 4-10). Which of the following is true regarding this diagnosis?

    A. Therapy instituted later than 72 hours after symptoms onset is of uncertain benefit
    B. Gabapentin is an effective treatment adjunct
    C. Pain occurring after the initial episode is seen in two-thirds of patients
    D. Abscess drainage should be performed after the second week of illness
    E. Laboratory testing should be performed to determine microbial load

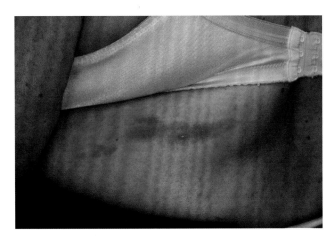

Figure 4-10

56. Which of the following is the most common relationship of the caregiver to the victim in Munchausen syndrome by proxy?

    A. Biologic father
    B. Stepfather
    C. Biologic mother
    D. Stepmother
    E. Nonparent guardian

57. The most common complication of peptic ulcer disease (PUD) is:

    A. Perforation
    B. Gastric adenocarcinoma
    C. Gastrointestinal bleeding
    D. Obstruction
    E. Penetration into an adjacent organ

58. A 6-year-old female is brought to the emergency room by her mother, who is concerned that she is being touched inappropriately by her ex-husband. The patient told her mother "daddy showed me how babies are made." Which of the following examination findings is most concerning for sexual assault?

    A. Annular hymen
    B. Anal fissure
    C. Complete transection of the hymen

D. Suprapubic tenderness
E. Hymenal bump

59. A 63-year-old male with a history of multiple myeloma presents with acute onset of generalized weakness, blurry vision, diffuse mucosal bleeding, and headache. A complete blood count and comprehensive chemistry panel is sent, but the laboratory is unable to perform the analysis, citing "inappropriate blood sample." Which of the following is the most appropriate definitive management?

    A. Hemodialysis
    B. Plasmapheresis
    C. Platelet transfusion
    D. Packed red blood cell (RBC) transfusion
    E. Erythropoietin

60. Which of the following best supports a diagnosis of pertussis in a child with cough?

    A. Pneumonia on chest x-ray
    B. Eosinophilia
    C. Prolonged course
    D. Age older than 7 years
    E. Fever >102°F

61. Which of the following is more characteristic of a subdural hematoma than an epidural hematoma?

    A. Lucid interval
    B. Coma
    C. Focal neurologic deficits
    D. Increased intracranial pressure
    E. Delayed presentation

62. A 28-year-old pregnant woman at 15 weeks presents to the ED in mid-summer with generalized malaise along with a high fever, headache, myalgias that are worse in her calves, and a rash. The rash, which started on her wrists and ankles, is petechial, and is somewhat diffuse, including her palms. She returned from visiting relatives who live in North Carolina approximately 4 days ago. Which of the following is the next best step in management?

    A. Doxycycline 100 mg IV
    B. Ciprofloxacin 500 mg IV
    C. Chloramphenicol (CAM) 500 mg IV
    D. Penicillin V 500 mg IV
    E. Gentamicin 1.5 mg/kg IV

63. Which of the following is true regarding acalculous cholecystitis?

    A. It tends to be diagnosed earlier in the disease course than calculous cholecystitis.
    B. It represents half of all cases of acute cholecystitis.
    C. It is most common in patients with hemolytic anemia.
    D. It responds to oral ursodeoxycholic acid therapy.
    E. It tends to have a more benign course than calculous cholecystitis.

64. Which of the following is rightly matched with the cause of visual loss?

    A. Cloudy vision with floaters due to vitreous hemorrhage
    B. Sudden painless loss of vision due to central retinal artery occlusion
    C. Pupil that dilates in swinging flashlight test and optic neuritis
    D. Curtain-like veil due to retinal detachment
    E. All of the above

65. After physiologic jaundice of the newborn (icterus neonatorum), which of the following is the most common cause of neonatal jaundice?

    A. Breast milk jaundice
    B. Cephalohematoma
    C. Sickle cell anemia
    D. Gilbert syndrome
    E. Biliary atresia

66. Which of the following is true regarding hypokalemia?

    A. Patients with a recent myocardial infarction (MI) are at increased risk for ventricular arrhythmias if the potassium concentration is less than 4.0 mEq/L.
    B. The presence of U waves and ST-segment depression on electrocardiograms (EKGs) correlates with the severity of hypokalemia.
    C. Neurologic problems are the most common manifestations of hypokalemia.
    D. Vomiting or nasogastric suctioning may lead to profound hypokalemia.
    E. Potassium is the most prominent extracellular cation.

67. You suspect that a lumbar puncture you performed to evaluate for subarachnoid hemorrhage (SAH) is a "traumatic tap." Which of the following CSF findings is most reliable for differentiating SAH from a traumatic lumbar puncture?

    A. A relative CSF leukocytosis will be present in cases of SAH.
    B. The presence of xanthochromia indicates SAH.
    C. A twofold or greater decrease in the number of RBCs from tube 1 to tube 4 is always due to a traumatic tap.
    D. A positive CSF clotting assay is consistent with a traumatic tap.
    E. All of the above are equally useful.

68. An otherwise healthy 12-year-old male is brought to the ED with a chief complaint of chest pain. The patient has been complaining of the pain over the past week. Which of the following is true?

    A. The friction rub of pericarditis is best heard when patients are lying supine.
    B. Cardiac causes of chest pain more commonly occur in the setting of exertion.
    C. In pediatric patients, myocardial infarction is most common in females.
    D. On physical examination, only diastolic murmurs are cause for concern of an underlying cardiac problem.
    E. Valve disorders are the most common cardiac causes of pediatric chest pain.

69. A 43-year-old otherwise healthy male presents with signs and symptoms of pneumonia. Antibiotics are ordered and the patient is admitted. An admission electrocardiogram (EKG) is ordered and is shown in Figure 4-11. Which of the following is most likely?

    A. The limb leads have been reversed.
    B. The patient is experiencing demand-ischemia and needs an emergent heart catheterization.
    C. An echocardiogram would likely reveal significant underlying structural heart disease.
    D. The patient has an increased risk for sudden cardiac death.
    E. The patient's calcium level is profoundly decreased.

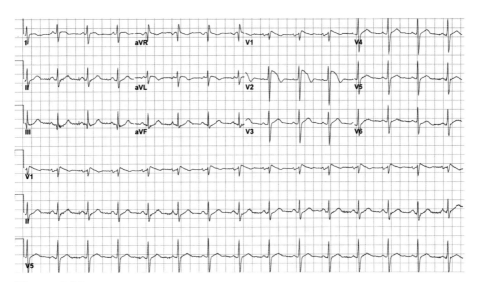

Figure 4-11

70. A 54-year-old male with a history of diabetes presents with 3 days of a slight red but extremely painful left lower extremity. He appears fatigued and ill. His vital signs are: 100.0, 122, 20, 100/70, 99% RA. The affected leg is swollen, warm, and only mildly erythematous. He has exquisite tenderness in the area. Strongly suspect necrotizing fasciitis. Which the following tests would be most helpful in evaluating that diagnosis?

    A. Platelets
    B. Potassium level
    C. C-reactive protein
    D. Procalcitonin
    E. Serum mycoplasma antigen

71. A 15-year-old male presents with progressively worsening groin and scrotal pain and swelling over the last 8 hours. He noticed a bulge in his scrotum the day before when he lifted a heavy object. Physical examination demonstrates an afebrile patient with moderate abdominal tenderness and fullness, with bowel sounds present in his right hemiscrotum. The testes are not tender or enlarged. Which of the following is the most appropriate next step in management?

    A. Ice pack to the groin and an attempt to reduce the mass
    B. Immediate operative reduction
    C. Outpatient urology referral
    D. Oral hydration
    E. Urinalysis

72. Which of the following is the most common risk factor associated with aortic dissection?

    A. Smoking
    B. Atherosclerosis
    C. Marfan syndrome
    D. Hypertension
    E. Bicuspid aortic valve

73. A 26-year-old previously healthy male construction worker is brought in by EMS after he fell approximately 20 feet while painting. He did not lose consciousness, but he complains of severe back and pelvic pain. His initial vital signs are HR 136, BP 86/46, RR 22, SaO_2 100% on a nonrebreather mask. Physical examination reveals multiple ecchymoses and abrasions over the low back, buttocks, and pelvis with an unstable pelvis on gentle lateral compression. Focused assessment with sonography for trauma (FAST) examination is negative. Pelvic x-ray reveals displaced fractures of the left anterior and posterior hemipelvis. Which of the following is the next best step?

    A. CT abdomen and pelvis
    B. Take to the OR for explorative laparotomy
    C. External fixation
    D. Endotracheal intubation
    E. Angiography for embolization

74. A 20-year-old male presents with a painful, ulcerated lesion on his penis. He noticed it 3 days before and the pain became progressively worse. Examination shows a tender, 1-cm ulcerated lesion at the base of his penis with a single, large, tender inguinal lymph node. Gram stain of the ulcer shows gram-negative bacilli. Which of the following is the most likely cause?

    A. Herpes simplex virus (HSV)
    B. *Chlamydia trachomatis*
    C. *Staphylococcus epidermidis*
    D. *Haemophilus ducreyi*
    E. *Treponema pallidum*

75. Which of the following has the greatest immediate effect on preload in the management of acute congestive heart failure (CHF)?

    A. Morphine
    B. Enalaprilat
    C. Digoxin
    D. Furosemide
    E. Nitroglycerin

76. Which of the following is characteristic of facial pain due to trigeminal neuralgia?

    A. It is most commonly bilateral.
    B. Attacks last for an average of 30 minutes.
    C. Patients demonstrate partial facial nerve palsy on examination.
    D. It most commonly involves the V2 and V3 branches of the trigeminal nerve.
    E. Most patients have concomitant dental disease.

77. Which of the following is the most commonly injured abdominal organ in pediatric blunt trauma?

    A. Liver
    B. Spleen
    C. Kidney
    D. Small intestine
    E. Large intestine

78. A 52-year-old female presents with right upper quadrant pain and fever for 2 days. The pain is unaffected by eating, but she states that it hurts to breathe and cough. Vital signs are 102.5°F, 110, 20, 165/92, 100% RA. She appears fatigued and in some pain. She does not have jaundice. Her lungs are clear. She has definite right upper quadrant tenderness without a positive Murphy sign. Chest radiography is normal. You order a right upper quadrant ultrasound, which shows a normal gall bladder, but a large, cavitary, fluid-filled lesion in her right hepatic lobe. Which of the following is the most likely etiology?

    A. Sterile inflammation
    B. *Entamoeba histolytica*
    C. *Streptococci*

D. *Candida*

E. Polymicrobial

79. Which of the following is the most common complication of acute sinusitis?

A. Maxillary cellulitis

B. Cavernous sinus thrombosis

C. Meningitis

D. Preseptal cellulitis

E. Orbital cellulitis

80. A 42-year-old female presents with progressive lower extremity numbness and weakness over several days. Her physical examination is remarkable for areflexia and weakness in her lower extremities. Which of the following findings is most likely to be present in this patient?

A. CSF with high leukocytes

B. CSF with high protein

C. Marked asymmetric weakness

D. Fever >102°F

E. Severe bowel or bladder dysfunction

81. Which of the following is true about acute diarrheal illnesses due to *Shigella* spp.?

A. Antimotility agents such as diphenoxylate are useful as monotherapy in patients with shigellosis.

B. Compared to infection with *Salmonella* spp., infection with *Shigella* spp. requires an unusually large inoculum.

C. Colicky abdominal pain with high fever and diarrhea is the most common presentation.

D. The treatment of choice is trimethoprim–sulfamethoxazole.

E. Fecal leukocytes are only rarely detected in patients with shigellosis.

82. A 64-year-old female presents with paresthesias in her hands and feet for the last few weeks. She is concerned that she has diabetes. She denies any past medical history. Physical examination reveals decreased vibratory sensation and proprioception in her hands and feet. Laboratory data demonstrate a normal glucose and macrocytic anemia. Which of the following is most likely to be present on further patient history?

A. Smoking history

B. Chronic aspirin use

C. Strict vegetarian diet

D. Chronic melena

E. Family history of thalassemia

83. Which of the following is true regarding acute salicylate toxicity?

A. Treatment should be instituted in strict accordance with the Done nomogram.

B. Initial symptoms of toxicity are tinnitus and altered hearing.

C. Metabolic alkalosis is characteristic.

D. Significant bleeding through the gastrointestinal (GI) tract is present in most patients.

E. Life-threatening hyperkalemia may occur.

84. A 19-year-old Mexican female with no past medical history is brought in to the emergency room after a witnessed generalized seizure. Head CT reveals a round brain mass. The most likely culprit is:

A. *Trypanosoma cruzi*

B. *Taenia solium*

C. *Taenia saginata*

D. *Trichuris trichiura*

E. *Leishmania braziliensis*

85. A 68-year-old male presents with headache and "acting like a jerk," according to the nursing staff. He has no reported past medical history and his family who are with him state that his personality is completely different from his usual pleasant one. Physical examination demonstrates an irritable man complaining loudly of a headache with altered attention, not oriented to place or time, and lacking in meningeal signs. His vital signs are: 100.2, 82, 20, 143/92, and 99% on RA. His urinalysis and chest x-ray are normal. Which of the following represents the next best step in management?

A. Discharge home with close outpatient follow-up

B. Empiric dexamethasone therapy

C. Chemical restraint with IV haloperidol

D. Empiric acyclovir therapy

E. MRI brain with contrast

86. The synovial white blood cell (WBC) count in cases of septic arthritis usually exceeds at least:

A. 250 per mm^3

B. 1,000 per mm^3

C. 25,000 per mm^3

D. 50,000 per mm^3

E. 100,000 per mm^3

87. A 34-year-old male presents with skin lesions shown (see Fig. 4-12). Which of the following is the most likely cause?

    A. *Mycoplasma pneumoniae*
    B. HSV
    C. HIV
    D. HPV
    E. HHV-3

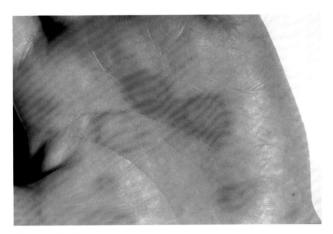

Figure 4-12

88. A 62-year-old male with a history of controlled hypertension presents to the ED with fever, headache, and vomiting. He is mildly somnolent on examination and has evidence of mild neck stiffness. Suspecting meningitis as the cause of his symptoms, which of the following empiric regimens should you start?

    A. Ceftriaxone, vancomycin
    B. Ceftriaxone, ampicillin
    C. Ceftriaxone, ampicillin, dexamethasone
    D. Ceftriaxone, vancomycin, ampicillin, dexamethasone
    E. Ceftriaxone, amphotericin, vancomycin, dexamethasone

89. A 55-year-old male is brought by his wife for confusion, memory loss, and impaired balance over the past several weeks. The patient's wife was concerned about a stroke, so she consulted the primary care physician, who ordered an outpatient noncontrast CT brain, which was normal. On examination, he has mild memory loss to recent events, nystagmus, and a wide-based gait. He has no focal weakness or altered sensation, and his cranial nerves, finger-to-nose, and heel-to-shin tests are normal.

Which of the following is most likely to reveal the cause of his symptoms?

    A. CT brain with IV contrast
    B. EEG
    C. Social history
    D. Cerebrospinal fluid (CSF) analysis
    E. Orthostatic vital signs

90. Which of the following tissues has the greatest resistance to electrical flow?

    A. Nerves
    B. Blood
    C. Fat
    D. Skin
    E. Muscle

91. A 67-year-old female with coronary artery disease (CAD) presents with dyspnea, which is her last anginal equivalent. She is known to have a pre-existing left bundle branch block. Which of the following EKG findings, when present in two contiguous leads, indicates the highest risk for acute MI?

    A. 4 mm of discordant ST elevation
    B. 4 mm of concordant ST elevation
    C. 2 mm of ST depression
    D. Tall T waves
    E. Inverted T waves

92. A 22-year-old female at 36 weeks of gestation is being treated with magnesium sulfate for pre-eclampsia while awaiting transfer to a nearby hospital for definitive management. Upon reevaluating the patient, you find her to be quite somnolent with markedly decreased deep tendon reflexes and a decreased respiratory rate. After managing the airway, the next best step in management is intravenous:

    A. Dexamethasone
    B. Lidocaine
    C. Labetalol
    D. Calcium gluconate
    E. Atropine

93. A 44-year-old male presents with chest pain after a motor vehicle collision. He receives an upright chest x-ray, which is shown in Figure 4-13. Which of the following is the most likely diagnosis?

    A. Pneumothorax
    B. Hemothorax
    C. Pulmonary contusion
    D. Traumatic aortic rupture
    E. Cardiac contusion

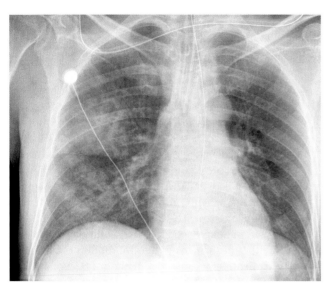

Figure 4-13

94. Which of the following elements is present in the new quick Sepsis-related Organ Function Assessment (qSOFA) score that may replace systemic inflammatory response syndrome (SIRS) criteria?

    A. Systolic blood pressure <100 mm Hg
    B. Glucose >100 mg/dL
    C. Temperature >99.0°F
    D. Hemoglobin >15 mg/dL
    E. Heart rate >90

95. Retrobulbar hemorrhage can result in what devastating complication?

    A. Corneal abrasion
    B. Hypopyon
    C. Central retinal artery occlusion (CRAO)
    D. Hyphema
    E. Corneal ulcer

96. A 45-year-old male presents with progressive scrotal pain for 3 days. He denies any swelling in the area, but reports mild dysuria. Physical examination demonstrates tenderness in the epididymis, normal descended testes, and normal bilateral cremasteric reflexes. Which of the following is the most likely cause of the symptoms?

    A. *Chlamydia*
    B. *Neisseria gonorrhoeae*
    C. *Escherichia coli*
    D. Chemical epididymitis
    E. Testicular torsion

97. The combination of ceftriaxone and azithromycin is a common dual-antibiotic regimen used in the empiric treatment of community-acquired pneumonia. For which of the following organisms is azithromycin included?

    A. *Haemophilus influenzae*
    B. *Staphylococcus aureus*
    C. *Legionella pneumophila*
    D. *Streptococcus pneumoniae*
    E. *Moraxella catarrhalis*

98. A 25-year-old female with a history of acne on doxycycline presents with several weeks of intermittent, diffuse, gradual onset headaches with occasional blurry vision episodes. She has had no fever. The week prior, she saw her primary care physician, who diagnosed her with migraines after obtaining a normal CT brain, with and without IV contrast. The patient complains that her migraine medicines have had only minimal effect on her headaches. Vital signs are 98.6°F, 82, 16, 110/70, 99% RA. Physical examination reveals an obese woman in no acute distress with a completely normal neurologic examination. Which of the following is the next best step in management?

    A. Repeat CT brain with IV contrast
    B. MRI brain
    C. Lumbar puncture
    D. EEG
    E. Psychiatry consultation

99. A 57-year-old male with a history of alcoholism and esophageal varices presents after two episodes of bloody emesis. Which of the following is true?

    A. The patient can be discharged if he has a negative nasogastric (NG) tube lavage, stable vital signs, and a normal initial hemoglobin level
    B. Antibiotics have no proven benefit
    C. IV fluids should be given cautiously to avoid overdilution of hemoglobin
    D. Patients requiring a transfusion should receive blood products to achieve a hemoglobin ≥10 g/dL
    E. Intravenous proton pump inhibitors and somatostatin analogues may be helpful

100. Which of the following is true regarding appendicitis?

    A. Nearly all patients with appendicitis younger than 3 years have evidence of perforation at the time of appendectomy.
    B. Most patients younger than 2 years have diffuse abdominal tenderness.
    C. An appendicolith is only seen in approximately 15% of cases.
    D. CT scan has better sensitivity and specificity than ultrasound.
    E. All of the above

TEST 4

ANSWERS AND EXPLANATIONS

1. Answer A. Roughly 70% of patients with meningococcemia have a rash which usually begins as petechiae of the wrists and ankles. However, the rash may also be composed of light pink macules that become petechial later in the disease course. Petechial lesions may have a "smudged" appearance although purpura may have a "gun-metal gray" center. Rubella and rubeola are maculopapular eruptions that tend to begin on the face and spread inferiorly. HSP is a vasculitis that is characterized by palpable purpura on the buttocks and lower extremities. Pityriasis rosea is a benign, self-limited rash characterized by patches and plaques that typically occur on the trunk.

2. Answer C. Uterine atony is the most common cause of immediate postpartum hemorrhage (defined as blood loss that occurs within the first 24 hours of delivery), as it is responsible for approximately 50% of cases. The risk factors for uterine atony are multiparity, prolonged labor, excessive uterine manipulation, and general anesthesia with halogenated anesthetic agents. Management involves abdominal or bimanual uterine massage as well as the use of oxytocic agents such as oxytocin, methylergonovine maleate or ergonovine maleate, or carboprost tromethamine. Tears of the maternal birth canal may also result in significant hemorrhage and are the second most common cause (as a group). Retained placental tissue accounts for roughly 10% of immediate postpartum hemorrhage. If uterine massage and oxytocic agents fail to control bleeding thought to be due to uterine atony, a meticulous search should be conducted for maternal birth trauma or retained placental tissue.

3. Answer D. Neonates with significant vital sign abnormalities, including fever or hypoxia, should be suspected of having a serious bacterial infection until proved otherwise. Even patients who exhibit strong signs of congenital heart disease should receive antibiotics and an evaluation for septic cause of the clinical findings. Cefotaxime and ampicillin are indicated for treatment of the most common pathogens in the neonatal period, Group B *streptococci*, gram-negative bacilli, pneumococcus, and *Listeria*. In the absence of a patient *in extremis,* therapy that affects ductus arteriosus patency such as indomethacin or prostaglandin should not be given until the exact congenital heart defect can be determined. Albuterol is indicated for reactive airways disease, and ribavirin is used in select patients with respiratory syncytial virus (RSV) bronchiolitis. Propanolol may be used in certain patients with tetralogy of Fallot during Tet spells to reduce right ventricular outflow obstruction.

4. Answer E. Abruptio placentae, or placental abruption, is the most common cause of third-trimester bleeding. Among patients with no prior history of abruption, there are myriad, poorly understood risk factors including advanced maternal age, cigarette smoking, hypertension, and pre-eclampsia. The incidence of abruption peaks between 24 and 26 weeks and then steadily declines as patients progress to term. Patients most commonly experience vaginal bleeding and abdominal pain although patients may present with only one or neither of these symptoms. Abruption often results in frequent, low-amplitude uterine contractions resulting in a uterus that is firm and frequently tender upon palpation. Disseminated intravascular coagulation is a dreaded complication. Ultrasonography must be performed in all patients with second- or third-trimester vaginal bleeding. However, ultrasonography is poorly sensitive for placental abruption, missing approximately 50% of cases. In contrast, ultrasonography is a very good modality for detecting placenta previa, the other major cause of second- and third-trimester vaginal bleeding. If placenta previa is present, abruption is less likely.

5. Answer C. In the classic surgical text, "Cope's Early Diagnosis of the Acute Abdomen," Cope states that "the diagnosis of gastritis or gastroenteritis is usually made in the emergency ward by a young physician who is "not impressed" by a patient's abdominal pain or physical findings." He goes on to write that, "the diagnosis of gastroenteritis in the emergency ward is so often incorrect as to raise a serious question whenever the emergency physician comes to this conclusion." Although this quote employs a bit of hyperbole, gastroenteritis *is* the most common misdiagnosis applied to cases of missed appendicitis. In contrast, many patients initially diagnosed with acute appendicitis have a normal appendix upon appendectomy. In fact, the rate of negative appendectomy has essentially remained unchanged. Among these patients, the most common diagnoses are unexplained abdominal pain (35.1%), mesenteric adenitis (22.8%), lymphoid hyperplasia (10.6%) or other diseases of the appendix (9.9%), gastroenteritis (4.4%), and ovarian cyst (3.3%).

6. Answer B. Two percent to 4% of patients with trigeminal neuralgia have MS. This patient's history of recurrent attacks of neurologic dysfunction in different regions suggests a diagnosis of MS. In addition, primary trigeminal neuralgia peaks in the sixth to seventh decade with an average onset of age 50 and >90% of patients who present are older than 40. Therefore, physicians need to have a higher suspicion for secondary causes in young patients with trigeminal neuralgia. The peak age at onset of MS is 25 to 30 years although women have a slightly younger age at onset than men. In addition, the incidence in women exceeds that in men by almost 2:1. Roughly 5% of cases are diagnosed before the age of 20 (early onset) and 10% are diagnosed after the age of 50 (late onset). Other than MS, posterior fossa tumors, and vascular or aneurysmal compression of the trigeminal nerve should be considered.

7. **Answer A.** Applying a magnet to the pulse generator causes the pacemaker to default to asynchronous pacing by turning off (or bypassing) the sense amplifier. In other words, a magnet "turns the sensing function off." The pacemaker will deliver impulses (pacer spikes) at its predefined default rate (sometimes called the "magnet rate") regardless of the heart's intrinsic electrical activity. Since the pacemaker began pacing the patient's heart appropriately after magnet application, it is clear that it is generating impulses appropriately, and that those impulses are appropriately captured by the heart (i.e., the pacer-spike–evoked ventricular depolarization in the patient's heart as intended). Thus, the problem lies in sensation. The patient's pacemaker was misinterpreting signal "noise" as actual native activity when none was present. Since it detected what it thought was a native beat, it inhibited its output generation. This is called oversensing and is more common in single-lead devices.

8. **Answer D.** The diagnosis of irritable bowel syndrome (IBS) is made when patients have at least 3 days of abdominal pain per month over 3 months along with changes in stool frequency and appearance. There are three main types of IBS, diarrhea-type IBS (IBS-D), constipation-type (IBS-C), and mixed-type (IBS-M). IBS is a syndrome of lower pain thresholds in the ileum, colon, and rectum, resulting in greater pain perception with even normal bowel stimuli. Affirmation of the diagnosis and reassurance have been proven effective in improving outcomes in patients with IBS. IBS is not associated with cancer, is not deforming or deteriorating, and doesn't reduce life expectancy. Surgery has no role in treatment of IBS, though patients with IBS often have a higher incidence of abdominal surgery due to chronic symptomatology and seeking health care services. IBS is not a type of thought disorder and antipsychotics have no current role in management. Weight loss, significant rectal bleeding, fever, onset after age 50, and unexplained anemia are not consistent with IBS and should be pursued further.

9. **Answer C.** This patient is presenting with acute CHF, likely due to virally mediated myocarditis. While patients with acute myocarditis often present in a more subtle manner than this patient, patients may present with a broad range of symptoms, from vague generalized malaise to fulminant heart failure. Therefore, the ED physician must maintain a high degree of suspicion in patients presenting to the ED with new symptoms in the convalescent phase of a viral illness. The most common arrhythmia in patients with myocarditis is sinus tachycardia. Patients rarely present with supraventricular tachycardia, but when present, the rate is typically 180 to 260 beats per minute. Though the CK-MB and troponin are frequently measured in adults with chest pain, CK-MB has not been shown to be either sensitive or specific for pediatric patients with myocarditis. Elevated troponin levels also demonstrate poor sensitivity (34%) but relatively high specificity (82%) for myocarditis. Therapy is not based on the levels of any biomarker. Since this patient is presenting with fulminant heart failure, loop diuretics (e.g., furosemide) and inotropes (e.g., dobutamine, milrinone) may be essential in her management. Vasodilators (e.g., nitroglycerin) are also a mainstay of therapy, but this patient's relative hypotension may limit their use. Early consultation with a pediatric cardiologist is also essential as the patient should be transferred to a center with the capability of providing extracorporeal membrane oxygenation, should that become necessary. The patient's lack of fever or cough points against pneumonia as a likely diagnosis. Echocardiography is an essential diagnostic tool, but patients only rarely have pre-existing, undiagnosed congenital heart disease. Most often, echocardiography reveals global left ventricular dysfunction, with variable degrees of left ventricular cavity enlargement.

10. **Answer B.** This patient has aspiration pneumonitis, which is a chemical pneumonitis caused by the aspiration of acidic gastric contents. The severity of lung injury increases as the pH drops, and most studies agree that the pH must be <2.5 to cause significant injury. Chemical aspiration most commonly occurs in patients who have depressed levels of consciousness, as in this patient, and in young persons. Aspiration is otherwise a common problem among elderly persons in nursing homes after strokes. Though they are widely used, antibiotics and corticosteroids are not routinely recommended in patients with aspiration pneumonitis. Gastric acid inhibits bacterial growth, so gastric contents are sterile under normal conditions. Unless the patient has a coexisting condition promoting gastric bacterial growth, antibiotics should not be used. Such conditions include patients on antacid therapy, patients receiving enteral feeding, and patients with known gastroparesis or small bowel obstruction. Corticosteroids are also widely used in patients with chemical aspiration, although they have not been proven to be beneficial. (Figure from Harris JH, Harris WH. *The Radiology of Emergency Medicine.* 4th ed. Philadelphia, PA: Lippincott Williams & Wilkins; 1999:547, with permission.)

11. **Answer A.** The patient has community acquired pneumonia (CAP). The location is likely in the lingula, as the left heart border is obscured. *S. pneumoniae* is still the most common cause in patients over 40 years of age. *H. influenzae* is a very common cause in patients with any chronic medical disease such as chronic obstructive pulmonary disease (COPD) or diabetes. *S. aureus* is primarily a nosocomial pathogen but is common in the setting of concomitant influenza infection. *Mycoplasma* is one of the most common causes of CAP in young adults (<40 years) and usually causes an interstitial pattern on chest x-ray. *Klebsiella* is seen far more often in the setting of COPD or alcoholism. (Figure from Harris JH, Harris WH. *The Radiology of Emergency Medicine.* 4th ed. Philadelphia, PA: Lippincott Williams & Wilkins; 1999, with permission.)

12. **Answer A.** In the setting of a headache and nonspecific symptoms, the onset of a petechial rash at the wrists and ankles with subsequent central spread is consistent with a diagnosis of Rocky Mountain spotted fever (RMSF). This tick-borne illness is caused by *R. rickettsii*. Treatment of RMSF is with doxycycline and admission to the hospital. *B. burgdorferi* is the causative bacterium of Lyme disease. Coxsackievirus causes herpangina and myocarditis. Gonococcus may cause a vesicular rash in association with septic arthritis, cervicitis, or pelvic inflammatory disease (PID). Meningococcus may cause a petechial rash with signs and symptoms of meningitis, but the onset is much more acute and severe than RMSF. (Figure courtesy of Arthur Eisen, MD. In: Council ML, Sheinbein D, Cornelius LA, eds. *The Washington Manual of Dermatology Diagnostics.* Philadelphia: Wolters Kluwer, 2016).

13. **Answer E.** Reactive arthritis is the name which is now given to arthritis, urethritis, and conjunctivitis that occurs after an infection (thus, "reactive") and which was formerly called Reiter syndrome. Patients with reactive arthritis frequently have conjunctivitis early in the disease course. Uveitis (or iritis) may also occur but is less common and unrelated. Roughly 10% of patients will develop keratoderma blennorrhagica, waxy plaques most commonly present on the palms and soles. Sausage-shaped inflammation of the digits (dactylitis) is another common occurrence in reactive arthritis. Finally, painless ulcers may develop in the mouth or on the penis (where they are called *balanitis circinata*), where they more frequently occur in uncircumcised men.

14. **Answer E.** Although >75% of patients with PE will have an abnormal chest x-ray, no single finding is diagnostic for PE. Westermark sign (decreased peripheral vascular markings in the lung field affected by the embolus) and Hampton hump (a wedge-shaped homogeneous density with its base along the pleural surface and its apex pointed toward the hilum representing pulmonary infarction) are the classic findings, but both findings have very low sensitivity and specificity. In addition to the other findings listed, parenchymal infiltrates, hilar or mediastinal enlargement, cardiomegaly, pleural effusions, pulmonary edema, and a prominent central pulmonary artery (Fleischner sign) may also be seen. None are sensitive or specific findings.

15. **Answer B.** Mallet finger is a disruption of the extensor tendon at the level of distal interphalangeal (DIP) joint with or without an associated avulsion fracture of the dorsal base of the distal phalanx. It is caused by a flexion force on the volar tip with an extended DIP joint and may commonly occur during ball sports in which the participant may describe it as a *jammed* finger. Patients should be splinted in extension with either a padded aluminum splint applied to the dorsal aspect of the distal phalanx or an unpadded aluminum splint applied to its volar aspect. There is some disagreement regarding the optimal management of mallet finger when it involves a fracture. Some advocate operative repair if subluxation is present whereas other authors opt for splinting in extension for 6 to 8 weeks. (Figure from Harris JH, Harris WH. *The Radiology of Emergency Medicine.* 4th ed. Lippincott Williams & Wilkins; 1999:430, with permission.)

16. **Answer D.** This patient presents with a peritonsillar abscess (PTA). Polymicrobial infections are the rule in PTAs. Although *Fusobacterium* sp. is isolated, so are numerous other bacteria, principally group A β-hemolytic *Streptococcus*, *S. aureus*, and numerous anaerobes. While many patients with PTAs received immediate tonsillectomy in the past, currently either needle aspiration or incision and drainage, in concert with antibiotics, is considered effective therapy. Most of the debate in the management of PTAs focuses on the best drainage strategy. To date, the evidence does not clearly favor one method, and both methods appear to be effective. Drainage has historically been performed with the patient sitting upright to reduce the chance of aspiration but recent literature also supports a supine approach in Trendelenberg with the physician at the edge of the stretcher beyond the patient's head (as is often done in dentistry). Suction equipment should also be assembled at the bedside to remove purulent debris. It is not possible to accurately differentiate between the presence of a PTA and peritonsillar cellulitis upon physical examination. Furthermore, because collections of pus may be highly viscous, a needle placed into the center of an abscess may not drain any material, resulting in a falsely negative aspirate. Patients with suspected PTAs but negative aspirates can undergo CT to determine if an abscess is present. Finally, trismus is a common finding among patients with a PTA, and its presence does not indicate extension of the infection to the deeper neck tissues.

17. **Answer C.** This image reveals uterine prolapse. There are no contraindications to the manual reduction of

uterine prolapse, although attempts at reduction may not be successful. The primary indication for reduction is symptomatic improvement. After reduction, the patient should be fitted with a pessary to prevent recurrence. The pessary is a short-term solution that may serve as a bridge to surgical repair. Pessaries should not be used in the setting of concomitant genital tract infection. (Figure from Evans RJ, Brown YM, Evans MK. *Canadian Maternity, Newborn & Women's Health Nursing.* 2nd ed. Philadelphia: Wolters, 2014.)

18. **Answer C.** In symptomatic individuals, the most common manifestation of infection with *B. pertussis* is a prolonged, spasmodic cough that may last for several weeks. In adolescents and adults, the mean duration of illness is between 36 and 48 days. Despite widespread belief that childhood vaccination confers lifelong immunity, the last booster is given at age 4 to 6 in the United States, and it generally provides immunity until the age of 10 to 12 years. As a result, the CDC and the US Advisory Committee on Immunization Practices (ACIP) now recommends an acellular pertussis booster for all adults. The booster is given as part of a vaccine with diphtheria and tetanus (Tdap, commercially available as Adacel or Boostrix). In children, the classical pertussis infection occurs in three discrete phases: the catarrhal phase, paroxysmal phase, and convalescent phase. In adults, however, prolonged cough may be the only manifestation of infection. Between 70% and 99% of adolescents and adults have paroxysmal cough, associated with an inspiratory whoop in 8% to 82% of patients (i.e., highly variable), coughing during the night in 65% to 87% of patients, and post-tussive vomiting in 17% to 50%. Patients may also experience episodes of choking, sweating attacks, syncope, or encephalopathy. Erythromycin is the treatment of choice for symptomatic patients and for prophylaxis of asymptomatic patients who have come into contact with infected individuals. Antibiotics *may* reduce both the severity and duration of symptoms if they are given to affected patients within 1 week of the onset of symptoms. However, because *B. pertussis* has been isolated from affected individuals who are 3 weeks into their illness, treatment is recommended for all individuals who have had symptoms for 4 weeks or less. Such treatment is thought to decrease the carriage rate and shedding of the bacterium, thereby reducing transmission. High-risk personnel, including health care workers, or persons who may come into contact with infants of pregnant women in the third trimester, may receive treatment up to 6 to 8 weeks after developing symptoms.

19. **Answer C.** A small degree of chronic hemolysis occurs in all patients, which in most cases is clinically insignificant if appropriate iron supplementation is instituted. Mechanical, not porcine, valves require anticoagulation with Coumadin, and the INR is generally kept between 2.5 and 3.5. Mechanical valves always have a metallic closure sound—*absence* of this sound indicates valve dysfunction. The risk of endocarditis depends on the length of time the valve is functioning but occurs in less than half the number of patients.

20. **Answer B.** The patient has frank blood at the urethral meatus, which is a sign of likely urethral injury. This precludes placement of a Foley catheter by anyone but a urologist. Initially, a retrograde urethrogram is performed to evaluate for urethral injury. If this is normal, a Foley catheter may be placed and retrograde cystogram performed to evaluate for bladder rupture. Urinalysis in a trauma patient with grossly bloody urine is not helpful. Aspiration of the corpora cavernosa is indicated only in patients with priapism. (Figure Courtesy of Figueroa TE. In: Chung EK, Atkinson-McEvoy LR, Boom JA, Matz PS, eds. *Visual Diagnosis and Treatment in Pediatrics.* 2nd ed. Philadelphia: Wolters Kluwer, 2010.)

21. **Answer D.** Patients with transverse myelitis usually have bilateral clinical findings referable to one or two discrete spinal levels. Children and younger adults represent the majority of cases. CSF is totally normal in about half of cases, and CSF glucose is almost always normal. Albuminocytologic dissociation, referring to elevated CSF protein in the absence of CSF pleocytosis, is seen more commonly in variants of Guillain–Barre syndrome than tranverse myelitis, which usually exhibits a mild–moderate, CSF lymphocytosis. A compressive lesion of the spinal cord by definition excludes the possibility of transverse myelitis.

22. **Answer C.** Electroencephalogram (EEG) changes last for an average of 59.9 seconds (standard deviation of 12 seconds), whereas behavioral changes last for 52.9 to 62.2 seconds (with a standard deviation of 14 seconds). Therefore, a seizure that has lasted for 5 minutes is more than 17 standard deviations longer than the "typical" seizure. This is partly why status epilepticus is now "operationally" defined as any seizure lasting 5 minutes. The traditional definition has been any seizure lasting 30 minutes or recurrent seizures without an interictal return to baseline mental status.

23. **Answer D.** Cocaine may be taken in a variety of routes, most commonly intranasal and inhalational (crack). Inhalational and intravenous use causes the quickest onset of action, followed by intranasal, and then oral. The duration of action is longest in oral, followed by intranasal, then intravenous/inhalational. The transdermal route is not used for cocaine abuse.

24. **Answer A.** The patients described in this vignette are suffering from a cholinergic syndrome. The nerve agents sarin, VX, tabun, and soman are all organophosphorus compounds that strongly inhibit acetylcholinesterase resulting in symptoms of acetylcholine excess. The

classic mnemonic used to recall the symptoms of a cholinergic toxidrome is SLUDGE: salivation, lacrimation, urination, defecation, gastrointestinal upset, and emesis. The "SLUDGE" mnemonic does not address the pulmonary muscarinic effects (bronchorrhea, bronchospasm), cardiac muscarinic effects (bradycardia), nor the *nicotinic* effects in the central nervous system (muscle weakness, fasciculations, and flaccid paralysis). For this reason, the "SLUDGE" mnemonic is sometimes appended as "SLUDGE/BBB" for bronchospasm, bronchorrhea, and bradycardia. There are several alternative mnemonics as well (e.g., DUMBELS). Since these drugs work through excessive acetylcholine action, atropine is the natural antidote and should be given immediately to any patient with evidence of moderate or more severe toxicity. The dose is titrated until the pulmonary symptoms are resolved (no shortness of breath, no wheezing, no excessive secretions). If initial doses of atropine are ineffective, the dose should be doubled every 3 to 5 minutes and repeated. 2-PAM is used to address the nicotinic effects of these agents, since atropine does not bind to nicotinic receptors. Like atropine, 2-PAM should be used liberally and should be given to any patient with evidence of toxicity. Even in the absence of significant acute toxicity, many nerve agents cause delayed neurologic effects which may be prevented by 2-PAM administration. In addition, 2-PAM should be given early because the nerve agents become irreversibly bound to acetylcholinesterase over time (called "aging"). Both atropine and 2-PAM can be given IV or IM. Since succinylcholine is metabolized by acetylcholinesterase, it should never be used for airway management in patients with organophosphate toxicity, as its use results in prolonged and excessive paralysis. Diazepam is used to treat the seizures that may occur. Sodium thiosulfate is used for cyanide intoxication while amyl and sodium nitrite are used for either cyanide or hydrogen sulfide exposure.

25. **Answer D.** Leukocytosis refers to an elevated number of WBCs in the peripheral blood. Hyperleukocytosis is a severely elevated number of WBCs and is variably defined as a WBC count $>50 \times 10^9$ per L or $>100 \times 10^9$ per L. While hyperleukocytosis occurs in several hematologic malignancies, leukostasis is a relatively uncommon phenomenon, with the exception of patients with AML. Leukostasis is technically a pathologic diagnosis reflecting microvasculature occlusion due to WBC plugs. The exact pathophysiology is not certain, but hyperviscosity is responsible for part of the phenomenon. Interestingly, however, while patients with ALL, CML, and CLL frequently have hyperleukocytosis *in excess* of 100×10^9 per L, they only rarely suffer from leukostasis, except in patients with CML who are in blast crisis (evolution to AML). Clinically, patients with leukostasis most commonly present with symptoms related to lung and brain involvement, such as short-

ness of breath with pulmonary infiltrates, and headache, vision and hearing changes, confusion, dizziness, ataxia, and variable degrees of mental status changes.

26. **Answer E.** IPA encompasses the following old terms—domestic violence, domestic abuse, and spousal abuse. It is likely to be vastly under-reported by both men and women. ED patients are at high risk for being victims of IPA, but large majority of patients will not report IPA unless specifically asked by a care provider in the absence of their intimate partners. Screening of all patients is the only way to accurately evaluate IPA among ED patients. Most violence against women is perpetrated by intimate partners, but most violence against men is perpetrated by strangers. Almost one-fourth of women and 10% of men of all sexual orientations report an incident of IPA. Victim substance abuse is a marker for IPA but is not thought to contribute to IPA—perpetrator substance is known to contribute to IPA.

27. **Answer A.** Scapular fractures occur in patients with high-force blunt trauma such as motor vehicle crashes or falls from heights. Because of its well-protected position, isolated fracture of the scapula is rare, and associated injuries to the chest and upper extremity are present in the large majority of cases. Operative repair of the scapular fracture is not usually necessary as most patients heal with conservative management and range-of-motion exercises. Patients with scapular fractures hold their ipsilateral arm in full adduction and any movement elicits extreme pain. Bilateral scapular fracture is uncommon and usually signifies life-threatening injuries.

28. **Answer A.** Even among close contacts of patients with meningitis caused by *N. meningitidis,* the approximate rate of transmission is only 1 in 250 (0.4%). While this rate is very small, it is 500 to 800 times larger than the likelihood of infection in the general population.

29. **Answer D.** Pelvic binders are a fast, easy, effective means to limit pelvic bleeding in patients with unstable pelvic fractures. Traditionally, a bedsheet wrapped around the pelvis has been used to compress the pelvis in an effort to limit bleeding. However, there are a number of commercial devices available as well. Binding the pelvis has been thought to reduce pelvic volume, which lays the groundwork for tamponade of ongoing venous bleeding. However, their use achieves relatively modest pelvic volume reduction and may disrupt the retroperitoneum which diminishes the tamponade effect. Thus, it is now thought that binders decrease hemostasis primarily by decreasing pelvic motion of unstable bony fragments by a splinting mechanism. Regardless of the exact etiology, binders are associated with decreased blood transfusions and shorter intensive care unit (ICU) stays and are at least as effective as external fixators in controlling venous hemorrhage. Neither modality is effective in

controlling arterial hemorrhage. Binders are placed over the greater trochanters to the iliac crests, such that the superior margin of the binder should lie inferior to the umbilicus. The use of military antishock trousers prevents vascular access and is associated with complications without clear benefit, so their use is discouraged.

30. **Answer A.** Choice B is seen in glaucoma, choice C in central retinal vein occlusion, choice D in vitreous hemorrhage, and choice E in macular degeneration.

31. **Answer B.** Most ingested isopropanol is converted to acetone by hepatic alcohol dehydrogenase. Acetone is a ketone body, but is not acidic or charged, and does not contribute to the anion gap. Ketosis without acidosis is the characteristic finding in patients with isopropanol poisoning. Serum creatinine, not BUN, may be falsely elevated because of laboratory interference by acetone. Choice D is seen with methanol poisoning. Fomepizole is not indicated, as the metabolites of isopropanol, like the parent compound, cause generalized central nervous system (CNS) depression without other major organ system effects. Dialysis may be indicated to treat extremely severe poisoning.

32. **Answer E.** The patient has clear evidence of meningitis. The acute onset, progressive nature, and severe symptoms all indicate a likely bacterial cause. With evidence of alteration in mental status, CT scan before lumbar puncture may be advisable. However, in cases where bacterial meningitis is clinically suspected, antibiotics should be administered before the patient is sent to CT scan or lumbar puncture is performed. Additionally, adult patients with suspected bacterial meningitis should receive dexamethasone with or before the first dose of antibiotics.

33. **Answer D.** Patients with ischemic stroke should not have their BP reduced unless they are either candidates for tPA, have concomitant aortic dissection, MI or renal failure, or their pressure is above 220/120 mm Hg. In fact, hypertension is probably neuroprotective in patients with ischemic stroke by ensuring that cerebral perfusion pressure is maintained. In contrast, patients with hemorrhagic stroke should have their BP reduced to a target SBP of 140 to 160 mm Hg (or the patient's prestroke level if it is higher). Lowering the BP in such patients may reduce the stimulus for bleeding and prevent hematoma expansion. Because prognosis in patients with intracerebral hemorrhage is tightly linked to hematoma volume, strict BP control may have a dramatic positive effect in such patients.

34. **Answer B.** The patient likely has pneumocystis pneumonia (PCP). *Pneumocystis* is a fungal opportunistic infection commonly seen in AIDS patients when the CD4 count drops below 250 cells per mcL. Exertional dyspnea (rather than dyspnea at rest), nonproductive cough, low-grade fevers, and malaise in an acute or subacute pattern are characteristic. Chest radiographs usually show an interstitial pneumonia pattern but can be completely normal in up to one-third of cases. First-line treatment of *Pneumocystis* pneumonia is with trimethoprim–sulfamethoxazole. Supplemental corticosteroid therapy is added to improve outcomes if the PaO_2 is less than 70 mm Hg. Clindamycin plus primaquine is third-line therapy, after pentamidine. Doxycycline represents excellent monotherapy for CAP in the young adult but does not adequately treat *Pneumocystis* pneumonia. Piperacillin–tazobactam possesses broad-spectrum coverage for most intra-abdominal and nosocomial infections but is not indicated for treatment of *Pneumocystis* pneumonia.

35. **Answer B.** This patient's AG is 12, which is normal. Assuming that the patient has a normal albumin concentration (the major contributor to the AG in healthy patients), the normal AG reflects a resolution of the ketoacidosis. If substantial ketoacids were still present, the AG would be persistently elevated and the patient would require an ongoing insulin infusion. The persistently low bicarbonate signifies that a metabolic acidosis is still present, but it is an HCMA (nonanion gap). The development of an HCMA is a common complication of DKA therapy. This is partly due to the infusion of a large volume of saline, which contains chloride in concentrations far greater than plasma (154 mEq/L). Another major contributor is the loss of ketoanions in the urine that would normally serve as precursors for bicarbonate regeneration. The development of HCMA is benign and requires no therapy. In the setting of normal renal function, it will resolve spontaneously over the next 24 hours due to increased renal acid secretion. Subcutaneous insulin should always be overlapped with an insulin infusion when discontinuing continuous insulin therapy.

36. **Answer B.** The patient has evidence of nephrotic syndrome with proteinuria accompanied by generalized fluid overload and nonspecific constitutional symptoms. Periorbital edema is often the first location where fluid overload is noted. Frank renal failure does not usually occur in patients with nephrotic syndrome. In children, minimal change disease is the most common cause. Hypoalbuminemia, thrombophilia, and hyperlipidemia are characteristic. Urinary tract infections (UTIs) are unrelated. Although microscopic hematuria may be present, gross hematuria is rare and suggests glomerulonephritis, infection, stone, tumor, or extrarenal cause. Acute management generally involves careful fluid resuscitation, systemic corticosteroid therapy, and admission for observation and possible renal biopsy.

37. **Answer A.** The presence of a large, expanding hematoma is a classic "hard sign" of vascular injury. When a hard sign of vascular injury is present, ancillary studies such as CT angiography, angiography, or ultrasound are unnecessary and delay definitive treatment. Other hard signs of injury include obvious pulsatile bleeding, a pulseless extremity, a bruit or thrill over the vessel, and shock with a presumed vascular injury and no alternative explanation. In the setting of an injured leg with "soft signs" of injury, such as a small, nonpulsatile hematoma, an associated peripheral nerve deficit (due to the proximity of nerves to vascular structures in the neurovascular bundle), or a diminished distal pulse or decreased ankle–brachial index (ABI), imaging should be performed. In such cases, CT angiography is rapidly becoming the gold standard, although ultrasound may be useful in select cases of pregnant women and children to avoid radiation.

38. **Answer C.** Fluoxetine is a type of selective serotonin reuptake inhibitor (SSRI). As a class, SSRIs are generally benign in overdose, causing mild GI and CNS symptoms and rarely leading to dysrhythmias. Cyproheptadine is a serotonin antagonist that has unproven clinical efficacy in most SSRI overdoses. Its use is mainly limited to patients with serotonin syndrome, a constellation of neurologic, GI, and cardiac findings. Dysrhythmia is rare and should be treated according to current ACLS guidelines. Unlike with tricyclic antidepressant overdose, there is no indication for routine use of sodium bicarbonate to treat dysrhythmias. As in virtually all overdoses, ipecac is not recommended as a method of gastric decontamination. Hemodialysis is not indicated in patients with SSRI overdose, as the drug is highly bound to plasma proteins.

39. **Answer A.** Uterine rupture may occur as a result of substantial maternal trauma. However, among typical pregnant women, the primary risk factor for uterine rupture is a prior cesarean delivery (c-section), particularly with a "classic" vertical incision. Patients may present with significant abdominal pain and vaginal bleeding or they may be relatively asymptomatic if only minor dehiscence has occurred. A more recent meta-analysis suggests that only the risk of dehiscence is increased among women with a prior cesarean-section (excluding women with a classic vertical incision). Oxytocin did not increase the risk of rupture. Emergent cesarean-section is indicated in all cases of uterine rupture.

40. **Answer B.** Digitalis toxicity causes lethal dysrhythmias, and treatment involves management of electrolytes, digitalis antibody (Fab) fragment therapy, and dialysis. The most important indications for Fab fragment therapy in acute digitalis toxicity are hyperkalemia, ventricular dysrhythmias, and coingestions of other cardiotoxic drugs. Elevated digoxin level and massive ingestion are other relative indications, but usually mandate additional rhythmic disturbance to warrant Fab fragment therapy. Supraventricular dysrhythmias are only an indication for Fab fragment therapy if the patient is hemodynamically unstable. Magnesium level aberrations may exacerbate hypokalemia or hyperkalemia, but in the absence of potassium abnormalities, they do not constitute an indication for Fab fragment therapy.

41. **Answer C.** The triad of anemia, thrombocytopenia, and renal insufficiency should prompt evaluation for either hemolytic uremic syndrome (HUS) or thrombotic thrombocytopenic purpura (TTP). Fever and neurologic signs and symptoms are more common in the latter, but the two are thought to be on the same spectrum of disease. The toxin-forming bacterium *E. coli* O157:H7 is responsible for most epidemic cases of HUS. Treatment is primarily supportive, aimed at preventing complications of severe anemia and thrombocytopenia. Plasmapheresis is used for cases of idiopathic HUS or TTP. *Shigella* is a less common precipitant of HUS than *E. coli*. *Salmonella* species and rotavirus are not implicated. Child abuse would be unlikely to cause these symptoms in an epidemic manner.

42. **Answer B.** Patients with kidney stones less than 5 mm who are minimally symptomatic usually pass the stones spontaneously and do not need further intervention other than nonsteroidal anti-inflammatory drug (NSAID) therapy, moderate fluid intake, and urologic follow-up. There is no proven benefit in outcomes to drinking large amounts of free water—this practice may actually cause harm (due to electrolyte shifts). Clonidine has no role in the management of kidney stones. Tamsulosin is often prescribed and may be more effective in larger stones (>5 mm). Emergent urologic consultation or admission is not generally indicated, unless patients have a solitary or transplanted kidney, sepsis, a significantly elevated creatinine, intractable pain or vomiting, or stones larger than 10 mm. (Annals, April 2016.)

43. **Answer C.** The patient likely has contact dermatitis from a nickel-containing belt buckle. Nickel sensitivity is seen in about 10% of the population. Treatment is simple removal of the offending agent and topical antihistamines as needed to manage pruritus. Arsenic does not typically cause contact dermatitis but can cause cancer if chronically exposed to the skin. Brass is an alloy of copper and zinc and does not usually cause dermatitis, unless it contains nickel. Dermatium is a made-up name. *Rhus* is the former name of the *Toxicodendron* species which cause poison ivy, oak, and sumac. It can certainly cause contact dermatitis, but the location is atypical and more likely related to a belt buckle containing nickel. (From Werner R. *Massage Therapist's Guide to Pathology.* 5th ed. Philadelphia, PA: Wolters Kluwer; 2012.)

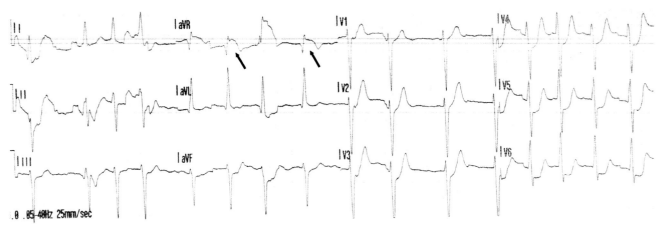

Figure 4-14

44. Answer C. After 6 hours of warm ischemia, 10% of patients will begin to develop irreversible damage to muscles and nerves. After 12 hours, 90% of patients will have irreversible damage.

45. Answer A. The patient's EKG demonstrates ST elevation in lead aVR with profound, diffuse ST depressions in the remaining leads (see Fig. 4-14). While lead aVR is routinely ignored in clinical practice, it provides useful information. In patients with chest pain, ST elevation in lead aVR, in concert with diffuse ST depressions, is a highly specific indicator of left main disease. While all of the interventions noted in the other answers may be appropriate, none of them favors immediate percutaneous coronary intervention (PCI) by cardiac catheterization, which is the standard of care among patients with STEMI.

46. Answer A. Drainage of a PTA is identical to drainage of any other abscess in that aspiration or incision should initially take place at the point of maximal fluctuance. While this is determined via digital palpation in other abscesses, physicians frequently use alternative devices to make this assessment within the oropharynx, such as a cotton swab or tongue blade, which diminishes the sensitivity of the examination. The use of ultrasound can be enormously helpful in locating the fluid collection. In some cases no fluid collection is found (peritonsillar cellulitis). When an abscess does occur, it most commonly develops at the upper pole of the tonsil, causing fluctuance superior to the tonsillar fossa. This is fortunate, since the carotid artery lies approximately 1.5 to 2.5 cm posterolateral to the tonsillar fossa. The actual distance from the mucosal surface overlying the abscess *may* be larger due to the anterior enlargement of the anterior pillar (palatoglossal arch) from the underlying purulent contents. However, aspiration should be done with caution, inserting the needle no more than 1 cm into the presumed abscess cavity.

47. Answer A. The most common complication of MS is atrial fibrillation, which puts the patient at high risk for thrombus formation and embolism. Atrial fibrillation occurs due to the severe atrial hypertrophy that results from the stenosed mitral valve preventing flow into the left ventricle.

48. Answer C. The patient has shingles, due to varicella zoster virus. Management involves antiviral therapy, which is especially effective for patients over 50 years of age. Valacyclovir is preferred to acyclovir due to the reduced frequency of dosing (3x/day vs. 5x/day). Supportive care is only considered in younger patients with mild symptoms. Antibiotics are not used for management of shingles and should only be used if a secondary bacterial cellulitis is suspected. A meta-analysis of five trials showed that routine use of adjunctive steroid therapy is not beneficial for any clinical endpoints in shingles. The risk–benefit profile of tricyclic antidepressants does not support their routine use, especially in older adults. (From Werner R. *Massage Therapist's Guide to Pathology.* 5th ed. Philadelphia, PA: Wolters Kluwer; 2012.)

49. Answer D. Patients with new-onset psychosis must be evaluated in the ED for treatable medical illness before being assigned a psychiatric diagnosis. Signs of a medical cause of the psychosis include acute onset, older patient, visual hallucinations, disorientation, and impaired consciousness. Abnormal physical examination findings, such as abnormal vital signs, aphasia, ataxia, and cranial nerve abnormalities usually indicate a medical cause. Many pharmacologic agents can also cause psychosis, including corticosteroids, antihistamines, antidepressants, and sedative hypnotic. True psychiatric disease is suggested by a young adult patient, auditory hallucinations, gradual progression, flat affect, and intact orientation and consciousness.

50. Answer C. Gentle, lateral compression of the iliac wings is the recommended physical examination approach to assess for pelvic instability. Rocking the pelvis by applying superior and posterior force on the bilateral ASIS is no longer recommended since doing so may worsen hemorrhage from an unstable fracture, and the procedure causes unnecessary pain. While pelvic fracture patterns on x-ray do not adequately predict hemodynamic stability, physical examination maneuvers may perform even worse, and such maneuvers may cause unnecessary pain or provoke further bleeding, as above. Thus, the role of "aggressive" pelvic physical examination maneuvers, particularly in hemodynamically unstable patients, is increasingly limited. In stable patients without overt evidence of severe trauma, physical examination is a more useful adjunct to identify those patients who need further investigation with radiologic studies.

51. **Answer C.** This patient most likely has a tubo-ovarian abscess (TOA) complicating PID. Her history suggests that she presented to her primary care doctor with symptoms of PID, but because she only received an antibiotic effective against *N. gonorrhoeae* and has not filled her prescription, she may still have untreated *C. trachomatis* infection. Interestingly, although *N. gonorrhoeae* and *C. trachomatis* are known to be instrumental in the development of a TOA, they are very rarely obtained at culture. Instead, the abscesses tend to be polymicrobial and include gram-negative enteric organisms as well as anaerobes, such as *Escherichia coli* and *Bacteroides fragilis*. It is thought that *N. gonorrhoeae* and *C. trachomatis* initiate the infection, whereas other organisms invade and take over once the initial damage allows them to gain entry and proliferate. All patients with a TOA should be admitted for broad-spectrum antibiotic therapy. Ampicillin, clindamycin, and gentamicin have been the antibiotic combination of choice. Abscesses between 4 and 6 cm in diameter respond to antibiotics alone 85% of the time. However, abscesses >10 cm often require surgical intervention. If untreated, abscesses continue to expand and may spontaneously rupture, resulting in secondary generalized peritonitis. Roughly 5% to 10% of women with acute PID will develop perihepatitis known as *Fitz–Hugh–Curtis syndrome*. This is primarily because of hematogenous or transperitoneal spread of *C. trachomatis* and is characterized by right upper quadrant pain and tenderness, pleuritic chest pain, and occasionally elevated liver enzymes.

52. **Answer D.** Only intravenous medications are appropriate for rapid, measured control of blood pressure. Nitroprusside is very easily titrated and extremely effective, making it the drug of choice for hypertensive crises. Nifedipine has been associated with severe side effects due to its unpredictable response. Isoproterenol is a β-agonist and will not decrease blood pressure. Phenoxybenzamine is an α-blocking agent used mostly in the prevention of catecholamine surge during therapy for pheochromocytoma. Hydrochlorothiazide is an oral medication appropriate for outpatient therapy for chronic hypertension.

53. **Answer E.** Patients wearing isolated lap-belt restraints may present with a "seatbelt syndrome," which classically consists of a transverse abdominal wall contusion, a chance fracture, and visceral trauma (e.g., hollow viscus rupture, of which jejunal rupture is most common, or solid organ injury, such as liver injury). Injury to the abdominal aorta has also been described but is rare. A chance fracture is an anterior compression fracture of the vertebral body with an associated transverse fracture of the posterior portion of the vertebral body as well as ligamentous disruption and possible vertebral body subluxation. Injury to the spinal cord is uncommon but can occur. Chance fractures occur when the spine is suddenly and forcefully flexed around the seatbelt, which serves as a fulcrum. Like the other injuries listed, chance fractures are most common among children in whom the seatbelt is improperly worn across the abdomen instead of low across the hips. These types of injuries are most common in 5- to 9-year olds, who are often too large to fit comfortably into a booster seat, yet too small to be adequately restrained by adult-sized shoulder harnesses.

54. **Answer D.** Emboli in the SMA account for 50% of the cases of acute mesenteric ischemia. Emboli usually originate in the left atrium or ventricle. Most emboli lodge just distal to a major branch point, and greater than 50% of SMA emboli are located just distal to the origin of the middle colic artery. Thrombosis of the SMA and mesenteric vein thrombosis each account for approximately 15% of cases.

55. **Answer A.** The rash is that of shingles, due to varicella zoster virus. Management involves antiviral therapy with valacyclovir, which is especially effective if given within 72 hours of symptom onset; after this time, benefit is uncertain. Gabapentin has been shown to be ineffective as adjunctive therapy. Postherpetic neuralgia is seen in about 15% of patients. Patients with shingles rarely develop abscesses and their presence should trigger an evaluation for alternate diagnosis. Viral load testing is not indicated in what is a purely clinical diagnosis. (Figure from Schalock PC, Hsu JT, Arndt KA. *Lippincott's Primary Care Dermatology*. Philadelphia, PA: Lippincott Williams & Wilkins; 2010.)

56. **Answer C.** Munchausen syndrome by proxy refers to the intentional faking or production of illness of a child by a caregiver. Virtually any type of illness is simulated by the caregiver in order to attain medical attention evaluation. The vast majority of caregivers who perpetrate Munchausen syndrome by proxy are biologic mothers, usually with a history of mood disorder or prior abuse. Fathers and nonparent guardians are much less likely to be involved. The victims are usually young children without gender predominance.

57. Answer C. PUD is the most common cause of upper gastrointestinal bleeding (UGIB), accounting for half of all cases. Bleeding is the most common complication of PUD, and perforation is the next most common. Gastric outlet obstruction occurs in only 2% of patients with known PUD.

58. Answer C. Sexual assault victims infrequently have significant genitourinary findings upon physical examination. Evidence of extragenital trauma, such as ecchymoses, erythema, or abrasions, is far more common (~65%) than evidence of vaginal, perineal, or anal trauma (~25%). Traumatic anogenital findings are more common among virgins, as well as victims of anal insertion. Among patients with an abnormal genitourinary examination, anal fissures are nonspecific and an annular hymen describes one of the many normal hymen variants, in which the hymen encircles the vaginal opening, forming a complete 360-degree ring. Hymenal bumps are normal elevations of hymenal tissue caused by an attachment of the hymen to the underlying intravaginal rugae. However, a deep hymenal cleft, or complete hymenal transection along the inferior hemisphere of the hymenal ring, for example at 6 o'clock, is abnormal and is specific for abuse.

59. Answer B. Patients with multiple myeloma are at risk for hyperviscosity syndrome, which is characterized by extremely high levels of pathologic proteins in the blood, causing increased viscosity and vascular sludging. Microinfarctions are common, especially in cerebral and ocular vessels. The triad of vision problems, neurologic symptoms, and mucosal bleeding in a patient with multiple myeloma or Waldenstrom macroglobulinemia strongly suggests the presence of hyperviscosity syndrome. Laboratory data, although helpful, often return with errors as most standard equipment may be unable to analyze the blood because of the elevated protein levels. Definitive treatment involves plasmapheresis. In patients with severely altered mental status, simple phlebotomy and saline replacement may rapidly improve the clinical condition. Hemodialysis is not used in dysproteinemias. Colloids such as platelets and packed RBC transfusions will likely exacerbate the viscosity. Erythropoietin has no role in the management of most acute conditions.

60. Answer C. Uncomplicated pertussis in an unvaccinated child is a clinical diagnosis. In children, the illness classically follows a three-stage pattern—the catarrhal phase, paroxysmal phase, and convalescent phase. The catarrhal phase usually lasts between 5 and 10 days but may last up to 3 weeks. During this phase, it is impossible to clinically differentiate these patients from patients with common cold. Unfortunately, patients are most contagious during this phase. Patients are typically afebrile or have only a minimal fever during this phase and throughout the illness. The presence of significant fever should prompt a search for a secondary infection. Additional typical symptoms include rhinorrhea, mild cough, sneezing, and occasionally conjunctivitis. These signs may be absent in very young infants. The paroxysmal phase is characterized by paroxysms of cough, often occurring during the night and associated with post-tussive emesis, especially in young infants. The inspiratory whoop, which is responsible for the common name, whooping cough, given to *Bordetella pertussis* infections, occurs at the end of a paroxysm, as air is inspired against a partially closed glottis. Due to the immaturity of their respiratory system, young infants are susceptible to developing apneic episodes during this phase, as well as choking or gasping for air. Apnea and choking may be sufficiently prolonged to cause hypoxia and cyanosis. Therefore, infants and toddlers presenting during the paroxysmal phase frequently require admission to an intensive care unit (ICU) setting where appropriate monitoring can be provided. Feeding may also be a problem during this phase, as it may provoke paroxysms of coughing and subsequent vomiting. Therefore, several infants and toddlers with this disease present with severe dehydration. The paroxysmal phase typically lasts from 1 to 6 weeks. During the convalescent phase, the paroxysms typically become less frequent and less distressing, although the cough may actually become louder. Although classical pertussis is a clinical diagnosis, lymphocytosis supports the diagnosis. Absolute lymphocyte counts >20,000 per mm^3 may be seen with a total WBC count >100,000 per mm^3. The chest x-ray is most often normal, although it may demonstrate a "shaggy" right-heart border. However, the presence of an infiltrate may indicate a secondary infection as bacterial pneumonia may complicate pertussis in up to 20% of patients. Although the incidence of *B. pertussis* is rising in the population as a whole, this rise is almost solely due to an increase in the number of adolescents and adults with the disease. However, children and infants still represent most cases of *B. pertussis*. Thirty-eight percent of cases occur in infants younger than 6 months and 71% of cases occur in children younger than 5 years. Additionally, adolescents and adults more often present with atypical signs and symptoms such as an isolated spasmodic cough without an associated inspiratory whoop. Previously vaccinated adults rarely demonstrate the lymphocytosis that is characteristic of pediatric infections.

61. Answer E. Subdural hematomas occur due to disruption of the cranial bridging veins from trauma, causing blood to collect deep to the dura. The elderly are at much higher risk than the average population due to brain atrophy, which causes these bridging veins to stretch and be susceptible to even minor trauma. Due to this low-pressure venous bleeding, patients with subdural hematoma may have a subacute or chronic presentation with mild initial clinical manifestations of injury.

Patients with epidural hematoma, on the other hand, usually have an arterial source and exhibit signs and symptoms almost immediately after the trauma. Some patients with subdural hematoma, especially the elderly and alcoholics, may not even recall their antecedent head trauma. Many patients with subdural hematoma have a lucid interval (where the mental status is completely normal before becoming altered again), which is more classically thought to be associated with epidural hematoma. Coma, focal neurologic deficits, and increased intracranial pressure are associated with both subdural and epidural hematomas.

62. **Answer C.** This patient has RMSF. Classically, patients with RMSF develop a maculopapular rash on the wrists and ankles 4 days after being bitten by an American dog tick (*D. variabilis*) or Rocky Mountain wood tick (*D. andersoni*) infected with *R. rickettsii*. Despite its name, North Carolina and Oklahoma account for more than one-third of RMSF cases. The rash rapidly spreads centrally to the trunk and extremities and becomes petechial and purpuric. However, up to 15% of patients do not develop a rash ("spotless fever"). Other common findings include a high fever (typically >102°F), myalgias (particularly of the gastrocnemius), headache, vomiting, and malaise. Doxycycline is the treatment of choice in all patients except for pregnant women, who should receive CAM. CAM is the drug of choice during pregnancy due to the effects of tetracyclines on fetal bones and teeth. However, CAM should be used with caution and should be avoided in near-term pregnancies or during the third trimester in order to avoid fetal bone marrow suppression, which results in the "gray baby syndrome." Doxycycline should be used in these cases. Previously, CAM was the recommended agent in children as well, but because doxycycline is more effective and the risk of teeth staining is low given the short duration of treatment, doxycycline is now the drug of choice for all patients except pregnant women.

63. **Answer A.** Acalculous cholecystitis comprises roughly 15% of acute cholecystitis cases. It is classically associated with critically ill patients in ICU settings. The presentation of acalculous disease in this population is often subtle, and may declare itself as an isolated and unexplained fever. This leads to a delay in diagnosis and contributes to its far more fulminant course. By the time it is diagnosed in this population, approximately half the number of patients would have experienced a major complication such as gangrene or perforation. The mortality rate ranges from 10% to 50%. However, recent studies suggest that many patients with acalculous cholecystitis develop symptoms and are diagnosed as outpatients, and they have a natural history that is similar to calculous disease. Some of these patients may be miscategorized, since microscopic calculi are evident in pathologic specimens, but there remain a large number of patients with true acalculous disease who are otherwise healthy.

64. **Answer E.** Optic neuritis usually causes slowly progressive painful visual loss over a few days, and is associated with an afferent pupillary defect (APD). This is diagnosed with the swinging flashlight test in which a light is quickly moved from left to right to examine the direct and consensual response to light. Since the efferent fibers of the affected eye work properly but the eye can't detect light (an afferent problem), the affected pupil will constrict when the light is shined into the unaffected eye. When the light is swung back to the affected eye, it doesn't detect the light so the pupil dilates back to its baseline. Along with retinal detachment, vitreous hemorrhage, posterior uveitis, and central retinal vein occlusion, central retinal artery occlusion is a painless event that causes monocular vision loss. Vitreous hemorrhage initially results in floaters but can progress to more significant vision loss depending on the amount of hemorrhage. Floaters are also common in retinal detachment along with flashes of light (photopsias) and classic "curtain-like" decreased vision with a field cut.

65. **Answer A.** Breast milk jaundice develops in 2% of breast-fed infants *after* the seventh day of life. Levels peak during the second to third week of life and may be as high as 10 to 30 mg/dL. Treatment is straightforward and involves stopping breast-feeding for 1 to 2 days and substitution of bottle feeding with formula. This results in a rapid decline in serum bilirubin after which nursing can be resumed without a recurrence of the prior hyperbilirubinemia. Breast milk jaundice is an unconjugated hyperbilirubinemia. Hyperbilirubinemia is described as "conjugated" when direct bilirubin exceeds 2 mg/dL or represents >20% of the total bilirubin level. Although breast milk jaundice is generally a benign process, phototherapy may be required if total bilirubin levels exceed 18 to 20 mg/dL. Finally, breast milk jaundice should be differentiated from breast-*feeding* jaundice, which is an early-onset unconjugated hyperbilirubinemia that occurs in the first week in breast-fed infants. The mechanism, as with breast milk jaundice, is unclear, but is thought to be related to decreased milk intake with dehydration or reduced caloric intake.

66. **Answer A.** Hypokalemia is more common and generally better tolerated than hyperkalemia. Diuretic therapy is the most common cause. Hypokalemia primarily affects the cardiac (arrhythmias), musculoskeletal (weakness, rhabdomyolysis), GI (ileus), and renal (nephrogenic diabetes insipidus, metabolic alkalosis) systems. Neurologic manifestations are not common. Cardiac dysrhythmias are the most serious complication, although patients without pre-existing heart disease *rarely* have any complications. In contrast, patients with acute or recent MI may develop ventricular fibrillation in the setting of even mild hypokalemia (five times

increased risk if the potassium concentration is less than 3.9 mEq/L. Therefore, recent recommendations are to maintain serum potassium levels greater than 4.5 mEq/L in such patients. The number or degree of EKG changes does not correlate with the severity of hypokalemia. Neither vomiting nor nasogastric suctioning causes significant potassium loss. Potassium is the most prominent intracellular cation, while sodium is the most prominent extracellular cation.

67. **Answer B.** Xanthochromia refers to the presence of a yellowish color to the supernatant of centrifuged CSF samples. It results from the breakdown of hemoglobin first to oxyhemoglobin and then to bilirubin. Methemoglobin may also be produced, but like bilirubin, it occurs after oxyhemoglobin is generated. These latter molecules have a yellowish tint and characteristic spectrophotometric absorption curves. Traditionally, oxyhemoglobin was thought to appear within 2 hours of SAH achieving a peak concentration between 24 and 46 hours. Bilirubin does not appear until approximately 10 hours after SAH. Although the presence of xanthochromia remains the most reliable method for differentiating between a traumatic lumbar puncture and an SAH, its presence is not pathognomonic for SAH. Recent studies have demonstrated that xanthochromia begins to develop immediately after mixing of blood and CSF as seen in traumatic lumbar puncture. The degree of xanthochromia correlates with the amount of bleeding induced by trauma. Clinically, recent studies have established that in the presence of a traumatic lumbar puncture and an RBC concentration of 10,000 RBC per μL, xanthochromia cannot be reliably used to confirm SAH. Conversely, xanthochromia in the setting of RBC concentrations <5,000 RBC per μL is a reliable indicator of SAH. The method of comparing RBC counts in the first and fourth tubes has been shown to be an unreliable means of differentiating these two entities. None of the other methods listed has been shown to be reliable.

68. **Answer B.** Chest pain is a frequent complaint among pediatric patients presenting to EDs. Fewer than 10% of patients are eventually diagnosed with a cardiac cause of chest pain. Most cases are caused by musculoskeletal etiologies (e.g., costochondritis) or are considered idiopathic. Among cardiac causes, pericarditis and arrhythmias are the most common. Valve disorders are uncommon and, when present, are more often diagnosed in early childhood. Recurrent chest pain that occurs with exertion, chest pain occurring prior to syncope, or a family history of sudden cardiac death each increases the likelihood of an underlying cardiac problem. Pericarditis is a common cardiac cause of pediatric chest pain. Patients with pericarditis typically feel better lying forward and worse when lying supine. However, the friction rub is best heard with the patient leaning for-

ward or even sitting on all fours. These positions bring the heart closer to the chest wall allowing for better auscultation. Myocardial infarction is rare in pediatric patients, but when it occurs, it is most common in males, and it is associated with smoking and substance abuse (primarily cocaine).

69. **Answer D.** This patient's EKG reveals classic or "type 1" Brugada syndrome. Brugada syndrome is characterized by a pseudo-RBBB and persistent ST elevation in V1–V3. There are three unique patterns of ST elevation consistent with Brugada syndrome. In type 1, the elevated ST segment is convex facing upward, and gradually descends to an inverted T wave. This is referred to as a "coved type" Brugada pattern, and is most common. Types 2 and 3 have identical patterns, in which the elevated ST segment (≥1 mm in type 2, <1 mm in type 3) first descends and then rises again after nearing the baseline, creating a "saddle back" appearance. It is associated with an upright or biphasic T wave. Brugada syndrome is not normally associated with any structural abnormalities. Most "standard" cardiac tests, including echocardiography, stress testing, and cardiac MRI are unrevealing. However, patients are at a much increased risk for sudden cardiac arrest due to ventricular arrhythmias. Unlike patients with hypertrophic obstructive cardiomyopathy, sudden cardiac arrest is not typically due to exercise and more commonly occurs in sleep. Most patients with Brugada syndrome undergo electrophysiology testing to determine their risk for cardiac arrest as well as the need for an automated implantable cardioverter-defibrillator.

70. **Answer C.** C-reactive protein is part of the Laboratory Risk Indicator for Necrotizing Fasciitis (LRINEC) score for screening of necrotizing fasciitis. An LRINEC score below a specific cutoff indicates that necrotizing fasciitis is extremely unlikely in patients with signs and symptoms of severe cellulitis. The LRINEC score contains the following variables: C-reactive protein, WBC, sodium level, creatinine level, hemoglobin, and glucose. Platelets are part of the qSOFA score for general sepsis. Procalcitonin is used to differentiate between bacterial and nonbacterial etiology in lower respiratory infections. Serum mycoplasma antigen is used to evaluate for *Mycoplasma pneumoniae* in patients with pneumonia, but mycoplasma is not a typical pathogen seen in necrotizing fasciitis.

71. **Answer A.** The patient has evidence of an incarcerated hernia. The presence of fullness and bowel sounds in the scrotum indicates a hernia, and tenderness with inability to easily reduce the hernia indicates incarceration. Ice packs should be applied to the area to reduce the attendant bowel edema and an attempt should be made to reduce the hernia, under procedural sedation if necessary. Operative reduction is required if the hernia

can't be reduced. Operative reduction and IV antibiotics would also likely be necessary if the patient presented with signs of strangulation such as fever, acidosis, and/or severe tenderness. Outpatient referral for an incarcerated hernia is not appropriate. Oral hydration may maintain euvolemia, but the possibility of procedural sedation or surgery should preclude any oral intake. Incarcerated hernia is a clinical diagnosis and urinalysis will not aid diagnostic accuracy.

72. **Answer D.** Although all the choices are risk factors for aortic dissection, the most common is hypertension. Though approximately half the number of patients with Marfan syndrome develop aortic dissections, <10% of all dissections are in Marfan patients.

73. **Answer E.** This patient has a mechanism of injury, physical examination, and x-ray consistent with an unstable pelvic fracture. While at least 50% of patients with unstable pelvic fractures experience major hemorrhage outside the pelvis, this patient has no evidence of intraperitoneal hemorrhage on FAST examination. Such patients should have a pelvic binder immediately applied and be taken to the angiography suite for control of possible arterial bleeding via embolization (binders are intended as adjuncts to control venous, not arterial, hemorrhage). If angiography is negative and the patient remains hemodynamically unstable, FAST examination should be repeated or the patient should simply be taken to the OR for a diagnostic laparoscopy or laparotomy.

74. **Answer D.** The patient has evidence of chancroid, caused by *H. ducreyi*, a gram-negative bacillus. A painful chancre-like lesion combined with a solitary tender unilateral lymph node which may also ulcerate is classic. Chancroid, unlike syphilis (caused by *T. pallidum*), is painful and tender. Treatment of chancroid is with azithromycin or ceftriaxone. HSV can cause ulcerated or vesicular lesions, but these are usually grouped and Gram stain of the lesions will be negative. *C. trachomatis*, a spirochete, may cause lymphogranuloma venereum, which is manifested by a painless ulcer combined with significant lymphadenopathy with a negative Gram stain. *S. epidermidis* may cause skin lesions in the genital region but Gram stain would show gram-positive cocci.

75. **Answer E.** Nitroglycerin directly dilates the great veins and reduces left ventricular preload. Afterload reduction by nitrates is much less prominent. Morphine and loop diuretics such as furosemide are also used for preload reduction but have a smaller effect than nitrates. While morphine has been used for years as part of the standard treatment of CHF for preload reduction, there have been few rigorously conducted randomized trials confirming its benefit. Morphine most likely exerts its preload reducing effect by reducing anxiety and subsequent catecholamine production and release. Loop diuretics

cause preload reduction by inhibiting renal sodium reabsorption thereby increasing urine volume and decreasing plasma volume. However, the elevated afterload in patients with CHF reduces renal perfusion and thereby limits the effectiveness of loop diuretics. Afterload reduction is most commonly achieved through the use of angiotensin converting enzyme (ACE) inhibitors such as enalaprilat, although nitroprusside and hydralazine may also be used to achieve this effect. Digoxin causes an increase in cardiac contractility without major changes on preload or afterload, and has no role in the management of acute CHF. In fact, prior digoxin use has been shown to correlate to increased in-hospital mortality among patients admitted with CHF.

76. **Answer D.** The pain of trigeminal neuralgia is characteristically explosive in onset, severe in intensity, brief, lasting 2 seconds to 2 minutes, and unilateral. It invariably involves either the V2 or V3 branch of the trigeminal nerve and sometimes involves both branches. It very rarely affects the V1 (ophthalmic) branch of the trigeminal nerve. Cranial nerve testing reveals completely normal function of the trigeminal nerve and remaining cranial nerves. Patients typically have normal dentition. In addition, patients with trigeminal neuralgia typically have "trigger zones" especially in the perioral area and near the nostril. Tapping or palpating these areas may provoke an attack. Other stimuli such as wind on the face, chewing, brushing teeth, and shaving may also provoke attacks of pain.

77. **Answer B.** The spleen and the liver (in that order) are the most commonly injured abdominal organs in children with blunt trauma. Liver lacerations tend to have higher mortality than splenic lacerations. Unlike the past, splenic lacerations are currently nonoperatively managed as much as possible, because of the deleterious immunologic effects of splenectomy. Renal injury is also common, given its proportionally larger size in children relative to adults. Bowel injury in blunt trauma is rare.

78. **Answer E.** The patient has evidence of liver abscess, with fever, right upper quadrant pain, and the ultrasound findings. Pleuritic pain and cough are common and can confuse the clinical picture by seemingly supporting a pulmonary etiology. Liver abscesses are usually pyogenic (80%) but can be amebic (10% to 15%) or fungal (<10%). Pyogenic liver abscesses are usually due to biliary obstruction or cholangitis but can be caused by other intra-abdominal infections such as diverticulitis or appendicitis. Pyogenic liver abscesses are usually polymicrobial, with concurrent gram-negative, gram-positive, and anaerobic offenders. Antibiotic treatment should therefore be broad-spectrum. Sterile liver abscesses are extremely uncommon, occurring rarely in cases of hepatic vasculitis or rheumatologic diseases. *E. histolytica* is the cause of amebic liver abscesses, which are suspected

in cases of foreign travel (often with a preceding intestinal illness) or oral–anal sexual contact causing fecal–oral contamination. *Streptococci* alone are not usually a cause of liver abscesses. Candidal infection represents less than 10% of all liver abscesses.

79. **Answer D.** Preseptal cellulitis is the most common complication of acute sinusitis. Orbital cellulitis may also occur and is often difficult to distinguish from preseptal sinusitis based on clinical examination alone. CT scans are generally able to differentiate between preseptal and orbital cellulitis. They also provide additional information about neighboring structures, including the sinuses. Cavernous sinus thrombosis is a rare, but life-threatening complication that results from extension of the infection through valve-free veins to the cavernous sinus. Patients typically present with severe headache as well as CN III and VI palsies along with retinal engorgement, chemosis, proptosis, and a high fever. Like cavernous sinus thrombosis, meningitis is another uncommon intracranial complication. Other complications include brain abscesses, subdural empyema, orbital abscesses, maxillary cellulitis, and localized osteomyelitis.

80. **Answer A.** The patient likely has the most common form of Guillain–Barre syndrome (GBS), called acute inflammatory demyelinating polyneuropathy (AIDP). AIDP represents about 90% of cases of GBS and usually causes symmetric motor weakness, hyporeflexia, elevated CSF protein in the absence of elevated CSF leukocyte count (albuminocytologic dissociation). Fever, asymmetric weakness, and severe bowel or bladder abnormalities are not common in AIDP. Other varieties of GBS include a motor axonal variety without sensory symptoms, a motor and sensory axonal variety, and Miller Fisher syndrome, characterized by ophthalmoplegia, ataxia, and areflexia.

81. **Answer C.** Abdominal pain and diarrhea occur in practically all cases of shigellosis and is often accompanied by fever. However, only 35% to 40% of patients have evidence of blood in their stools. Resistance to trimethoprim–sulfamethoxazole is widespread, making fluoroquinolones the drug of choice. Antimotility drugs may be safely given if antibiotics are also administered but are contraindicated when used alone as they may actually worsen the clinical course. Most infections are caused by *Shigella sonnei*, with only a minority of infections caused by *Shigella dysenteriae*. Although *Salmonella* spp. requires a very large inoculum to cause disease, infection with *Shigella* spp. requires a very small inoculum, making *Shigella* the most efficient enteric human pathogen known. Fecal leukocytes are almost universally detected in patients with shigellosis, as *Shigella* invades the mucosa resulting in local destruction and

inflammation. Seizures may occur in children infected with *Shigella*.

82. **Answer C.** Neurologic symptoms of paresthesias combined with dorsal column findings in the face of macrocytic anemia are indicative of vitamin B_{12} deficiency. Ataxia, depression, and paranoia may also accompany these symptoms. Pain and temperature are usually spared, as these sensations are not carried by the dorsal spinal columns. Causes of vitamin B_{12} deficiency include chronic malabsorption, strict vegetarian diet, chronic alcohol use, ileal disease, and pernicious anemia. Chronic smoking can cause COPD, which may lead to polycythemia rather than anemia. Chronic aspirin use and melena can predispose patients to iron-deficiency anemia, which is either microcytic or normocytic. Family history of thalassemia may be a risk factor for younger patients to develop a well-compensated microcytic anemia but has little relevance in an older adult.

83. **Answer B.** Otic symptoms are the earliest symptoms observed in salicylate toxicity. The Done nomogram is not predictive of serious pathology in salicylate toxicity and is not used clinically (unlike the Rumack–Matthew nomogram for acetaminophen toxicity). Metabolic acidosis due to uncoupling of oxidative phosphorylation is much more likely to be observed than metabolic alkalosis. Despite the clear role of chronic aspirin and NSAID use in GI bleeding, acute toxicity causes far less serious GI bleeding. Hypokalemia is far more common than hyperkalemia with salicylate toxicity, due to a variety of renal and extrarenal mechanisms. Therapy with bicarbonate may further exacerbate this potassium loss.

84. **Answer B.** The pork tapeworm, *T. solium*, causes neurocysticercosis, an extremely common cause of seizures worldwide. Infection occurs after humans eat contaminated pork. The parasite multiplies in the small intestine and eventually enters the bloodstream and brain. The tapeworm produces cysts in the brain, which appear as ring-enhancing lesions on contrast CT scan. Seizures are the most common serious manifestation of disease. Praziquantel and corticosteroids are the medical treatment. Neurosurgical consultation is required in all cases to evaluate and manage increased intracranial pressure. *T. cruzi* causes Chagas disease, a cardiomyopathy due to parasitic infection occurring primarily in Latin America. *T. saginata*, the beef tapeworm, causes a self-limited gastroenteritis. *T. trichiura*, the whipworm, also causes gastroenteritis, which may lead to iron-deficiency anemia due to malabsorption. *L. braziliensis* causes chronic cutaneous ulcerations.

85. **Answer D.** The patient is exhibiting evidence of acute herpes simplex encephalitis. Fever, headache, and

personality changes are the most common symptoms. Empiric antiviral treatment for herpes simplex encephalitis is indicated, as early therapy improves mortality and has few side effects and definitive diagnostic testing can take significant time. Discharging a patient with fever and delirium home is decidedly suboptimal therapy. Dexamethasone therapy may play a role in herpes simplex encephalitis, but it is not yet proven to be of definite benefit in these patients and is not as important as antiviral therapy at this time. Chemical restraint with haloperidol should not be instituted given the side effect profile in the geriatric population as well as the simple fact that the patient has not demonstrated a harm to himself or others. MRI brain with contrast would be a very reasonable study in the evaluation of herpes simplex encephalitis, but the duration of the test in most EDs would likely worsen outcomes if empiric treatment is not given first.

86. **Answer D.** In septic arthritis, the synovial WBC usually exceeds 50,000 WBC per mm³ and often exceeds 100,000 per mm³, with >75% polymorphonuclear cells. However, patients with gout, pseudogout, and rheumatoid arthritis may also have WBC counts in this range with a similar differential. Therefore, when the WBC is elevated approximately 50,000 per mm³, septic arthritis must be presumed until ruled out.

87. **Answer B.** The patient has target lesions, which are a common sign of erythema multiforme. The most common cause overall is HSV. *Mycoplasma pneumoniae* is the most common bacterial cause. HIV and HPV do not usually cause erythema multiforme. HHV-3 (human herpesvirus-3) is also known as varicella zoster virus, causing shingles and chickenpox rather than target lesions or erythema multiforme. (Figure from Rubin E, Reisner H, eds. *Essentials of Rubin's Pathology.* 6th ed. Philadelphia, PA: Wolters Kluwer; 2013.)

88. **Answer D.** Patients older than 50 years are at risk for *S. pneumococcus* and *N. meningitidis,* as well as *L. monocytogenes.* Ceftriaxone covers pneumococcus, whereas vancomycin is necessary for resistant pneumococcus. However, in older patients at risk for *Listeria* infection, ampicillin is also necessary. Patients younger than 50 who are immunocompromised or who are alcoholic are also at risk for *Listeria* infection and should be covered with ampicillin. All patients with suspected meningitis should be given 10 mg of dexamethasone IV just before or with the first dose of antibiotics. Adjunctive dexamethasone reduces mortality and neurologic sequelae. The reduction is most marked in patients with intermediate disease severity, defined as those patients with a Glasgow Coma Scale rating of 8 to 11, as well as in patients with pneumococcal meningitis. Amphotericin is used for confirmed fungal infections.

89. **Answer C.** The triad of confusion, ataxia, and oculomotor dysfunction is indicative of Wernicke encephalopathy, which is usually due to alcohol use. Pathology is likely due to thiamine deficiency and affected areas of the brain include the thalamic nuclei, mammillary bodies, and cerebellar vermis. In Wernicke encephalopathy, balance is abnormal more often than coordination testing such as finger-to-nose because the cerebellar vermis is involved more often than the cerebellar hemispheres. Oculomotor dysfunction can be as simple as nystagmus; frank ophthalmoplegia is not required for the diagnosis. CT brain with IV contrast reveals major blood vessel pathology such as dissection or dural sinus thrombosis, but these would reveal focal neurologic deficits or headache with possible fever, respectively. Vertebral artery dissection can certainly cause nystagmus and gait disturbances but almost always causes another focal neurologic symptom (such as weakness or paresthesias) or neck pain or headache. EEG can evaluate for seizure activity, but the subacute, constant nature of symptoms without discrete episodes would be unlikely. CSF analysis could reveal a subacute encephalitis or even malignancy, but lumbar puncture should not be performed without a thorough history to ensure no other cause is likely. Orthostatic vital signs are rarely helpful in evaluation of most emergency conditions, partly due to unproven guidelines of what constitutes a positive change in heart rate or blood pressure and what duration of time the examiner should wait between testing positional changes.

90. **Answer C.** Fat, tendons, and bones have the greatest resistance to electrical flow (bones have the highest resistance of all), whereas nerves, blood, mucous membranes, and muscle have the least resistance. The resistance of dry skin is intermediate, although it varies greatly depending on the skin surface involved. Tissues with high resistance tend to heat up and coagulate in response to electrical flow.

91. **Answer B.** The Sgarbossa criteria were devised to assess the likelihood of infarction in patients with a left bundle branch block. Three different electrocardiographic criteria are given specific scores: A total score of 3 or greater indicates that the patient likely has acute MI. Concordant (in the same direction as the QRS complex) ST elevation >1 mm is given 5 points, ST depression >1 mm in V1–V3 is given 3 points, and discordant ST elevation >5 mm (in the opposite direction as the QRS complex) is given 2 points.

92. **Answer D.** Calcium gluconate antagonizes the effect of magnesium and should be given immediately in all patients with any sign of respiratory depression. The magnesium infusion is discontinued, and 1 g of calcium gluconate is infused over 2 to 3 minutes.

93. Answer C. The patient has air-space consolidation in the right mid-lung field in the setting of trauma, which is consistent with a pulmonary contusion. Management is directed at adequate oxygenation and ventilation and prevention of secondary complications such as acute respiratory distress syndrome (ARDS) and pneumonia. There is no obvious pneumothorax present, although an occult pneumothorax may be picked up if CT chest is performed. On an upright chest x-ray, hemothorax would appear as a pleural effusion around the lower lung segments. Chest radiography is not specific for the diagnosis of traumatic aortic rupture, which requires CT angiography for definitive diagnosis. Cardiac contusion is an older term to describe blunt cardiac injury, which is diagnosed by a combination of EKG, echocardiography, and sometimes cardiac markers. (Figure courtesy of Robert Hendrickson, MD, In: Greenberg MI, Hendrickson RG, Silverberg M, et al., eds. *Greenberg's Text-Atlas of Emergency Medicine.* Lippincott Williams & Wilkins; 2004:634, reprinted with permission.)

94. Answer A. The qSOFA score is a modified version of the full SOFA score, which was advocated by the Society of Critical Care Medicine in 2016. The SIRS criteria were felt to be not sufficiently sensitive or specific for the definition of sepsis. The qSOFA score includes: systolic blood pressure <100 mm Hg, Glasgow Coma Scale (GCS) <14, and respiratory rate >21 per minute. The full SOFA score is a more complex scoring system and includes: PaO_2/FiO_2 ratio, platelets, bilirubin, blood pressure, GCS, and creatinine. It is unclear at the present time whether the qSOFA will replace SIRS, but it is unlikely that the full SOFA will be in widespread use in the prehospital or ED setting due to its complexity. The wrong answer choices can be guessed by their overly insensitive cutoffs (e.g., a glucose >100 is very common in all patients, not just septic ones). Heart rate >90 is an element of the SIRS criteria rather than the qSOFA. (Annals, May 2016.)

95. Answer C. Retrobulbar hemorrhage is a result of ocular trauma that causes pressure on the posterior portion of the eye. The globe is pushed outward, and proptosis may be seen on physical examination. Increased pressure in the orbit can compress the central retinal artery or vein and cause loss of vision. Choices A, B, D, and E are all pathologic processes involving the anterior portion of the eye and are not usually caused by a retrobulbar hematoma. Secondary glaucoma may occur as a result of increased overall pressure in the globe, including in the anterior chamber. Treatment of a retrobulbar hemorrhage involves emergent lateral canthotomy and drainage of the hematoma out of the temporal border of the globe. Failure to perform lateral canthotomy for acute retrobulbar hemorrhage may result in irreversible vision loss in as little as 90 minutes.

96. Answer C. The patient has evidence of acute epididymitis, an infection of the epididymis causing local tenderness and lacking findings suggestive of testicular torsion (unilateral testicular tenderness or edema or absent cremasteric reflex). The etiologies in sexually active men younger than 35 years of age are *Chlamydia* or gonococcus. In men older than 35 years, *E. coli* is the most common cause. Antibiotic therapy is directed to the causative organism.

97. Answer C. *Legionella* spp., along with *Chlamydia* spp. and *Mycoplasma* spp. all respond to macrolide therapy. The remaining organisms are usually treated with cephalosporins or fluoroquinolones.

98. Answer C. The patient has evidence of idiopathic intracranial hypertension (IIH, also known as pseudotumor cerebri), a syndrome likely caused by increased CSF production combined with decreased CSF resorption. IIH should be considered in any case involving obese women of childbearing age with diffuse headaches and visual symptoms. Drugs such as oral contraceptives, tetracyclines, and vitamin A can increase predisposition to IIH. Diagnosis rests on exclusion of mass lesion (and dural sinus thrombosis in suspected cases) with CT brain in conjunction with a CSF opening pressure of greater than 20 cm water. Treatment consists of withholding suspected causative medications, acetazolamide with loop diuretics to decrease CSF production and possibly a ventriculoperitoneal shunt in recalcitrant cases. Initial evaluation with lumbar puncture can also serve as a temporary treatment modality by draining off CSF to normal opening pressure levels. Repeating the CT brain with IV contrast is unlikely to yield an answer after one has already been performed and increases risks of contrast administration. MRI brain may be pursued in the outpatient setting if lumbar puncture is unrevealing. EEG in the outpatient setting would be useful if seizures were suspected, but intermittent headache is an uncommon sign of seizure. Psychiatric consultation should not be performed in the ED before organic causes are ruled out.

99. Answer E. There are few differences in the ED management of patients with presumed variceal upper GI hemorrhage compared to other causes of upper GI bleeding. The initial focus is on stabilizing unstable patients with intravenous fluids and blood products as needed to maintain a target hemoglobin >7 g/dL unless patients are at high risk for, or have evidence of, cardiac ischemia or other end-organ dysfunction attributable to anemia. NG tube lavage has not been clearly shown to be useful. While a frankly positive lavage predicts high risk lesions, a negative lavage does not conclusively rule them out. IV fluids may dilute the hemoglobin concentration but they don't diminish the actual hemoglobin content (and thus, the oxygen carrying capacity of blood). While intravenous proton pump inhibitors and somatostatin analogues may not offer a significant mortality benefit to patients, they are well tolerated with few significant side effects. Their use may be helpful, possibly in consultation with a gastroenterologist who will be performing esophagoduodenoscopy.

100. **Answer E.** The incidence of perforation at the time of appendectomy has an inverse correlation with the age of the patient. More than 90% of patients younger than 3 years have evidence of perforation in the operating room. In contrast, only 15% of adolescents have perfora-tion at the time of appendectomy. This difference relates to the difficulty and subsequent delay in making a diagnosis in infants and toddlers. Most patients younger than 2 years have diffuse tenderness rather than focal tenderness over the right lower quadrant. Appendicoliths are considered pathognomonic for appendicitis but are only present in roughly 15% of cases. On the basis of the few studies performed to date, most authors recommend CT as superior to ultrasonography for the diagnosis of appendicitis. However, more data need to be collected before CT is routinely recommended as the standard of care as ultrasound may perform nearly as well, particular in pediatric centers with appropriately selected patients.

1. A 47-year-old noncompliant male with hypertension and hyperlipidemia presents with a history of 10 minutes of weakness on the right side of his body that has since resolved. His workup in the emergency department (ED) is normal and he is admitted for further evaluation. Which of the following should be included in his treatment in the ED?

   A. Clopidogrel
   B. Ticlopidine
   C. Heparin
   D. Aspirin
   E. Warfarin

2. Which of the following disease states are all patients with continuous flow left ventricular assist devices assumed to have?

   A. Vitamin D deficiency
   B. Hypoproteinemia
   C. Cirrhosis
   D. Renal failure
   E. Acquired von Willebrand deficiency

3. A 26-year-old male presents concerned he has suffered a brown recluse spider bite. He has a 1-cm red lesion on his forearm without scaling or vesicular fluid. Which of the following is the most appropriate next step in management?

   A. Reassurance and education
   B. Dapsone 100 mg PO
   C. Calcium gluconate 1 amp IV
   D. Latrodectus antivenin
   E. Bactrim DS

4. A 6-year-old female presents with abdominal pain. She has had moderate, constant periumbilical pain for several hours with associated nausea. Her parents noted a rash on her legs and buttocks for several days, which they attributed to poison ivy. Physical examination demonstrates an afebrile, uncomfortable patient, diffuse abdominal tenderness without true rebound or guarding, a maculopapular rash on the legs and buttocks, and diffuse joint tenderness. Which of the following is the most important next step in evaluation?

   A. Urinalysis
   B. CT scan of the abdomen/pelvis
   C. Antistreptolysin O antibodies (ASO) titer
   D. Blood cultures
   E. Meckel scan

5. A 5-year-old male is brought by his mother for a rash on his lower abdomen (Fig. 5-1). You suspect contact dermatitis from the metal on his jean button. Which of the following is the most likely cause?

   A. Silver
   B. Platinum
   C. Copper
   D. Nickel
   E. Zinc

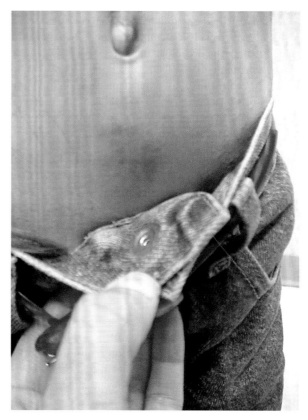

Figure 5-1

6. The preferred method of hand splinting is:

   A. The position of greatest comfort for the patient

   B. Wrist extended to 30 degrees, metacarpophalangeals (MCPs) in full extension, intraphalangeal (IP) joints flexed to 60 degrees

   C. Wrist neutral, MCPs flexed to 60 degrees, IP joints free

   D. Wrist extended to 30 degrees, MCPs flexed to 90 degrees, IP joints extended

   E. Wrist extended to 30 degrees, MCPs flexed to 30 degrees, IP joints flexed to 30 degrees

7. Which of the following is true regarding the diagnosis of aortic dissection?

   A. Magnetic resonance imaging (MRI) is more specific than CT or transesophageal echocardiogram.

   B. Chest x-ray is normal in most cases.

   C. Transthoracic echocardiogram is useful to confirm the diagnosis.

   D. Aortography is the best screening test.

   E. EKG has excellent specificity.

8. Which of the following statements about *Pseudomonas aeruginosa* is correct?

   A. Most patients with cystic fibrosis (CF) are ultimately colonized with *P. aeruginosa* and are susceptible to infection.

   B. Ceftriaxone plus azithromycin, a common front-line regimen for community-acquired pneumonia (CAP), provides antipseudomonal coverage.

   C. *P. aeruginosa* is less common among patients admitted to the intensive care unit (ICU) with severe pneumonia.

   D. *P. aeruginosa* is an important cause of malignant otitis media.

   E. *P. aeruginosa* has only a small role in causing nosocomial infections.

9. A 47-year-old previously healthy male presents to the ED with a chief complaint of fever, severe body aches, headache, and fatigue after recently returning from a family vacation in the Caribbean. Which of the following is the most likely cause of his symptoms?

   A. Amebiasis

   B. Dengue

   C. Chikungunya

   D. Zika

   E. Malaria

10. A 10-year-old male presents with fever, diarrhea, pallor, and weakness. Renal function is abnormal and the patient is anemic. A peripheral blood smear reveals schistocytes. Which of the following is the most likely diagnosis?

    A. Henoch–Schönlein purpura

    B. Hemolytic uremic syndrome (HUS)

    C. Disseminated intravascular coagulation (DIC)

    D. Idiopathic thrombocytopenic purpura

    E. Nephrotic syndrome

11. A 9-month-old male is brought by his parents for evaluation of an abdominal mass that they noticed while changing his diaper. Physical examination demonstrates a nontoxic, active infant with a palpable, nontender mass measuring 4×6 cm. Which of the following studies is most likely to reveal the diagnosis?

    A. Gall bladder ultrasonography

    B. Scrotal ultrasonography

    C. Renal ultrasonography

    D. Urinalysis

    E. Meckel scan

12. Which of the following is true regarding physostigmine?

    A. It is the drug of choice to treat most anticholinergic crises.

    B. It affects muscarinic, but not nicotinic receptors.

    C. It affects nicotinic, but not muscarinic receptors.

    D. It is able to cross the blood–brain barrier.

    E. It should be rapidly pushed to achieve clinical effect.

13. Which of the following is used in addition to acetaminophen concentration to determine severity in overdose?

    A. Lipase

    B. Amylase

    C. Gamma glutamyl transpeptidase (GGT)

    D. Aspartate aminotransferase (AST)

    E. Alkaline phosphatase

14. Which of the following muscles is most commonly injured in rotator cuff tears?

    A. Supraspinatus

    B. Infraspinatus

    C. Subscapularis

    D. Teres minor

    E. Deltoid

15. An 85-year-old female presents with right shoulder stiffness. She was diagnosed with a shoulder sprain 3 weeks ago after a fall, and has been wearing a sling since then. Physical examination demonstrates an afebrile patient with painful, restricted range of motion of the shoulder in all directions. Which of the following is the most likely diagnosis?

    A. Rotator cuff tear

    B. Adhesive capsulitis

    C. Septic arthritis

    D. Associated scapular fracture

    E. Rheumatoid arthritis

16. A 28-year-old previously healthy male presents to the ED with severe medial left upper leg pain × 1 day. The pain was mild at first but has "become unbearable" and is making it difficult for him to walk. He denies any recent trauma, or excessive exercise involving the leg. He initially noted minimal redness over the site which has started to become a "little purplish in spots." He also complains of fever, fatigue, myalgias, and nausea. Examination of his leg reveals a large area of moderate erythema with scattered ecchymotic areas and a few clear bullae. There is no crepitus. X-ray of the leg is unrevealing. His vital signs are T 102.4°F, P 122, BP 98/64, RR 20, SaO₂ 96% on RA. Which of the following is the most appropriate next step?

A. IV fluids, IV ampicillin–sulbactam and clindamycin, surgical consultation

B. IV fluids, IVIG, IV vancomycin

C. IV fluids, IV vancomycin and metronidazole, stat MRI

D. IV fluids, IV ampicillin–sulbactam and clindamycin, IV high-dose corticosteroids, IVIG

E. IV fluids, IV clindamycin, and penicillin G

17. A 35-year-old female presents with severe weakness, lightheadedness, and chest pain. Her blood pressure is 70/40 and her pulses are weak. The EKG is shown in Figure 5-2. Which of the following is the most important next step in management?

A. Adenosine 6 mg IV

B. Diltiazem 20 mg IV

C. Amiodarone 300 mg IV

D. Synchronized cardioversion at 50 J

E. Defibrillation at 200 J

18. Which of the following signs and symptoms may accompany a cluster headache?

A. Ptosis

B. Lacrimation

C. Miosis

D. Nasal congestion

E. All of the above

19. A 68-year-old male with a history of chronic obstructive pulmonary disease (COPD) presents to the emergency department (ED) with worsening dyspnea, cough, and subjective intermittent fevers. He tells you that he spent 1 week in the intensive care unit (ICU) 6 months ago after being intubated for a similar episode and states "I don't ever want to be intubated again." You discuss the use of noninvasive positive pressure ventilation (NIPPV) with him (bilevel positive airway pressure [BiPAP]) and he is agreeable. With which of the following comorbidities is BiPAP safe to use?

A. Excessive secretions

B. Decreased sensorium

C. Severe hypertension

D. Midfacial trauma

E. Uncooperative patient

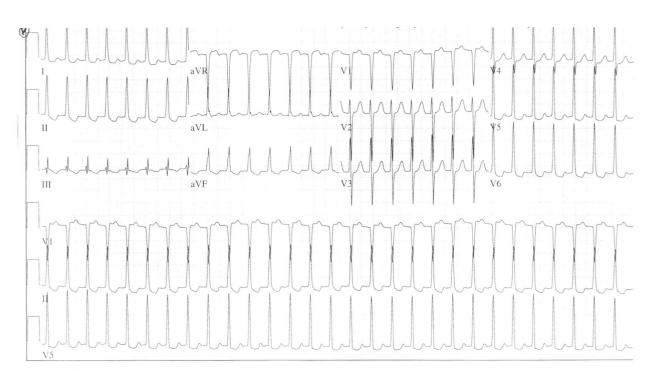

Figure 5-2

20. Which of the following is an element of the NEXUS criteria for cervical spine imaging?

    A. Absence of paraspinal tenderness
    B. Absence of smoking
    C. Absence of focal neurologic deficit
    D. Presence of forehead injuries
    E. Presence of scalp laceration

21. An 82-year-old female with a history of hypertension presents with generalized weakness and alteration of mental status for 2 days. Her vital signs are: 101.4, 110, 22, 85/45, 94% RA. Urinalysis shows >100 WBC and her chest x-ray is unremarkable. Appropriate antibiotics are already ordered. Which of the following is the most appropriate next step in her management?

    A. Intravenous fluid bolus 30 mL/kg
    B. Norepinephrine 5 mcg/kg/minute
    C. Milrinone 0.5 mcg/kg/minute
    D. Dobutamine 5 mcg/kg/minute
    E. Dopamine 5 mcg/kg/minute

22. A 42-year-old female is brought to the ED after she rear-ended a tractor trailer while driving a small sedan which partially submarined under the tractor trailer's rear bumper. Airbags were deployed, and she states she was "out for a second." She complains of headache, neck pain, back pain, as well as transient numbness over her "entire right side" that has since resolved. Her physical examination reveals multiple contusions over her face and scalp, mild left-sided ptosis, as well as abrasions over her extremities and a seatbelt sign over her left neck, chest, and abdomen. Subsequent CT scans of her head, cervical spine, chest, abdomen, and pelvis are unrevealing. Which of the following is the best next step?

    A. Admission for observation
    B. CT angiography of the neck
    C. MRI of the brain with gadolinium
    D. Discharge with outpatient follow-up
    E. Neurology consultation

23. A 45-year-old female with a history of arthritis presents with weakness in her arms and hands after being involved in a motor vehicle crash in which her head hit the windshield. She is able to walk, but has 3/5 strength in her bilateral upper extremities. Which of the following is the most likely diagnosis?

    A. Complete cord transection
    B. Anterior cord syndrome
    C. Central cord syndrome
    D. Brown–Sequard syndrome
    E. Spinal shock

24. A 34-year-old male is brought to the ED by paramedics after collapsing due to extreme exhaustion while running a marathon. Which of the following features indicate a diagnosis of heat stroke rather than simple heat exhaustion?

    A. Temperature >103.5°F
    B. Myalgia
    C. Altered mental status
    D. Syncope
    E. Paresthesias

25. A 22-year-old female presents in anticholinergic crisis. She is delirious, agitated, and requires sedation. Which of the following medications would be most appropriate to sedate this patient?

    A. Thorazine
    B. Fluphenazine
    C. Lorazepam
    D. Etomidate
    E. Ketamine

26. A 65-year-old smoker presents with sudden onset of shortness of breath for 2 hours. He denies chest pain, fever, productive cough, or lower extremity edema. Vitals signs are 99°F, 95, 24, 200/95, 92% on RA. He has bilateral wheezes. Which of the following best differentiates between obstructive lung disease and congestive heart failure (CHF)?

    A. Clinical response to albuterol
    B. D-dimer
    C. B-type natriuretic peptide (BNP)
    D. Troponin I
    E. Angiotensin-converting enzyme

27. A 21-year-old female presents to the ED for a "recheck" of her β-hCG level. She was evaluated in the ED 2 days ago after presenting with crampy low abdominal pain and vaginal spotting. Her β-hCG level at that time was 1,350 mIU/mL but her ultrasound was not diagnostic. She states that she continues to have intermittent crampy pain but she is no longer spotting. Her β-hCG level is currently 1,900 mIU/mL. What is the best next step in management?

    A. Discharge her home with a diagnosis of pregnancy.
    B. Order a pelvic ultrasound.
    C. Consult an obstetrician (OB) for a probable missed abortion.
    D. Discharge her home with a diagnosis of threatened abortion.
    E. Discharge her with instructions to follow-up with OB in 2 days for serial β-hCG levels.

28. A positive head impulse test, nystagmus that changes direction with different positions of gaze, or positive skew deviation on eye testing indicate which of the following?

    A. A hemiplegic migraine
    B. Benign paroxysmal peripheral vertigo

C. Vetebral artery dissection

D. A brainstem or cerebellar lesion

E. A vestibular nerve lesion

29. A 52-year-old female with no past medical history presents with fever, right lower quadrant pain, and occasional diarrhea for the past several days. She takes no medications and has not traveled internationally recently. Her CT scan reveals terminal ileitis. Which of the following is the most likely cause?

A. Ulcerative colitis

B. *C. difficile*

C. *Yersinia*

D. Irritable bowel syndrome

E. Giardiasis

30. A 45-year-old female with a history of asthma presents with her typical acute asthma exacerbation. She has had a runny nose and a sore throat but denies fever or productive sputum. Examination reveals bilateral wheezes. Her vital signs are 98.6°F, 110, 24, 156/95, 99% RA. She feels slightly better after an albuterol nebulizer treatment. You send off labs, and the white blood cell (WBC) count returns elevated at 13.5K. Which of the following is the next best course of action?

A. Treat community-acquired pneumonia (CAP) with azithromycin

B. Treat CAP with moxifloxacin

C. Treat airway inflammation with prednisone

D. Obtain arterial blood gas sample

E. Observe for 2 more hours, then discharge with outpatient follow-up

31. Which of the following statements about joint pathology is true?

A. Viscosity of synovial fluid increases in inflammatory or infectious arthritis.

B. Osteoarthritis (OA) classically affects the metacarpophalangeal (MCP) and proximal interphalangeal (PIP) joints.

C. A cardiac rub in the setting of arthralgias suggests systemic lupus erythematosus (SLE).

D. Sausage-shaped swelling of the fingers or toes suggests pseudogout.

E. An abducted, externally rotated hip in a neonate suggests an occult hip fracture.

32. Which of the following is true of vitreous hemorrhage?

A. Symptoms progress from floaters to visual loss.

B. The red reflex is enhanced.

C. Sudden onset of unilateral pain is typical.

D. Valsalva can be helpful in management.

E. Treatment involves recumbent position.

33. A 34-year-old male presents with acute onset of penile pain and swelling, which occurred during sexual intercourse. His penis is shown in Figure 5-3. Which of the following is the most appropriate definitive management?

A. Observation

B. Foley catheterization

C. Surgical repair

D. Penile splinting

E. Penile pressure dressing

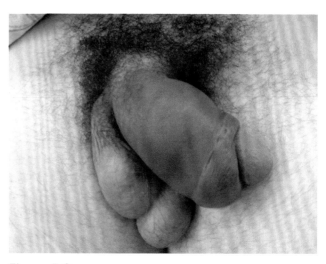

Figure 5-3

34. A 55-year-old male presents with severe chest pain radiating to the back. A CT scan of the chest reveals both ascending and descending aortic dissections. Which of the following is true regarding this patient?

A. Early, aggressive BP control is likely to be detrimental to outcome.

B. Emergent surgery is warranted.

C. Aspirin should be given in case the dissection has extended to the coronary arteries.

D. HR should be kept >100 to maximize cardiac output.

E. Transthoracic echocardiogram has the best specificity to make the diagnosis.

35. A 22-year-old female presents with acute onset of right eye discharge 3 hours before presentation. The discharge reaccumulates almost immediately after wiping it away. She does not wear contact lenses. Physical examination demonstrates normal visual acuity and copious greenish-yellow discharge in the right eye. Conjunctival injection and chemosis are prominent. Which of the following is the most likely cause?

A. *S. pneumoniae*

B. *H. influenzae*

C. *M. catarrhalis*

D. *Klebsiella pneumoniae*

E. *N. gonorrhoeae*

36. A 33-year-old male is bitten on his hand by his friend's pet rattlesnake. Which of the following is the most important next step in management?

A. Heat packs
B. Caregiver-initiated oral venom suction
C. Patient-initiated oral venom suction
D. Splint immobilization
E. IV methylprednisolone

37. Which of the following is true regarding irritable bowel syndrome (IBS)?

A. It is more common in men than in women.
B. Pain associated with IBS is usually relieved with defecation.
C. IBS is a psychiatric diagnosis.
D. IBS is most commonly caused by unrecognized food allergies.
E. All of the above

38. The most common cause of death in recipients of a solid-organ transplant is:

A. Recurrent organ failure
B. Infection
C. Drug toxicity
D. Organ rejection
E. Effects of the primary disease process

39. Which of the following correctly matches the clinical entity and its effects on phosphate metabolism?

A. Rhabdomyolysis causes hypophosphatemia.
B. Respiratory alkalosis causes hyperphosphatemia.
C. Hyperparathyroidism causes hyperphosphatemia.
D. Chronic renal insufficiency causes hypophosphatemia.
E. Treatment of diabetic ketoacidosis (DKA) causes hypophosphatemia.

40. A 46-year-old female presents with right ankle pain after a car accident. Her x-ray is shown. Which of the following is true (Fig. 5-4)?

A. A femoral nerve block provides the best anesthesia for further treatment
B. Flexing the patient's knee will make ED manipulation easier
C. The patient can be splinted for follow-up the following day
D. The patient should receive hip films to ensure there is no occult fracture
E. All of the above

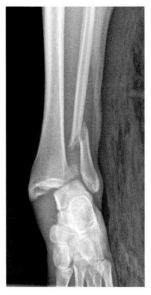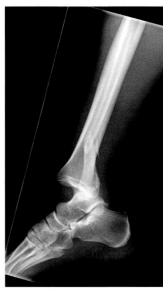

Figure 5-4

41. The drug of choice for sedation in the setting of acute delirium is

A. Haloperidol
B. Diazepam
C. Diphenhydramine
D. Morphine
E. Promethazine

42. Which of the following is the most common cause of duodenal perforations?

A. Foreign body
B. Neoplasia
C. Crohn disease
D. Tuberculosis
E. Peptic ulcer disease

43. A 76-year-old female presents to the ED in the middle of summer complaining of swelling of her ankles and feet. The daily high temperature has exceeded 100°F for the last 10 days. Which of the following is true?

A. She should be treated with furosemide.
B. Her condition may resolve with acclimation.
C. She should be treated with hydrochlorothiazide.
D. An echocardiogram should be performed to exclude heat-induced congestive heart failure.
E. Her condition is actually most common in the pediatric population.

44. A 53-year-old male with a history of alcohol abuse and chronic back pain presents to the emergency department from an alcohol treatment center for evaluation of diaphoresis and vomiting. The patient sought treatment for alcohol use after binge drinking for 2 months. His last drink was about 24 hours prior to your evaluation. While waiting for evaluation at the treatment center, he began to feel sick with multiple episodes of nonbloody emesis and abdominal pain. Staff at the treatment center sent him to the ED for further evaluation. His vitals are: T 99.4°F P 113, RR 18, BP 119/76, SaO$_2$ 97% on RA. His abdominal examination was unremarkable despite his complaints of pain. His blood tests and urinalysis are significant for:

WBC 14,200 mm^3

Hgb 13.5 g/dL

Na$^+$, 129 mEq/L

K$^+$, 3.8 mEq/L

Cl$^-$, 90 mEq/L

HCO$_3^-$, 13 mEq/L

BUN, 24 mg/dL

Cr, 1.3 mg/dL

Glucose, 86 mg/dL

Urine ketones 4+

Which of the following is the best next step?

A. IV thiamine, bolus infusion of 5% dextrose in normal saline
B. IV insulin infusion, IV thiamine, IV infusion of 5% dextrose with 20 mEq of potassium chloride in normal saline over 1 hour
C. IV insulin infusion, IV infusion of 5% dextrose with 40 mEq of potassium chloride
D. Bolus of normal saline over 1 hour
E. All of the above regimens will be equally effective

45. A 27-year-old male being treated for a performance anxiety disorder with propranolol is brought to the ED with profound hypotension. He admits to taking "the entire bottle" of tablets because he has been feeling depressed recently and "couldn't take it anymore." He started to regret the decision later, and confided in his girlfriend who called EMS. EMS found the patient somewhat somnolent and complaining of lightheadedness with a BP of 70/47, P 46, RR 18, and SaO$_2$ 98% on RA. In the ED, the patient's BP is 65/43, without any significant change in his other vital signs. Over the next 2 hours, a central venous catheter is placed, and he is given aggressive IV hydration, intravenous atropine, glucagon, calcium, and

an epinephrine drip. Despite these therapies, he remains hypotensive. Which of the following is the best next step?

A. Intravenous lipid emulsion therapy
B. Emergent hemodialysis
C. Intravenous milrinone infusion
D. High-dose intravenous insulin infusion and intravenous glucose infusion
E. Intra-aortic balloon pump and temporary transvenous pacing

46. Which of the following characteristics of warfarin is an advantage over the novel oral anticoagulants (inhibitors of Factors IIa and Xa) in the treatment of venous thromboembolism?

A. No need for monitoring of drug levels
B. Less frequent major bleeding episodes
C. Lower myocardial infarction risk
D. Reduced early pro-thrombotic effect
E. Reduced risk of venous thromboembolism recurrence

47. Which of the following physical examination findings is consistent with a relative left-sided afferent papillary defect when a penlight is swung between the two eyes in a darkened room?

A. The left pupil dilates when light is shined into the left eye.
B. The left pupil constricts when light is shined into the left eye.
C. The left pupil does not respond to light when light is shined into the left eye.
D. The left pupil dilates when light is shined into the right eye.
E. The left pupil constricts when light is shined into the right eye.

48. Which of the following is true regarding inflammatory bowel disease?

A. Toxic megacolon is more common in patients with Crohn disease than ulcerative colitis.
B. Perianal complications are most common in patients with Crohn disease.
C. Crohn disease always involves the rectum.
D. Erythema nodosum is most common in male patients with ulcerative colitis.
E. Anal fissures in patients with Crohn disease tend to be located in the posterior midline.

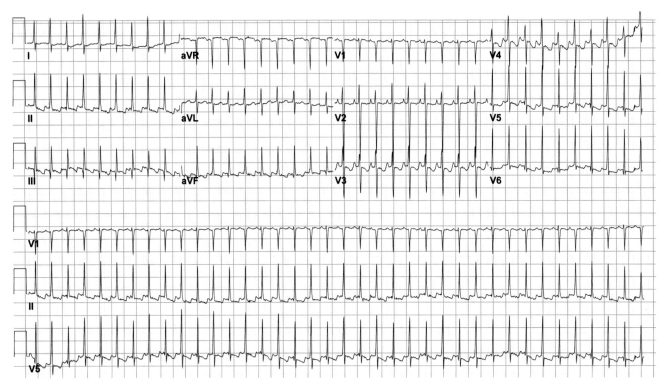

Figure 5-5

49. A 4-week-old infant is brought in by his parents breathing fast and appearing sweaty. His respiratory rate is 54, BP 88/60, P 200. His skin is pink and capillary refill is about 2 seconds. His EKG is shown. Which the following is true (Fig. 5-5)?

   A. A bag of ice should be held over the infant's nose and mouth for 30 seconds
   B. The baby has Wolff Parkinson White (WPW) syndrome
   C. Adenosine should be avoided
   D. Electrical cardioversion should be performed immediately
   E. Verapamil is the intravenous agent of choice

50. Which of the following is true about peptic ulcer disease?

   A. Pain that wakes patients in the middle of night is typical of duodenal ulcers.
   B. The incidence of bleeding from gastric ulcers is approximately two times that of duodenal ulcers.
   C. *Helicobacter pylori* is the major risk factor linked to the development of duodenal ulcers but has almost no role in the development of gastric ulcers.
   D. Barium contrast is the diagnostic study of choice to diagnose peptic ulcer disease.
   E. Only 50% of those people infected with *H. pylori* will develop a peptic ulcer in their lifetime.

51. A 4-day-old term neonate with an uncomplicated birth history is brought to the ED by his parents who complain he seems very yellow. He is feeding normally and seems active. Which of the following is true?

   A. If indicated, phototherapy is the initial treatment of choice
   B. Severe hyperbilirubinemia primarily causes cardiac complications
   C. The patient will probably need an exchange transfusion
   D. The patient has "bronze baby" syndrome
   E. The bilirubin level can be roughly determined by physical examination

52. Which of the following is the major pathophysiologic mechanism in gastroesophageal reflux disease (GERD)?

   A. Increased gastric acid production
   B. Decreased lower esophageal sphincter tone
   C. Increased gastric emptying time
   D. Increased gastric pressure
   E. Decreased gastric mucosal barrier

53. A 63-year-old male with a history of nephrolithiasis presents to the ED with acute onset right flank pain. He receives an uncontrasted CT scan which is unrevealing, and he has no hematuria. A repeat study with contrast is performed, a slice of which is shown in Figure 5-6. The patient feels better and has minimal pain. His vital signs are T 98.4, P 84, RR 16, BP 156/82, SaO_2 98% on RA. Which of the following is true (Fig. 5-6)?

   A. His blood pressure is already at the treatment goal.
   B. More than 90% patients have a diagnosis of hypertension.

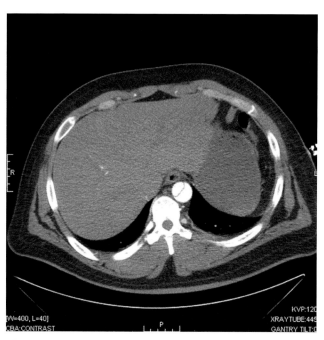

Figure 5-6

C. EKGs are helpful in discriminating this from myocardial infarction.

D. Elevated D-dimer levels increase the likelihood of the diagnosis.

E. An upper extremity pulse deficit is the most specific physical examination finding.

54. A 76-year-old female presents after a fall from standing height onto a countertop. She landed on the right side of her ribcage and complains of pain in that area and difficulty taking a deep breath. Vital signs are normal and physical examination is remarkable only for point tenderness in the right lateral fourth and fifth ribs. A chest x-ray done in the ED is normal. Which of the following is the most appropriate next step in management?

A. Admit to the intensive care unit (ICU)
B. Discharge home
C. Discharge home with pain medication
D. Discharge home with pain medication and incentive spirometer
E. Discharge home with pain medication, incentive spirometer, and antibiotics

55. Which of the following is true regarding renal injury in trauma?

A. In penetrating trauma, absence of hematuria rules out renal injury.
B. In blunt trauma, microscopic hematuria alone is rarely associated with renal injury.

C. Most renal injuries require operative repair.
D. Renal injuries are extremely uncommon in children with blunt trauma.
E. Plain radiography is the imaging test of choice for diagnosis.

56. Which of the following is the most common symptom in patients with spinal cord compression?

A. Urinary retention
B. Saddle anesthesia
C. Motor weakness
D. Bowel incontinence
E. Ascending paresthesias

57. A 1-year-old presents with sudden onset of high fever for several days, followed by defervesence and the rash seen on the image (Fig. 5-7). Which of the following is true regarding this condition?

A. It is caused by human herpesvirus-6
B. Concomitant lymphadenopathy is rare
C. Seizures are seen in most cases
D. Management involves intravenous antibiotics
E. A "slapped cheek" appearance is the initial manifestation

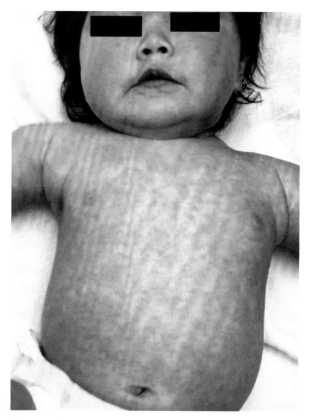

Figure 5-7

58. Which of the following is true about volvulus?

    A. Plain films are more often diagnostic in cases of cecal volvulus than sigmoid volvulus.
    B. Reduction of cecal volvulus is best achieved endoscopically.
    C. Cecal volvulus is diagnosed by visualizing a massively dilated cecum in the left upper quadrant on x-ray.
    D. Cecal volvulus is more common than sigmoid volvulus.
    E. Cecal volvulus is most common in patients aged 25 to 35 years.

59. Which of the following is true regarding heart transplant recipients?

    A. The resting heart rate is decreased from their pretransplant baseline.
    B. Tamponade cannot occur in a transplanted heart.
    C. Acute rejection is usually diagnosed by endomyocardial biopsy.
    D. There is no increased risk of endocarditis with invasive procedures.
    E. The heart rate increases only minimally with exercise or stress.

60. A 74-year-old female presents with acute onset of severe, diffuse abdominal pain and nausea. Her vitals are: 100.5, 112, 18, 100/67, 99% on RA. Her heart reveals an irregular rhythm, but her abdominal examination exhibits only mild tenderness. You order comprehensive labs, an upright chest x-ray, and a CT of the abdomen with IV contrast. Which of the following is the next best step in management?

    A. Broad-spectrum antibiotics
    B. Tissue plasminogen activator
    C. Barium enema
    D. HIDA scan
    E. Norepinephrine

61. A 46-year-old female presents with a chief complaint of painless flashes and floaters. She has not noted any trouble reading or other changes to her vision. Which of the following examination findings increases the likelihood of an associated retinal detachment?

    A. A wavy hyperechoic line anterior to the retina on bedside ultrasound
    B. Visual field deficit on confrontation testing
    C. Vitreous hemorrhage on slit-lamp examination
    D. Decreased visual acuity
    E. All of the above

62. A 57-year-old male smoker with hypertension, hypercholesterolemia, and peripheral vascular disease presents unable to walk due to pain. He has had progressive worsening of pain in both his legs on walking for several weeks, and the left calf has been extremely painful for 2 days. Vital signs are T 98.2, HR 90 regular, BP 175/90, RR 20, SpO$_2$ 98% RA. Examination reveals a regular heart rate, 1+ dorsalis pedis (DP)/posterior tibialis (PT) pulses on the right, absent DP/PT pulses on left, ABI 0.55 on the right and 0.40 on the left, no bruits, and no signs of infection. Which of the following is the most likely pathophysiologic mechanism?

    A. In situ thrombosis
    B. Arterial embolism
    C. Inflammation
    D. Vasospasm
    E. Arteriovenous (AV) fistula

63. Which of the following pediatric heart diseases causes cyanosis?

    A. Mitral stenosis
    B. Coarctation of the aorta
    C. Transposition of the great vessels
    D. Atrial septal defect (ASD)
    E. Ventricular septal defect (VSD)

64. A 23-year-old female presents with shortness of breath. She is 3 days postpartum after a term, normal spontaneous vaginal delivery. She describes bilateral leg swelling, orthopnea, and cough with frothy sputum. She denies chest pain. Physical examination demonstrates presence of S3, bilateral pulmonary crackles, and pitting edema of her lower extremities. Which of the following is true regarding this condition?

    A. Cardiac catheterization is the next step in management.
    B. It occurs in approximately 10% of all pregnancies.
    C. Patients who survive do not develop the condition in subsequent pregnancies.
    D. Mortality is as high as 30%.
    E. Aspirin is the mainstay of therapy.

65. Which of the following is an expected finding in pregnancy?

    A. Increased tidal volume
    B. Decreased RBC mass
    C. Decreased WBC count
    D. Increased respiratory rate
    E. Decreased glomerular filtration rate

66. A 47-year-old male presents with erythema of his left foot for several days with intermittent chills. Examination reveals a warm, erythematous, and tender dorsal foot consistent with cellulitis. He indicates that he has had methicillin-resistant *Staphylococcus aureus* skin infection in the past. Which of the following is the best treatment for this patient?

    A. Doxycycline
    B. Azithromycin
    C. Dicloxacillin

D. Cephalexin

E. No antibiotics—watchful waiting

67. The pictured deformity in Figure 5-8 occurs in:

A. Rheumatoid arthritis

B. Osteoarthritis

C. Systemic lupus erythematosus

D. Reactive arthritis

E. Psoriatic arthritis

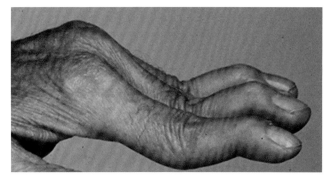

Figure 5-8

68. What is the sensitivity of plain abdominal radiographs for the diagnosis of small bowel obstruction (SBO)?

A. 10%

B. 25%

C. 50%

D. 75%

E. 90%

69. Which of the following is a unique aspect of tarantulas?

A. Their abdominal hairs can become embedded in the skin resulting in subsequent allergic reactions.

B. In addition to venom, they serve as a vector for *Borrelia* spp. and may transmit Lyme disease.

C. Their venom triggers widespread mast cell degranulation resulting in diffuse flushing and pruritus.

D. Tarantula envenomation may result in anaphylaxis and rapid respiratory failure.

E. Envenomation of an extremity can cause transient paralysis distal to the wound.

70. A 25-year-old male presents with paralysis of the right side of his face on waking this morning. On examination, you note that the upper half of his face on the right side is functioning normally, but the lower half is completely paralyzed. He does not have a rash and has not traveled recently. Which of the following is the most appropriate next step in management?

A. Prednisone PO

B. Valacyclovir PO

C. Prednisone PO + valacyclovir PO

D. Doxycycline PO

E. CT brain

71. What is the most commonly encountered anorectal problem in infants?

A. Anal fissure

B. Hemorrhoids

C. Fistula

D. Ischiorectal abscess

E. Pilonidal cyst

72. Which of the following is true in alcoholic ketoacidosis (AKA)?

A. In addition to glucose, insulin is useful in management.

B. The alcohol level is usually >100 mg/dL.

C. The osmolal gap is usually elevated.

D. β-hydroxybutyrate is the primary ketone responsible for the acidosis and is produced due to inadequate glucose stores.

E. All of the above

73. Oropharyngeal dysphagia:

A. Results in more difficulty swallowing solids than liquids

B. Is a common result of stroke

C. Is almost never associated with myasthenia gravis (MG)

D. Is characterized by progressive, unremitting dysphagia

E. Commonly presents with neck pain and torticollis

74. Which of the following is a classic symptom of a hydatidiform mole?

A. Pregnancy-induced hypertension occurring during the first trimester

B. Uterine enlargement greater than expected for gestational dates

C. Abnormal vaginal bleeding

D. Hyperemesis gravidarum

E. All of the above

75. A 38-year-old female presents with progressive, lower extremity weakness and numbness for 1 week. Her physical examination reveals decreased strength, sensation, and deep tendon reflexes in both lower extremities. CSF would most likely reveal which of the following?

A. Significant elevations in protein and cells

B. Significant elevation in protein, mild elevation in cells

C. Mild elevation in protein, significant elevation in cells

D. Significant elevation in protein, significant decrease in glucose

E. Mild elevation in protein, significant decrease in glucose

76. A 69-year-old male with diabetes, hypertension, hyperlipidemia, and COPD presents with signs and symptoms of sepsis. A chest x-ray reveals pneumonia. A lactate level is measured. At what lactate level does patient mortality rise significantly?

    A. Lactate >0.5 mmol/L
    B. Lactate >1 mmol/L
    C. Lactate >2 mmol/L
    D. Lactate >4 mmol/L
    E. Lactate >6 mmol/L

77. Which of the following is true about vertigo?

    A. Purely vertical nystagmus is almost always consistent with peripheral vertigo.
    B. Nystagmus in central vertigo may change direction.
    C. Patients with central and peripheral causes of vertigo generally have equal difficulty with gait (ataxia).
    D. Nausea and vomiting are classically more prominent in central vertigo.
    E. Nystagmus in central vertigo is inhibited with fixation.

78. A 44-year-old male with AIDS presents with chronic diarrhea, flatulence, and generalized malaise for 1 month. Which of the following is the most likely cause of his symptoms?

    A. *Cryptosporidium* spp.
    B. *Campylobacter* spp.
    C. *Giardia lamblia*
    D. *Escherichia coli*
    E. *Enteromonas hominis*

79. Which of the following areas is susceptible to thermal burns that are often deeper than they initially appear?

    A. Ears
    B. Medial thighs
    C. Volar surfaces of the forearms
    D. Perineum
    E. All of the above

80. A 44-year-old male is struck on the head with a baseball bat. A CT scan of the brain is shown in Figure 5-9. Which of the following is the most likely diagnosis?

    A. Epidural hematoma
    B. Subdural hematoma
    C. Subarachnoid hemorrhage
    D. Cerebral contusion
    E. Diffuse axonal injury (DAI)

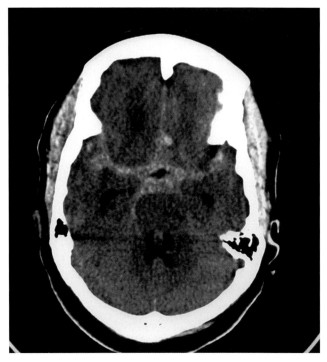

Figure 5-9

81. Parents of a 3-year-old male bring him to the ED with a yellowish, crusting facial rash, as shown in Figure 5-10. Which of the following is true?

    A. The lesions are not easily transmitted to other patients.
    B. Most cases are caused by group A *Streptococcus*.
    C. Antibiotic therapy reduces the incidence of post-streptococcal glomerulonephritis.
    D. Regional lymphadenopathy is a common finding.
    E. The lesions are typically painful.

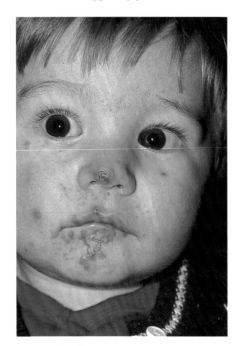

Figure 5-10

82. A 42-year-old healthy male experiences crampy abdominal pain and persistent, violent recurrent retching, and vomiting 3 hours after eating a hamburger, corn, and potato salad at a backyard picnic. Which of the following is true about his illness?

    A. The disease is caused by rapid invasion of the intestinal mucosa
    B. Antibiotics are instrumental in management
    C. Most cases are caused by *Bacillus cereus*
    D. A heat-stable toxin is responsible for his symptoms
    E. This syndrome is the most common cause of acute food poisoning in the United States

83. Which of the following animals confers the highest risk of transmitting rabies?

    A. Squirrel
    B. Raccoon
    C. Hamster
    D. Bat
    E. Rabbit

84. Which of the following is the major complication of ischemic central retinal vein occlusion (CRVO)?

    A. Conjunctivitis
    B. Iritis
    C. Glaucoma
    D. Lens dislocation
    E. Corneal ulcer

85. A 23-year-old previously healthy female is brought in for evaluation after a house fire. The patient had been sleeping when she was pulled out of a burning bedroom by her father. She is awake but somnolent, and complains of a headache as well as a burning sensation to her arms and face. EMS reports her CO level was 20% on initial assessment. What is the best means to determine if she has concomitant cyanide toxicity?

    A. Send a STAT cyanide level
    B. Test for methemoglobinemia
    C. Send a venous blood gas with a lactate level
    D. Order coximetry
    E. Administer empiric amyl nitrite and look for a positive effect

86. A 34-year-old male presents after a high-speed motor vehicle crash. Chest x-ray is performed and shown in Figure 5-11. Which of the following is the most likely diagnosis?

    A. Pneumothorax
    B. Small bowel rupture
    C. Duodenal hematoma
    D. Diaphragmatic rupture
    E. Hemothorax

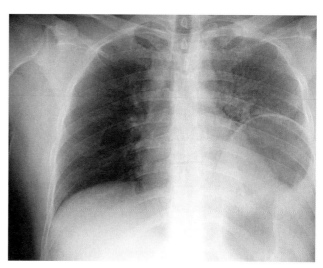

Figure 5-11

87. The most common cause of bacterial arthritis in adults is:

    A. *Staphylococcus aureus*
    B. *Neisseria gonorrhoeae*
    C. *Streptococcus pyogenes*
    D. *Hemophilus influenza*
    E. Polymicrobial

88. A 41-year-old female with fibromyalgia syndrome presents with an acute flare of her pain. Her only daily medication is gabapentin, and she takes acetaminophen as needed for pain. Her vital signs are unremarkable. Which of the following is the most appropriate therapy to add to acetaminophen for pain?

    A. Oxycodone
    B. Tramadol
    C. Aspirin
    D. Ibuprofen
    E. Prednisone

89. A 55-year-old female presents with wrist pain after falling on her outstretched right hand. A lateral wrist radiograph is shown in Figure 5-12. Which of the following is the most likely diagnosis?

    A. Scaphoid fracture
    B. Lunate dislocation
    C. Perilunate dislocation
    D. Distal radius fracture
    E. Thumb metacarpal fracture

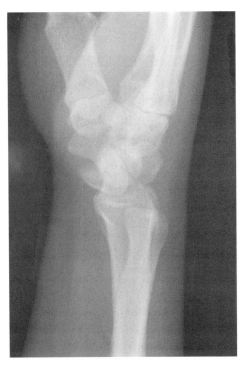

Figure 5-12

90. A 24-year-old male presented to the ED with an acute asthma exacerbation that was refractory to optimal treatment. A few minutes after intubating him, the resuscitation nurse tells you that the patient is waking up and "fighting the vent." Your best initial course of action is to

    A. Paralyze the patient with cisatracurium to ensure that he "synchronizes" with the vent.
    B. Give the patient a bolus of IV propofol and place the patient on a propofol drip.
    C. Infuse ketamine at a dose of 1.5 mg/kg.
    D. Paralyze the patient with succinylcholine to ensure that he "synchronizes" with the vent.
    E. Check a stat metabolic panel to ensure that the patient is not hyperkalemic.

91. A 62-year-old male presents after a motor vehicle collision with severe ankle pain after his left foot got caught under the accelerator. His foot is shown in Figure 5-13. Which of the following is likely to be true regarding this patient?

    A. Ankle sprain is the most likely diagnosis.
    B. Accompanying bony fracture is extremely likely.

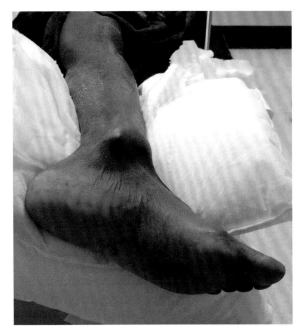

Figure 5-13

    C. Sciatic nerve injury is likely to be involved.
    D. Nonemergent reduction is the most appropriate treatment option.
    E. Pain control is rarely needed due to associated nerve injury.

92. Which of the following is the most effective treatment for lithium poisoning?

    A. Activated charcoal
    B. Sodium bicarbonate
    C. Glucagon
    D. Potassium chloride
    E. Hemodialysis

93. A 26-year-old primigravida is diagnosed with a spontaneous abortion at 6 weeks' gestation. She asks you, "why did this happen?" Which of the following is the most common cause of first-trimester miscarriage?

    A. Fetal chromosomal trisomy
    B. Uterine structural abnormality
    C. Maternal stress
    D. Minor trauma, e.g., falls
    E. Cigarette smoking

94. A 46-year-old female presents with a large amount of bright red bloody stool. In the ED she experiences another episode of significant rectal bleeding. The most likely underlying cause is:

    A. Angiodysplasia
    B. Diverticulosis
    C. Ischemic colitis
    D. Colon cancer
    E. Inflammatory bowel disease

95. A 35-year-old female presents after a high-speed MVC. She was unrestrained and there was considerable damage to the vehicle. She complains of chest pain and right leg pain. Paramedics report that the right ankle is visibly deformed. The patient is brought in on a backboard and in a C-collar. Primary survey in the ED is intact. Secondary survey reveals normal pulses and sensation in the deformed right ankle. Vital signs are T 99.0°F, P 90, RR 22, BP 144/92, PO$_x$ 95% RA. Which of the following is the most appropriate next step in management?

   A. Chest x-ray
   B. Lateral cervical spine x-ray
   C. Right ankle x-ray
   D. CT scan of the abdomen/pelvis
   E. CT scan of the head

96. A 54-year-old male presents with a 4-hour history of chest pain, which has resolved at presentation. He also complains of diaphoresis, shortness of breath, and orthopnea. Vital signs are 98.6, 60, 22, 97/60, 92% on RA. Physical examination demonstrates an S$_3$ and bilateral crackles to the midlung fields. The EKG is shown in Figure 5-14. Which of the following is the most appropriate definitive management?

   A. Admit for immediate percutaneous transluminal coronary angioplasty
   B. Admit for immediate fibrinolytic therapy
   C. Admit for immediate upper endoscopy
   D. Admit for immediate heparin, G2b3a inhibitor, and cardiac care unit admission
   E. Discharge home for outpatient stress test

97. Neglect or "hemi-inattention" usually indicates a stroke in which of the following distributions?

   A. Frontal lobe
   B. Occipital lobe
   C. Left hemisphere
   D. Right hemisphere
   E. Brainstem

98. The Ottawa knee rules:

   A. Should never be used in children
   B. State x-rays are not needed in patients with isolated patella tenderness
   C. State x-rays are required in patients complaining of knee pain who walk with a significant limp
   D. Are nearly 100% sensitive in identifying patients with knee fractures
   E. Were developed to determine which patients need x-rays among those with chronic knee pain

99. A 32-year-old female with a history of systemic lupus erythematosus (SLE) presents with chest pain. EKG shows sinus tachycardia. Which of the following is the most likely cause?

   A. Coronary artery atherosclerosis
   B. Coronary artery vasculitis
   C. Pericarditis
   D. Myocarditis
   E. Endocarditis

100. An 18-day-old term neonate, weighing 5 kg is brought in by his parents with vomiting and poor feeding. The patient has a seizure in the emergency room and a point of care blood glucose reading is 30 mg/dL. The next best step is to infuse:

   A. 5 mL/kg of 10% dextrose in water (D10)
   B. 1 mL/kg of 50% dextrose in water (D50)
   C. 25 mcg/kg of glucagon
   D. 5 mL/kg of 5% dextrose in water (D5)
   E. All of the above are reasonable choices

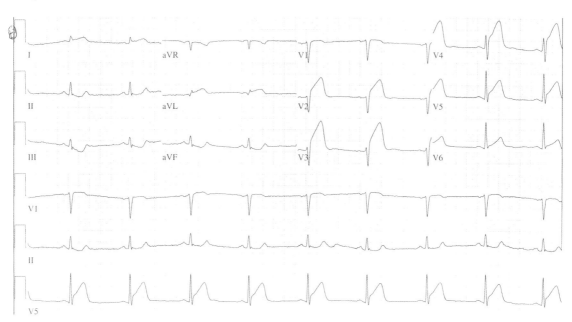

Figure 5-14

ANSWERS AND EXPLANATIONS

1. **Answer D.** Although no trial has definitively evaluated the effect of aspirin when given immediately after a transient ischemic attack (TIA), aspirin has been shown to reduce the long-term risk of stroke and cardiovascular events by 22%. No other agent has been studied as thoroughly as aspirin. The optimal dose of aspirin has yet to be determined, as doses ranging from 75 to 1,300 mg demonstrate similar reductions in vascular events (although the risk of intracerebral bleeding increases at high doses). Regular strength aspirin (325 mg) is probably adequate for most patients. The data regarding the immediate initiation of heparin for patients with TIA and atrial fibrillation are mixed. Finally, patients who are already taking aspirin and who experience a TIA may be candidates for additional drug therapy such as clopidogrel. Consultation with a neurologist is suggested before starting such therapy.

2. **Answer E.** Patients with continuous flow left ventricular assist devices (LVADs) have continuous shearing of the blood, cleaving von Willebrand factor multimers into smaller, less active pieces. Von Willebrand factor is responsible for platelet adhesion and reduction in its active form due to LVAD cleavage usually causes skin and mucosal bleeding and easy bruising. More serious bleeding can occur, including epistaxis and gastrointestinal (GI) bleeding. Desmopressin or platelet transfusion may be necessary to manage bleeding. None of the other disease states are almost always seen in patients with LVADs, although renal failure may be more common than A, B, or C.

3. **Answer A.** The vast majority of people who claim to have a spider bite usually have either a developing abscess due to methicillin-resistant *Staphylococcus aureus* (MRSA) or self-limited minor, local skin irritation. To make the diagnosis of a spider bite, the patient actually has to witness the spider biting them and the spider has to be one that is known to bite humans. Treatment for minor skin lesions (such as the one described in the question) involves education and reassurance. Human-biting spiders that are known to cause significant disease include the brown recluse (*Loxosceles reclusa*) and the black widow (*Latrodectus mactans*). Brown recluse bites can sometimes cause large necrotic skin lesions. Dapsone has unclear benefits though some experts recommend its use in the setting of true skin necrosis. Most brown recluse bites should be managed with supportive care only. Black widow spider bites rarely cause skin lesions. Calcium gluconate is a somewhat outdated therapy for black widow spider bites based on the finding that many patients with black widow bites presented

with hypocalcemia. This electrolyte abnormality was more likely a result of (rather than a cause of) constant muscle contraction, including the classic "pseudoperitoneum" of the abdomen that occurs with some black widow spider bites. Black widow bites should be treated with supportive care and benzodiazepines. Bactrim can be a useful adjunct in patients with abscesses presumed secondary to MRSA.

4. **Answer A.** The patient has evidence of Henoch–Schonlein purpura (HSP), an immune-mediated vasculitis of idiopathic origin. Young children are the highest risk group. Dermatologic, gastrointestinal, renal, and musculoskeletal findings are seen. The rash of HSP is characteristic: A maculopapular eruption on the legs and buttocks and almost never involving the upper extremities or trunk. Abdominal pain is due to intestinal vasculitis or intussusception, which occurs with higher frequency in patients with HSP than the normal population. Renal involvement may be due to glomerulonephritis, which is detected as hematuria on urinalysis. In addition, patients may have mild to nephritic range proteinuria. While the long-term prognosis of children with renal involvement is good, persistent renal dysfunction accounts for a significant portion of the morbidity associated with HSP. Current management of HSP involves potential administration of corticosteroids or intravenous immunoglobulin (IVIG) to prevent and treat glomerulonephritis. Abdominopelvic CT scan is not indicated, as HSP is a clinical diagnosis. Despite the possibility of HSP as an immune-mediated response to streptococcal infection, ASO titers are not routinely indicated, as they do not change management. Blood cultures are not necessary in these patients except when systemic infection is suspected by fever and focal abdominal tenderness. A Meckel scan is used to detect the presence of Meckel diverticulum, which usually presents with painless rectal bleeding rather than the constellation of signs seen in HSP.

5. **Answer D.** Nickel is the most common overall cause of contact dermatitis in the world and the second most common cause in the United States (after poison ivy/oak). Nickel is found in many metals on clothes, and many silver and gold chains use nickel as a filler metal. Notably, "sterling silver" chains do not contain significant amounts of nickel. Symptoms of allergic contact dermatitis include a pruritic, maculopapular rash. Treatment involves avoiding nickel substances and mild topical corticosteroids. (Figure courtesy of Robert Hendrickson, MD, In: Greenberg MI, Hendrickson RG,

Silverberg M, et al., eds. *Greenberg's Text-Atlas of Emergency Medicine.* Lippincott Williams & Wilkins; 2004:51, with permission.)

6. **Answer D.** The position described is called the intrinsic plus position or the safe hand position. When the MCP joint is extended, the collateral ligaments are relatively flaccid, while they are stretched during flexion. If patients are splinted with the MCP joints in extension, contraction of the collateral ligaments occurs and patients may not be able to fully flex their digits once the splint is removed. In contrast, extension of the IP joints ensures that its collateral ligaments will also be taut.

7. **Answer A.** MRI is the most specific test for the diagnosis of aortic dissection. Logistic difficulties prevent routine use of MRI in this setting—for this reason, CT aortogram is the most commonly used test and has excellent sensitivity and specificity. Chest x-ray is abnormal in most cases, but the sensitivity is not high enough to rule out the diagnosis in high-risk patients. Transesophageal, not transthoracic, echocardiography may provide useful structural information about the descending aorta, heart, and pericardium, but CT aortogram and MRI are far more specific. Aortography is used only in confirmatory settings. Electrocardiography is useful only in ruling out other causes of the patient's symptoms and has no utility in confirming the diagnosis of aortic dissection.

8. **Answer A.** *P. aeruginosa* is a common nosocomial pathogen, especially in ICUs. It rarely causes infection in healthy hosts but it has an increasingly appreciated role in community-acquired infections. Most patients with *P. aeruginosa* infections have known risk factors, including patients who are mechanically ventilated, immunocompromised, HIV+, as well as patients with underlying malignancies. Among these, patients with neutropenia and those under mechanical ventilation are at highest risk. This is why empiric coverage for neutropenic fever has, in the past, included two antibiotics with activity against *Pseudomonas. P. aeruginosa* is also the most prominent pathogen in patients with CF. Some studies have demonstrated that as many as 97% of children with CF were colonized with *P. aeruginosa* by the age of 3. It is known that *P. aeruginosa* has a prominent role in the progression of CF, resulting in significant morbidity and mortality. However, the exact mechanisms by which it achieves this are not entirely elucidated. Ceftriaxone and azithromycin do not provide any coverage against pseudomonas infections. Antibiotics that have antipseudomonal activity include some cephalosporins, such as ceftazidime and cefepime, β-lactam/β-lactamase inhibitor combinations (e.g., piperacillin/tazobactam), monobactams (e.g., aztreonam), carbapenems (e.g., imipenem, meropenem), aminoglycosides, and fluoroquinolones. Resistance patterns will vary depending on the local community. *P. aeruginosa* is an important cause of malignant otitis externa, not media, in patients with diabetes.

9. **Answer B.** Dengue is a viral infection endemic to the Caribbean that is also the most prevalent mosquito-borne disease worldwide. Few patients are symptomatic, but patients with "classic" dengue fever complain of fever, headaches, fatigue, and severe myalgias and arthralgias, a syndrome which is sometimes called "break bone fever." There are no effective antiviral medications for dengue so treatment is supportive. Chikungunya and Zika are also mosquito-borne viral infections which are usually asymptomatic and for which treatment is supportive. Chikungunya is more widely distributed in Africa while a Zika virus outbreak recently took place in the Americas and Caribbean. Malaria is a more virulent mosquito-borne parasitic illness that is treated with specific antimalarial drugs. Finally, amebiasis is most commonly an asymptomatic infection caused by a protozoan, *Entamoeba histolytica,* that spreads through contaminated food or water. Symptomatic patients present with dysentery from colitis or sometimes amebic liver abscesses.

10. **Answer B.** In the setting of renal dysfunction, anemia, and diarrhea, schistocytes suggest a diagnosis of hemolytic uremic syndrome (HUS). The triad of anemia, thrombocytopenia, and renal insufficiency should prompt evaluation for either HUS or thrombotic thrombocytopenic purpura (TTP). Fever and neurologic signs and symptoms are more common in the latter, but the two are thought to be on the same spectrum of disease. The toxin-forming bacterium *E. coli* O157:H7 is responsible for most epidemic cases of HUS. Treatment is primarily supportive, aimed at preventing complications of severe anemia and thrombocytopenia. Plasmapheresis is used for cases of idiopathic HUS or TTP. Henoch–Schönlein purpura is a vasculitis heralded by renal dysfunction in the setting of lower extremity palpable purpura, abdominal pain, and arthralgias. DIC is due to distortion of the clotting cascade from severe associated illness. Idiopathic thrombocytopenic purpura causes thrombocytopenia without schistocyte formation. Nephrotic syndrome causes renal dysfunction without hematologic abnormalities.

11. **Answer C.** Abdominal masses in infants are usually renal in origin, most commonly benign tumors or cysts. Both neuroblastoma, most often arising from the adrenal glands, and Wilms tumor, the most common renal malignancy, are frequent causes of abdominal masses. Renal ultrasonography or CT of the abdomen and pelvis should be performed to better evaluate the mass. Gall bladder tumors and stones are rare in infants. Scrotal ultrasonography will help to evaluate groin and testicular

pathology but is not useful for abdominal evaluation. Urinalysis is commonly normal in patients with renal cysts or tumors. A Meckel scan is useful to evaluate a Meckel diverticulum, which usually presents with painless rectal bleeding rather than mass.

12. **Answer D.** Physostigmine is an acetylcholinesterase inhibitor that serves to antagonize the effect of anticholinergic agents. It affects both nicotinic and muscarinic receptors and crosses the blood–brain barrier. Potential toxicity may occur during rapid administration, severely limiting its clinical use. It is absolutely contraindicated in patients with tricyclic overdose due to its potential for causing seizures and asystole. Supportive care is more beneficial than physostigmine therapy in most anticholinergic crises.

13. **Answer D.** Acetaminophen is metabolized by a variety of pathways, the most important of which is through the cytochrome P-450 system, which produces *N*-acetyl-*p*-benzoquinoneimine which is the toxic metabolite causing hepatocyte necrosis. The drug *N*-acetylcysteine reduces the amount of acetaminophen metabolized by this route by replenishing glutathione, the reducing agent which induces sulfation of acetaminophen to a nontoxic compound. Severity of acetaminophen overdose is measured by a 4-hour acetaminophen concentration as well as markers of liver damage, the most important of which is AST. Amylase and lipase are important indicators of pancreatic damage. Although GGT and alkaline phosphatase are present in the biliary ductal epithelium, they are less specific for hepatocellular damage than AST or ALT.

14. **Answer A.** The rotator cuff is a group of muscles composed of the supraspinatus, infraspinatus, teres minor, and subscapularis (SITS). Its primary function is to stabilize the shoulder joint. It is most commonly injured chronically with repetitive motions or acutely with a fall on an outstretched hand. The supraspinatus is the most common of the rotator cuff muscles to be injured. Physical examination of patients with supraspinatus tears indicates inability to maintain active abduction at 90 degrees without limitation in passive range of motion. Diagnosis may be confirmed with MRI and acute tears may require early surgery. The deltoid muscle is not technically part of the rotator cuff.

15. **Answer B.** Limited range of motion in the shoulder in patients with preceding trauma is most likely to be due to adhesive capsulitis (also called *frozen shoulder*). Adhesive capsulitis is characterized by stiffness with or without pain in all directions of shoulder movement. Prevention and treatment of adhesive capsulitis after shoulder injury are accomplished by range of motion exercises. Rotator cuff tear is usually heralded by significant pain when the arm is moved in a particular direction. Septic

arthritis usually involves a febrile patient with extreme pain on any movement of the joint. Scapular fracture is rare in patients without high-force mechanisms such as motor vehicle crashes or falls from height. Rheumatoid arthritis would be unlikely in an 85-year-old without prior history.

16. **Answer A.** This patient is presenting with findings most consistent with type II necrotizing fasciitis caused by group A *Streptococcus* (GAS). Type I necrotizing fasciitis is a polymicrobial infection caused by a mixture of aerobes and anaerobes that most commonly occurs in diabetic and postsurgical patients. In contrast, type II necrotizing fasciitis is a monomicrobial infection, primarily caused by GAS that occurs in previously healthy patients. Regardless of the cause, necrotizing fasciitis is a rapidly progressive, severe infection associated with a significant mortality rate, even with optimal treatment. While there is no single, wholly reliable finding in the setting of early necrotizing fasciitis, extreme pain with minimal cutaneous findings is often the first manifestation. Once the initial mild erythema develops into ecchymoses with vesicles and bullae, extensive damage has already taken place in the subcutaneous tissues. The primary treatment is immediate surgical debridement. While antibiotics are also essential, the mortality rate is close to 100% without surgery. Though a monomicrobial infection is likely, broad antibiotic coverage including anaerobes is recommended until an agent is identified. Clindamycin is the recommended therapy for GAS (as opposed to penicillin) and anaerobic coverage, while ampicillin–sulbactam broadens the coverage to include more anaerobes and gram-negative coverage. Recently hospitalized patients may need broader gram-negative coverage with other agents. Neither corticosteroids nor IVIG has any role in treatment, though some small studies of IVIG show early promise. As with other imaging studies, MRI is most useful when gas is present in the tissue, though this is an uncommon finding in GAS fasciitis. MRI also tends to overestimate the degree of deep tissue involvement. Ultimately the diagnosis and decision to operate is primarily made based on clinical grounds.

17. **Answer D.** The EKG shows a regular, narrow complex tachycardia at a rate of 175, most likely paroxysmal atrioventricular (AV) nodal re-entrant tachycardia (AVNRT). The patient is hemodynamically unstable and synchronized cardioversion at 50 J is indicated after appropriate sedation. In contrast to patients with AVNRT and atrial flutter, patients with rapid atrial fibrillation, which can appear regular at high rates, do not typically respond to 50 J for cardioversion. Thus, if the patient does not respond at 50 J, the energy level should be immediately stepped up to 100 J and then 200 J, or to the equivalent energy dose if using biphasic equipment.

Adenosine is the next best option, but hypotension and severe symptoms warrant more emergent conversion to sinus rhythm. Diltiazem and amiodarone can be used to convert the rhythm, but will cause further hypotension. Defibrillation is only indicated in patients who lack pulses (ventricular fibrillation, pulseless ventricular tachycardia).

18. **Answer E.** Cluster headaches may be associated with ipsilateral autonomic instability reflecting both sympathetic dysfunction such as ptosis, miosis, and forehead as well as facial sweating and parasympathetic activation, such as rhinorrhea, lacrimation, and nasal congestion. Due to the combination of these findings in concert with the distribution of pain, it is thought that the area responsible for cluster headaches is the cavernous sinus. In the cavernous sinus, the trigeminal nerve, sympathetic and parasympathetic fibers converge.

19. **Answer C.** NIPPV has revolutionized the treatment of COPD, cardiogenic pulmonary edema, as well as neuromuscular disease (e.g., myasthenia gravis). Contraindications for NIPPV include noncompliance (which is the most common reason for treatment failure), midfacial trauma (preventing an appropriate fit for the mask), excessive secretions or retention of secretions, decreased sensorium with absent cough and pharyngeal reflexes, recent gastric surgery (because of possible gastric distension), and vasopressor-dependent hypotension. Hypertension does not affect, nor is it affected by NIPPV.

20. **Answer C.** The NEXUS criteria include *absence* of the following: focal neurologic deficit, posterior midline neck tenderness, intoxication, altered mental status, distracting injury. The NEXUS criteria have a sensitivity between 90% and 99% for ruling out clinically significant fractures. The Canadian C-spine criteria, which focus on excluding high-risk mechanisms and instituting an assessment on range of motion, may be more sensitive and specific than the NEXUS criteria.

21. **Answer A.** The patient has clear evidence of septic shock. She meets 2/4 systemic inflammatory response syndrome (SIRS) criteria, has definite evidence of an infection, and exhibits end-organ dysfunction with her acute encephalopathy and hypotension. Intravenous antibiotics and adequate fluid resuscitation are crucial. Without a history of severe congestive heart failure, this patient should receive a 30 mL/kg bolus of 0.9 normal saline as the preferred initial resuscitation. The remainder of the choices are all vasoactive agents which will increase blood pressure, but are only indicated after fluid resuscitation has been optimized.

22. **Answer B.** This patient presents with findings concerning traumatic carotid artery dissection leading to a partial ipsilateral Horner syndrome with concomitant contralateral hypoesthesia. Patients experiencing sudden, compressive forces to the neck may develop traumatic carotid artery dissection. The sympathetic fibers that innervate the face and eye are also damaged by direct compression since they travel within the wall of the artery, resulting in an ipsilateral Horner syndrome (miosis, ptosis, anhidrosis, and enophthalmos). Horner syndrome may be the only indication of underlying carotid artery dissection. This patient also experienced transient contralateral hypoesthesia indicating ischemia of the ipsilateral brain in the middle cerebral artery distribution, likely because of internal carotid artery dissection. Thus, the patient should receive either CT angiography or magnetic resonance angiography (MRA) to further elucidate the vascular anatomy. MRI of the brain *may* demonstrate an acute infarct in the middle cerebral artery distribution, but without an angiographic study, carotid dissection would be missed.

23. **Answer C.** Central cord syndrome is caused by a hyperextension mechanism of the cervical spine where the ligamentum flavum is pushed into the spinal cord, causing central cord compression. Because of the distribution of motor fibers, upper extremity weakness is more profound than lower extremity weakness. Central cord syndrome is the most common of all partial cord injuries. Complete cord transection results in total loss of motor and sensory function below the level of injury. Anterior cord syndrome results from hyperflexion injury and causes paralysis and decreased pain and temperature sensation below the level of illness but with preserved vibration and position sense. The dorsal columns are spared in anterior cord syndrome. Brown–Sequard syndrome, or hemisection of the cord, is usually due to penetrating trauma and causes ipsilateral paralysis and loss of position and vibration sensation and contralateral loss of pain and temperature sensation. Spinal shock is a temporary loss of all motor and sensory function below the level of the lesion lasting from several hours to several days. Onset of recovery is usually marked by return of the bulbocavernosus reflex.

24. **Answer C.** Heat stroke is defined as the presence of elevated temperature (generally >104°F) due to some heat stress combined with alteration of mental status. The degree of temperature elevation by itself does not signify the presence of heat stroke; there must be some measure of alteration of mental status such as agitation, confusion, delirium, or frank somnolence. Myalgias, syncope, paresthesias, edema, rash, fatigue, and other nonspecific symptoms are categorized under heat exhaustion. Treatment of heat exhaustion requires aggressive fluid therapy along with passive cooling measures. Treatment of heat stroke mandates undressing the patient and aggressive active and passive cooling measures such as cooled IV fluids, fanned cool mist, and ice water immersion.

25. **Answer C.** Benzodiazepines are recommended for sedation of patients in anticholinergic crises due to their antiepileptic activity and absence of anticholinergic activity. Neuroleptic agents may exacerbate seizures and anticholinergic symptoms. Etomidate is too short acting for sedation due to agitation and may cause rapid respiratory insufficiency. Ketamine increases blood pressure and will exacerbate delirium, especially with its potential for the emergence phenomenon.

26. **Answer C.** The patient presents with symptoms of either obstructive lung disease or flash pulmonary edema with reactive bronchospasm, also called cardiac asthma. The two entities can be clinically indistinguishable. BNP is released in response to ventricular stretch during CHF. Normal BNP levels significantly reduce the likelihood of CHF exacerbation. Both obstructive lung disease and cardiac asthma may respond to albuterol therapy. D-dimer has a high negative predictive value for pulmonary embolism (PE) but has no role in the diagnosis of CHF or obstructive lung disease. Troponin I has high specificity for acute myocardial infarction and would not be elevated in CHF exacerbations without infarction. Angiotensin-converting enzyme levels are used to evaluate sarcoidosis.

27. **Answer B.** The minimal rise in the β-hCG level of a viable intrauterine pregnancy is >50% over a 2-day period, although 85% of women will have an increase of >66%. However, 21% of patients with ectopic pregnancy will exhibit a rise in their β-hCG level that mimics a normal intrauterine pregnancy. This patient's β-hCG level rose 41% in the 2 days since her previous visit which is inappropriately low and she continues to have pelvic pain. Therefore, transvaginal ultrasound should be performed to ensure there is no ectopic pregnancy.

28. **Answer D.** The head impulse test, evaluation for bidirectional nystagmus, and tests for skew deviation make up the HINTS (head impulse, nystagmus, test of skew) battery of tests used to differentiate between central and peripheral causes of vertigo. When all three tests are normal, a peripheral nerve lesion is likely. However, when any of the three tests is positive, a central lesion is more likely and an MRI should be performed. The HINTS battery is most useful in differentiating central versus peripheral causes in patients with unremitting rather than episodic vertigo. The head impulse test is a bedside test to assess the patient's vestibule–ocular reflex (VOR). The patient is asked to fix their gaze on a distant object while the provider turns their head to the left and right. Patients with a normal VOR are able to maintain their fixed gaze when their head is turned to the left and right. Testing patients with a vestibular lesion demonstrates that their eyes are "dragged" off target before marching back to the target in a saccadic fashion. Counterintuitively, a "normal" test in which the patient demonstrates

normal fixation is more concerning for a central lesion and those patients should receive an urgent MRI. Abnormal tests indicate a peripheral lesion affecting vestibular nerve (cranial nerve VIII) which is more reassuring. While both central and peripheral lesions produce nystagmus, peripheral lesions typically produce nystagmus that is fixed in one direction regardless of gaze. Nystagmus that changes direction, so-called bidirectional nystagmus, is concerning for a central lesion. Finally, skew deviation is a test in which one eye is covered while the other is open, fixating on a distant object, and the provider evaluates for vertical shift in the covered eye when it is then abruptly uncovered. A positive test in which the covered eye shifts its position to fixate on the object suggests a central lesion.

29. **Answer C.** *Yersinia enterolitica* can cause a terminal ileitis which is very similar to Crohn disease. Symptoms are virtually identical to Crohn disease and can also resemble appendicitis. In mild cases, *Yersinia* colitis can be treated supportively, but in more severe cases, fluoroquinolone or doxycycline therapy may be used (trimethoprim–sulfamethoxazole in children). Ulcerative colitis almost never involves the terminal ileum and is limited to the colon. *C. difficile* usually causes a colitis due to antibiotic use and doesn't usually affect the terminal ileum. Irritable bowel syndrome does not cause objective abnormalities on imaging. Giardiasis generally causes a watery diarrhea on exposure to infected water without evidence of terminal ileitis.

30. **Answer C.** The patient has a typical acute asthma exacerbation. The mainstays of treatment are bronchodilators for bronchospasm and corticosteroids for airway inflammation. Despite her upper respiratory symptoms and the presence of leukocytosis, she has no signs of superimposed pneumonia, so empiric treatment is not indicated. A chest x-ray could be obtained to further evaluate the possibility of pneumonia. Arterial blood gas sampling is only helpful in patients who are deteriorating despite aggressive bronchodilator therapy and should not routinely be obtained in the evaluation of most acute asthma exacerbations. Patients with asthma exacerbations should not be discharged without providing either systemic or inhaled corticosteroid therapy.

31. **Answer C.** Viscosity decreases with any inflammatory process of the joint because of decreased hyaluronic acid, which is the main contributor to synovial fluid viscosity. RA classically affects the metaphalangeal and PIP joints of the hand, whereas OA affects the first carpometacarpal joint as well as the PIP and distal interphalangeal (DIP) joints. SLE may cause inflammation of serosal surfaces such as the pleura or pericardium. Pericarditis in a patient with SLE may result in an audible cardiac

friction rub. Reiter syndrome may cause sausage-shaped swelling of the digits. An abducted, externally rotated hip in a neonate suggests infection, even in patients who are afebrile.

32. **Answer A.** Vitreous hemorrhage is usually caused by diabetic retinopathy, posterior vitreous detachment with or without retinal detachments, or trauma. Symptoms are similar to retinal detachment, with floaters early in the course and painless visual loss later. The red reflex is usually diminished or darkens into a black reflex. As in most acute ophthalmologic disorders, Valsalva maneuvers and recumbent positioning are to be avoided. The presence of an afferent pupillary defect indicates a concomitant retinal detachment. Ophthalmologic consultation should be sought in the ED in patients with suspected retinal detachment or traumatic vitreous hemorrhage.

33. **Answer C.** The patient has ecchymosis and deformity of his penile shaft indicative of penile fracture. Although important ancillary studies such as ultrasonography, retrograde urethrography, and cavernosography may be necessary for further evaluation, definitive management almost always requires urgent urologic repair. Conservative management with penile splinting and pressure dressings has an unacceptably high risk of complications such as deformity and impotence. Foley catheterization may be performed in patients without urethral injuries to help guide the surgical repair. (Figure from Graham SD, Keane TE. *Glenn's Urologic Surgery*. 8th ed. Philadelphia: Wolters Kluwer, 2015.)

34. **Answer B.** The patient has a Stanford class A aortic dissection—a tear involving the ascending aorta. Management involves emergent surgical repair along with early, aggressive BP control. Patients with aortic dissection often complain of severe chest pain radiating to the back or both arms. Aspirin should not be given to any patients suspected of having an aortic dissection, as this may increase the degree of bleeding into the false lumen. HR should be kept well below 100 to minimize the shear stress on the wall of the aorta that is related to the number of beats per minute. Transesophageal, not transthoracic, echocardiography may provide useful structural information about the descending aorta, heart, and pericardium, but CT aortogram and MRI are far more specific.

35. **Answer E.** Hyperacute bacterial conjunctivitis is usually caused by *Neisseria* species. It is differentiated from ordinary bacterial conjunctivitis by the rapidity of onset. Populations at risk include neonates and sexually active adults. Prompt diagnosis is essential because of the rapid course and the ability of gonococci to invade

intact corneal epithelium. Treatment generally involves systemic and topical antibiotics covering both *Neisseria* and *Chlamydia,* as 30% of patients are coinfected. Choices A, B, and C are common causes of bacterial conjunctivitis in children. *Klebsiella* is not a common cause of conjunctivitis.

36. **Answer D.** Rattlesnakes are part of the crotalid family of snakes whose venom contains cytotoxic compounds that cause direct skin necrosis and sometimes are severe enough to result in disseminated intravascular coagulation and delayed compartment syndrome. Signs of envenomation generally occur within 6 hours of the bite, unlike elapid envenomation, which can be delayed up to 12 hours. Management of crotalid envenomation involves immobilization with a loose-fitting splint to minimize skin and soft-tissue destruction, tetanus prophylaxis, and antivenin. Home remedies such as heat, ice, electric shock therapy, and tourniquets are rarely helpful and can easily worsen tissue necrosis. Oral suction is never indicated and usually seed the open wound with oral flora, which can cause considerable morbidity. Commercial suction devices have not been shown to improve clinical outcomes or remove sufficient quantities of venom in vivo. Corticosteroid therapy is not indicated in cases of envenomation and can increase the risk of secondary infectious complications.

37. **Answer B.** IBS is a common, chronic GI illness characterized by abdominal pain or discomfort, bloating, and either constipation or diarrhea. Although it is not a psychiatric diagnosis, patients with IBS more commonly have a concomitant psychiatric diagnosis (most commonly anxiety or depression). The cause of IBS is not known, but it is not related to food allergies. It is at least twice as common in women as in men. Although there are several clinical criteria for the disease, one well-known set of criteria (the Rome II criteria) includes abdominal pain that is relieved after defecation as necessary for a diagnosis of IBS.

38. **Answer B.** Due to the need for powerful immunosuppressant agents, all solid-organ transplant recipients are at increased risk for infection. Infections are divided into three time periods—those occurring within the first month of transplantation, those occurring between 1 and 6 months after transplantation, and those occurring >6 months after transplantation. Nosocomial agents are prominent in the first month, although cytomegalovirus (CMV) is the most prevalent infection between 1 and 6 months (particularly CMV pneumonitis).

39. **Answer E.** The most common causes of hypophosphatemia in the ED are probably respiratory alkalosis, treatment of DKA, and alcoholism. The most common mechanism is an intracellular shift of phosphate

(respiratory alkalosis, treatment of DKA). Renal insufficiency leads to phosphate retention, whereas hyperparathyroidism causes increased renal excretion.

40. **Answer B.** The patient's x-ray reveals an ankle fracture dislocation. Ankle dislocations are sometimes relatively easy to reduce because they tend to occur as a result of high-energy mechanisms of injury that result in considerable damage to connective tissues creating laxity within the joint. However, in muscular patients with less disruption, flexing the knee to 90 degrees is helpful as it releases the tension on the gastrocnemius making ankle reduction easier. This is best achieved by having the patient sit up on the side of the bed or by flexing the hip and knee with the patient supine, while having an assistant hold counter traction in the popliteal fossa. The best regional nerve block for ankle procedures is a sciatic nerve block performed at the level of the popliteal fossa. The femoral nerve block is most commonly used for knee surgery and procedures of the upper leg. While nearly any injury affecting the ankle can be splinted for follow-up, an ankle dislocation with skin tenting must be reduced emergently to avoid skin necrosis which creates an open fracture.

41. **Answer A.** Haloperidol is a potent dopamine antagonist, which does not have anticholinergic or hypotensive effects. Phenothiazines, such as prochlorperazine and chlorpromazine, cause orthostatic hypotension, lower the seizure threshold, and have strong anticholinergic properties that can exacerbate delirium. Diphenhydramine, while sedating, also shares these anticholinergic properties. Opioids may induce dysphoria and can exacerbate brain dysfunction. Diazepam has a long half-life due to its metabolites and may result in hypotension and respiratory depression. Promethazine is primarily an antihistamine that also has strong anticholinergic properties.

42. **Answer E.** Peptic ulcer disease is the most common cause of both duodenal and gastric perforations. The other answer choices are less common causes. Crohn disease tends to cause distal small bowel perforations more often than duodenal. Diverticulitis and neoplasia are the most common causes of large bowel perforations.

43. **Answer B.** Acclimation or acclimatization is a collection of physiologic changes that occur in response to repeated heat stress. Physiologic changes typically occur over a 7- to 14-day period presuming consistent, daily exposure. Physiologic changes include increased plasma volume, a lower threshold for sweating (earlier onset), increased rate and volume of sweating with decreased electrolyte content of sweat, increased aldosterone secretion, decreased heart rate, and increased capacity for peripheral vasodilation. This patient has heat edema, which is a benign condition most commonly seen in the elderly and in nonacclimatized individuals. It is thought to be due to a combination of orthostatic pressure and vascular leak. Diuretic therapy is not beneficial and may cause dehydration. Although a minimal workup for other common conditions resulting in lower extremity edema may be necessary, an echocardiogram is not required. Generally, heat edema resolves with acclimation or upon return to a patient's baseline climate and may be treated with simple measures such as leg elevation and support stockings.

44. **Answer A.** This patient is presenting with alcoholic ketoacidosis (AKA). Though patients with diabetic ketoacidosis (DKA) can present with a normal blood glucose level (euglycemic DKA), most patients with DKA present with elevated glucose levels and often have a history of diabetes. Differentiating between the two disorders is usually straightforward but in patients presenting with an elevated glucose level, a hemoglobin A1C may be helpful. Patients with AKA are typically chronically malnourished with a history of chronic alcohol abuse. Thiamine is given before glucose-containing fluids since thiamine is a cofactor in glucose metabolism and many patients with AKA are thiamine deficient so glucose administration without thiamine could theoretically precipitate Wernicke–Korsakoff syndrome.

45. **Answer D.** The majority of beta-blocker overdoses are successfully managed with supportive care. The front-line agents for managing the cardiovascular complications evident in this patient include aggressive IV fluids, and atropine, with glucagon and calcium (either chloride or gluconate) used if initial measures are ineffective. Epinephrine is the vasopressor of choice if all these measures fail. In patients refractory to these treatments, high-dose insulin and glucose is the therapy of choice. Insulin circumvents the beta-receptor, inducing increased levels of cyclic AMP production through its own receptor, thus mirroring the effect of the G-protein-coupled beta-receptor. To be effective, insulin must be used at extremely large doses. The commonly used protocol calls for 1 unit per kg of regular insulin as a bolus, followed by a 0.5 unit per kg insulin infusion. Dextrose infusions are required to maintain euglycemia. The effects of this therapy are delayed 30 to 60 minutes after initiation. Lipid emulsion therapy remains experimental, but there are positive case reports of its use in some beta-blocker overdoses. Dialysis is not used in beta-blocker overdose, and propranolol is not removed by hemodialysis. Phosphodiesterase inhibitors such as milrinone, intraaortic balloon pumps, and temporary transvenous pacing may be helpful in patients who are refractory to all other therapies.

46. **Answer C.** In several meta-analyses, the novel oral anticoagulants (NOACs) have exhibited a higher risk of

causing myocardial infarction than warfarin. It is unclear why this occurs (or whether this risk will continue), but it is currently one of the only advantages that warfarin has over the NOACs. Choices A, B, and D actually represent advantages that the NOACs have over warfarin. Venous thromboembolism recurrence rates are about the same with both classes of drugs. (Annals, April 2016.)

47. **Answer A.** The "swinging penlight" test is used to diagnose afferent papillary defects. In the test, a light is swung between the two eyes in a darkened room, spending approximately 1 second per eye to determine pupillary response. An afferent pupillary defect is present when the affected eye appears to dilate in response to light. The presence of an afferent pupillary defect reflects a problem with light perception from the eye. This could reflect a problem anterior to the retina (e.g., blood in the anterior or posterior chamber), within the retina, or in the optic nerve. It most commonly reflects optic nerve lesion on the affected size. Whatever the cause, the pupil of the affected eye will not respond correctly when exposed to light. Since the efferent pathways (from brain to eye) are not affected, light shined into the unaffected, contralateral eye results in a normal, constrictive response. Furthermore, since the efferent pathways are normal, the two pupils are always the same size as each other. However, since the affected eye does not sense as much light as the unaffected eye, exposing the affected eye to light produces a weaker constrictive response than light exposure in the normal eye. When a penlight is swung between the two eyes, this gives the appearance of dilation when the light is swung to the affected eye.

48. **Answer B.** Although rectal involvement is uncommon in patients with Crohn disease and nearly universal in patients with ulcerative colitis, perianal complications are much more common in patients with Crohn disease. The anal canal is the most terminal segment of the large intestine. In approximately 25% of patients with Crohn disease, perianal complications may occur before the onset of overt disease. Toxic megacolon is more common in patients with ulcerative colitis. Erythema nodosum occurs most often in women patients with Crohn disease. Anal fissures associated with Crohn disease are typically eccentrically located. In patients without Crohn disease, more than 90% of fissures are located in the posterior midline.

49. **Answer A.** This patient has supraventricular tachycardia (SVT). Since the diving reflex is very effective in neonates, the first step is to hold a bag of ice or a frozen towel over the patient's nose and mouth for 30 seconds. If the infant fails to convert, the next step is to use adenosine. Verapamil is avoided in infants because it may cause significant hypotension. Digoxin, on the other hand, may be effective, but has a slow onset. Electrical

cardioversion is effective, but is reserved for patients with refractory symptoms or who are in shock. Given that this patient has good perfusion and is maintaining his blood pressure, electrical cardioversion is not needed. Finally, while WPW can lead to SVT, it is not possible to determine if WPW underlies the patient's SVT until after cardioversion.

50. **Answer A.** The pain of duodenal ulcers is usually described as a burning or gnawing epigastric sensation that is decreased with food or antacids. The pain typically occurs 2 to 3 hours after a meal. Classically, two-third of patients with duodenal ulcers describe pain that wakes them from sleep in the middle of the night, although few patients have pain on waking in the morning. The pain of gastric ulcers tends to occur more quickly after meals and may even be precipitated by food in some patients. Therefore, anorexia and weight loss occur in approximately 50% of patients with gastric ulcers but rarely occur in patients with duodenal ulcers. Duodenal ulcers are twice as likely to be complicated by bleeding as gastric ulcers. *H. pylori,* although more commonly found in the setting of duodenal ulcers, is the major risk factor for the development of either type of ulcer. Flexible endoscopy is the diagnostic study of choice for peptic ulcer disease. Finally, only 15% to 20% of patients colonized with *H. pylori* will develop a peptic ulcer in their lifetime.

51. **Answer A.** Neonatal jaundice is a common and normal part of neonatal life as more than half of term neonates will develop jaundice in the first week of life. However, severe hyperbilirubinemia places infants at risk for irreversible neurologic disease as bilirubin is a neurotoxin. There are several online calculators based on the nomogram developed by Bhutani et al. that can be used to determine whether or not an infant is at risk for developing dangerous levels of bilirubin. Phototherapy is the first-line treatment when treatment is indicated except in the rare cases in which an infant presents with hyperbilirubinemia and clinical evidence of neurologic compromise (e.g., lethargy). In addition, any infant with a bilirubin level of 25 mg/dL is in danger of developing neurologic injury and should be admitted for emergent treatment. The bronze baby syndrome is an uncommon side effect of phototherapy treatment characterized by a grayish-brown skin color. Bilirubin levels can't be reliably determined by physical examination and should always be checked with blood testing, when needed.

52. **Answer B.** While all mechanisms contribute to GERD, lower esophageal dysfunction is the major one. This underscores the importance of behavioral changes in the management of GERD. While proton pump inhibitors and antihistamines are important to reduce acid production, reduction in smoking, alcohol intake, caffeine use,

fatty foods, and large meals, exercise and lying down immediately after eating is also necessary for successful treatment.

53. **Answer E.** Acute aortic dissection is a hypertensive emergency (see Fig. 5-15). Initial treatment should focus on reducing the patient's blood pressure to a systolic blood pressure of 100 to 120 mm Hg using parenteral beta-blockers (labetalol, esmolol, propranolol). Beta-blockers are the preferred agent because they also reduce heart rate and aortic wall stress by reducing the rate of systolic blood pressure rise. While hypertension is the most common risk factor, approximately 25% of patients have no history of hypertension and approximately one-third are normotensive at presentation. EKGs are not usually helpful to differentiate acute aortic dissection from myocardial infarction as most EKGs in patients with either condition are nonspecific. There are ongoing investigations into the use of low D-dimer levels as a means of excluding aortic dissection. However, there are no validated prediction rules to determine the exact pretest probability in patients with suspected aortic dissection, and no outcome studies have demonstrated the safety of using "negative" D-dimer levels as a means to rule out aortic dissection. As with pulmonary embolism, elevated D-dimer levels do not significantly increase the likelihood of acute aortic dissection. An upper extremity blood pressure disparity is a classically described, though somewhat unreliable finding in patients with aortic dissection. A pulse deficit between the upper extremities is the most reliable physical examination finding, and pulses should always be assessed to determine whether there are discrepancies. Unfortunately,

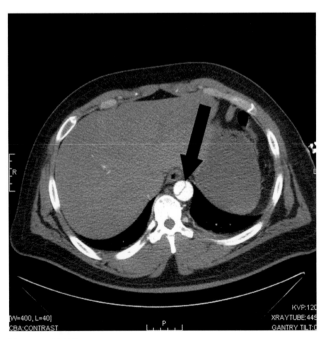

Figure 5-15

the sensitivity of this finding is low, as only 15% of patients in the International Registry of Acute Aortic Dissection (IRAD) study had such a deficit.

54. **Answer D.** Elderly patients with even mild blunt chest trauma are at high risk for pulmonary complications, including atelectasis, delayed contusion, infection, and acute respiratory distress syndrome (ARDS). Aggressive pain management and pulmonary toilet is mandatory for these patients to maintain proper lung expansion in order to prevent the complications mentioned earlier. Most patients are successfully managed on an outpatient basis—admission is indicated if the patient has significant chest wall or pulmonary injury revealed on chest x-ray or chest CT, or has hypoxia, or other severe symptoms. Prophylactic antibiotics are not recommended in the absence of clinical and radiographic findings of infection.

55. **Answer B.** Significant renal injury in blunt trauma rarely occurs in the absence of other organ injury. Gross hematuria is the standard indication for further evaluation of the urologic tract, and CT scan with IV contrast is the best imaging tool to evaluate renal injuries. In stable patients with microscopic hematuria due to blunt trauma, significant renal injury is uncommon. Penetrating trauma to the back or abdomen may cause renal injury in the absence of either gross or microscopic hematuria and should be evaluated with CT imaging. The vast majority of renal injuries do not require operative management; exceptions include large renal lacerations and major vascular injuries. The kidneys are among the most commonly injured abdominal organs in blunt abdominal trauma in children.

56. **Answer C.** Sixty percent to 85% of patients have motor weakness at the time of presentation. The most common pattern of muscle weakness is symmetric lower extremity weakness although any pattern can be seen. Bladder and bowel findings occur late in the course of the disease. Although it also occurs late in the course of compression, any patient with saddle anesthesia should be considered to have cauda equina syndrome until proven otherwise. Back pain is the most common symptom of epidural spinal cord compression, occurring in 83% to 95% of patients, and characteristically precedes neurologic symptoms by approximately 2 months.

57. **Answer A.** The rash and clinical history describe roseola, caused by human herpesvirus-6 (known as sixth disease, for this reason). It occurs most commonly in the first 2 years of life and supportive care is all that is required for management. Lymphadenopathy is extremely common, seen in almost all cases. Seizures are seen only in a small minority of cases. The "slapped cheek" rash is actually due to erythema infectiosum, caused by parvovirus B-19. (Figure from Kyle T, Susan

Carman S, eds. *Essentials of Pediatric Nursing.* 3rd ed. Philadelphia, PA: Wolters Kluwer, 2016.)

58. **Answer C.** Sigmoid volvulus accounts for 75% of volvulus cases, whereas cecal volvulus accounts for the remaining 25%. Although patients with cecal volvulus are younger than patients with sigmoid volvulus, they are not *young*, as affected patients are typically in their late fifties. Plain films are diagnostic in 80% of cases of sigmoid volvulus but <50% of cases of cecal volvulus. The classic findings of cecal volvulus include a massively dilated cecum typically in the left upper quadrant or epigastrium (i.e., not within the right abdomen). Although selected patients with sigmoid volvulus may be candidates for endoscopic reduction, patients with cecal volvulus almost always require surgical repair due to the difficulty of accessing this area endoscopically and the need for cecopexy to prevent recurrence.

59. **Answer C.** Due to denervation in the transplanted heart and the consequent lack of vagal tone, the resting heart rate averages between 100 and 110 beats per minute. However, the heart rate can increase up to 70% of the maximum for age due to circulating endogenous catecholamines and upregulation of β-adrenergic receptors. Although rare, tamponade can occur in the transplanted heart because of scar tissue formation and its ability to contain pericardial fluid or blood under pressure. Before the advent of cyclosporine, acute rejection presented as acute-onset CHF or atrial dysrhythmias with a new S3 and diffusely decreased QRS voltage on EKG. These features are now only present in cases of *severe* failure, and typical acute rejection, which occurs in 75% to 85% of patients, is diagnosed by endomyocardial biopsy. There is an increased risk of endocarditis with invasive procedures, so antibiotic prophylaxis should be used in any procedure expected to produce bacteremia.

60. **Answer A.** Given her age, pain out of proportion to physical examination findings, and presumed atrial fibrillation, the patient likely has acute mesenteric ischemia, which is usually caused by an arterial embolism. Acute mesenteric ischemia carries with it the possibility of infarcted or necrotic bowel, and all patients strongly suspected of this condition should receive early broad-spectrum antibiotics, intravenous hydration, and anticoagulation with heparin. Tissue plasminogen activator is not indicated, as surgery is a very possible treatment strategy. Barium enema is used to diagnose and treat intussusception and would not be appropriate here. HIDA scan is a confirmatory test for biliary pathology when ultrasound is nondiagnostic. Norepinephrine and other vasopressors should not be used in the setting of acute mesenteric ischemia as this may further constrict an already narrowed blood vessel.

61. **Answer E.** In a meta-analysis of 17 studies, subjective vision reduction (LR+ = 5) was the most important symptom associated with retinal detachment among patients with flashes and floaters. On examination, bedside ultrasound is a simple, useful tool that reveals a thick membrane that appears to have lifted away from the retina as it "floats" in the vitreous anterior to the retina. Vitreous hemorrhage or vitreous pigment (unlikely to be diagnosed by an ED physician) upon slit-lamp examination also greatly increases the likelihood of associated detachment, even if one is not seen. Vitreous pigment is unfortunately named, since its presence reflects *retinal* pigment *within* the vitreous (thus, vitreous pigment). A progressive visual field deficit in the setting of flashes and floaters also indicates retinal detachment until proven otherwise.

62. **Answer A.** The patient has chronic peripheral vascular disease leading to acute in situ arterial thrombosis in the left leg. Ankle–brachial index (ABI) is >0.9 in patients without peripheral vascular disease, and bilateral reduction in the ABI indicates chronic in situ disease. Arterial embolism is also a very common cause of acute arterial occlusion, but the history of progressively worsening claudication before the acute event is more often seen with in situ thrombosis. Isolated inflammation, vasospasm, and fistulas may also cause arterial occlusion but are far less common than thrombosis and embolism.

63. **Answer C.** The cyanotic heart diseases in children can be remembered by the fact that each begins with the letter "T"—truncus arteriosus, transposition of the great vessels, tricuspid atresia, tetralogy of Fallot, and total anomalous pulmonary venous return. Another common mnemonic is to think of the five cyanotic heart lesions as easy as 1, 2, 3, 4, 5.

One big trunk: Truncus arteriosus.

Two interchanged vessels: Transposition of the great vessels.

Three: TRIscuspid atresia.

Four: TETRAlogy of Fallot.

Five words: Total anomalous pulmonary venous return.

Cyanosis generally indicates the presence of right-to-left shunting, causing bypass of the pulmonary circuit and infusion of deoxygenated blood into the systemic circulation. Cyanosis due to cardiac disease is generally central (truncal and facial), unlike dehydration or hypothermia, which usually causes peripheral cyanosis (in the extremities).

64. **Answer D.** The patient has peripartum cardiomyopathy, which occurs in approximately 0.03% of all pregnancies and almost one-third of patients die. Risk factors

include greater maternal age, multiparity, and twin pregnancies. Clinical characteristics and acute management are the same as that of congestive heart failure due to dilated cardiomyopathy. ECG, not cardiac catheterization, is usually the first step in assessing structural cardiac abnormalities. Patients are at high risk of developing peripartum cardiomyopathy in subsequent pregnancies. Aspirin plays no role in management, although patients may benefit from heparin prophylaxis due to the thromboembolic risk.

65. **Answer A.** The diaphragm elevates during pregnancy, resulting in decreased total lung capacity and functional residual capacity. However, diaphragmatic excursion actually increases resulting in an increased tidal volume and mild alveolar hyperventilation despite the fact that the respiratory rate remains unchanged. The RBC mass and hemoglobin increase throughout pregnancy. RBC mass rises steadily to term, as it increases 18% without iron supplementation. In contrast, the plasma volume, which also increases during pregnancy, plateaus at 30 to 34 weeks of gestation. The peripheral WBC count steadily rises during pregnancy and may be as high as 20,000 to 30,000 mm^3 during labor after which it returns to normal in approximately 1 week. Finally, the glomerular filtration rate increases throughout pregnancy.

66. **Answer A.** Methicillin-resistant *Staphylococcus aureus* (MRSA) is amenable to treatment only with specific antibiotics. Doxycycline *usually* covers MRSA adequately and is the best choice among the options presented. Azithromycin and cephalexin do not cover MRSA and are responsible for treatment failure. Dicloxacillin is the drug of choice for methicillin-sensitive *Staphylococcus aureus* but not for MRSA. Avoiding antibiotics is not a proper treatment strategy for a clinically significant cellulitis with early signs of systemic involvement (chills).

67. **Answer A.** This is the swan neck deformity. It is caused by hyperextension at the proximal interphalangeal (PIP) joint and flexion at the distal interphalangeal (DIP) joint. The DIP joint flexion occurs due to elongation or rupture of the extensor tendon attachment to the distal phalanx (i.e., similar to a mallet injury). Left untreated, PIP hyperextension occurs as a consequence of the distal mallet deformity. However, the deformity can begin in the PIP joint as well due to synovitis of the volar capsule resulting in PIP hyperextension. In the latter case, DIP flexion occurs as a secondary effect. Both the swan neck and boutonniere deformities are common in rheumatoid arthritis. (Figure reprinted with permission from Oatis CA. *Kinesiology: The mechanics and Pathomechanics of Human Movement.* Philadelphia, PA: Lippincott Williams & Wilkins; 2004.)

68. **Answer D.** Abdominal radiography is generally considered the first-line imaging modality to evaluate patients with suspected SBO. The sensitivity of plain radiography is about 75%. If radiographs are normal, but the diagnosis of SBO is still suspected clinically, then CT abdomen/pelvis, with both sensitivity and specificity of over 85%, can be used to confirm the diagnosis. CT also identifies many causes of SBO (such as volvulus or intussusception), other diagnoses in the differential of SBO, and complications such as closed-loop obstruction. To avoid unnecessary ionizing radiation, use of abdominal radiography is most efficient in patients with known prior SBOs who present with typical signs and symptoms without systemic toxicity or severe focal tenderness (which could indicate a closed-loop process).

69. **Answer A.** Although tarantula bites may inflict a significant amount of pain, there is usually minimal erythema and swelling at the bite site. Severe envenomation is extremely uncommon and fatalities have not been described in the United States. However, tarantulas are covered with "urticating hairs" that it can cast out toward a victim. The hairs become embedded in the skin and may cause an intense inflammatory response, resulting in pruritus and occasionally erythematous papules. After rubbing the area, patients may also unintentionally transfer the hairs to their eyes resulting in a severe keratoconjunctivitis that requires ophthalmologic referral for treatment and hair removal.

70. **Answer E.** The patient has evidence of an upper motor neuron facial palsy. Sparing of the upper half of the face implies a lesion in the cerebrum or facial *nucleus* (rather than a facial *nerve*). Neuroimaging, either with CT or MR, should be pursued in these cases. The other answer choices all assume the diagnosis of a facial nerve (rather than nucleus) lesion. Prednisone plus an antiherpetic agent is the generally accepted treatment for Bell palsy, the most common cause of facial nerve palsy. Doxycycline is used to treat Lyme disease, which is a common cause of facial nerve palsy in endemic areas (Northeast, Mid-Atlantic, Wisconsin, Minnesota).

71. **Answer A.** Anal fissures are actually the most commonly encountered anorectal problem in all of pediatrics. However, they are especially common in infants.

72. **Answer D.** AKA is an elevated anion gap metabolic acidosis that usually occurs in chronic alcoholics after a recent binge of alcohol results in vomiting, starvation, dehydration, and acidosis. Due to complex pathophysiology, the acidosis is dominated by β-hydroxybutyrate, which is not detected by standard urinary ketone tests. Furthermore, as the acidosis resolves, β-hydroxybutyrate is converted to acetoacetate and acetone resulting in a paradoxical (or false) "worsening" of the acidosis

evidenced by increased detection of acetoacetate in the urine. Traditionally, the osmolal gap is normal, although there are case reports of patients with AKA and an elevated osmolal gap. It may be difficult to differentiate patients with AKA from chronic alcohol abusers with toxic alcohol ingestion. Toxic alcohol ingestion should always be in the differential of AKA and should be the top consideration whenever the osmolal gap is elevated. The alcohol level is typically zero as AKA is primarily a starvation ketosis. Glucose levels are not usually elevated and insulin is unnecessary. Treatment is with saline and glucose solutions as well as electrolyte replacement.

73. **Answer B.** Oropharyngeal dysphagia is due to difficulty in the initiation of swallowing. Approximately 80% of cases are due to neuromuscular diseases, strokes being chief among them. Polymyositis and dermatomyositis are the second most common causes. Two-third of patients with MG have dysphagia, but because MG is a rare disease, they do not account for a large number of patients with oropharyngeal dysphagia. Liquids usually result in more dysphagia than solids, particularly when the liquids are extremely hot or cold. Symptoms tend to be intermittent rather than progressive.

74. **Answer E.** Hydatidiform moles are placental abnormalities characterized by enlarged and edematous placental villi and trophoblastic tissue (into grape-like structures) as well as loss of fetal blood vessels. The two types of hydatidiform moles are complete and incomplete. Complete moles almost always have a 46, XX karyotype that is paternally derived (due to duplication of a paternally derived haploid genome), whereas incomplete moles have a complete trisomy with a karyotype of 69, XXX or 69, XXY. Incomplete moles have two sets of paternal chromosomes (again due to duplication of a paternally derived haploid genome) and one set of maternally derived chromosomes. Complete moles are so named because of complete absence of fetal parts (no fetus, umbilical cord, or amniotic membrane) and swelling of all placental villi. In contrast, incomplete moles have partial placental villi swelling, and may have a few fetal parts present and occasionally a complete fetus. The classic features associated with hydatidiform moles are more common in the setting of complete moles. These include pregnancy-induced hypertension occurring in the first trimester, uterine enlargement greater than expected for dates, hyperemesis and very high β-hCG levels, as well as theca lutein ovarian cysts. Vaginal bleeding is the most common presenting symptom and ultrasonography will reveal the diagnosis in both cases (molar pregnancy in the case of a complete mole, and possibly missed abortion or intrauterine fetal demise in the case of an incomplete mole). The classic ultrasonographic appearance of a complete molar pregnancy is described as a "snowstorm."

75. **Answer B.** Patients with Guillain–Barré syndrome (GBS) exhibit significant elevations of protein with only mild (if any) elevation in cells in their CSF. This is known as albumino-cytologic dissociation. The presence of more cells (also known as pleocytosis) in the CSF argues more for an infectious or inflammatory cause other than GBS. The principal symptoms of GBS are progressive, symmetric muscle weakness accompanied by absent or depressed deep tendon reflexes. The weakness most often begins in the legs and "ascends." More than 80% of patients complain of associated extremity paresthesias, though sensory findings on examination are minimal as GBS is primarily a motor disease.

76. **Answer D.** Though definitions of severe sepsis have been changing, it's clear that an initially elevated lactate level and a persistently elevated lactate level (inadequate lactate clearance) are predictors of increased mortality. An initial lactate level >4 mmol/L predicts a 27% mortality rate, versus only 7% mortality in septic patients with lactate levels of 2.5 to 4.0 mmol/L and <5% mortality for patients with a lactate level <2.5 mmol/L.

77. **Answer B.** It may be difficult to clinically differentiate between patients with central and peripheral vertigo. However, peripheral vertigo is classically associated with marked nausea and vomiting. Furthermore, peripheral vertigo more commonly occurs along with auditory symptoms such as hearing loss, tinnitus, or a feeling of pressure or fullness in the ear. Although all patients with vertigo may have some difficulty walking, many patients with central lesions cannot even stand or take a single step without falling. In contrast, patients with peripheral vertigo can usually walk, even in the acute phase of their illness. This is why it is important to encourage patients with vertigo to walk during bedside examination. Finally, nystagmus is an important physical examination finding in patients with vertigo. Spontaneous nystagmus of peripheral origin does not change direction with gaze to either side. Nystagmus in such patients, however, does increase in amplitude when patients look in the direction of the fast phase (known as the *Alexander law*). In patients with central lesions, nystagmus generally changes direction when the patient looks in the direction of the fast phase. Nystagmus that is purely vertical (upbeat or downbeat nystagmus) is almost always caused by a central lesion, typically of brainstem vestibular pathways. Finally, nystagmus due to peripheral lesions typically fatigues or ceases when the patient fixates his or her vision on a target object. Fixation does not generally affect nystagmus due to central lesions.

78. **Answer A.** *Cryptosporidium* is the most common cause of chronic diarrhea in patients with AIDS. However, it is much less common in the era of successful antiretroviral

therapy. Cryptosporidiosis is usually self-limited in immunocompetent patients as well as in patients with AIDS when the CD4 count is >180 per μL. In contrast, patients with CD4 counts <100 may develop a chronic course of diarrhea and weight loss. Patients with CD4 counts <50 may experience fulminant diarrhea.

79. **Answer E.** All of these areas are characterized by thin skin which is easily damaged when exposed to heat. Thus, physicians who initially manage these wounds should presume that burns to these areas are deep and take a very conservative approach to therapy and follow-up.

80. **Answer C.** The CT scan shows diffuse, bilateral bright signal consistent with acute hemorrhage in the subarachnoid space. Epidural and subdural hematomas are usually focal, unilateral, and often cause midline shift. Cerebral contusion appears as blood in the parenchyma rather than the cisterns. DAI usually does not appear on an emergent brain CT and requires clinical evaluation and MRI for diagnosis. (Figure from Wiesel SW. *Operative Techniques in Orthopaedic Surgery.* Philadelphia: Wolters Kluwer, 2010.)

81. **Answer D.** This patient has impetigo, which is initially a superficial vesicular eruption that later develops into multiple honey-crusted lesions. In the United States, *S. aureus* is the most common cause, whereas group A *Streptococcus* is responsible for the bulk of the remainder. In cases caused by *Streptococcus*, antibiotic therapy does not reduce the incidence of poststreptococcal glomerulonephritis. Furthermore, topical therapy with mupirocin is as effective as systemic therapy, although systemic therapy is recommended when a large area is involved or when the involvement is near the mouth (allowing topical antibiotics to be licked away). The lesions are not painful even though they may be pruritic. However, regional lymphadenopathy is a common associated finding. The lesions are highly contagious and easily transmitted to other children. (Figure reprinted with permission from Pilliterri A. *Maternal and Child Health Nursing.* Lippincott Williams & Wilkins; 2006.)

82. **Answer D.** This patient experienced acute food poisoning due to *Staphylococcus*. The illness is not caused by infection of the bacteria but by a heat-stable enterotoxin produced by the bacteria before ingestion. *Staphylococcus* proliferates with ease in foods with a high protein content, such as ham, eggs, poultry, custard-based pastries as well as potato or egg salads. The illness occurs 1 to 6 hours after ingestion and is typically acute in onset. Abdominal pain and vomiting are the most prominent symptoms although occasionally a mild diarrhea may also be present. Symptoms are self-limited, typically resolving within 8 hours and only rarely lasting for a full day. Because the disease is caused by a heat-stable toxin, cooking will not remove the toxin once it is formed, and antibiotics have no role in treatment. Although *B. cereus* causes a similar illness by virtue of a heat-stable toxin it produces, it almost always occurs after ingestion of fried rice. Of note, *B. cereus* may produce a second, different syndrome characterized primarily by diarrhea and abdominal pain. This latter syndrome results from the production of a heat-labile toxin that is released in vivo after ingestion of live organisms. It is clinically similar to food poisoning caused by *Clostridium perfringens* and results from ingestion of meats or vegetables colonized with the bacterium.

83. **Answer B.** Rabies is a virus that carries virtually 100% mortality. Humans contract the virus from being bitten by infected animals. Raccoons are the number one vector though bats, skunks, coyotes, and foxes all may carry rabies. Dogs and cats may also carry rabies, but the vast majority of domesticated animal bites do not cause rabies, due to vaccination programs. The virus is transmitted from the animal's saliva through open skin into the victim's bloodstream. It then invades peripheral nerves and travels up the spinal cord to the brain. The incubation period in humans lasts 1 to 3 months. A nonspecific viral prodrome affects most patients. Specific symptoms of rabies include altered mental status and hydrophobia (inability to swallow water or saliva due to hyperactive airway reflexes). Coma and death are inevitable, and no effective treatment exists once rabies is clinically evident. Postexposure prophylaxis, consisting of local wound care, human rabies immune globulin (HRIG), and rabies vaccine, is essential to prevent rabies infection.

84. **Answer C.** CRVO causes backup of blood flow into the eye and carries the potential for increased intraocular pressure, eventually leading to glaucoma. The classic history is acute or subacute painless loss of vision, although pain may occur in some cases. Risk factors include hypertension, diabetes, thrombophilia, funduscopic examination reveals disc edema with tortuous veins and retinal hemorrhages. ED management is supportive in conjunction with ophthalmologist consultation. Choices A, B, D, and E may be caused by trauma or anterior eye disorders.

85. **Answer C.** Unfortunately, cyanide levels are not available at the point of care. Instead, lactate is frequently used as a surrogate for cyanide intoxication, as lactate levels >10 mmol/L are strongly suggestive of cyanide poisoning. In addition, patients will have a severe metabolic acidosis with a significant anion gap. Thus, a lot of useful information can be learned quickly with a venous blood gas. Co-oximetry could verify EMS' report of carboxyhemoglobin

as well as the methemoglobin level, but neither of these things will change presumed cyanide management in this setting. Amyl nitrite (or other nitrites) is contraindicated in combined CO and CN poisoning since induced methemoglobinemia will further decrease oxygen carrying capacity and worsen tissue hypoxia.

86. **Answer D.** The chest x-ray demonstrates presence of the gastric bubble inside the thoracic cavity, indicating a large diaphragmatic rupture from blunt trauma. The left diaphragm is much more likely than the right to rupture due to protection on the right from the liver. Management involves nasogastric decompression and surgical repair. Patients with penetrating thoracoabdominal trauma may have delayed abdominal herniation into the thorax as far out as decades after the initial injury. Right-sided diaphragmatic injuries are less likely to have abdominal herniation into the thorax, also because of the presence of the liver. Diaphragmatic injuries may be very subtle and diagnosed only on direct visualization with laparoscopy or thoracoscopy. Diagnostic peritoneal lavage (DPL), focused assessment of sonography in trauma (FAST), and CT scan all lack sufficient sensitivity for ruling out the diagnosis. (Figure courtesy of Mark Silverberg, MD. In: Greenberg MI, Hendrickson RG, Silverberg M, et al., eds. *Greenberg's Text-Atlas of Emergency Medicine.* Lippincott Williams & Wilkins; 2004:654, with permission.)

87. **Answer A.** *S. aureus* remains the most common cause of septic arthritis, accounting for 37% to 56% of infections. It causes 80% of the infections in patients with underlying diabetes or rheumatoid arthritis. Group A β-hemolytic streptococci are the second most common cause of septic arthritis. The remainder is caused by other streptococci, gram-negative organisms, and gonococcus. *N. gonorrhoeae* accounts for only 20% of monoarticular septic arthritis, although it accounts for a larger proportion of polyarticular septic arthritis, which is its usual presentation. Gram-negative organisms are the most common cause of septic arthritis in newborns and in children younger than 5 years old, although vaccination programs have nearly eliminated *H. influenzae* as a cause.

88. **Answer B.** Tramadol is a useful adjunct to acetaminophen for treatment of fibromyalgia. It has been shown to decrease pain better than acetaminophen alone. It should be used in caution in patients who are on a selective serotonin reuptake inhibitor, as it may theoretically increase the risk of serotonin syndrome. Without a history of chronic opiate use and opioid tolerance, starting oxycodone therapy from the ED is not the best possible management for the patient's health. Aspirin should no longer be used as first-line analgesic therapy for any condition. Furthermore, no anti-inflammatories (including all NSAIDs and steroids) work effectively in fibromyalgia

pain management as the primary pathophysiology is not inflammatory—rather, it is pain hypersensitivity.

89. **Answer B.** The lateral wrist radiograph demonstrates volar displacement and angulation of the lunate relative to the radius, indicating a lunate dislocation. The "spilled teacup" sign is present with the lunate appearing as a teacup that is tilted forward. Treatment involves orthopedic consultation and urgent surgical repair. Scaphoid fractures are best seen on an anteroposterior (AP) wrist or dedicated scaphoid view. Perilunate dislocation involves the capitate dislocating relative to the lunate and radius. Distal radius fractures and metacarpal fractures are best seen on AP views. (Figure courtesy of Mark Silverberg, MD. In: Greenberg MI, Hendrickson RG, Silverberg M, et al., eds. *Greenberg's Text-Atlas of Emergency Medicine.* Lippincott Williams & Wilkins; 2004, with permission.)

90. **Answer B.** Inadequate sedation of recently intubated patients is a common problem in the ED. Although the common initial response to the waking patient is to infuse paralytics, such action is typically not necessary. Usually, all that is required is adequate sedation with propofol or with benzodiazepines (such as midazolam) with or without narcotic agents such as morphine or fentanyl. It is critical to provide adequate analgesia, as many patients who require mechanical ventilation have suffered significant, painful traumatic injuries, which may be the cause of their distress. Paralytics should be reserved for the patient with persistently high plateau pressures despite optimal ventilatory management and sedation. In such patients, paralysis ensures that the patient's intrinsic respiratory effort will not interfere with the ventilator's attempts at delivering breaths. However, because paralysis increases the risk of aspiration and subsequent pneumonia, paralytics should not be routinely used. Ketamine would be effective but is short acting and would need to be followed by another agent. Hyperkalemia is not likely to cause the patient's agitated mental status.

91. **Answer B.** The appearance of the foot and ankle is highly indicative of an ankle dislocation. The skin between the foot and the ankle appears tented and the foot is rotated relative to the rest of the leg. Ankle dislocations almost always involve a fracture of one or more of the bones in the mortise (malleoli, talus). With this degree of deformity, simple ankle sprain is highly unlikely. Nerves injured in ankle dislocation include the tibial, superficial peroneal, and sural. Emergent closed reduction with splinting is the most appropriate initial management. If there is no neurovascular compromise, it is reasonable to wait for plain radiographs to perform closed reduction. Definitive care usually requires operative management. Pain control is absolutely indicated as total anesthesia with ankle dislocations is rare.

92. **Answer E.** Lithium toxicity generally causes gastrointestinal (nausea, vomiting, abdominal pain), renal (diabetes insipidus), and neurologic (tremor, ataxia, coma) dysfunction. Management involves whole bowel irrigation with polyethylene glycol, intravenous saline rehydration, and dialysis in severe cases. Activated charcoal does not bind lithium. Bicarbonate is used to treat tricyclic antidepressant overdoses. Glucagon is used to treat β-blocker overdoses. Potassium chloride is not useful for management of lithium toxicity except in cases of severe hypokalemia.

93. **Answer A.** By far, chromosomal abnormalities are the most common cause of first-trimester spontaneous miscarriage. *At least* 50% of first-trimester pregnancy losses are related to fetal chromosomal abnormalities. Autosomal trisomy is the most common abnormality, with trisomy 16 being the most common specific chromosomal defect. Polyploidy is the next most common defect, with tetraploidy being most common. Uterine structural abnormalities, cigarette smoking, and trauma may all contribute to fetal loss. However, minor trauma such as a fall or strike to the abdomen, is very unlikely to cause fetal loss. Other factors include corpus luteum failure, antiphospholipid antibody syndrome, and maternal endocrine diseases such as diabetes mellitus and hypothyroidism.

94. **Answer B.** Diverticulosis is the most common cause of lower gastrointestinal bleeding (LGIB), which may be massive in 5% of cases. However, most cases of LGIB due to diverticulosis are mild and resolve without intervention. Interestingly, although most diverticula are located in the left (descending) or sigmoid colon, most *bleeding* diverticula are located in the right colon. This is fortuitous, because most cases of angiodysplasia, a common cause of severe LGIB in the elderly, are also located in the right colon. Angiographic studies performed to localize bleeding, therefore, canalize the superior mesenteric artery (SMA) first.

95. **Answer A.** As this patient is complaining of both chest pain and leg pain, radiographs of the chest and pelvis are indicated after the primary survey to rule out important causes of immediate death, including pneumothorax, hemothorax, and pelvic fracture. Ultrasonography in the form of a FAST scan may also be performed to evaluate for significant intraperitoneal hemorrhage. After these initial studies are performed (or in conjunction with them) the secondary survey is conducted to identify injuries that may cause significant morbidity without mortality. Obvious external injuries may distract the trauma leader from identifying the immediate life threat. In this patient's case, the broken right ankle, though impressive, is unlikely to be the cause of death.

If the initial chest x-ray is omitted, however, the potential pneumothorax missed on physical examination may be lethal. This is the main reason for the stepwise, algorithmic approach to trauma which is targeted to identify immediate life threats first and other injuries later. Cervical spine radiographs may be left until after the secondary survey, assuming appropriate spine precautions are used when moving the patient. CT scans should not be initiated until the primary and secondary surveys are complete, except in special circumstances of isolated, severe head injury.

96. **Answer A.** The patient has acute anterior ST-segment elevation myocardial infarction (STEMI) with evidence of congestive heart failure (CHF) due to cardiogenic shock. In these patients, immediate angioplasty has been shown to reduce mortality more than fibrinolytic therapy and is the preferred definitive therapy. Choices C and E are not appropriate for patients with acute STEMI. Choice D represents treatment of a non-ST-segment elevation myocardial infarction (NSTEMI).

97. **Answer D.** Neglect or hemi-inattention results from an infarction of the parietal lobe in the nondominant hemisphere. In most people, the left hemisphere is the dominant hemisphere whether they are right handed or left handed. In left-sided lesions, a milder neglect typically results on the patient's right side.

98. **Answer D.** The Ottawa knee rules were derived to help physicians determine which patients need x-rays in the setting of acute knee trauma. The rules state that a patient needs imaging if *any* of the following are present:

- Age ≥55
- Isolated patella tenderness
- Isolated tenderness of the fibular head
- Inability to flex the knee to 90 degrees
- Inability to bear weight or walk four steps both at the time of the accident and in the emergency room (limping is allowed)

The criteria have been prospectively validated and are nearly 100% sensitive in identifying patients with clinically significant fractures. Successive studies have validated the use of the rules in children as young as 2 years old, though given the difficulty in examining very young children, the clinical utility of the rules in children younger than 5 has been questioned.

99. **Answer C.** Pericarditis is the most common cardiac complication of SLE. While not usually serious by itself, associated pericardial effusions can potentially cause hemodynamic compromise. Chest pain is the most common symptom of pericarditis in SLE patients. Myocarditis also commonly occurs in patients with SLE, but it is often clinically silent and overt symptoms are more likely to be related to signs of CHF such as shortness of

breath or peripheral edema. Coronary artery disease can complicate SLE as well but is less common than either pericarditis or myocarditis. Noninfective endocarditis (also known as Libman–Sacks endocarditis) is present in a minority of patients with SLE. Lesions can get super-infected and cause valvular insufficiency, often without frank chest pain. The most common overall cause of chest pain in patients with SLE is likely musculoskeletal disease.

100. **Answer A.** Though there is scant evidence to sup-port it, in neonates with hypoglycemia, D10 and D5 (or D25) are preferred to treat hypoglycemia because D50 is thought to provoke rebound hypoglycemia in hyperinsulinemic infants. Furthermore, D50 has much higher osmolarity than the lower concentration fluids which could cause tissue damage if extravasation occurs. While the exact dextrose dose can deviate from this rule, the easiest way to remember the amount of dextrose to deliver in acutely hypoglycemic, symptomatic neo-nates is to follow the "rule of 50." The basic formula is % dextrose $\times$ mL/kg volume = 50. So:

D5 $\times$ 10 mL/kg = 5 $\times$ 10 = 50. For a 5-kg child, bolus 10 mL/kg or 50 mL of D5

D10 $\times$ 5 mL/kg = 10 $\times$ 5 = 50. For a 5-kg child, bolus 5 mL/kg or 25 mL of D10 (this scenario)

D25 $\times$ 2 mL/kg = 25 $\times$ 2 = 50. For a 5-kg child, bolus 2 mL/kg or 10 mL of D25

Glucagon is a reasonable rescue therapy if the neonate remains hypoglycemic despite appropriate therapy.

QUESTIONS

1. Which of the following is an indication for replantation after amputation?

   A. Amputation of the thumb in the nondominant hand.
   B. Ring finger amputation distal to the distal interphalangeal (DIP) joint.
   C. A 58-year-old diabetic factory worker with an amputation of his index finger at the metacarpophalangeal (MCP) joint.
   D. A 23-year-old laboratory worker with a middle finger amputation at the level of his middle phalanx who stored his finger packed in dry ice for the last 12 hours.
   E. All of the above.

2. A 3-year-old previously healthy female is brought to the emergency department (ED) by her parents with a complaint of fever and cough. Her physical examination findings and chest x-ray are consistent with pneumonia. She is tolerating PO without difficulty and appears nontoxic. Which of the following is the most appropriate antibiotic regimen?

   A. Doxycycline
   B. Erythromycin
   C. Levofloxacin
   D. Trimethoprim–sulfamethoxazole
   E. High-dose amoxicillin

3. A 29-year-old male emergency medicine resident physician presents immediately after a needlestick from performing a procedure on a known chronic hepatitis B (HB) virus carrier. He has not ever received vaccination for HB. Which of the following is the next best step in management?

   A. Ribavirin
   B. Test for hepatitis B e antibody (HBeAb)
   C. HB vaccine
   D. Hepatitis B immunoglobulin (HBIG)
   E. HB vaccine plus HBIG

4. Which of the following findings is seen in most patients with meningococcemia?

   A. Bilateral adrenal infarction
   B. Skin lesions

C. Hypothermia
D. Seizure
E. Arthritis

5. One week after returning from India, the parents of a previously healthy 9-year-old female bring her to the emergency room for evaluation of a 3-day history of progressive fever, headache, malaise, nausea without vomiting, and generalized abdominal pain with minimal loose stools but no frank diarrhea. In addition to completing the CDC's routine vaccination series, she received additional vaccinations for hepatitis A and yellow fever prior to her trip and she took mefloquine for malaria prophylaxis throughout her visit. In the emergency room, she is noted to appear dehydrated but has a pulse in the low 50s. There is also a faint, blanching, erythematous rash over her chest and upper abdomen. Blood testing reveals anemia with a minimally elevated white blood cell (WBC) count, and moderately elevated liver function tests. Which of the following is true?

   A. She requires admission for likely dengue fever, and IV clindamycin should be started.
   B. Her relative bradycardia in the setting of a high fever may indicate typhoid fever.
   C. She most likely contracted a strain of malaria that is resistant to mefloquine.
   D. Her WBC differential most likely reveals a prominence of eosinophils.
   E. Her presentation is most consistent with yellow fever, as the vaccine produces incomplete immunity.

6. A 10-year-old male presents with chest pain. Which of the following is the most likely cause?

   A. Cardiac
   B. Gastrointestinal (GI)
   C. Psychogenic
   D. Musculoskeletal
   E. Endocrine

7. The classic sequence of color changes in the fingers of patients experiencing Raynaud phenomenon is:

   A. Blue to white to red
   B. Red to white to blue
   C. White to red to blue
   D. White to blue to red
   E. Blue to red to white

8. Which of the following treatments has been shown to be effective in the prevention of acute mountain sickness (AMS)?

   A. Propranolol
   B. Acetazolamide
   C. Furosemide
   D. Caffeine
   E. Nifedipine

9. Which of the following is the best rationale for using the primary survey in trauma?

   A. Cranio-caudal direction ensures a uniform approach
   B. Early identification of the most immediate life threats
   C. Ease of documentation
   D. Complete physical examination to maximize sensitivity
   E. Early identification of relevant medications and allergies

10. A 26-year-old female presents with a rash on her legs. She states that she has been feeling somewhat tired lately and notes generalized body and joint aches, as well as a sore throat. Over the last day or so, she has noted a rash developing over her anterior shins. The rash is very tender to the touch and is nonpruritic (Fig. 6-1). Which of the following is true?

   A. She should be referred to a dermatologist for a biopsy.
   B. First-line treatment is with aspirin or nonsteroidal anti-inflammatory drugs (NSAIDs).
   C. These lesions do not occur in children.
   D. The rash tends to be nontender and pruritic.
   E. These lesions tend to be recurrent over a patient's lifetime.

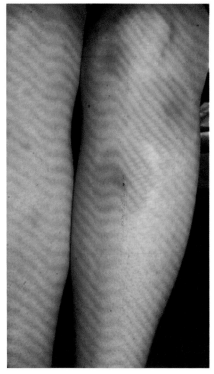

Figure 6-1

11. A 24-year-old male is brought to the emergency room by emergency medical services (EMS) after being assaulted in a robbery with an unknown blunt object. He does not know if he lost consciousness, but he complains of a severe left-sided headache and left ear pain. His secondary survey reveals left-sided hemotympanum. Which of the following is also most likely present?

   A. Epidural hematoma
   B. Cervical spine injury
   C. Nasal fracture
   D. Dissection of the internal carotid artery
   E. Cranial nerve palsy

12. A 78-year-old male admitted for urinary tract infection and dementia becomes increasingly agitated while boarding in your ED for 5 hours. Which of the following is the most appropriate next step in management?

   A. Reassessment and verbal redirection
   B. Lorazepam 1 mg IV
   C. Diphenhydramine 12.5 mg IV
   D. Diphenhydramine 25 mg IV
   E. Haloperidol 2 mg IV

13. A 28-year-old female at 29 weeks gestation is brought to the ED by ambulance after a minor motor vehicle accident. She was the restrained driver of a car traveling approximately 20 mph when she lost control on "black ice" and collided with a road sign. There was minimal damage to the car according to EMS but they placed her in a cervical spine collar and on a backboard for transport. She has no complaints in the ED except for discomfort related to the board and collar. After finding that her primary and secondary survey is intact, she is asking to go home. Which of the following is the next best step in management?

A. Discharge the patient with close obstetric follow-up.
B. Document fetal heart tones before discharge.
C. Perform a transabdominal ultrasonography to ensure fetal viability and absence of placental abruption.
D. Perform 4 hours of cardiotocographic monitoring before discharge.
E. Admit her for 23 hours of cardiotocographic monitoring in labor and delivery.

14. Treatment of group A beta-hemolytic streptococcal throat infection (GAS pharyngitis) with antibiotics is intended to prevent which of the following complications?

A. Erythema marginatum
B. Endocarditis
C. Migratory arthritis
D. Glomerulonephritis
E. A, B, and C

15. A 10-year-old male presents with elbow pain after falling off the bed. Radiographic visualization of which of the following usually indicates an occult elbow fracture?

A. Anterior fat pad
B. Posterior fat pad
C. Baumann angle of 75 degrees
D. Bilaterally equal Baumann angles
E. Anterior humeral line bisecting the capitellum

16. Which of the following is a risk factor for completed suicide?

A. Women younger than 50 years
B. Antisocial personality disorder
C. Family history of suicide
D. Generalized anxiety disorder
E. Arachnophobia

17. A 30-year-old female presents for evaluation of left elbow pain after a fall on an outstretched hand. She reports her arm was "locked" at the time of the fall. She rested the elbow overnight but awoke in the morning with increased pain, swelling, and decreased range of motion (Fig. 6-2). Which of the following is the most likely injury?

A. Supracondylar fracture
B. Olecranon fracture
C. Radial head fracture
D. Radial–ulnar dislocation
E. Sprain of the ulnar collateral ligament

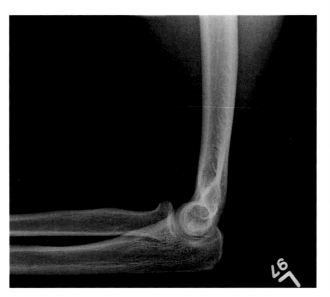
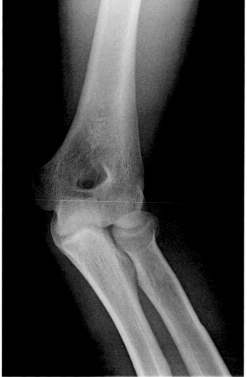

Figure 6-2

18. A 23-year-old male presents with flaccid bilateral lower extremity paralysis 1 day after being assaulted. An anterior lumbar spinal cord injury is identified. Which of the following is the most appropriate therapy at this time?

    A. Normal saline hydration
    B. Naloxone
    C. Methylprednisolone
    D. Vancomycin
    E. Vasopressin

19. A 56-year-old diabetic male presents to the ED after a brief episode of chest pain. His initial EKG reveals no ischemia and his troponin is negative. Which of the following is true about coronary CT angiography (CCTA) in this patient?

    A. If the HEART score stratifies the patient as low risk, the CCTA provides no additional useful information
    B. CCTA is most useful in very high risk patients
    C. Bradycardia will result in higher absorbed radiation doses
    D. CCTA may provide useful prognostic information to help with risk stratification
    E. CCTA is contraindicated because of the substantial radiation dose

20. A 55-year-old female presents with a laceration on her arm after falling from her bicycle. She does not know the last time she had a tetanus booster, but wants to know why she should have one. Which of the following is true regarding tetanus?

    A. Mortality for clinically evident tetanus is almost 50%.
    B. All patients with tetanus have a history of preceding injury.
    C. Wound cultures are helpful for diagnostic screening.
    D. Cardiac dysrhythmia is the most common cause of death.
    E. Tetanus boosters should be updated every year with clean wounds.

21. A 56-year-old male presents with postoperative bloating. The consulting surgeon suspects an ileus. Which of the following lab findings is most likely contributing to the patient's symptoms?

    A. Lactic acidosis
    B. Hypokalemia
    C. Hypomagnesemia
    D. Hypercalcemia
    E. Uremia

22. A 39-year-old male with a surgical history of appendectomy presents with abdominal pain and vomiting. You strongly suspect small bowel obstruction. Which of the following abdominal examination findings is most likely to be present?

    A. Distention
    B. Focal tenderness
    C. High-pitched bowel sounds
    D. Rebound tenderness
    E. Percussion tenderness

23. A 70-year-old female is brought in by EMS with right-sided rib pain and painful breathing after a fall against a dresser. Her SaO$_2$ is 96% on room air. A chest x-ray reveals a solitary right 7th rib fracture but no pneumothorax. Which of the following is true?

    A. She may be safely discharged home
    B. Chest x-rays detect >75% of rib fractures
    C. Elastic chest binders are helpful to reduce pain without impacting respiration
    D. Elderly patients with rib fractures can be discharged home unless they have ≥6 rib fractures
    E. A dedicated rib series is the gold standard to detect rib fractures

24. A 19-year-old female, accompanied by her college roommate, presents to the emergency room for evaluation of "an eating problem." The patient's roommate states that the already thin patient began losing excessive weight after she decided to become a vegetarian because she thought she "was too fat" 2 months ago. The patient is awake and alert, but is a reluctant historian, though she willingly came to the ED for evaluation. She is a self-described "perfectionist." Her vitals are T 97.6°F, P 42, RR 16, BP 90/58. She is 5 ft 6 in tall, and weighs 43 kg (95 lb), which puts her in the third percentile for weight based on her age and gender. An EKG reveals sinus bradycardia. Which of the following is the next best step in her evaluation and management?

    A. Initiation of paroxetine (Paxil) and referral to an outpatient psychiatrist
    B. Completion of involuntary commitment paperwork since she is starving herself to death
    C. Referral for outpatient cognitive–behavioral psychotherapy
    D. Referral to a cardiologist for evaluation of bradycardia
    E. Admission to the hospital for emergent refeeding

25. Which of the following is true regarding laboratory testing in patients with abdominal trauma?

    A. Liver enzymes are used to help distinguish minor contusions from high-grade lacerations.
    B. Elevated serum amylase and lipase are always indicative of pancreatic injury.
    C. Microscopic hematuria may indicate a need for abdominal CT scanning in pediatric blunt trauma patients.
    D. The hematocrit is only useful when serial measurements are conducted.
    E. None of the above.

26. Which of the following is the most common cause of multiple rib fractures in children?

    A. Motor vehicle collision
    B. Child abuse
    C. Fall
    D. Sports injury
    E. Gunshot wound

27. A 26-year-old male is brought to the ED after a motor vehicle accident. He was the restrained passenger in a jeep traveling 45 mph when the driver lost control and struck a tree. The patient's left knee struck the dashboard and he is now complaining of pain in his left knee and hip (Fig. 6-3). Which of the following is the most likely diagnosis?

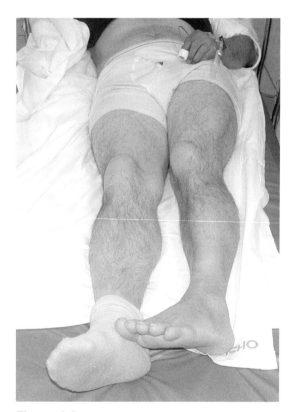

Figure 6-3

A. Femoral neck fracture
B. Open book pelvis fracture
C. Ischial tuberosity fracture
D. Posterior hip dislocation
E. Greater trochanter fracture

28. Which of the following is the most common lead point in cases of pediatric intussusception?

    A. Meckel diverticulum
    B. Lymphoma
    C. Intestinal polyp
    D. Mucosal hemorrhage in Henoch–Schönlein purpura
    E. Peyer patches

29. Which of the following is the leading cause of legal blindness in the United States?

    A. Cataracts
    B. Glaucoma
    C. Diabetic retinopathy
    D. Macular degeneration
    E. Retinal detachment

30. Which of the following is true about neonatal seizures?

    A. They are usually absence seizures
    B. They are most often due to hyponatremia
    C. Treatment with barbiturates is avoided
    D. They are usually caused by inadequate breast-feeding
    E. They tend to be more subtle than seizures in older children and adults

31. Among the elderly, which of the following is the most common cause of delirium?

    A. Stroke
    B. Electrolyte abnormalities
    C. Infection
    D. Medication interactions or side effects
    E. Trauma

32. A 26-year-old pregnant woman at 8 weeks presents to the ED with a chief complaint of nausea and vomiting. Her abdomen and pelvic examinations are normal and her ultrasonogram reveals a normal live intrauterine pregnancy at 8 weeks. Her urine reveals no ketones. Which of the following is the best recommendation for reducing her symptoms?

    A. Diazepam
    B. Promethazine
    C. Vitamin B_6
    D. Ondansetron
    E. Dexamethasone

33. What is the most common cause of lower gastrointestinal (GI) bleeding (LGIB) in children?

    A. Anal fissure
    B. Hemorrhoids

C. Henoch–Schönlein purpura

D. Food allergy

E. Meckel diverticulum

34. A 19-year-old female presents with worsening unilateral purulent discharge from her left eye that started the day before presentation. She has blurry vision that resolves when wiping the drainage out of her eye. She also notes nausea and intermittent fevers for the past few days, lower abdominal pain, and dysuria. Slit lamp examination demonstrates purulent discharge, but no corneal or anterior chamber abnormalities. Which of the following is the most appropriate management strategy?

A. Topical antibiotics, follow-up with ophthalmology in 2 days

B. Topical antivirals, follow-up with ophthalmology in 2 days

C. Systemic antibiotics, admission to hospital

D. Systemic antivirals, admission to hospital

E. Topical and systemic antibiotics, admission to hospital

35. A 63-year-old female presents with low-grade fever, nasal congestion, malaise, cough, and sore throat for 3 days. She is fairly certain she has sinusitis and states that her primary care doctor always gives her antibiotics for these symptoms. Her vitals are: 99.7, 85, 16, 123/72, 99% RA. Her physical examination is normal, including no facial tenderness, periorbital edema, or cranial nerve abnormalities. Which of the following is the next best step in management?

A. Nasal culture

B. Sinus aspiration

C. Prednisone 40 mg for 5 days

D. Amoxicillin–clavulanic acid for 10 days

E. Supportive care

36. Which of the following is indicated for treatment of a stable, wide-complex regular tachycardia at a rate of 200 in a patient with Wolff–Parkinson–White (WPW) syndrome?

A. Adenosine

B. Amiodarone

C. Esmolol

D. Digoxin

E. Procainamide

37. A 24-year-old diabetic male presents with rapid, deep breathing in the setting of severe hyperglycemia. Lungs are clear and SaO_2 is 100% on RA. His urine dipstick is only mildly positive for ketones. Which of the following is the likely explanation?

A. β-hydroxybutyrate, which is poorly detected by dipsticks, is the predominant ketone

B. His rapid breathing is likely due to pulmonary pathology not a metabolic acidosis

C. Acetoacetate interferes with the dipstick analysis

D. He has lactic acidosis from sepsis not detected by dipsticks

E. None of the above

38. Which of the following is true regarding imaging of patients with suspected sinusitis?

A. Plain films are more accurate in diagnosing frontal and ethmoid than maxillary sinusitis.

B. Waters view plain film is the most sensitive test for maxillary sinusitis.

C. Computed tomography (CT) scans are able to differentiate between acute bacterial and viral sinusitis.

D. CT scans are both highly sensitive and highly specific in the diagnosis of sinusitis.

E. Most patients with viral upper respiratory infections (URIs) have abnormal CT scan findings.

39. A 65-year-old male presents with a syncopal event without prodromal symptoms. His vital signs are 98.6, 60, 18, 142/75, 99% RA. The EKG is shown in Figure 6-4. Which of the following is the most appropriate next step in management?

A. Admit for observation

B. Cardioversion at 50 J

C. Defibrillation at 200 J

D. Amiodarone 150 mg IV

E. Admission and pacemaker placement

40. A 29-year-old G1P0 is brought in by EMS in active labor. The patient attempted a home birth but the midwife called EMS after a prolonged, unsuccessful labor. Upon arrival, the patient spontaneously delivers a male infant who then begins to seize. What is the most likely etiology?

A. Hypoxia

B. Hydrocephalus

C. Intracranial hemorrhage

D. Down syndrome

E. Hypoglycemia

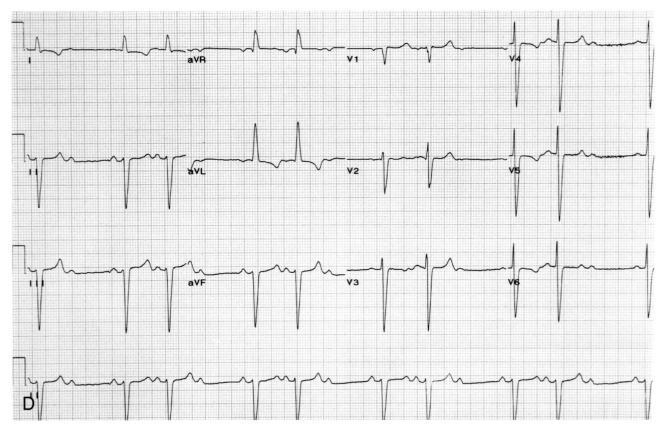

Figure 6-4

41. A 45-year-old male presents with locking and clicking of his knee for several days. He twisted it several weeks ago and did not seek medical care at the time. Physical examination demonstrates no knee instability or patellar tenderness. His knee clicks with flexion and occasionally gets locked just before full extension. Which of the following structures is most likely injured?

    A. Anterior cruciate ligament
    B. Posterior cruciate ligament
    C. Medial meniscus
    D. Patella tendon
    E. Medial collateral ligament

42. Which of the following is a known effect of haloperidol?

    A. Lowers the seizure threshold
    B. Dopamine D2-receptor antagonist
    C. α-1 receptor agonist
    D. Histamine receptor agonist
    E. Agranulocytosis

43. A 22-year-old male presents to the ED with a left posterior hip dislocation sustained in a car accident. Which of the following neurologic findings is most likely present?

    A. Ipsilateral Babinski sign
    B. Erectile dysfunction
    C. Ipsilateral foot drop
    D. Numbness over the ipsilateral anterior thigh
    E. Weakness of contralateral hip adduction

44. A 22-year-old G1 at 9 weeks gestation with proven intra-uterine pregnancy presents to the ED with severe nausea and vomiting for 3 days. She has been unable to eat and can drink only minimal fluids. Which of the following suggests a diagnosis of hyperemesis gravidarum?

    A. Bilious vomiting
    B. Hypokalemia
    C. Metabolic alkalosis
    D. Ketonuria
    E. White race

45. A 15-year-old male is brought in by his parents with a chief complaint of bloody stools. They describe the stools as coated with bloody material and report blood on the tissue paper. The patient reports a history of chronic constipation and straining but has no complaints. He has a benign abdominal examination, normal vital signs, and a hemoglobin value of 14.5 g/dL. Which of the following is true?

    A. Anal fissures are usually painless
    B. Anal hemorrhoids are the likely source of bleeding
    C. Diverticulosis is a common cause of pediatric lower GI bleeding
    D. The patient should be admitted for a 99m technetium pertechnetate infusion
    E. The patient should be referred for outpatient GI evaluation for possible juvenile polyps

46. A 17-year-old basketball player collapses and dies while playing a game. Which of the following is the most likely cause?

    A. Coronary artery disease
    B. Pulmonary embolism
    C. Hypertrophic cardiomyopathy
    D. Subarachnoid hemorrhage (SAH)
    E. Spontaneous pneumothorax

47. A 45-year-old female with a history of hypertension presents with lower lip swelling, as shown in Figure 6-5. She was recently started on a new blood pressure medication. Despite therapy with steroids, antihistamines, and epinephrine, her condition continues to worsen. In addition to measures for airway control, which of the following is most likely to be helpful in this patient?

    A. Verapamil
    B. Metoprolol
    C. Fresh frozen plasma
    D. Danazol
    E. Aldosterone

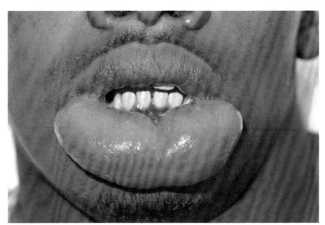

Figure 6-5

48. When compared with adults, which of the following is true when evaluating infants and children for cervical spine (c-spine) injuries?

    A. There are no clinical decision rules available to assist with clinical c-spine clearance in children
    B. C-spine injuries in infants tend to occur at higher c-spine levels than in adults
    C. MRI is an important adjunct in patients with a negative c-spine CT
    D. Plain x-rays are not useful in pediatric c-spine evaluation
    E. C-spine injuries are more common in children than in adults

49. Which of the following is the most important factor in determining the risk of rupture of an abdominal aortic aneurysm (AAA)?

    A. Age of the patient
    B. Hypertension
    C. Size of the aneurysm
    D. Location of the aneurysm
    E. Male gender

50. A 78-year-old previously healthy woman presents with right hip pain after a fall. Her hip x-ray reveals a right femoral neck fracture. Which of the following is the most important factor in returning the patient to optimal mobility?

    A. Suicidality screening in the ED
    B. Preoperative physical therapy
    C. Preoperative medication reconciliation
    D. Minimizing time to surgical repair
    E. Postoperative primary care follow-up

51. A 50-year-old male develops acute-onset severe right flank pain. A CT scan demonstrates a calculus in the bladder. The patient has never had a kidney stone before. He asks you what his risk of getting another stone is. You tell him that the lifetime risk of recurrence is approximately:

    A. <1%
    B. 10%
    C. 25%
    D. 50%
    E. >99%

52. A 23-year-old male presents with shoulder pain after falling on his left shoulder. Physical examination demonstrates tenderness in his lateral clavicle. He is able to touch his opposite shoulder with his left hand. There are no neurovascular deficits (Fig. 6-6). Which of the following is the most likely diagnosis?

    A. Anterior shoulder dislocation
    B. Inferior shoulder dislocation
    C. Posterior shoulder dislocation
    D. Acromioclavicular separation
    E. Sternoclavicular dislocation

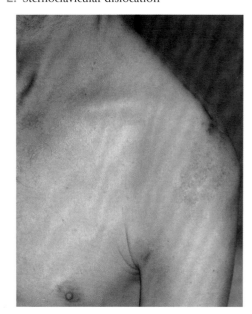

Figure 6-6

53. Which of the following fractures is most suggestive of child abuse?

    A. Supracondylar humerus fracture
    B. Spiral tibia fracture
    C. Distal radius fracture
    D. Posterior rib fractures
    E. Tibial plateau fracture

54. Which of the following is a negative symptom of schizophrenia?

    A. Delusions
    B. Hallucinations
    C. Flat affect
    D. Disorganized speech
    E. Disorganized behavior

55. A 28-year-old male presents to the ED stating that he drank a whole bottle of antifreeze 4 hours before presentation. He had drunk a fifth of liquor just before drinking the antifreeze. Except for moderate intoxication, he is asymptomatic and his vital signs and physical examination are normal. Which of the following is the most appropriate next step in management?

    A. Discharge him without further testing.
    B. Check the oxalic acid level and discharge him if <50 mg/dL.
    C. Check urine for crystals and discharge him if negative.
    D. Check urine for fluorescence and discharge him if negative.
    E. Check the ethanol level and administer fomepizole if negative.

56. A 26-year-old previously healthy male presents with a chief complaint of a 2-day history of abdominal cramps and multiple episodes of watery brown nonbloody diarrhea. Which of the following is most likely?

    A. *Campylobacter* spp.
    B. *Salmonella* spp.
    C. *Shigella* spp.
    D. *Escherichia* spp.
    E. *Yersinia* spp.

57. What is the most common dysrhythmia in hypothyroid cardiovascular disease?

    A. Atrial fibrillation
    B. Long QT syndrome
    C. Junctional escape rhythm
    D. Sinus rhythm with left or right bundle branch block
    E. Sinus bradycardia

58. Which of the following is a criterion for the systemic inflammatory response syndrome (SIRS)?

    A. Systolic BP <90
    B. Diastolic BP <60
    C. HR <90
    D. Temperature <36°C
    E. RR <20

59. A 44-year-old male presents to the ED with a 3-day history of a painful rash on his right buttock and leg (Fig. 6-7). He has a history of inflammatory bowel disease and is on immunosuppressive therapy with 6-mercaptpurine and low-dose methotrexate. He first presented to his primary care physician who referred him to the emergency room due to concern for disseminated varicella zoster virus (VZV) infection. Which of the following is true?

    A. Lung involvement (pneumonitis) is the most common presentation of disseminated VZV.
    B. The patient will likely be resistant to standard treatment with acyclovir.
    C. Given the time since onset, the patient should receive corticosteroids without antiviral treatment.
    D. Mortality is most often caused by sepsis from bacterial superinfection of skin lesions.
    E. Even in immunocompromised patients, disseminated VZV is rarely fatal.

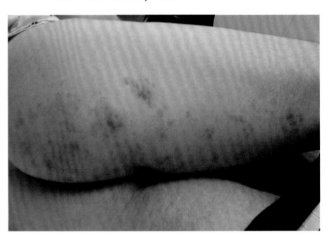

Figure 6-7

60. Which of the following is more characteristic of transverse myelitis than acute inflammatory demyelinating polyneuropathy, the most common variant of Guillain–Barre syndrome?

    A. Albuminocytologic dissociation
    B. Equal weakness in upper and lower extremities
    C. Normal spinal MRI
    D. Hemodynamic instability
    E. Association with *Campylobacter* infection

61. Which of the following represents the approximate proportion of acute myocardial infarctions (MIs) that occur without a history of chest pain?

    A. 1%
    B. 5%
    C. 10%
    D. 25%
    E. 50%

62. A 35-year-old male complains of progressively worsening right leg pain 2 hours after undergoing a closed reduction in the ED for a mid-shaft tibia fracture. After the splint is removed, physical examination reveals a firm, tender compartment of his right anterior leg with diminished sensation in the area. Pulses in the foot are 2+. Compartment pressure is 30 mm Hg. The patient's vital signs are T 98.8°F, P 98, RR 18 BP 110/55 SaO_2 98% on RA. Which of the following is the most appropriate course of action?

    A. Elevate the leg and recheck compartment pressure in 1 hour.
    B. Resplint with a looser wrap, discharge with next-day follow-up.
    C. Order an MRI of the leg.
    D. Check ankle/brachial index and discharge patient if the index is >0.9.
    E. Consult orthopedics for a possible fasciotomy.

63. A 61-year-old male smoker recently performed some repairs on several air-conditioning units during the late summer. He is now brought in by his family confused, with high fevers, chills, a dry cough, and diarrhea. The test that will best determine the likely specific cause of his illness is which of the following?

    A. Urine antigen testing
    B. Blood cultures
    C. Sputum cultures
    D. Chest x-ray
    E. Serology testing

64. A 5-year-old female without past medical history presents with fever and pruritic rash on several areas of her trunk. The parents report a sick contact with similar symptoms at school and think the rash may be chicken pox. There is no reported cough, shortness of breath, headache, or stiff neck. Physical examination demonstrates a nontoxic, playful child with a crop of vesicles in one area and dried crusted lesions in other areas. Which of the following is the most appropriate next step in management?

    A. Aspirin
    B. Acetaminophen
    C. IV acyclovir
    D. Varicella zoster vaccine
    E. Varicella zoster immune globulin

65. A 51-year-old male with a history of end-stage renal disease who recently started continuous ambulatory peritoneal dialysis (CAPD) presents to the ED with a chief complaint of abdominal pain and fever for 1 day. He has noted a cloudy effluent which is a change from the baseline clear character of the dialysate. A presumptive diagnosis of peritonitis is made. Which of the following empiric strategies is best?

    A. Intraperitoneal vancomycin plus gentamicin
    B. Intravenous vancomycin plus gentamicin combined with intraperitoneal vancomycin plus gentamicin
    C. Intravenous vancomycin, gentamicin, and voriconazole
    D. Intraperitoneal vancomycin plus cefepime, followed by catheter exchange
    E. Monotherapy with intravenous cefepime

66. A 65-year-old female presents in out-of-hospital cardiac arrest with ventricular fibrillation. Which of the following is the most effective management for this condition?

    A. Defibrillation
    B. Pericardiocentesis
    C. Epinephrine IV
    D. Amiodarone IV
    E. Invasive mechanical ventilation

67. Which of the following patients most likely has giant cell arteritis?

    A. An 18-year-old male with chronic daily headaches and a family history of lupus
    B. A 55-year-old female with diabetes without vision complaints referred by her optometrist for evaluation of a dilated right pupil
    C. A 20-year-old female with a temporal headache and an erythrocyte sedimentation rate of 26 mm/hour
    D. A 74-year-old female with jaw pain after chewing food
    E. A 37-year-old male with a parietotemporal headache and a family history of berry aneurysms

68. A 22-year-old female presents to the ED after a domestic dispute with a boyfriend in which she was stabbed in the neck just lateral to her thyroid cartilage. Which of the following is an indication for mandatory operative exploration?

    A. Palpable thrill
    B. Subcutaneous emphysema
    C. Violation of the platysma
    D. Bruit upon auscultation
    E. All of the above

69. Which of the following is true regarding traumatic iridocyclitis?

    A. It is generally painless.
    B. Findings include a fixed and dilated pupil.
    C. Treatment involves long-acting cycloplegics.
    D. Steroids play no role in management.
    E. Resolution generally occurs 1 month after the onset of symptoms.

70. Which of the following is the narrowest portion of the pediatric airway?

   A. Nasopharynx
   B. Oropharynx
   C. True cords
   D. False cords
   E. Cricoid cartilage

71. Which of the following is true regarding concussions?

   A. Loss of consciousness is required to meet the technical definition.
   B. CT brain is acutely abnormal in half of all cases.
   C. MRI brain is almost always acutely abnormal.
   D. Postconcussive anosmia may be permanent.
   E. On the field of play, simple orientation questions are adequate to detect concussion.

72. When evaluating a trauma patient with a focused assessment with sonography in trauma (FAST) scan, which of the following views is ideally performed first?

   A. Right flank
   B. Left flank
   C. Pericardial
   D. Suprapubic
   E. Thoracic

73. An 18-year-old intoxicated appearing male is brought in by EMS after ingesting some windshield wiper fluid on a dare from his drunk friend. In addition to fomepizole, which of the following is an important component of treatment?

   A. Cobalamin
   B. Folate
   C. Niacin
   D. Vitamin D
   E. Vitamin K

74. A 75-year-old male with a history of hypertension, diabetes, and ischemic stroke causing mild residual left-sided hemiparesis presents with sudden onset of complete left-sided arm and leg paralysis with mild confusion. The symptoms occurred 1 hour prior to arrival. His vital signs are 98.5°F, 75, 16, 168/92, 99% RA. Physical examination reveals a regular heart rhythm and 0/5 strength on the left side. Which of the following is the most appropriate next step in management?

   A. EKG
   B. Blood glucose level
   C. PO aspirin
   D. IV tissue plasminogen activator (TPA)
   E. Arterial blood gas

75. Which of the following is true regarding viral hepatitis?

   A. Ten percent of adult patients infected with acute hepatitis A become chronic carriers.
   B. Pregnant women infected with acute hepatitis E are more susceptible to fulminant hepatitis.
   C. Children infected with hepatitis A virus develop symptoms more often than adults.
   D. Hepatitis B is the most common cause of viral hepatitis worldwide.
   E. Although hepatitis A primarily undergoes fecal–oral transmission, percutaneous transmission occurs at rates similar to hepatitis B.

76. A 75-year-old male presents with a fall on an outstretched hand. Radiographs demonstrate a distal radius fracture with dorsal displacement of the distal segment. Which of the following is the most likely nerve injury?

   A. Median
   B. Radial
   C. Ulnar
   D. Axillary
   E. Vagus

77. Which of the following is most effective in reducing mortality from acute MI?

   A. Metoprolol
   B. Aspirin
   C. Nitroglycerin
   D. Abciximab
   E. Morphine

78. Upon examining a patient with a rash, applying light manual pressure to the skin adjacent to the skin lesions of the rash causes the top layers of skin to peel away and rub off. Which of the following is the likely underlying diagnosis?

   A. Roseola infantum
   B. Bullous impetigo
   C. Pemphigus vulgaris
   D. Tinea corporis
   E. Erysipelas

79. A 43-year-old female presents with a painful area in her calf for several days. She read on the internet about deep venous thromboses and is worried she has one. She does not take oral contraceptive therapy and is a nonsmoker. She has a definite, focal area of tenderness in her calf without obvious cellulitis. A duplex ultrasound reveals a 1.5-cm superficial vein thrombosis below the knee. Which of the following is the next best step in management?

   A. CT angiogram of the chest to evaluate for pulmonary embolism (PE)
   B. Repeat duplex ultrasound in 3 hours to assess progression
   C. NSAID therapy, rest, and gentle warmth
   D. Warfarin
   E. Intravenous tissue plasminogen activator

80. A 23-year-old male is bitten on his forearm by a raccoon. Which of the following is the most appropriate anatomical region to administer human rabies immune globulin (HRIG)?

   A. Deltoid
   B. Gluteus maximus
   C. At the wound site
   D. Contralateral forearm
   E. Corpora cavernosum

81. What is the half-life of carboxyhemoglobin with a 100% oxygen nonrebreather mask?

   A. 6 hours
   B. 3 hours
   C. 90 minutes
   D. 60 minutes
   E. 30 minutes

82. Which of the following is the most common complication of diverticulosis?

   A. Perforation
   B. Bleeding
   C. Obstruction
   D. Diverticulitis
   E. None of the above

83. Which of the following helps to differentiate a sympathomimetic crisis from an anticholinergic crisis?

   A. Tachycardia
   B. Mydriasis
   C. Diaphoresis
   D. Seizures
   E. Altered mental status

84. Which of the following is true regarding foreign body removal from the external auditory canal?

   A. Vegetable matter should be removed by irrigation with water.
   B. Smaller instruments are more likely to cause damage to the ear canal.
   C. The central portion of the external auditory canal is the smallest segment.
   D. Insects should be removed while still alive.
   E. Button batteries are best removed by irrigation with mineral oil.

85. A 29-year-old male presents with an extremely pruritic rash several hours after running through a forest (Fig. 6-8). Which of the following is the next best step in management?

   A. Supportive care
   B. Prednisone
   C. Methotrexate
   D. Cephalexin
   E. Trimethoprim–sulfamethoxazole

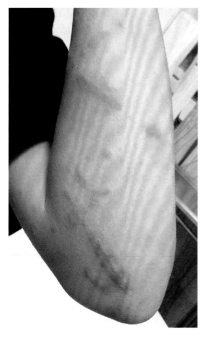

Figure 6-8

86. Which of the following is true regarding hip fractures?

   A. The highest incidence of avascular necrosis (AVN) occurs in patients with intertrochanteric fractures.
   B. Isolated fractures of the lesser trochanter are most commonly seen in young adults.
   C. Femoral nerve block is contraindicated in the setting of a hip fracture.
   D. The development of acute respiratory distress in a patient with an acute femoral shaft fracture but no other trauma is most likely due to blood loss into the soft tissues of the thigh.
   E. All of the above.

87. Which of the following is the most common cause of superior vena cava syndrome (SVCS)?

   A. Lung cancer
   B. Deep venous thrombosis (DVT) of the superior vena cava
   C. Tuberculosis
   D. Non-Hodgkin and Hodgkin lymphoma
   E. Aortic aneurysm

88. A patient presenting to the ED with which of the following is *least* likely to have audible wheezes on physical examination?

   A. Congestive heart failure (CHF)
   B. Chronic obstructive pulmonary disease (COPD)
   C. Aspirated foreign body
   D. Asthma
   E. Sarcoidosis

89. A 55-year-old female presents with uncontrollable twisting movements of her face and tongue. She has been on an antipsychotic for 25 years for treatment of schizophrenia. Which of the following is true regarding this condition?

    A. Patients with concomitant depression are at higher risk.
    B. Symptoms usually start within the first week of treatment.
    C. It is 100% reversible if the medication is stopped.
    D. Young men are the highest risk group.
    E. Treatment with anticholinergics is usually successful.

90. Which of the following is true regarding treatment of acute lead toxicity?

    A. Acute lead encephalopathy is generally self-limited and requires no specific therapy.
    B. Dimercaprol should be given before calcium disodium ethylenediamine tetra-acetic acid (EDTA).
    C. Activated charcoal is the mainstay of GI decontamination.
    D. Succimer should be the first chelator given in patients with severe lead poisoning.
    E. Penicillamine is more effective than succimer in chelation of lead.

91. A 24-year-old female previously unvaccinated presents with progressively worsening sore throat and fever for 3 days. Her oropharyngeal examination reveals an extensive grayish membrane extending between both tonsils. Which of the following is the most appropriate management?

    A. Piperacillin–tazobactam
    B. Acyclovir plus rifampin
    C. Penicillin plus antitoxin
    D. Amikacin plus methylprednisolone
    E. Vancomycin plus methylprednisolone

92. A 12-year-old male presents with progressive testicular swelling (Fig. 6-9). Which of the following is the most common complication of this condition?

    A. Testicular torsion
    B. Epididymitis
    C. Infertility
    D. Malignancy
    E. Deep venous thrombosis

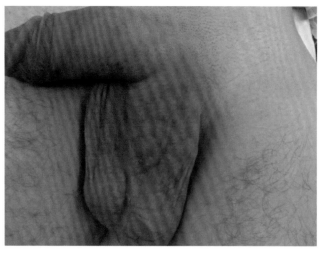

Figure 6-9

93. A 68-year-old female presents with a chief complaint of severe weakness, general malaise, and fever. The patient is hypotensive, and is found to have pneumonia on chest x-ray. The patient received broad-spectrum antibiotics but remains hypotensive despite 5 L of fluids. Which of the following is the best next step?

    A. Norepinephrine
    B. Vasopressin
    C. Dopamine
    D. Dobutamine
    E. Phenylephrine

94. A 22-year-old male presents with palpitations. He reports no chest pain, shortness of breath, or lower extremity edema. He states that he "got really drunk" the night before. He denies any past medical history, family history, or illicit drug use. His examination is unremarkable except for irregular tachycardia (Fig. 6-10). Which of the following is the most likely etiology?

    A. Myocardial infarction (MI)
    B. Pulmonary embolism
    C. Alcohol use
    D. Hypertension
    E. Diabetes

95. Which of the following is true regarding retinal detachment?

    A. It is usually painful.
    B. Presbyopia is a risk factor.
    C. Visual acuity may be normal.
    D. The elevated retina often appears dark red.
    E. Ophthalmologic follow-up is indicated in 1 week.

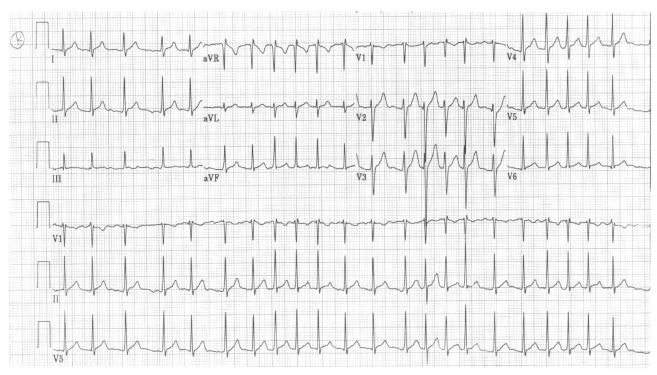

Figure 6-10

96. A 72-year-old male develops acute-onset shaking chills and shortness of breath a few days after an URI. His past medical history is significant for diabetes and stable coronary artery disease. Vital signs are 101°F, 115, 24, 144/95, 90% RA. Physical examination reveals a patient with rigors and right lower lobe crackles. Which of the following is the most appropriate next step in management?

   A. Doxycycline PO and discharge
   B. Azithromycin PO and discharge
   C. Ceftriaxone and azithromycin IV and admit
   D. Clindamycin IV and admit
   E. Piperacillin–tazobactam IV and admit

97. Which of the following is true about upper gastrointestinal bleeding (UGIB) due to peptic ulcer disease (PUD)?

   A. In patients with normal GI anatomy, hematochezia will not occur.
   B. Bleeding will stop spontaneously in 70% to 80% of patients.
   C. Most patients will present with isolated melena.

D. The mortality rate of bleeding due to a peptic ulcer is 25%.
E. Perforation may be accompanied by hemorrhage in 50% of cases.

98. The manifestations of hyperphosphatemia are related to its effects on:

   A. Sodium
   B. Potassium
   C. Magnesium
   D. Calcium
   E. Chloride

99. A 55-year-old patient presents with palpitations for 1 week (Fig. 6-11). The patient is sent to the emergency room (ER) for further evaluation. Which of the following is the most appropriate next step in management?

   A. Diltiazem 20 mg IV
   B. Esmolol 50 μg/kg/minute IV
   C. Enoxaparin 1 mg/kg SC
   D. Amiodarone 150 mg IV
   E. Adenosine 6 mg IV

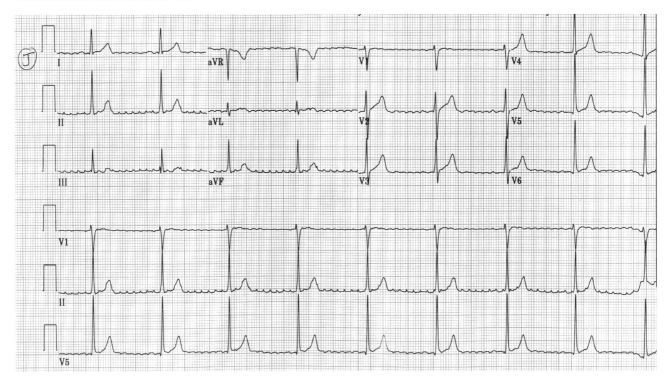

Figure 6-11

100. A 23-year-old male reaches into a snake cage at a zoo and is bitten by the snake pictured (Fig. 6-12). Which of the following is the most likely effect?

   A. Abdominal muscle spasms
   B. Disseminated intravascular coagulation (DIC)
   C. Compartment syndrome
   D. Neurotoxicity
   E. Renal failure

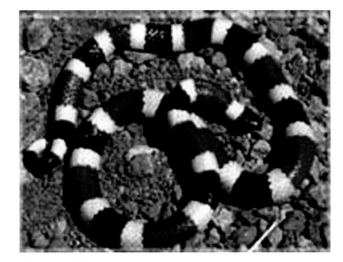

Figure 6-12

1. **Answer A.** In general, indications for replantation include multiple digit amputations, thumb amputations, wrist and forearm amputations, single digit amputations between the proximal interphalangeal (PIP) and distal interphalangeal (DIP) joints, and any pediatric amputation. Amputations distal to the DIP joint are typically debrided and closed along with amputations proximal to the PIP. Amputations that are between the PIP (distal to the flexor digitorum superficialis insertion) and DIP joints tend to do well. However, single digit amputations are often considered unnecessary to replant. In addition, patients with underlying vascular disease, diabetes, congestive heart failure, or other medical problems may not have a good outcome even when the characteristics of the amputation are encouraging for replantation. Finally, all patients with amputation should wrap the amputated digit in saline-soaked gauze, place the gauze in a ziplocked bag, and place the bag on ice or in an ice-water bath. Freezing the digit should be avoided as it results in irreversible damage to cellular structures due to ice crystal formation.

2. **Answer E.** Viruses are the predominant etiology of pneumonia in children between the ages of 4 months and 4 years. However, *S. pneumoniae* is the most common bacterial cause of pneumonia in this age group. Although chest x-rays are not reliable in distinguishing between viral and bacterial pneumonias, this patient has an infiltrate, so it seems prudent to treat the patient with an antibiotic with antipneumococcal activity. Doxycycline and levofloxacin are contraindicated in children. Erythromycin, a macrolide antibiotic, would be a better choice for children older than 5 years or younger than 4 months since *M. pneumoniae* and *C. trachomatis* are the most common bacterial causes of pneumonia in these respective groups.

3. **Answer E.** The patient has never received vaccination for HB virus. Therefore, the best step in management is to provide active immunization (with vaccine) as well as passive immunization (with immunoglobulin). Ribavirin is used in the treatment of hepatitis C infection in combination with interferon alpha. HBeAb demonstrates immunologic response to HBe antigen, a marker which connotes a higher infectivity. Testing for HBeAb has no role in the evaluation of acute hepatitis exposure. Vaccine or immunoglobulin alone is insufficient protection against exposure in an unvaccinated patient. If the patient had ever been vaccinated, then testing his blood for HB surface antibody (if positive indicates immunity) before treatment with vaccine and immunoglobulin is reasonable.

4. **Answer B.** *Meningococcemia* refers to systemic infection with *Neisseria meningitidis*, a gram-negative diplococcus. Mortality is as high as 50%, due to multiorgan failure from septic shock which can occur within hours. Fever and rash occur in most patients. Fifty percent of patients present with true petechiae, and another 20% to 30% exhibit a maculopapular rash which later turns into petechiae or purpura. Bilateral adrenal infarction, part of a constellation of signs known as the *Waterhouse–Friderichsen syndrome*, occurs in approximately 10% of cases. Hypothermia, seizure, and arthritis each occurs <10% of the time. Laboratory studies may demonstrate a significant leukocytosis (although leukopenia, when present, is a poor prognostic indicator), thrombocytopenia, and DIC. Treatment is with a third-generation cephalosporin and aggressive management of shock (fluids, vasoactive agents, intensive care unit [ICU] monitoring).

5. **Answer B.** This patient's presentation is most consistent with typhoid fever, a bacterial infection caused by *Salmonella typhi*. It is contracted through oral ingestion of contaminated food or water. While there are two vaccines for typhoid fever (an injectable, unconjugated polysaccharide vaccine, and an oral, live attenuated vaccine), they cumulatively provide only about 55% immunity, and this patient did not receive a vaccination prior to travel. In contrast, the vaccine for yellow fever confers near complete immunity. Ingestion of the organism is followed by a 1- to 2-week asymptomatic period. Patients then typically develop a fever, generalized fatigue and malaise, nausea, anorexia, generalized abdominal pain, and a headache. Children may have diarrhea, but adults frequently have constipation. Nearly a third of patients also have rose spots, which comprise a blanching, faint erythematous maculopapular rash over the chest and abdomen. A relative bradycardia in the setting of fever and dehydration is considered a classic finding, but no studies have determined exactly how often it is present. Complete blood count (CBC) typically reveals anemia and either leukopenia (more common in adults) or leukocytosis (more common in children). Liver enzymes are elevated in more than 80% of patients and may create a clinical picture consistent with acute hepatitis. Fluoroquinolones remain the treatment of choice in adults (bactericidal, concentrated in the bile), while third-generation cephalosporins are preferred in children. Because of the vague presentation, other causes of bacterial gastroenteritis or infections which may include gastroenteritis, such as malaria, dengue fever, amebiasis, or leishmaniasis, must be considered. Although this patient's presentation could be consistent with malaria, her compliance

with appropriate prophylactic therapy makes it unlikely. Mefloquine is very effective, providing 91% efficacy in preventing malaria. Dengue fever is a viral illness that is not treated with antibiotics. It is the most common mosquito-borne viral infection. Patients classically present with fever, malaise, and severe myalgias and arthralgias ("break-bone fever"). Among returned travelers with a fever, eosinophilia is most likely a manifestation of helminthic infection such as ascaris or hookworm.

6. **Answer D.** Musculoskeletal and pulmonary etiologies combine for roughly half of all cases of pediatric chest pain. GI, cardiac, and psychogenic conditions each account for approximately 10%. Idiopathic cases comprise a large minority. Endocrine causes are rare. As in adults, most pediatric patients with acute chest pain should have a screening chest x-ray and EKG to evaluate for pulmonary and cardiac causes, respectively. Although cardiac causes of pediatric chest pain tend to not be immediately life threatening, they often radically alter management and are not as rare as once believed.

7. **Answer D.** Raynaud phenomenon occurs in three phases. Initially, digital pallor (white) results from total closure of the palmar and digital arteries causing a cessation in digital blood flow. When mild relaxation occurs, a trickle of blood is able to perfuse the ischemic digit but the hemoglobin is rapidly desaturated resulting in cyanosis (blue). Finally, arterial spasm resolves and restores blood flow to baseline, resulting in a reactive hyperemia (red).

8. **Answer B.** Only acetazolamide and dexamethasone have been shown to be effective for the prevention of AMS. Acetazolamide is a carbonic anhydrase inhibitor, which prevents the reabsorption of bicarbonate in the proximal tubule. The resulting bicarbonate diuresis causes a metabolic acidosis within 1 hour of ingestion, which stimulates ventilation and speeds ventilatory acclimatization. In addition, acetazolamide reduces periodic breathing during sleep, thereby eliminating the associated apnea and hypoxia. Dexamethasone has also been shown to reduce the symptoms of AMS, although its mechanism of action is not known. Furthermore, patients can experience a rebound phenomenon upon stopping the drug, so it is generally reserved for the treatment of AMS rather than prophylaxis. Nifedipine is useful for prophylaxis of high-altitude pulmonary edema (HAPE), but it has no role in AMS. Caffeine stimulates the hypoxic ventilatory response but has not specifically been shown to reduce the incidence of AMS.

9. **Answer B.** The primary survey in trauma is designed to identify and address the most immediate life threats. This includes airway obstruction, pneumothorax or hemothorax, hemorrhage, and brain and spinal cord

abnormalities. Although the primary survey does tend to follow a cranio-caudal direction, this is not the main reason for the elements of the primary survey. Documentation should be tailored around the primary survey, not vice versa. The complete physical examination is important during the secondary survey, as this will identify important, but not emergent, issues. Medication and allergy history can be done either immediately after the primary survey or concomitantly with the secondary survey.

10. **Answer B.** The patient has erythema nodosum, which is thought to be a hypersensitivity reaction to a number of different antigens. It most commonly occurs in women (female:male ratio of 5:1) during the third decade but it frequently occurs in children as well. Patients often experience a vague prodrome of fever, malaise, and arthralgias, followed by the development of painful oval erythematous nodules typically over the shins. Individual lesions are not pruritic and are usually self-limited, lasting approximately 2 weeks, although new lesions may continue to appear such that the entire illness lasts up to 6 weeks. The most common cause is streptococcal infection in children and streptococcal infection and sarcoidosis in adults. Other causes include tuberculosis (TB), coccidioidomycosis, *Yersinia* or *Chlamydia* infection, inflammatory bowel disease, Hodgkin lymphoma, pregnancy, and drugs including oral contraceptives and sulfonamides. The lesions usually respond to high-dose aspirin (650 mg every 4 hours) or NSAIDs (e.g., naproxen or indomethacin) and bed rest. Occasionally, patients are treated with supersaturated potassium iodide (mechanism is uncertain). Corticosteroids are effective but are rarely used and may worsen the underlying infection if one is present. (Figure from Ayala C, Brad Spellberg B, eds. *Boards & Wards for USMLE Steps 2 & 3.* 5th ed. Philadelphia, PA: Wolters Kluwer; 2012.)

11. **Answer A.** Hemotympanum is one of the signs of a basilar skull fracture. Of the five bones that make up the base of the skull, the temporal bone is by far the most frequently injured, typically due to a direct blow from an assault or motor vehicle collision (MVC). Due to the relative weakness of the lateral aspect of the temporal bone, direct trauma may result in disruption of the middle meningeal artery leading to an epidural hematoma. This patient's questionable history of temporary loss of consciousness with subsequent awakening is a classically described feature of epidural hemorrhage known as the "lucid interval." Patients subsequently become increasingly symptomatic and experience a progressive decline in mental status over the next several hours. This patient's mechanism of injury and symptoms do not support a diagnosis of a cervical spine injury or nasal fracture. Carotid artery dissection has been described after blunt trauma to the temporal bone but is a rare

occurrence. Finally, patients with temporal bone trauma occasionally present with cranial nerve palsies. However, such palsies are not evident until 2 to 3 days after the initial injury and are due to compression or contusion. They typically resolve with time and may benefit from treatment with steroids. Acute facial nerve palsies are rare as they are due to complete nerve transection. Such injuries do not respond to steroids and typically lead to significant, permanent deficits.

12. **Answer A.** The first-line management for delirium is to reassess the patient to ensure that there is no untreated medical cause and redirect with verbal reassurance and environmental improvements. Expediting patient transport up to an inpatient bed by involving hospital administration is a key component in a comprehensive strategy to manage this patient. Benzodiazepines and anticholinergics are strongly discouraged as part of the Beers list of potentially inappropriate medications for geriatric patients. Benzodiazepine clearance is significantly slowed in older adults and anticholinergic drugs cause significant side effects and can worsen delirium. Haloperidol used to be suggested as the first-line treatment for acute delirium, but increasing reports of side effects have rendered this a second-line (or even third-line) option.

13. **Answer D.** All pregnant patients with a viable fetus (defined as 24 weeks of gestation and beyond) should undergo continuous cardiotocographic monitoring for 4 hours before discharge after possible abdominal and pelvic trauma. This duration has not been validated, and some experts recommend shorter observation periods of only 2 hours. Even in the setting of "minor" trauma, approximately 4% of pregnant patients will develop placental abruption. In the setting of major trauma or in the presence of vaginal bleeding or any uterine contractions, patients should be admitted for 24 hours of cardiotocographic monitoring. Cardiotocographic monitoring is the most sensitive indicator of trauma-related fetal distress. Furthermore, as the fetus is more sensitive than the mother to decreases in maternal blood pressure and blood flow, fetal distress can be an early indicator of occult maternal shock. Most fetal losses in trauma occur due to placental abruption and cardiotocographic monitoring is the most sensitive marker of fetal distress due to abruption. In contrast, ultrasonography is notoriously insensitive, detecting only 50% of placental abruptions. Finally, in patients with a *nonviable* fetus, intermittent documentation of fetal heart tones, as well as ultrasonography to assess fetal viability are probably adequate.

14. **Answer E.** Although acute pharyngitis is a common reason for presentation to the emergency room, GAS is the cause of a minority of infections, ranging from 5% to 30% (estimated to be 5% to 10% in adults, as it is a less common cause of adult pharyngitis than pediatric pharyngitis). GAS is, however, the most common *bacterial* cause of the disease and, regardless of the etiology, it is the only common cause that requires treatment. As the pharyngitis is self-limited with or without treatment, the reason for treating GAS pharyngitis is to prevent the sequelae of the disease, primarily acute rheumatic fever. Acute rheumatic fever is a nonsuppurative complication of GAS pharyngitis. The other rare nonsuppurative complications include poststreptococcal glomerulonephritis (PSGN) and streptococcal toxic shock syndrome. Suppurative complications include peritonsillar cellulitis or abscess, otitis media, sinusitis, necrotizing fasciitis, and meningitis. The ability of antibiotic therapy to prevent the development of suppurative complications is not well defined, but the effect is thought to be small. However, antibiotics are thought to be more effective in reducing the rate of acute rheumatic fever, and they have been shown to decrease the length and severity of acute GAS pharyngitis. There is no definitive evidence that antibiotic therapy reduces the rate of PSGN. Acute rheumatic fever typically occurs 2 to 4 weeks after acute pharyngitis develops, and most commonly occurs in children 4 to 9 years old. The diagnosis of rheumatic fever is made in the presence of one or more of the five major Jones criteria in association with an antecedent GAS pharyngitis. The major Jones criteria include: pancarditis, migratory arthritis, CNS involvement (classically Sydenham chorea), erythema marginatum (diffuse rash sparing the face), and subcutaneous nodules.

15. **Answer B.** Initial radiographs of pediatric patients with elbow trauma may not clearly demonstrate a fracture. The posterior fat pad, which is closely applied to the posterior portion of the humerus, is normally invisible in the intact elbow. Blood in the elbow joint due to fracture will cause this fat pad to show up as a dark line just posterior to the supracondylar region of the humerus. The anterior fat pad may be present in the intact elbow as a dark line, but enlargement of this into a sail shape indicates likely injury. On anteroposterior view, the Baumann angle is formed by a line parallel to the capellar growth plate and a line parallel to the long axis of the humerus. A normal Baumann angle is 75 degrees, and bilaterally equal Baumann angles reduce the likelihood of unilateral fracture. On a lateral view of the normal elbow, the anterior humeral line should bisect the capitellum. With a supracondylar fracture, the anterior humeral line lies anterior to the midpoint of the capitellum.

16. **Answer C.** Family history of suicide is an independent risk factor for completed suicide. Other risk factors include depression, schizophrenia, substance abuse, prior attempts, presence of a firearm in the home, and feelings of hopelessness and long-term loneliness.

Young women have the lowest rate of completed suicide but have the highest rate of suicide attempts. Patients with antisocial personality disorder do not have higher rates of suicide completion unless there is comorbid substance abuse. Generalized anxiety disorders and simple phobias do not confer a higher risk of completed suicide in the absence of depression or substance abuse.

17. **Answer C.** Radial head fractures are common fractures in adults who have fallen on an outstretched hand. The force of the injury is directed axially through the radius, impacting the radial head against the capitellum of the humerus. In children, these injuries most frequently result in supracondylar fractures, but supracondylar fractures are rare in adults, in whom the radial head is the weakest link in the chain. The patient's x-ray reveals both an anterior and posterior fat pad sign indicative of a hemarthrosis as well as a subtle lucency at the radial head suggestive of an undisplaced fracture (Fig. 6-13). Even in the absence of the subtle fracture on x-ray, a radial head fracture should be suspected based on the patient's symptoms and the anterior and posterior fat pads on x-ray. A child with the same symptoms and x-ray most likely has a supracondylar fracture. Olecranon fractures usually result from a direct blow to the elbow, while a sprain of the ulnar collateral ligament typically results from a throwing injury. (Figure from Bucholz RW and Heckman JD. *Rockwood & Green's Fractures in Adults,* 5th ed. Philadelphia, PA: Lippincott, Williams & Wilkins, 2001.)

18. **Answer A.** Acute spinal cord injuries may benefit from high-dose corticosteroid therapy if given within 8 hours of injury. However, their use and efficacy is constantly debated, and neither administering nor withholding glucocorticoids can be considered the standard of care. If they are administered, a longer delay than 8 hours may actually result in worsened outcomes. Normal saline or lactated Ringer hydration should be given to all trauma patients. Naloxone may be given to patients with altered mental status as empiric therapy for opioid intoxication but is not generally used in patients with spinal cord injury. Vancomycin and other antibiotics are not routinely indicated in trauma patients, except in clinically evident cases of post-traumatic infection. Vasopressin may be used in patients with medical causes of shock who do not respond to crystalloid or colloid administration but is unlikely to be useful in patients with traumatic shock.

19. **Answer D.** Radiation exposure in coronary CT angiography (CCTA) has historically been substantial but has begun to significantly decline with newer generation, multidetector scanners, and new protocols. Patients with relative bradycardia can get high-quality images with minimal radiation exposure. In the ED, CCTA is most useful for low- and intermediate-risk patients to help with further risk stratification. Studies predict that patients with completely negative CCTA (no calcified or uncalcified coronary artery disease) studies will have no significant cardiac events for 2 full years. This greatly

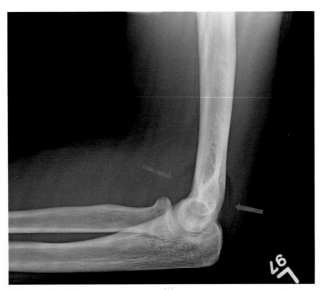
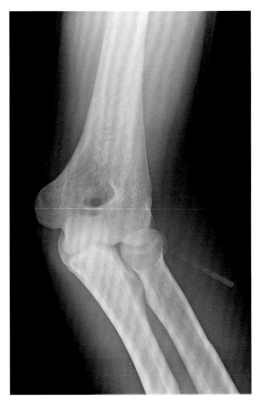

Figure 6-13

exceeds the performance of the HEART score, which measures much shorter term risk. The next generation scanners are also able to yield information about plaque composition which may help stratify plaques into high- and low-risk lesions.

20. **Answer A.** Tetanus is a serious, toxin-mediated disease with a mortality of up to 50%. *Clostridium tetani*, a ubiquitous, gram-positive anaerobic bacterium, is the causative organism, producing tetanospasmin toxin, which is responsible for the pathologic effects. Though clinical tetanus is rare in the United States, the underimmunized population is steadily increasing with immigration. Patients are inoculated with the bacteria during any break in the skin, such as simple wounds. Approximately one-third of the patients with clinically evident tetanus do not recall a preceding injury. Skeletal muscle spasm affecting the upper respiratory tract is the most common cause of death. Diffuse muscle rigidity, autonomic instability, hyperthermia, and rhabdomyolysis all accompany the pharyngeal and facial muscle spasm. Tetanus is a clinical diagnosis and cultures have no role in acute diagnosis or screening. Tetanus prophylaxis is initiated in childhood with a series of three vaccines, followed by boosters every 10 years for clean, uncontaminated wounds (or 5 years for wounds with significant contamination). Tetanus immunoglobulin is given to patients with dirty wounds who have never undergone primary vaccination. Treatment of clinically evident tetanus involves antibacterial therapy with penicillin and/or metronidazole, tetanus immunoglobulin, and aggressive supportive care with early intubation and tracheostomy placement.

21. **Answer B.** Postoperative ileus is a common, expected outcome after laparotomy. However, multiple electrolyte abnormalities may also cause or exacerbate the condition. Hypokalemia is the most common electrolyte abnormality responsible for ileus, though hypomagnesemia, hyponatremia, hypocalcemia, and uremia may also contribute.

22. **Answer A.** About two-thirds of patients with small bowel obstruction exhibit abdominal distention, making it the most common physical examination finding seen. Focal tenderness is uncommon, as are rebound or percussion tenderness—these are more indicative of peritonitis. High-pitched bowel sounds are certainly consistent with small bowel obstruction, but are not as commonly seen as distention.

23. **Answer A.** Given their decreased cardiopulmonary reserve, elderly patients more often suffer complications from rib fractures. However, in the absence of hypoxia or a clinically significant hemothorax, pneumothorax, or pulmonary contusion, even elderly patients with isolated rib fractures may be safely discharged home.

Pain control and incentive spirometry are important components of treatment to avoid atelectasis and possible pneumonia. Chest x-rays detect less than 50% of rib fractures. Dedicated rib series detect about 75% of fractures, while chest CT is considered the gold standard. Still, in most adult patients only a chest x-ray is needed after minor trauma since detecting injuries not seen on chest x-ray usually doesn't change treatment or outcome. In patients older than 65, however, rib fractures lead to higher rates of pulmonary complications such as atelectasis and pneumonia so understanding the exact extent of thoracic injury is more important. Older patients with ≥6 rib fractures have a 30% mortality rate and should be admitted. In fact, the mortality rate really begins to climb once elderly patients have suffered ≥3 fractures and most such patients should be admitted for observation to ensure they don't develop a pulmonary contusion and respiratory decompensation.

24. **Answer E.** This patient is presenting with profound weight loss due to anorexia nervosa. There are both psychiatric and medical indications for admission of patients with anorexia nervosa. The psychiatric indication for admission is primarily limited to those patients who have a high degree of suicidality, or active suicidality, or comorbid depression that may interfere with their ability to comply with treatment. Medical indications for admission are described by both the Society for Adolescent Medicine and the APA, and include body weight <75% of average body weight for age, height, and gender, bradycardia <50 or any significant arrhythmia, hypotension (<80/50), hypothermia (<96°F), severe orthostatic changes, severe electrolyte disturbances (e.g., severe hypophosphatemia, hypokalemia, or hypomagnesemia), or other medical complications of anorexia, including pancreatitis, heart failure, syncope, or seizures. Committing a patient to inpatient therapy may be needed if they refuse admission, but this patient arrived willingly and has given no indication that she intends to refuse therapy.

25. **Answer C.** Laboratory testing has a limited, but an important role in the evaluation of patients with abdominal trauma. The hematocrit is primarily important because it establishes a baseline value before resuscitation and redistribution. However, although the hematocrit is primarily useful for following serial levels in the setting of solid organ injury, it is also valuable in any patient who presents with a very low hematocrit in the setting of trauma because it most likely indicates that significant blood loss has already occurred. Liver enzymes are not helpful and are not used to distinguish between minor and major liver contusions or lacerations. Although often elevated in the setting of pancreatic injury, serum amylase and lipase are nonspecific and poorly sensitive. Therefore, normal levels do

not exclude pancreatic injury and high levels may be due to a host of other causes. Conflicting data exist regarding the utility of microscopic hematuria in pediatric blunt trauma patients. Low-risk patients have <5 RBCs/ HPF, while patients complaining of abdominal pain or patients who provide other reasons to be suspicious of injury in the setting of microscopic hematuria >5 RBCs/ HPF should receive a CT.

26. **Answer B.** Nonintentional blunt thoracic injury in children rarely causes multiple rib fractures, due to the compliance of the pediatric chest wall. For this reason, external injury is often absent, although pulmonary and cardiac injuries may be prominent. Multiple rib fractures are usually caused by child abuse, especially rib fractures that are observed radiographically to be in various stages of healing. Falls and sports injuries rarely cause rib fractures in children. Gunshot wounds are much more likely to cause thoracic organ damage than serious chest wall injuries.

27. **Answer D.** This patient has a posterior hip dislocation. Posterior hip dislocations account for 90% of all hip dislocations. The most common mechanism of injury is a "dashboard injury," in which a seated patient strikes the dashboard with a flexed knee, driving the femur posteriorly. Due to the force required to dislocate the well-protected hip joint, posterior hip dislocations are often associated with multisystem trauma. Patients will present with a shortened leg, with the hip internally rotated, adducted, and slightly flexed. Posterior hip dislocations must be reduced emergently due to the high risk of avascular necrosis of the femoral head. Radiographs should be obtained before reduction, unless a pulse deficit is present. (Figure courtesy of Robert Hendrickson, MD. In: Greenberg MI, Hendrickson RG, Silverberg M, et al., eds. *Greenberg's Text-Atlas of Emergency Medicine*. Philadelphia, PA: Lippincott Williams & Wilkins; 2004:515, with permission.)

28. **Answer E.** Recognizable lead points other than Peyer patches are found in only 2% to 8% of patients. All of the listed choices may serve as lead points in intussusception. However, most cases are thought to occur when an enlarged Peyer patch telescopes into adjoining bowel. The most common location is ileocolic.

29. **Answer D.** Age-related macular degeneration is the most common cause of blindness in the industrialized world. It occurs primarily because of retinal damage from unknown causes. Almost one-fourth of all Americans older than 90 are affected by macular degeneration.

30. **Answer E.** Neonatal seizures are often subtle, with less motor activity than seizures that occur in older children or adults. Seizures may involve sucking or chewing, lip smacking, random and unusual eye movements, rowing, swimming or leg pedaling movements, and unusual

sounds. They may be associated with apnea. This constellation of signs is formally referred to as "subtle" seizures as opposed to more traditional generalized tonic–clonic events. Absence seizures don't typically occur until age 4. Seizures can be due to hyponatremia in which case congenital adrenal hyperplasia (CAH) should be considered. Barbiturates have long been the first-line therapy for neonatal seizures although there is no evidence that one particular antiepileptic agent is better than another.

31. **Answer D.** Twenty-two percent to 39% of cases are caused by medications. Delirium that begins while patients are taking a drug usually ceases once the drug is discontinued. All of the other findings listed can cause delirium in elderly patients.

32. **Answer C.** Nausea and vomiting are common in pregnancy, with symptoms usually developing between 4 and 7 weeks' gestation and resolving by 16 weeks' gestation. All of the agents listed have been used in pregnant women suffering from nausea or vomiting in early pregnancy. However, only vitamin B_6 has been demonstrated to be beneficial among those agents listed. Although vitamin B_6 has been proven to be of use in reducing symptoms of nausea, its ability to reduce vomiting related to pregnancy is less clear. More recently, ginger supplementation has been shown to reduce both nausea and vomiting related to pregnancy and may be superior to vitamin B_6. The mutagenic effects of ginger are not known, but it is presumed to be safe.

33. **Answer A.** Anal fissures are the most commonly encountered anorectal problem in children and they are the most common cause of LGIB in this population, particularly in the first 2 years of life. Meckel diverticulum is the most common cause of substantial GI bleeding in this population.

34. **Answer E.** The patient likely has gonococcal conjunctivitis. The patient has signs and symptoms of pelvic inflammatory disease and urethritis and systemic antibiotic therapy is warranted. Treatment should include ceftriaxone, doxycycline or azithromycin, topical antibiotics, and saline irrigation. Admission is not absolute—however, the presence of nausea, vomiting, or fevers generally warrants in-hospital management.

35. **Answer E.** The patient likely has rhinitis or other nonbacterial upper respiratory infection. Sinusitis occurs with facial pain or tenderness and is only likely to be bacterial in the presence of fever >102°F, duration of 10 days or greater, or clinical worsening after initial improvement. Supportive care is indicated in the vast majority of cases of upper respiratory infection, as viral etiology is most likely. Nasal culture is not a useful test given low yield and absence of management change based on results. Sinus aspiration is overly invasive for

this patient who is not clinically toxic. Empiric oral steroids are not indicated in most viral syndromes. Antibiotics should be reserved in cases with strong suspicion of bacterial etiology as noted above.

36. **Answer E.** WPW syndrome is the most frequently occurring accessory pathway syndrome. Patients have an accessory conductive pathway (bundle of Kent) from the atria to the ventricles which pre-excites the ventricular myocytes before the AV node conducts the normal sinoatrial depolarization wave. As a result, patients with WPW have a shortened PR interval and a delayed QRS upstroke, called the δ *wave*. Patients with WPW syndrome can have re-entrant dysrhythmias, in which the accessory pathway can either conduct in a retrograde fashion producing an "orthodromic" pattern (in which the AV node conducts in the normal direction, which results in a narrow QRS complex) or an anterograde fashion forming an "antidromic" pattern (in which forward [or anterograde] conduction occurs through the accessory pathway first before cycling around to pass through the AV node backward, which produces a wide QRS complex since the initial conduction does not utilize the Purkinje system). A patient with WPW syndrome, tachycardia, and wide QRS complexes suggests the presence of an antidromic conduction pattern (where the accessory pathway conducts anterograde and the AV node conducts retrograde). Agents with relatively "pure" or isolated AV nodal activity such as adenosine or verapamil (which are the preferred agents in orthodromic re-entrant tachycardias in the setting of WPW) are contraindicated in this circumstance, as inhibition of the AV node will promote faster conduction through the anterograde accessory pathway, which may cause degeneration into an unstable rhythm such as ventricular tachycardia. The treatment of choice in stable antidromic or irregular tachycardias in WPW patients is procainamide, while amiodarone is considered a second-line agent. Unstable patients require cardioversion.

37. **Answer A.** β-hydroxybutyrate, which isn't detected by standard nitroprusside urine dipsticks, is the predominant ketone in diabetic ketoacidosis (DKA), especially in severe cases. That can yield false negative or weakly positive results and can cause confusion. Nitroprusside reacts with acetoacetate and to a lesser degree, with acetone. In DKA, the ratio of β-hydroxybutyrate:acetoacetate can be as high as 10:1.

38. **Answer E.** Sinus imaging has very little role in the ED except in the evaluation of patients with suspected complications of sinusitis (e.g., orbital cellulitis, cavernous sinus thrombosis). However, in the modern era it is clear that plain films have such a low sensitivity for sinus disease that they are virtually never requested. When plain films are used, they are best used for the diagnosis of maxillary sinusitis as their sensitivity drops when used to image other sinuses. CT scans are currently the most useful imaging modality in the evaluation of sinusitis. Although they are highly sensitive tests, they have a poor specificity (high false positive rate). Several studies have demonstrated that asymptomatic patients with uncomplicated viral URIs have abnormalities of one or both maxillary sinuses on CT scan. The same is true for asymptomatic patients with seasonal allergies. Therefore, CT scans should never stand alone in the diagnosis of sinusitis. A diagnosis of sinusitis should be supported with clinical findings of facial or dental pain, headache, and purulent nasal discharge, often preceded by a viral URI.

39. **Answer E.** The patient has Mobitz type II second-degree AV block, which is an indication for admission to a telemetry unit and possible pacemaker placement. The PR interval is prolonged and does not show any observable pattern of increasing prolongation as in Mobitz type I second-degree AV block (Wenckebach phenomenon). Dropped QRS complexes do not occur in any predictable pattern like they do in Mobitz type I. Cardioversion and amiodarone are not indicated in stable bradydysrhythmias, and defibrillation of an awake patient is never indicated. (Figure from Fowler NO. *Clinical Electrocardiographic Diagnosis: A Problem-Based Approach.* Philadelphia, PA: Lippincott Williams & Wilkins; 2000, with permission.)

40. **Answer A.** Intrapartum or antepartum asphyxia resulting in either global or focal brain ischemia is the most common cause of seizures in the term neonate. Intracranial hemorrhage accounts for approximately 15% of cases (most commonly intraventricular or intraparenchymal). Sepsis, inborn errors of metabolism, metabolic abnormalities (primarily hypoglycemia, hypocalcemia, and hypomagnesemia), and toxins account for an additional 10%. Neonatal seizures are rarely idiopathic, so an extensive diagnostic workup must be performed.

41. **Answer C.** Locking or clicking of the knee is often due to a meniscal injury, usually medial. Patients may not recall a specific traumatic event and chronic, repeated trauma may predispose to the injury. The medial meniscus is less mobile and therefore more predisposed to injury than the lateral. Knee locking from medial meniscal tears may be relieved by applying valgus stress and gentle extension.

42. **Answer B.** Haloperidol is a high-potency antipsychotic agent whose primary therapeutic action is to block dopamine-2 receptors in the basal ganglia to cause rapid sedation and control of psychotic behavior. Haloperidol is commonly given with benzodiazepines for this use. Although haloperidol is often mistakenly considered to be part of the phenothiazine class of drugs (which lower

the seizure threshold), it is actually part of the butyro-phenone category, which does not affect the seizure threshold. Antipsychotics are α-1 antagonists (causing orthostatic hypotension) and antihistaminergic (causing sedation). Agranulocytosis is a side effect peculiar to clozapine, a newer generation antipsychotic.

43. **Answer C.** Ninety percent of hip dislocations are posterior hip dislocations, typically caused by high-velocity MVCs in which a patient's knee strikes the dashboard, resulting in posterior directed forces through the hip. Approximately 10% of cases are complicated by a sciatic nerve palsy, which travels posterior to the hip joint. The peroneal division of the nerve is more commonly affected than the tibial branch, though both are commonly affected. This results in weakness of ankle dorsiflexion and foot eversion, as well as decreased sensation along the entire posterior lower leg (below the knee). The skin of the posterior upper leg is innervated by the posterior femoral cutaneous nerve, which is derived from the lumbosacral plexus. With timely reduction, patients with sciatic nerve palsies typically recover without any residual deficits. The femoral nerve innervates most of the remainder of the leg via its many branches, including cutaneous innervations to the anterior thigh and lower leg, as well as the posteromedial lower leg via the saphenous nerve.

44. **Answer D.** Hyperemesis gravidarum (HG) is a severe variant of vomiting related to pregnancy. There are no strict clinical criteria to make the diagnosis, but persistent vomiting causing ketonuria as well as >5% weight loss by weight loss are commonly used. It peaks at 8 to 12 weeks. It occurs in about 1% of all pregnancies. Risk factors include non-white race, age less than 30, and first pregnancy. Pathophysiology is unknown but elevated human chorionic gonadotropin (HCG) levels have been implicated. Treatment for HG involves IV hydration, glucose administration (to reduce ketosis created by fatty acid oxidation), nausea control, and electrolyte and vitamin supplementation. HG is more serious than simple nausea and vomiting of pregnancy, because weight loss and dehydration can have fetal effects. Ketosis has also been shown in animal data to cause birth defects—however, this is unproven in humans. Ketones in the urine have served as a marker for efficacy of therapy. Bilious vomiting is not characteristic of either HG or nausea and vomiting of pregnancy and another cause should be aggressively sought. Hypokalemia and metabolic alkalosis can occur with any vomiting illness (due to loss of gastric acid and intracellular exchange of potassium) and does not reliably distinguish between the two diagnoses in question.

45. **Answer B.** Hemorrhoids are a common cause of lower GI bleeding in adolescents and adults. Among other risk factors, hemorrhoids are associated with both diarrhea and constipation though the exact pathophysiology is not clear. Anal fissures are also a frequent cause of lower GI bleeding but are most often accompanied by pain. The pain associated with anal fissures may be less prominent in patients with chronic anal fissures. A 99m technetium pertechnetate infusion, also called a "Meckel scan" is a test to determine if a patient has a Meckel diverticulum. Meckel diverticula are uncommon, present in roughly 2% of the population. Of those who have a diverticulum, only 2% develop complications. GI bleeding can occur because of the acid produced by ectopic gastric tissue within the diverticulum. Given that this patient has formed stools coated with blood, a Meckel diverticulum is unlikely. Diverticulosis and polyps are also uncommon in pediatric patients.

46. **Answer C.** Hypertrophic cardiomyopathy is the most common cause of atraumatic sudden death in young athletes. Choices A, B, and D are far less common in this age-group. Choice E can occur in tall, thin athletes, and although death may result from tension physiology, it is almost never sudden or without preceding symptoms.

47. **Answer C.** The patient has severe lower lip swelling, likely from angiotensin-converting enzyme (ACE) inhibitor-induced angioedema given the history of new antihypertensive medication. Pathophysiology involves buildup of bradykinin due to inhibition of ACE. Acute treatment with epinephrine, steroids, and antihistamines is generally ineffective. Fresh frozen plasma contains kininase II, which can cleave bradykinin and reduce the angioedema. Verapamil, metoprolol, and aldosterone have no role in the management of angioedema. Danazol is used for angioedema due to hereditary C1 esterase inhibitor deficiency, but its role is generally limited to prophylaxis rather than acute treatment. (Figure courtesy of Lawrence, B. Stack, MD. In: Plantz SH, Martin HM, eds. *Step-Up to Emergency Medicine.* Philadelphia, PA: Wolters Kluwer, 2015, with permission.)

48. **Answer B.** Infants with c-spine injuries tend to be injured at C1-4 while older children, teenagers and adults tend to have lower c-spine injuries. This occurs because the c-spine fulcrum lies at C2-3 at birth and moves inferiorly as the child grows, reaching C5-6 by age 8. While the NEXUS study did not include many young children with c-spine injuries in their study, there is a PECARN c-spine rule which is similar as well as guidelines from the American Association for the Surgery of Trauma (AAST) that allow clinical c-spine clearance without imaging. Furthermore, as the incidence of significant c-spine trauma is very low in children, plain films are very useful to evaluate the c-spine when patients present after a low-energy mechanism of injury

with a low clinical suspicion for serious injury on examination. CT is best used when the suspicion for injury is at least moderate and modern CT scanners detect all serious injuries. MRI is reserved for patients with neurologic findings and should not be used routinely in patients with persistent neck pain after a negative c-spine CT.

49. **Answer C.** Aneurysms >5 cm in size are at greatest risk of rupture, although smaller aneurysms may also rupture. Debate exists as to the optimal time of elective repair of asymptomatic aneurysms, but patients presenting to the ED with symptomatic aneurysms should always be aggressively evaluated.

50. **Answer D.** Minimizing the time to operation for geriatric patients significantly improves their postoperative outcomes and is the basis for geriatric fracture programs throughout the country. Screening questions targeted to suicidality, depression, HIV, and others in the ED have not been shown to improve the outcome of patients with such obvious serious pathology and can delay access to care. Preoperative physical therapy or medication reconciliation will likely have little effect on outcomes compared to early surgical management for these patients. Postoperative primary care follow-up is certainly necessary but will not likely be more effective than postoperative orthopedic or physical therapy follow-up.

51. **Answer D.** Kidney stones most commonly occur in middle-aged patients, usually men. Recurrence occurs in approximately half the number of patients. Risk factors include age, male gender, family history, and conditions which increase serum and urinary calcium levels. Kidney stones are divided into four main categories—calcium, magnesium-ammonium-phosphate, uric acid, and cystine. Calcium stones represent approximately two-third of all stones and occur more often in patients with common precipitants of hypercalcemia, including hyperparathyroidism, milk–alkali syndrome, laxative abuse, and sarcoidosis. Inflammatory bowel disease (IBD) also causes the formation of calcium oxalate stones, due to hyperoxaluria. Magnesium-ammonium-phosphate (struvite) stones account for one-fifth of all calculi and occur in patients with urinary tract infections due to *Proteus, Klebsiella,* and *Pseudomonas.* Uric acid stones occur in patients with hyperuricemia, often due to gout. They are usually radiolucent and missed on plain radiographs. Cystine stones are the least common and are due to hypercystinuria, an inborn error of metabolism usually diagnosed at birth.

52. **Answer D.** The patient has a prominent lateral clavicular border with the deltoid and humeral margin displaced inferiorly. The most likely cause for this is an acromioclavicular separation due to a torn acromioclavicular ligament. Radiographs will demonstrate this injury more definitively. Acute management involves sling immobilization and orthopedic follow-up. If there were a shoulder dislocation, it would be impossible for the patient to touch his opposite shoulder with the affected hand. A sternoclavicular dislocation is not apparent due to the lack of abnormalities noted on the medial sternal border. (Figure from Berg D, Worzala K. *Atlas of Adult Physical Diagnosis.* Philadelphia, PA: Lippincott Williams & Wilkins, 2006, with permission.)

53. **Answer D.** There are no fractures that are pathognomonic for abuse. However, rib fractures, particularly posterior rib fractures, are more than twice as likely to be due to abuse then other fractures. Femur and skull fractures are also common in the setting of abuse. Concerning skull fracture patterns include multiple fractures, bilateral fractures, and fractures that cross suture lines. Many physically abused patients will have suffered more than one fracture. It is important to remember that while rib fractures are commonly associated with abuse, chest x-rays are a poor screening modality for such fractures. Dedicated rib series should be obtained for patients in whom there is suspicion for a rib fracture due to abuse.

54. **Answer C.** Schizophrenia is a chronic, progressive thought disorder present in 1% of the population. It is characterized by the presence of both positive symptoms (choices A, B, D, and E) and negative symptoms—flat affect, lack of speech, and inability to perform goal-directed activities. Although the positive symptoms are often managed successfully by pharmacotherapy, the negative symptoms are often refractory.

55. **Answer E.** Toxic alcohol ingestions often present with delayed morbidity and mortality, especially when ethanol is coingested. Ethylene glycol is the main toxic alcohol present in antifreeze, and its half-life without coingestants is up to 9 hours. In the presence of ethanol, the half-life roughly doubles. Therefore, patients who have ingested both ethanol and ethylene glycol may be asymptomatic on presentation (other than inebriation). Diagnosis involves cardiac monitoring, basic chemistry labs, ethanol level, blood gas, EKG, urinalysis, and creatine phosphokinase (CPK). Fomepizole, a pharmacologic alcohol dehydrogenase inhibitor, is administered if there is suspicion of ethylene glycol overdose, especially if the ethanol level is negative, which indicates that alcohol dehydrogenase is free to convert ethylene glycol to its toxic metabolites. Fomepizole does not detoxify the parent compound—it simply buys time for the definitive removal of the toxic alcohol by dialysis. Choices A and B are inappropriate because they fail to consider the delayed toxicity of coingested toxic alcohol and ethanol. Regarding choices C and D, only approximately half the number of patients with ethylene glycol poisoning develop urine crystals or urinary fluorescence on presentation.

56. **Answer A.** *Campylobacter* spp. is found in the stools of 5% to 14% of patients presenting with a chief complaint of diarrhea. The exact incidence in the United States is not known due to under-reporting and sporadic testing.

57. **Answer E.** The most common dysrhythmia in hypothyroid cardiac disease is sinus bradycardia. Cardiomegaly and depressed cardiac contractility are other manifestations.

58. **Answer D.** The SIRS was devised to be able to formally describe basic vital sign and laboratory abnormalities associated with severe inflammation, such as infection, trauma, burns, and severe medical illness. SIRS is said to be present when two out of the following four criteria are present:
   - Temp >38°C or <36°C.
   - WBC >12 K or <4 K or >10% bands.
   - RR >20 or Pa_{CO_2} <32.
   - HR >90.
   - Sepsis is the presence of SIRS with a suspected or proven infectious cause. *Septic shock* is defined as sepsis plus inadequate tissue perfusion, which may be manifested as hypotension or end-organ dysfunction. Note that hypotension is *not* a criterion for SIRS or sepsis, but is present in most cases of septic shock.

59. **Answer E.** Patients with disseminated VZV most often present with widely distributed vesicles outside the initially involved dermatome. Visceral involvement can occur, and includes pneumonitis, hepatitis, and meningoencephalitis. Though bacterial superinfection of skin lesions occurs, most deaths caused by disseminated VZV are due to VZV pneumonitis. In VZV pneumonitis, patients develop respiratory failure which is often refractory to treatment, even when it is started early. There is no firm evidence that corticosteroids are beneficial in the treatment of VZV (either dermatomal or disseminated), or in the prevention of postherpetic neuralgia. However, some experts still recommend their use, especially in patients with pain syndromes refractory to other treatments. While the benefit of acyclovir has not been established among immunocompetent patients presenting after 72 hours of symptoms, it should be used in *any* immunocompromised patient, as well as in patients in whom new lesions are actively appearing. There is no evidence of significant resistance. Ultimately, disseminated VZV is rarely fatal, even among patients with disseminated disease.

60. **Answer B.** Patients with transverse myelitis usually have one or two discrete spinal levels where inflammation occurs. If the spinal level is in the cervical region, patients will exhibit equal upper and lower extremity weakness. If the spinal level is in the thoracic region, patients will exhibit no upper extremity weakness at all. By contrast, the inflammation in acute inflammatory demyelinating polyneuropathy (AIDP) causes weakness that is more marked in the lower extremities than the upper extremities in virtually all cases. Albuminocytologic dissociation, referring to elevated CSF protein in the absence of CSF pleocytosis, is seen more commonly in AIDP than tranverse myelitis, which usually exhibits a mild–moderate, CSF lymphocytosis. Spinal MRI is usually abnormal in patients with transverse myelitis as a discrete inflamed spinal level is the cardinal pathophysiology. Spinal MRI is normal in patients with AIDP. Hemodynamic instability and antecedent *Campylobacter* infection are seen more often in AIDP; bowel and bladder malfunction is seen more often in transverse myelitis.

61. **Answer D.** Elderly patients, diabetic patients, and women with acute MIs may have atypical symptoms without the classic history of left-sided chest pain. Dyspnea, nausea, and diaphoresis may be anginal equivalents in many patients. Additionally, patients may deny "pain"—rather, they may describe their symptoms as "pressure" or "discomfort."

62. **Answer E.** Compartment syndrome refers to ischemia that occurs in the extremities when pressure in the soft tissues exceeds that of the microcirculation. Most experts use a definition based on the difference between the diastolic pressure and the compartment pressure. When the diastolic pressure minus the compartment pressure (called the acute compartment syndrome [ACS] delta pressure) is <30, a fasciotomy should be considered. This patient's ACS delta pressure is 25 (55 − 30 = 25). Normal compartment pressure is zero, and pressures >30 mm Hg are usually enough to predispose to compartment syndrome. Long bone fractures are the usual reason for compartment syndrome, causing extravasated blood and soft tissue edema to accumulate. The tibia is the most commonly affected bone. The most common symptoms are pain and paresthesias. Diminished pulses generally occur only in extremely advanced cases, as pressure in compartment syndrome is usually well below arterial pressure. For this reason, ankle–brachial indices are usually normal in compartment syndrome unless there is simultaneous arterial insufficiency. Patients with compartment syndrome should not be discharged. Imaging may help delineate the cause of the compartment syndrome, but diagnosis is still clinical. Diagnosis is made by directly measuring compartment syndromes with a Stryker needle device. Treatment is with urgent fasciotomy.

63. **Answer A.** *L. pneumophila* is an important cause of severe community-acquired pneumonia (CAP). In patients with more severe symptoms due to CAP, the percentage of *Legionella* spp. isolates increases. Epidemiologic studies have exposed links of legionellosis to exposure to contaminated water sources, such as air-conditioning

units and cooling towers. Furthermore, older patients with a history of alcoholism, tobacco use, and COPD as well as patients on immunosuppressive therapy appear to be at higher risk. Although the role of *Legionella* spp. is still being defined in the setting of more benign illness, legionellosis is classically described as a severe infection, associated with high fevers, a dry cough which may turn productive late in the course, pleuritic chest pain, and prominent GI symptoms including abdominal cramps and diarrhea. However, several studies have demonstrated that the clinical and radiographic features of the disease are nonspecific. Therefore, to make the diagnosis, laboratory testing is required. Urinary antigen testing is the test of choice as it is both highly sensitive (>90%) and specific (>99%) and is also quite rapid. Although antibiotic therapy should be started empirically before such results are obtained, urine testing can be initiated in the ED to guide the patient's further therapy and to provide useful information about prognosis.

64. **Answer B.** Chicken pox is an acute illness caused by varicella zoster virus (VZV) causing fever, myalgias, and a maculopapular rash progressing to vesicles which then rupture and form dry crusted lesions. Children are the most common group affected, and serious disease can occur in adults. Immunocompetent children are treated symptomatically with acetaminophen for fever. Aspirin should be avoided in children with viral illnesses, as this may predispose to Reye syndrome. Acyclovir is used in adults, immune-compromised patients, and when there are signs of encephalitis or pneumonitis. VZV vaccine is indicated for prevention and has no role in acute management of evident disease. VZV immune globulin is only indicated in immune-compromised patients in conjunction with acyclovir.

65. **Answer A.** Patients with peritoneal dialysis (PD) associated peritonitis rarely develop bacteremia which forms the basis for intraperitoneal (as opposed to intravenous) antibiotic therapy, which can frequently be performed as an outpatient presuming the patient is otherwise stable and has adequate pain control. The infection is almost always limited to the peritoneal cavity and a few cellular layers of the peritoneum. Gram-positive infections are most common, and due to the increasing prevalence of methicillin resistance among *Staphylococcus* isolates, vancomycin is typically recommended. However, 15% of infections are due to gram-negative organisms, so a third- or fourth-generation cephalosporin, an aminoglycoside or a carbapenem, is also needed. While the third- and fourth-generation cephalosporins also have significant activity against gram-positive organisms, they are inadequate for methicillin-resistant organisms, so they are not recommended for monotherapy. Catheter removal or catheter exchange is not typically needed unless the peritonitis proves to be refractory. Due to the ease of drug delivery

and, more importantly, the higher intraperitoneal drug concentrations achieved with intraperitoneal dosing, it is preferred over intravenous dosing. However, intraperitoneal drug delivery results in significant systemic absorption such that blood levels of vancomycin and gentamicin require monitoring when their use is prolonged. Fortunately, fungal peritonitis is rare, occurring in less than 2% of patients. When present, it is difficult to treat and often requires catheter removal.

66. **Answer A.** Patients in ventricular fibrillation require electrical defibrillation for optimal management. In certain cases, a cycle of chest compressions before defibrillation may be reasonable, but the emergency physician should err on the side of defibrillation first. Pericardiocentesis may be pursued in cases of pulseless electrical activity—with the advent of ultrasound, a rapid pericardial view can exclude the need for blind pericardiocentesis. No medication, including epinephrine or amiodarone, improves survival to hospital discharge in out-of-hospital cardiac arrest. Invasive mechanical ventilation is not absolutely indicated in cardiac arrest and can be delayed in favor of early defibrillation and high-quality chest compressions.

67. **Answer D.** Giant cell arteritis (GCA, formerly called temporal arteritis) is a vasculitis of large- and medium-sized vessels that occurs almost exclusively in adults older than 50. That fact alone rules out three of the patients in this question. Though the disease is systemic, it most commonly produces symptoms when it involves the cranial branches of arteries originating from the aortic arch. Temporal arteritis, which may lead to vision loss, is one of the most classic and dangerous manifestations. Symptoms that increase the likelihood of GCA include new headaches, jaw claudication (jaw pain after chewing), new visual changes, an elevated erythrocyte sedimentation rate (the ESR increases with age, but the increase is actually quite modest), unexplained fever, and symptoms of polymyalgia rheumatica. Though the 20-year-old female has temporal headache and an elevated ESR, an elevated ESR is nonspecific with a broad differential and the patient's age makes GCA very unlikely. The 74-year-old female has classic jaw claudication and fits the epidemiologic profile. The 55-year-old female likely has microvascular ischemia affecting cranial nerve III, resulting in relative weakness of the pupillary constrictors. This is common in diabetics and most often resolves without treatment over several months.

68. **Answer C.** This patient has an injury to zone II of the neck defined as the region of the neck superior to the cricoid cartilage and inferior to the angle of the mandible. Trauma to zone II is most common but also most amenable to repair due to relatively uncomplicated surgical exposure and vascular control. Traditionally, all patients

with violation of the platysma have been taken to OR for exploration. In the modern era of rapidly improving radiologic testing, operative repair may increasingly be deferred in favor of diagnostic testing such as helical CT angiography (e.g., to evaluate vascular injury indicated by a bruit or thrill), laryngoscopy, or esophagoscopy (e.g., to evaluate subcutaneous emphysema).

69. **Answer C.** Inflammation of the iris caused by trauma causes constant pain and photophobia, especially consensual photophobia (light exposure to the unaffected eye causes pain in the affected eye due to consensual constriction). Long-acting cycloplegics and steroids are the mainstay of treatment. The pupil is reactive and constricted, and ciliary flush (conjunctival injection in a circular rim around the limbus) is prominent. Resolution should occur within 1 week.

70. **Answer E.** Unlike the adult, the narrowest portion of the pediatric airway is the cricoid cartilage, necessitating the use of uncuffed tubes in children younger than 8 years. Other important considerations for the pediatric airway are the proportionally larger tongue, floppier epiglottis, more anterior airway position, and shorter tracheal length. These anatomic differences require slightly different techniques from those used with adult airway management, including an adjunctive oral airway, frequent use of a straight blade, and more anteriorly directed laryngoscopic technique. Most children older than 12 years have airway characteristics similar to adults.

71. **Answer D.** Concussion is defined as a clinical syndrome following mild traumatic brain injury with or without loss of consciousness. The symptoms are most commonly confusion, amnesia surrounding the traumatic event, headaches, and nausea. Other neurologic signs such as slurred speech, attention deficits, incoordination, mild personality changes, and disorientation may occur in conjunction with amnesia and confusion. Acute neuroimaging is usually normal as concussion is characterized by functional, rather than structural findings. MRI may detect subtle signs of cerebral contusion or axonal injury a few days after the injury in a minority of cases. Generally accepted guidelines indicate that athletes who have had a concussion should not return to sports until approximately 1 week after symptoms have resolved. Simple orientation tests are inadequate to detect concussion. The Standardized Assessment of Concussion (SAC) is a point-based tool meant to be used on the field of play. It assesses short-term memory, concentration, delayed recall, neurologic testing, and exertional tests such as sprints and sit-ups in addition to orientation. Anosmia, the absence of the sense of smell, may occur in concussions and may be permanent, also causing alterations in taste.

72. **Answer C.** Following the principle of trauma management that the most immediate life threats should be addressed earliest, the pericardial view is the ideal first view during the FAST scan. This will identify cardiac tamponade. The other views can be done after the pericardial view in the following order: right flank, left flank, suprapubic, and thoracic.

73. **Answer B.** This patient is presenting with methanol intoxication as windshield wiper fluid often contains methanol. Methanol toxicity results in the formation of formic acid due to the effects of alcohol dehydrogenase. Formic acid accumulates in the brain and causes blindness and death. Ethanol and fomepizole are temporizing measures to inhibit alcohol dehydrogenase from catalyzing the conversion of toxic alcohols, such as methanol, into their toxic metabolites. Folate is a cofactor for the conversion of methanol's toxic metabolite, formic acid, to carbon dioxide and water. Once formic acid is produced, significant toxicity is probably inevitable, but the addition of folate to the standard treatment of methanol overdose (bicarbonate, alcohol dehydrogenase inhibitors, and dialysis) may attenuate further injury.

74. **Answer B.** The patient presents with a focal neurologic deficit in the setting of pre-existing residual stroke symptoms. The differential diagnosis includes not only stroke but also any process that can disrupt the metabolic supply–demand balance for nutrients or oxygen, including hypoglycemia or infection. More than three-quarters of all strokes are ischemic and can be treated within 3 hours (4.5 hours in selected cases) with IV TPA. However, differentiating ischemic stroke from hemorrhagic stroke is difficult without neuroimaging. The most important initial test, therefore, is noncontrast CT of the brain. However, among the answer choices, the only choice that can be easily performed and would change immediate management in this clinical setting is checking the blood glucose level. While obtaining an EKG is important, it is unlikely to reveal findings that will change immediate management. Oral aspirin and IV TPA should never be given before hemorrhagic stroke is excluded. Arterial blood gas is rarely required in the evaluation of focal neurologic deficit.

75. **Answer B.** Patients with hepatitis A never develop chronic disease. Approximately 100% of patients recover from acute illness within 6 months, although fulminant hepatitis leading to death rarely occurs. The mortality rate of hepatitis E infection during pregnancy depends on the trimester during which a woman is infected. The maternal mortality rate is only 1.5% for infections in the first trimester, 8.5% for those in the second trimester, and 21% for those in the third trimester. Roughly 5% of children infected with hepatitis A are symptomatic at presentation versus 70% to 80% of adults.

In endemic areas, such as Southeast Asia, most of the population is infected as children, and most of the community is immune by age 10. Hepatitis A is the most common cause of viral hepatitis worldwide. Hepatitis A is transmitted through the fecal–oral route. Although percutaneous transmission may occur (e.g., through a needlestick injury), it is very rare because the concentration of the virus in the blood is quite low and the duration of viremia is brief.

76. **Answer A.** The patient has a Colles fracture, which puts him at risk for median nerve injury. Injury to this nerve can result from either the fracture itself or during therapeutic reduction. Falling on an outstretched hand is the most common mechanism for Colles fracture. A volarly displaced distal radius fracture is referred to as reverse Colles or Smith fracture, which usually results from trauma to the dorsum of the hand. Smith fracture also involves the median nerve more often than other peripheral nerves of the upper extremity. An intra-articular fracture of the distal radius with displacement of the carpal bones is referred to as a Barton fracture.

77. **Answer B.** Antiplatelet therapy with aspirin is still the most effective and cheapest medical therapy for treatment of acute MI. No other single pharmacologic agent can boast of as large a mortality reduction, including metoprolol and abciximab. Nitroglycerin and morphine do not reduce mortality in acute MI, but they are effective in managing symptoms of angina.

78. **Answer C.** A positive Nikolsky sign occurs when pressure applied to the margin of a blistered or ulcerated lesion expands the lesion into the adjacent apparently normal skin. This is also known as *marginal modification*. In addition, direct pressure applied to normal-appearing skin that is distant from any blistered lesions may also result in erosion or ulceration. This is known as *direct* modification. These findings occur because of intraepidermal acantholysis (separation of keratinocytes from their neighbors within the epidermis). Nikolsky sign is most commonly associated with pemphigus vulgaris but may also be found in staphylococcus scalded skin syndrome and toxic epidermal necrolysis. There are also multiple reports of other disease associations, but the finding (particularly of direct modification) is very specific for pemphigus vulgaris.

79. **Answer C.** The patient has superficial thrombophlebitis, which can be managed supportively with NSAIDs, rest, and heat. Without symptoms or signs of or risk factors for a pulmonary embolism, evaluation for pulmonary embolism with a CT is not warranted. Repeat ultrasound is usually undertaken several days to a week after the initial evaluation of DVT. Warfarin therapy is not usually initiated alone due to its early prothrombotic effect. Furthermore, anticoagulation is only considered for large superficial thromboses (>5 cm) and thromboses above the knee, as these are more likely to progress to deep venous thromboses. Intravenous tissue plasminogen activator is only indicated for large pulmonary emboli with hemodynamic effect.

80. **Answer C.** Raccoons are the most common wild animals with rabies. HRIG should be administered as close to the bite site as possible. When this is not suitable (such as in the digits), give as much HRIG as possible at the bite site and the remainder at any skeletal muscle distant from the site. Choices A, B, and D are all reasonable choices. The distal extremities, especially the penis, should not be used as HRIG sites. Rabies vaccine should be administered at a site distant from both the bite and HRIG. Along with passive and active immunization, local wound care is extremely important, as soap and povidone–iodine cleansing solutions are 100% virucidal when used early enough.

81. **Answer C.** The half-life of carboxyhemoglobin is 6 hours on room air, 90 minutes on 100% nonrebreather, and 30 minutes on hyperbaric oxygen.

82. **Answer D.** Diverticulitis occurs in 10% to 30% of patients with diverticulosis. Severe bleeding occurs in only 3% to 5% of patients with diverticula. Most bleeding is minor and resolves spontaneously without intervention.

83. **Answer C.** Sympathomimetic and anticholinergic crises may be very difficult to distinguish on clinical grounds. Both toxidromes exhibit tachycardia, delirium, mydriasis, and hyperthermia. The presence of diaphoresis indicates that a sympathomimetic cause is far more likely, as patients with anticholinergic crises have inhibition of their sweat glands. However, the absence of diaphoresis is not necessarily diagnostic of an anticholinergic syndrome, as patients with sympathomimetic crises may have profound dehydration. Seizures may occur in either toxidrome, although it is probably more common in sympathomimetic states.

84. **Answer B.** The majority of aural foreign bodies can be easily removed in the ED without otolaryngology referral. There are several effective means of foreign body removal, including irrigation, or mechanical removal with a curette, right-angled loop, forceps, suction catheters, or cyanoacrylate (Dermabond) affixed to the blunt end of a cotton swab. One guiding principle is that smaller instruments have a greater potential for damage, given their often sharp tips. Thus, the largest, most blunt instrument that will still fit into the ear canal should be used. Furthermore, sedation or referral should be considered in uncooperative patients to avoid mechanical

trauma to the ear. Irrigation should never be used in cases of vegetable matter or button battery impaction since the former will swell and increase obstruction, and the latter may leak. Insects should first be killed, preferably with mineral oil, though alcohol or 1% lidocaine can also be used. Living insects tend to skip and flutter in the ear canal which is a distressing sensation for patients that may lead to less cooperation. The external auditory meatus is the smallest portion of the ear canal.

85. **Answer B.** The patient has evidence of poison ivy, or *Toxicodendron* dermatitis. The pathogenesis is due to an allergic contact dermatitis to urushiol, a substance found in poison ivy, sumac, and oak. Symptoms can develop in as little as a few hours, but can also be delayed for several days after exposure. While supportive care alone is reasonable, an oral prednisone course of 2 to 3 weeks can improve symptoms significantly. Methotrexate is too strong an immune-suppressant for management of poison ivy. Antibiotics are not indicated except in cases of secondary cellulitis. (Figure courtesy of Darren Fiore, MD. In: Nicol N, ed. *Dermatology Nursing Essentials.* 3rd ed. Philadelphia, PA: Wolters Kluwer; 2016.)

86. **Answer B.** Femoral neck fractures and intertrochanteric fractures account for 90% of all hip fractures. They both most commonly occur in osteoporotic elderly patients after a low-energy fall. In contrast, young patients develop these fractures in the setting of high-energy trauma such as in high-speed motor vehicle accidents. Therefore, many of those patients have evidence of multisystem trauma. The intertrochanteric femur has a better blood supply than the femoral neck, resulting in a much smaller incidence of AVN. As many as 40% of patients with femoral neck fractures may develop AVN. The use of a femoral nerve block in the setting of a femur fracture is an attractive means of delivering adequate pain control to patients. Although it has not been widely used in the United States, several recent papers demonstrate that it is an effective, safe means of pain control in both pediatric and adult patients. Isolated fractures of the lesser trochanter almost always occur in young adults. The fracture represents an apophyseal avulsion due to a forceful contraction of the iliopsoas muscle. A similar injury can occur at the greater trochanter. Patients with isolated lesser trochanter fractures are normally able to ambulate, although they will complain of pain. Physical examination will demonstrate a patient's inability to lift the affected leg from the floor while in a seated position (iliopsoas insufficiency). Patients will also have pain when they are asked to flex their hip against resistance. PE is most common in the postoperative patient. Acute respiratory distress is most likely because of fat embolism, which complicates 2% to 23% of patients with isolated femoral shaft fractures. Acute respiratory distress, associated

with altered mental status, tachycardia, and fever are hallmarks of the illness. Although diffusely scattered petechiae are nearly pathognomonic for the syndrome, they do not normally occur until late in the course of the illness and only occur in 50% of patients.

87. **Answer B.** While historically, syphilitic aortic aneurysms and tuberculosis accounted for the majority of cases of SVCS, the majority of cases today are due to DVT of the SVC in patients with an indwelling catheter such as a PICC line or Port-a-Cath. Many of these patients have such devices because of cancer treatment, but their cancers are not the primary cause of SVC obstruction. Such patients are managed with anticoagulation and may need to have the device removed. Among patients without indwelling catheters, lung cancer (primarily nonsmall cell) is the most common cause while lymphoma is the next most common. The symptoms include head and facial edema, as well as edema of the neck and arms. The edema is often associated with plethora, cyanosis, and visibly distended subcutaneous vessels. The course is typically indolent, and patients rarely present with acute airway compromise. Patients with SVCS due to a malignancy are typically managed with palliative chemotherapy and radiation since the long-term prognosis is poor.

88. **Answer E.** Wheezes are continuous, high-pitched, musical sounds that can be heard on inspiration or expiration. They are caused by high-velocity airflow through a narrowed airway (in much the same way that a murmur is caused by high-velocity blood flow through a narrowed vessel or valve). Any pulmonary disease characterized by obstruction can result in audible wheezes on physical examination. A good, short mnemonic for obstructive airway disease is **LACE**:

Local airway obstruction

Asthma

Chronic bronchitis

Emphysema

Unilateral or localized wheezes should prompt a consideration of local airway obstruction, caused by an aspirated foreign body, endobronchial cancer, lymphadenopathy, or infection. Diffuse bilateral wheezes are generally caused by asthma or COPD. Patients with CHF exacerbations may also have diffuse wheezes caused by relative airway obstruction as a result of airway congestion from the transudation of fluid and cellular debris from the interstitium and epithelium. However, patients with CHF usually have other historical and physical findings that help to differentiate them from pulmonary diseases. Pulmonary sarcoidosis is a *restrictive* disease that results primarily from interstitial fibrosis. Physical examination frequently reveals *dry* rales or *fine* crackles.

89. **Answer A.** The patient has evidence of tardive dyskinesia, a syndrome of uncontrollable contractions of the facial muscles because of long-term therapy with neuroleptic medications. The risk for development of this disorder is increased with longer duration of treatment, total cumulative dosage of medication, concomitant mood disorder, and patient age. Symptoms do not usually start until several years into the neuroleptic therapy. Tardive dyskinesia is only rarely reversible if the causative medication is stopped. Elderly women are the highest risk group. Specific treatment does not exist for the condition, although benzodiazepines and the newer atypical antipsychotic medications have reduced the incidence.

90. **Answer B.** Chelation therapy for acute lead toxicity is indicated in patients with worsening clinical course or severe CNS or GI symptoms. Several chelation therapies exist for lead. Dimercaprol (or British antilewisite) should be the first chelator given in patients with severe poisoning. It should be given before calcium disodium EDTA, as the latter, if given first, will cause chelated lead to cross the blood–brain barrier. Acute lead encephalopathy should be treated aggressively with chelation and management of attendant cerebral edema (hyperventilation and mannitol). Activated charcoal does not bind lead or other heavy metals. Patients deemed stable enough for outpatient chelation therapy should be given oral succimer. Penicillamine is a less effective alternative to succimer and should be given only if succimer is not tolerated due to GI side effects.

91. **Answer C.** The patient has diphtheria pharyngitis, due to the gram-positive facultative anaerobe, *Corynebacterium diphtheriae*. It occurs most commonly in unvaccinated individuals. The bacteria release diphtheria toxin, which helps the formation of pseudomembranes in the tonsils, potentially obstructing the airway. Treatment involves close airway monitoring and antitoxin administration. Penicillin and erythromycin are first-line agents, but antibiotics are useful mostly for reducing transmission rates and have little effect on the course of this toxin-mediated disease. Piperacillin–tazobactam may help reduce transmission rates but will not affect the clinical course. Acyclovir, rifampin, amikacin, and vancomycin have little effect. Corticosteroids have not been shown to improve outcomes.

92. **Answer C.** The patient has a large left-sided varicocele. Varicoceles are caused by abnormal dilation of the testicular vein and pampiniform plexus of the scrotum due to venous pooling from impaired drainage of the left internal spermatic vein into the left renal vein. Large varicoceles substantially increase the risk of infertility due to impaired blood flow and temperature of the ipsilateral testis. Testicular torsion may occur in patients with varicoceles but is not as common as infertility. Epididymitis and malignancy do not occur at appreciably higher rates in patients with varicoceles. Deep venous thrombosis due to inferior vena cava thromboses may cause varicoceles, but this is rare. (Figure Courtesy of Figueroa, TE. In: Chung EK, Atkinson-McEvoy LR, Lai NL, Terry M, eds. *Visual Diagnosis and Treatment in Pediatrics.* 3rd ed. Philadelphia, PA: Wolters Kluwer, 2014, with permission.)

93. **Answer A.** Norepinephrine is beneficial in sepsis because in addition to causing aterial vasoconstriction, it also causes venoconstriction increasing preload and it has positive inotropic effects which improves cardiac output and organ perfusion (including renal perfusion). Furthermore, there is increasing data that delayed vasopressor administration is associated with worse outcomes in septic patient. Put another way, norepinephrine infusions should be considered as part of early therapy for sepsis. To hasten vasopressor delivery, norepinephrine can be delivered peripherally while central venous access is obtained. Delays in administration may lead to worsened outcomes.

94. **Answer C.** The EKG demonstrates atrial fibrillation with rapid ventricular response. The most likely cause in this young adult with no medical history except for alcohol abuse is "holiday heart syndrome," which can occur within 2 days of an alcohol binge. It often resolves spontaneously but may require rate control therapy and possibly anticoagulation. In the absence of cocaine use, MI would be extremely unlikely in an otherwise healthy 22-year-old. Pulmonary embolism is an important cause of atrial fibrillation but is not likely in the absence of chest pain, dyspnea, or risk factors. The physical examination is unremarkable, so hypertension is unlikely. Diabetes does not confer an increased risk of atrial fibrillation.

95. **Answer C.** Floaters with or without painless visual loss is the usual clinical presentation of retinal detachment. Direct funduscopy and visual acuities may be completely normal if the detachment is peripheral or small. The elevated retina will appear out of focus and as a hazy gray membrane. Ophthalmologic consultation should be emergent since reattachment is often successful if performed early in the disease course.

96. **Answer C.** The patient has evidence of moderately severe community-acquired pneumonia, with tachycardia, tachypnea, and hypoxia. Accordingly, the patient should be admitted to the hospital for intravenous antibiotics and fluids and oxygen. Community-acquired pneumonia in this age-group is most commonly due to pneumococcus, atypical organisms, and gram-negative bacilli. Among the choices in the preceding text, C is the most appropriate. Other acceptable regimens could

include a fluoroquinolone or ampicillin–sulbactam. Oral medications and discharge would not be appropriate because of the vital sign abnormalities and comorbidities. Clindamycin possesses little gram-negative coverage and would not be adequate therapy. Piperacillin-tazobactam is a potent, broad-spectrum, antipseudomonal antibiotic used only for nosocomial pathogens causing severe illness.

97. **Answer B.** Hemorrhage occurs in approximately 15% of patients with PUD, although it is twice as likely in patients with duodenal ulcers as in patients with gastric ulcers. Roughly half the number of patients with UGIB due to PUD present with melena and hematemesis. Isolated melena occurs in only 20% of patients and isolated hematemesis occurs in only 30% of patients. The mortality rate has remained relatively unchanged over the last 30 years, and is between 6% and 10%. Perforation is accompanied by hemorrhage in roughly 10% of cases. Therefore, these entities are not usually confused upon evaluation.

98. **Answer D.** Like hypermagnesemia, hyperphosphatemia is rare in patients without renal insufficiency. Its manifestations are related to its effects on calcium and its rate of rise. A rapid rise in phosphate levels results in calcium chelation and subsequent hypocalcemia, which may present as tetany. When the calcium phosphate product is greater than 70, precipitation of calcium phosphate can occur in a variety of tissues (e.g., renal stones). Apart from renal failure, any process that results in rapid, extensive cell damage may cause phosphate to be released into the extracellular space in large amounts.

Examples of this include rhabdomyolysis, tumor lysis syndrome, and hemolysis.

99. **Answer C.** The EKG demonstrates atrial flutter at a ventricular rate of 50. The risk of atrial thrombus increases with the amount of time the patient is in atrial fibrillation or atrial flutter. Emergent management of atrial fibrillation or flutter involves reduction of rate to below 100 and anticoagulation if the duration of the dysrhythmia is longer than 48 hours, unless echocardiogram indicates no cardiac thrombus. This patient is not tachycardic and requires no rate controlling agents such as diltiazem or esmolol. Amiodarone is not indicated as this may actually terminate the atrial flutter and put the patient back into sinus rhythm and at risk for thromboembolus. Adenosine is indicated for paroxysmal supraventricular tachycardia—it may be used in unclear cases of narrow-complex tachycardia but has no role in obvious atrial flutter.

100. **Answer D.** The snake pictured is the coral snake, part of the elapid family of snakes whose venom contains potent neurotoxins. The red-on-yellow coloration indicates that it is definitely venomous—however, snakes not native to the United States without the red touching the yellow can also be venomous. Bites can cause paralysis and diaphragmatic weakness, leading to respiratory failure. Abdominal muscle spasms are seen with black widow spider bites. DIC and compartment syndrome can occur with crotalid snake envenomations. Renal failure is not a common sequela of envenomation. (Figure from Fleisher GR, Ludwig S, Baskin MN. *Atlas of Pediatric Emergency Medicine*. Philadelphia, PA: Lippincott Williams & Wilkins; 2004.)

QUESTIONS

1. A 50-year-old male presents with inability to swallow his secretions and feeling like something is stuck in his throat after swallowing a piece of steak. You suspect an esophageal food impaction. Which of the following is true regarding this patient?

    A. The patient likely has a predisposing anatomic abnormality of his esophagus.
    B. Nitroglycerin will likely be effective in resolving his impaction.
    C. Glucagon will likely be effective in resolving his impaction.
    D. Concomitant alcohol ingestion puts patient at lower risk for impaction.
    E. A trial of papain as a meat tenderizer can be attempted before moving to endoscopy.

2. An 8-year-old female is brought in by EMS for evaluation of a depressed level of consciousness after an MVC. The girl was the restrained rear seat passenger in a car that hit a tree. She was initially acting normally but complained of a headache and subsequently became increasingly sleepy such that she can't be aroused upon arrival to the emergency department (ED). Her examination reveals anisocoria with a right-sided dilated pupil. CT reveals an epidural hematoma. What is the cause of her dilated pupil?

    A. Traumatic mydriasis from an associated direct blow to the eye
    B. Compression of the optic chiasm
    C. Diffuse axonal injury affecting the occipital lobe
    D. Compression of the oculomotor nerve
    E. Compression of the brainstem

3. A 24-year-old male came to the ED with dyspnea and pleuritic chest pain for 10 days, complaining that his breathing is getting worse. You are surprised to find a 40% right-sided pneumothorax and you immediately place a chest tube, connecting it to wall suction. Although the patient initially improved, 1 hour later he began coughing vigorously, and he appears tachypneic and dyspneic. Assuming he has not experienced a recurrence or worsening of his pneumothorax, what is the most likely cause of his problem?

    A. Hemothorax caused by intercostal artery laceration
    B. Development of empyema
    C. Asthma exacerbation triggered by the procedure
    D. Re-expansion pulmonary edema (REPE)
    E. Pulmonary embolism (PE)

4. A 42-year-old female presents for evaluation of headaches and horizontal diplopia. Her examination reveals normal vital signs, mild papilledema, and she is unable to move her right eye outward. Her head CT is normal. Which of the following is the most likely finding on lumbar puncture?

    A. Elevated protein
    B. Opening pressure of 320 mm H_2O
    C. Low glucose
    D. Increased lymphocyte predominant white blood cells
    E. Oligoclonal bands

5. A 63-year-old female presents with a chief complaint of progressive tingling and burning in her bilateral lower legs and feet. Recently, she has also noted some numbness. She says a neurologist diagnosed her with distal symmetric polyneuropathy. Which of the following is the most likely cause of these symptoms?

    A. Amyotrophic lateral sclerosis
    B. Guillain–Barré syndrome
    C. Alcoholism
    D. Diabetes mellitus
    E. Paraneoplastic syndrome

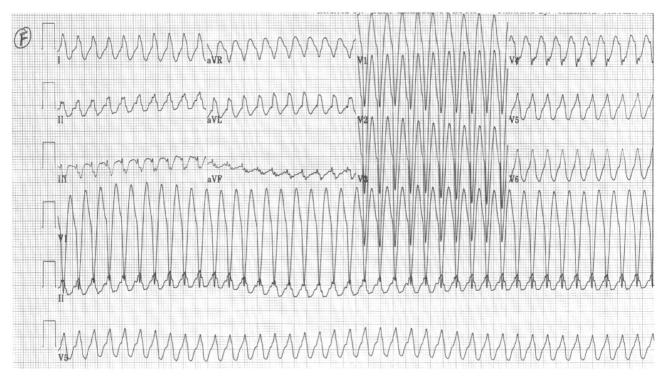

Figure 7-1

6. A 65-year-old female presents with lightheadedness. She denies chest pain or shortness of breath. Vital signs are 99.0°F, 160, 20, 144/75, 96% RA (Fig. 7-1). Which of the following is the most appropriate next step in management?

A. Adenosine
B. Diltiazem
C. Amiodarone
D. Cardioversion at 50 J
E. Cardioversion at 200 J

7. A 7-year-old female is brought in by her father after choking on a plastic toy. She was coughing violently and gasping in the car, so the father tried the Heimlich maneuver and a blind finger sweep but she seemed to get worse. His daughter is now unconscious and cyanotic. After performing a jaw-thrust maneuver, you fail to locate the foreign body. Attempts to place an endotracheal tube fail, as the tube seems to be striking an object. What is the best next step?

A. Laryngeal mask airway
B. Surgical cricothyroidotomy
C. Back blows to dislodge the foreign body
D. Blind finger sweeps to remove the foreign body
E. Needle cricothyroidotomy

8. Which of the following studies has the highest sensitivity for traumatic pericardial tamponade?

A. Anteroposterior (AP) chest x-ray
B. Lateral chest x-ray
C. Electrocardiogram (EKG)
D. Focused assessment with sonography in trauma (FAST) scan
E. Diagnostic peritoneal lavage (DPL)

9. Which of the following is true regarding treatment for acute aspirin toxicity?

A. A urinary pH goal of 7.5 to 8 is desirable.
B. Forced diuresis is an effective adjunctive therapy.
C. Activated charcoal is ineffective.
D. Whole bowel irrigation is contraindicated.
E. Hemodialysis plays no role in management.

10. A 47-year-old male with a history of alcohol abuse presents with a 1-day history of constant, dull, nonradiating epigastric pain. He recently drank more alcohol than usual. His vital signs are 98.5°F, 100, 18, 145/85, 99% RA. He is tender in the epigastrium without rebound or guarding. Serum lipase is significantly elevated. Which of the following is the next best step in evaluation?

A. Triphasic CT pancreas
B. HIDA scan
C. MR cholangiopancreatography (MRCP)
D. Endoscopic retrograde cholangiopancreatography (ERCP)
E. No specific imaging test needed

11. A 47-year-old female with a history of factor V Leiden mutation presents for evaluation of a 3-day history of an unremitting, moderate, right-sided headache. Which of the following is true?

   A. She will likely have papilledema on funduscopic examination
   B. CT head with contrast is the preferred test
   C. Magnetic resonance venography (MRV) is the test of choice
   D. A negative D-dimer test prevents the need for neuroimaging
   E. Seizure is the most common initial presentation

12. A 42-year-old previously healthy woman presents with a "bad" sore throat and painful swallowing. She is febrile, but nontoxic and in no respiratory distress (Fig. 7-2). Which of the following is the cause of this patient's illness?

   A. Retropharyngeal abscess (RPA)
   B. Epiglottitis
   C. Peritonsillar abscess (PTA)
   D. Bacterial tracheitis
   E. Ludwig angina

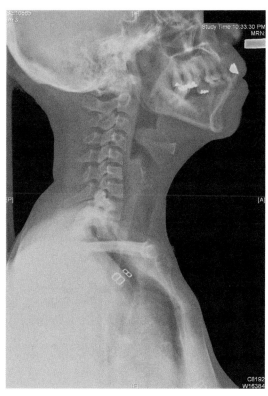

Figure 7-2

13. A 60-year-old male presents with painless hematuria. Which of the following is the most likely cause?

   A. Renal carcinoma
   B. Bladder carcinoma
   C. Urinary tract infection (UTI)
   D. Glomerulonephritis
   E. Nephrotic syndrome

14. A mother brings her 3-year-old daughter to the ED for evaluation of a persistent, foul-smelling, bloody vaginal discharge. The patient has been complaining of "itching down there" and her mother noted that she has been frequently placing her hands in her perineal region. Which of the following is the most likely cause of her symptoms?

   A. *Trichomonas* vaginitis
   B. Poor perineal hygiene
   C. Dysfunctional uterine bleeding (DUB)
   D. *Candidal* vaginitis
   E. Vaginal foreign body

15. A 54-year-old male with a history of chronic alcohol abuse is brought in by his wife because of a "big stomach" and confusion. She tells you his stomach has been big for 1 year but over the last month she adds that he seems to be forgetting things, has had difficulty sleeping, and has not been tending to his own appearance. Which of the following is true?

   A. Ammonia levels correlate with the severity of his illness.
   B. The most common finding on CT of the brain is hydrocephalus.
   C. Spontaneous bacterial peritonitis is the most common precipitant.
   D. Gastrointestinal (GI) bleeding may exacerbate or trigger this condition.
   E. The treatment of choice is ceftriaxone.

16. A 34-year-old male presents with chest pain for 4 hours, resolved at presentation. He has been smoking marijuana, which he obtained from an unknown source. His vital signs are 98.6°F, 115, 20, 167/95, 98% RA. His physical examination reveals pupillary dilation, tachycardia, and diaphoresis. His electrocardiogram (EKG) demonstrates ST depressions in V3–V5. Initial troponin level is 0.20 ng/mL. Which of the following is the most appropriate therapy at this time?

   A. Percutaneous transluminal coronary angioplasty (PTCA)
   B. Tissue plasminogen activator (tPA)
   C. Abciximab
   D. Metoprolol
   E. Aspirin

17. Which of the following is the most common area to be affected in compartment syndrome?

   A. Upper arm
   B. Forearm
   C. Hand
   D. Thigh
   E. Lower leg

18. A 34-year-old female presents with fever, headache, and blurry vision. Physical examination reveals complete oculomotor paralysis bilaterally and mild proptosis. Imaging reveals cerebral venous thrombosis (CVT). Which venous sinus is most likely affected?

    A. Cavernous sinus
    B. Sagittal sinus
    C. Sphenoid sinus
    D. Occipital sinus
    E. Straight sinus

19. A 60-year-old male presents with testicular pain for 2 days and fever of 101°F. He also complains of dysuria, but denies scrotal edema, flank pain, nausea, or vomiting. Physical examination demonstrates moderate tenderness with mild edema and erythema in the scrotal area. Cremasteric reflexes are present bilaterally. A testicular ultrasound is performed and is negative for torsion. Which of the following is the most likely etiology of the patient's symptoms?

    A. Viral
    B. *Chlamydia*
    C. *N. gonorrhoeae*
    D. *E. coli*
    E. *Pseudomonas aeruginosa*

20. A 62-year-old female with a history of hypertension presents with sudden onset of severe chest pain with radiation to the back. Her vital signs are: 98.7, 100, 18, 195/90, 99% RA. You suspect the diagnosis of aortic dissection. Her EKG and chest x-ray are normal. Which of the following is the next best step in evaluation?

    A. D-dimer
    B. Coronary angiogram
    C. CT aortogram
    D. V-Q scan
    E. Transthoracic echocardiogram

21. A 58-year-old female with a history of diabetes, hypertension, and hyperlipidemia presents to the ED with a chief complaint of diplopia. Examination reveals the patient's left eye is turned outward and appears to be looking down. Pupillary response is normal. Which of the following is the next step?

    A. MRI and MRA of the brain
    B. CT brain without contrast
    C. MRA of the neck vessels
    D. Carotid duplex ultrasound
    E. Brain angiogram

22. A 55-year-old male presents from his doctor's office with nausea, vomiting, right upper quadrant pain, and abnormal outpatient labs. Which of the following is consistent with alcoholic hepatitis?

A. AST >20 × upper limit of normal
B. ALT >20 × upper limit of normal
C. Hypermagnesemia
D. Leukocytosis
E. Elevated partial thromboplastin time (PTT)

23. The most common etiology of an intracranial tumor is:

    A. Meningioma
    B. Astrocytoma
    C. Medulloblastoma
    D. Metastases
    E. Pituitary adenoma

24. Which of the following is the most appropriate outpatient management for mechanical corneal abrasions?

    A. Eye patching
    B. Topical anesthetic
    C. Topical steroids
    D. Topical antibiotics
    E. Topical saline solution

25. Cold allodynia, the sensation of pain or dysesthesia when coming into contact with cool or cold objects (often called *cold reversal*) is virtually pathognomonic for which of the following causes of acute food poisoning?

    A. Scombroid
    B. Shigellosis
    C. *Clostridium perfringens*
    D. Ciguatera
    E. *Bacillus anthracis*

26. A 65-year-old male presents with fever, chills, and dysuria for 2 days. He denies vomiting or back pain. Physical examination reveals a patient in mild discomfort, with normal cardiac, pulmonary, and abdominal examinations. He lacks costovertebral angle tenderness, but rectal examination reveals a boggy, tender prostate. Which of the following is the most appropriate therapy?

    A. Ceftriaxone 125 mg IM and doxycycline 100 mg PO b.i.d. for 10 days
    B. Azithromycin 1 g PO
    C. Ciprofloxacin 500 mg PO b.i.d. for 3 days
    D. Ciprofloxacin 500 mg PO b.i.d. for 7 days
    E. Ciprofloxacin 500 mg PO b.i.d. for 30 days

27. Which of the following is true of Prinzmetal angina?

    A. It is not relieved by nitroglycerin.
    B. It may be relieved by exercise.
    C. The pathophysiology involves acute plaque rupture with thrombosis.
    D. Characteristic EKG changes usually distinguish Prinzmetal angina from acute myocardial infarction (MI).
    E. β-blockers are contraindicated.

28. Most cases of pseudogout are:

    A. Due to hyperparathyroidism
    B. Due to hemochromatosis
    C. Due to hypomagnesemia
    D. Due to hypothyroidism
    E. Idiopathic

29. Which of the following is true regarding patients with sternal fractures?

    A. Coexisting aortic injury occurs in half of cases.
    B. Mortality is close to 50% even in isolated cases of sternal fracture.
    C. Lateral chest radiography is diagnostic.
    D. Spinal fracture is the most common associated bony injury.
    E. Unrestrained passengers are at higher risk than restrained passengers.

30. Which of the following is true regarding cluster headaches?

    A. The pain is typically bilateral.
    B. They occur more commonly in men.
    C. The average age of onset is 45 years.
    D. The average cluster period lasts for 1 week.
    E. Pain typically occurs in the V2 distribution of the trigeminal nerve.

31. A 22-year-old male presents for substernal chest burning for several weeks which is worse after eating. He denies fever, cough, or shortness of breath. He does not smoke, drink alcohol, drink caffeine, or take over-the-counter nonsteroidal anti-inflammatory drugs (NSAIDs). His only medication is a pill for acne. His physical examination, chest x-ray, and EKG are normal. Which of the following is the most likely cause?

    A. Atypical pneumonia
    B. Asthma
    C. Pericarditis
    D. Pill esophagitis
    E. Psychogenic

32. Which of the following is true regarding urethritis in men?

    A. Gonococcal infection is almost always symptomatic.
    B. Gonococcal and chlamydial infection rarely coexist.
    C. Gram-negative intracellular diplococci on urine Gram stain indicate *Escherichia coli* infection.
    D. Chlamydial infection is more common in men older than 35 years.
    E. First-line therapy is with amoxicillin.

33. A 25-year-old male with schizophrenia presents with acute agitation. According to a family member, he was seen by a psychiatrist during the previous week, diagnosed with schizophrenia, and started on a new medication. He is extremely agitated, tachycardic, diaphoretic, febrile, and exhibits muscle rigidity. Which of the following is the most appropriate next step in management?

    A. Acetaminophen
    B. Lorazepam
    C. Amantadine
    D. Bromocriptine
    E. Haloperidol

34. A 45-year-old female presents with depressed mental status, hypothermia, hypotension, and bradycardia. She has not been taking her thyroid replacement therapy. Which of the following findings is most likely to be present?

    A. Hyperglycemia
    B. Hypernatremia
    C. Hypercapnia
    D. Hyper-reflexia
    E. Polycythemia

35. A 38-year-old female presents to the ED with a complaint of extreme hand and finger pain, which she says is exacerbated any time her fingers are exposed to the cold. She first noticed the problem when reaching into the freezer to grab a frozen dinner. She notes that her fingers become "ghost white" or blue at the tips and have a painful ache. Which of the following is the most common underlying disorder that produces these symptoms?

    A. Systemic lupus erythematosus (SLE)
    B. Rheumatoid arthritis (RA)
    C. Scleroderma
    D. Polyarteritis nodosa (PAN)
    E. Inflammatory bowel disease

36. Which of the following is more characteristic of migraine headaches than cluster headaches?

    A. The pain is unilateral.
    B. Pain is of moderate to severe intensity.
    C. The pain is throbbing in quality.
    D. The pain responds to sumatriptan.
    E. The patient has a concomitant upper respiratory infection.

37. A 58-year-old female with no prior history of abdominal surgery presents with progressive abdominal bloating and distension over the past several days as well as a 1-day history of nausea and vomiting (Fig. 7-3). Which of the following is most likely responsible?

    A. Incarcerated hernia
    B. Intussusception
    C. Cancer
    D. Volvulus
    E. Gallstone ileus

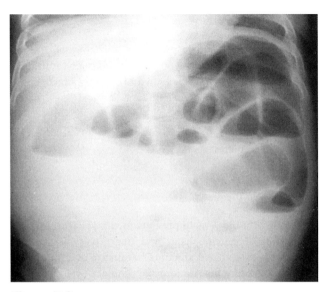

Figure 7-3

38. A 22-year-old intoxicated male is brought in by EMS in hemorrhagic shock after a major motor vehicle accident. Which of the following is true?

    A. Tranexamic acid may reduce the patient's mortality
    B. Tranexamic acid is only helpful if given within 1 hour after injury
    C. Tranexamic acid may substantially increase the patient's risk of a life-threatening blood clot
    D. Tranexamic acid has no role in this patient's care
    E. Tranexamic acid is only useful if the patient requires operative intervention

39. Which of the following personality disorders is seen in most patients with somatization disorder?

    A. Histrionic
    B. Antisocial
    C. Schizoid
    D. Schizotypal
    E. Narcissistic

40. Which of the following is true regarding *Bordetella pertussis* infections?

    A. Prophylaxis with erythromycin is recommended for adults who come into contact with pertussis-infected individuals.
    B. Almost all cases of pertussis in adolescents and adults occur in previously unvaccinated patients.
    C. Immunization against *B. pertussis* confers lifelong immunity.
    D. Older children infected with *B. pertussis* have the most severe disease.
    E. The clinical course in symptomatic adults is characterized by a mild cough that resolves within 3 to 7 days.

41. A 5-year-old male is brought by his mom for a "rash" on his back. His back is shown with close-up of the left flank lesion. The remainder of his physical examination is normal (Fig. 7-4). Which of the following is the most likely cause?

    A. Henoch–Schönlein purpura
    B. Idiopathic thrombocytopenic purpura (ITP)
    C. Lyme disease
    D. Child abuse
    E. Roseola

42. Which of the following is true regarding thyroid storm?

    A. Glucocorticoids may be useful in management.
    B. Supersaturated potassium iodide (SSKI) should be given before thionamides (propylthiouracil and methimazole).
    C. Most patients have underlying Hashimoto thyroiditis.
    D. Atrial fibrillation is the most common dysrhythmia.
    E. Beta-blockers are contraindicated unless there is concomitant hypertension.

43. Which of the following is the most common arrhythmia in patients with pulmonary embolism (PE)?

    A. Multifocal atrial tachycardia
    B. Sinus tachycardia
    C. Atrial fibrillation
    D. Sinus rhythm with atrial premature contractions
    E. Ventricular fibrillation

44. A 26-year-old female presents with eye pain after she was hit in the face with a softball (Fig. 7-5). Which of the following is the best therapeutic regimen?

    A. Topical antibiotics
    B. Topical steroids
    C. Eye patching
    D. A and C
    E. A, B, and C

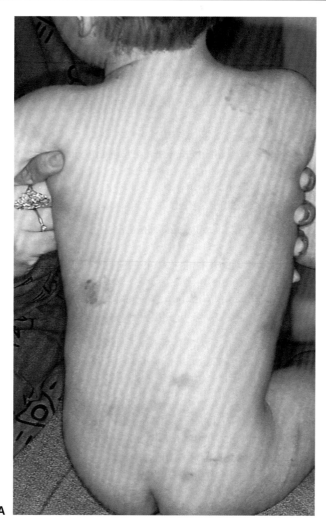

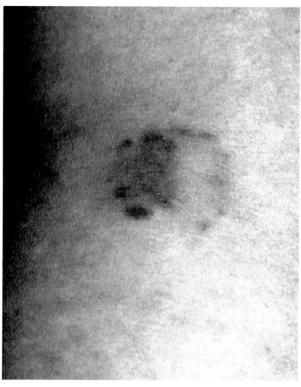

A   B

Figure 7-4

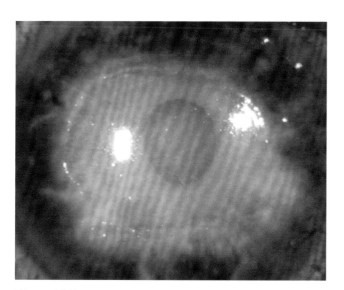

Figure 7-5

45. You decide to intubate a 54-year-old male with severely altered mental status. Your favorite induction agent for rapid-sequence intubation is etomidate. The respiratory therapist asks you whether etomidate is safe for this patient because of the potential for septic shock. You tell him:

    A. "Etomidate can cause increased intracranial pressure and laryngospasm, but this is uncommon."
    B. "Etomidate transiently reduces adrenal function but doesn't cause increased mortality."
    C. "Good point, I'll try thiopental instead—I've never tried it and this is a good time to test it out."
    D. "Etomidate has no side effects and should be used as an induction agent for all patients."
    E. "You should go to pharmacy school, medical school, PA school, or nursing school before providing advice on pharmacotherapy."

46. A 49-year-old female presents with chronic intermittent myalgias for several months. She discussed the diagnosis of fibromyalgia syndrome with her primary care physician and was going to be sent for evaluation with a rheumatologist when her pain suddenly became worse. Her vital signs are normal. Which of the following is most consistent with a diagnosis of fibromyalgia syndrome?

    A. Creatine phosphokinase (CPK) 22,000 units/L
    B. Erythrocyte sedimentation rate (ESR) 110 mm/hr
    C. C-reactive protein (CRP) 8.5 mg/dL
    D. Jaw claudication
    E. Fatigue

47. In patients with tibial shaft fractures, which of the following is the most common associated finding?

    A. Fibular fracture
    B. Common peroneal nerve injury
    C. Posterior tibial nerve injury
    D. Dorsalis pedis artery injury
    E. Posterior tibial artery injury

48. Hypernatremia …

    A. Almost never occurs in alert patients with an intact thirst mechanism.
    B. May occur after the administration of a single dose of charcoal.
    C. Is most commonly due to increased body stores of sodium (or sodium gain).
    D. Is best treated with normal saline.
    E. May result in central pontine myelinolysis if not treated within 72 hours.

49. Posterior hip dislocations:

    A. Are less common than anterior hip dislocations.
    B. Most commonly result in compression of the femoral nerve.
    C. Are more commonly associated with fractures of the femoral head than anterior dislocations.
    D. Are associated with an inability to see the lesser trochanter on an anterior–posterior view.
    E. Cause the patient to have an externally rotated, abducted, and shortened leg.

50. EMS arrives in the ED with a 26-year-old female G2P1 in active labor. In preparing for delivery, you discover that the baby is at the introitus, with the umbilical cord wrapped tightly around its neck. If unable to slip the cord over the baby's head, you should:

    A. Cut the cord without clamping and deliver the baby as rapidly as possible
    B. Deliver the baby as rapidly as possible
    C. Push the baby back into the vaginal canal
    D. Double-clamp and cut the cord and deliver the baby as rapidly as possible
    E. Suction the baby's mouth and give ventilated breaths while in the birth canal

51. A 45-year-old female with alcoholic cirrhosis presents with abdominal distention and pain with low-grade fever. You suspect spontaneous bacterial peritonitis (SBP) and perform a paracentesis. The total cell count is 300 cells per mm^3 with 60% neutrophils. Which of the following is the most appropriate next step in management?

    A. Discharge home
    B. Search for alternate cause for symptoms
    C. IV cefotaxime
    D. IV vancomycin
    E. IV metronidazole

52. Which of the following is true regarding cerebral venous thrombosis (CVT)?

    A. CT with IV contrast is the current "gold standard" for diagnosis of CVT.
    B. The most common presentation is lethargy.
    C. In most cases the outcome of CVT is worse than arterial stroke.
    D. Men are more commonly affected than women.
    E. Most seizures that occur are focal seizures.

53. A 47-year-old diabetic male is being treated for septic shock. After receiving 4 L of fluid, a passive leg raise test is performed and results in no change in his blood pressure. Which of the following is the next step?

    A. An additional 1 L fluid bolus
    B. Broad-spectrum antibiotics
    C. Vasopressors
    D. Jugular vein central line placement to assess central venous pressure (CVP)
    E. Lactate measurement

54. A 4-year-old female presents with signs and symptoms of cystitis. Which of the following is the most appropriate initial treatment?

    A. Amoxicillin–clavulanic acid
    B. Ciprofloxacin
    C. Doxycycline
    D. Cefixime
    E. Trimethoprim–sulfamethoxazole (TMP-SMX)

55. A 72-year-old female presents with fever, stiff neck, and headache. You strongly suspect bacterial meningitis. Which of the following is the most appropriate treatment strategy?

    A. Dexamethasone
    B. Vancomycin and ceftriaxone
    C. Ampicillin
    D. A and B
    E. A, B, and C

56. A 22-year-old male is brought to the ED after a near-drowning episode. He was at a party on his friend's yacht and fell off the boat while trying to impress his friends. He was submerged for about a minute and briefly lost consciousness before being transported to the ED. He currently complains of mild shortness of breath. His vital signs are 99°F, 100, 18, 120/70, 95% RA. His physical examination is unremarkable. Chest x-ray is normal. Which of the following is the most appropriate next step in management?

    A. Discharge home
    B. Admission for observation
    C. IV methylprednisolone
    D. IV piperacillin–tazobactam
    E. Endotracheal intubation with mechanical ventilation

57. What is the most commonly injured ligament during ankle sprains?

    A. Anterior talofibular
    B. Calcaneofibular
    C. Posterior talofibular
    D. Anterior inferior tibiofibular
    E. Deltoid

58. A 36-year-old female presents to the ED with a chief complaint of finger pain and swelling. She had previously been treated for an acute paronychia a few months ago, but states it "won't go away." Examination reveals a dystrophic nail, loss of the cuticle, as well as an area of tender, erythematous swelling along the proximal nail fold, without abscess formation. This chronic paronychia is best treated with:

    A. Topical corticosteroids
    B. Oral antibiotics
    C. Oral antifungals
    D. Warm water soaks
    E. Oral antivirals

59. A 23-year-old female without past medical history presents with acute onset of watery diarrhea and abdominal cramping 3 hours after eating dinner at a local restaurant. She has no nausea, vomiting, or fever. Her vital signs are 98.6°F, 85, 18, 115/70, 99% RA. She is nontoxic, and her abdominal examination shows minimal diffuse tenderness. Which of the following is the most appropriate next step in management?

    A. Oral ciprofloxacin
    B. Oral metronidazole

    C. Check stool leukocytes
    D. Check stool ova and parasites
    E. Supportive care only

60. A 21-year-old male is brought to the ED by his ex-girlfriend because she is concerned about his suicidal ideation. While the patient has a history of depression, he states that he "spiraled downhill" after his recent breakup with her. In the course of his evaluation, however, he answers questions appropriately and directly, and he verbally "contracts for safety." Such contracts:

    A. Are encouraged by the American Psychiatric Association (APA) as an effective means of establishing trust and rapport with patients
    B. Do not afford clinicians any increased liability protection
    C. Have been shown to decrease the rate of future completed suicide
    D. Should only be used and discussed by psychiatrists or psychologists
    E. Are less effective than written contracts containing similar content

61. An 85-year-old female presents from a nursing home with fever and hypotension. According to the paramedic, she began to have lethargy and refused to get out of bed 1 day ago. There is no reported history of cough, shortness of breath, diarrhea, headache, or rash. Her vital signs are: 102.4°F, 122, 22, 72/44, 95% RA. The patient's physical examination is nonfocal, and routine laboratory work is sent. Which of the following is the most appropriate empiric antibiotic therapy at this time?

    A. Ampicillin
    B. Ampicillin and gentamicin
    C. Vancomycin and piperacillin–tazobactam
    D. Vancomycin, piperacillin–tazobactam, metronidazole
    E. Vancomycin, piperacillin–tazobactam, clindamycin

62. What is the most reliable early indicator of shock in a pregnant patient after blunt abdominal trauma?

    A. Hypotension
    B. Elevated lactate
    C. Tachycardia
    D. Peritoneal signs on examination
    E. Cool, clammy skin

63. An 8-year-old male presents with wrist pain after a fall on his outstretched right hand (Fig. 7-6). Which of the following is the correct type of injury?

    A. Salter–Harris I
    B. Salter–Harris II
    C. Salter–Harris III
    D. Salter–Harris IV
    E. Salter–Harris V

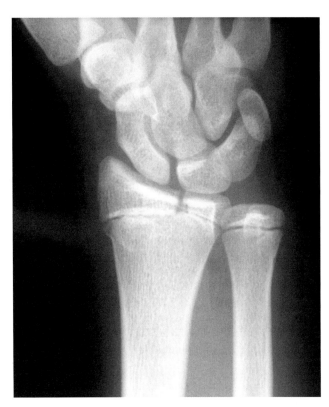

Figure 7-6

64. A 16-year-old previously healthy male presents for evaluation of difficulty breathing, throat swelling, nausea, and vomiting after eating cake at a birthday party. He is successfully treated with epinephrine and his vital signs are stable. Which of the following is true regarding biphasic anaphylactic reactions?

    A. They are more common when initial treatment is suboptimal
    B. They tend to occur in the first 4 to 6 hours after resolution of symptoms
    C. They tend to be more severe than the initial episode
    D. They require treatment with high-dose steroids
    E. They are most common after anaphylaxis due to hymenoptera envenomation

65. A mother brings in her 7-year-old daughter with a chief complaint of a rash, colicky abdominal pain, and achy ankles. The rash is palpable upon physical examination (see Fig. 7-7). Which of the following is true?

    A. When present in adults, this tends to be a much more severe disease.
    B. Her prognosis is primarily dependent on the presence of gastrointestinal bleeding.
    C. Intussusception complicating this condition is most commonly ileocecal in location.
    D. This patient should receive a short course of high-dose intravenous corticosteroids.
    E. None of the above.

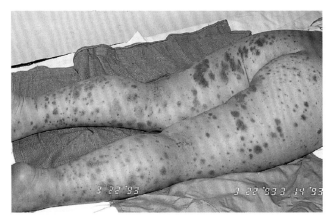

Figure 7-7

66. Which of the following is true regarding *Mycoplasma pneumoniae* infections?

    A. The presence of bullous myringitis is central to making a diagnosis of *M. pneumonia*.
    B. Outbreaks are common in institutional settings such as camps and military bases.
    C. Neurologic complications occur in up to 30% of patients.
    D. Cold agglutinin titers rise within 1 to 2 days of infection with *M. pneumoniae*.
    E. Mycoplasma is the most frequent cause of community-acquired pneumonia in elderly patients older than 65.

67. A 45-year-old female with a history of untreated hyperthyroidism presents with acute onset of left foot pain. Physical examination reveals normal vital signs, an irregular heart rhythm, clear lung sounds, and loss of pulses in the left foot with decreased capillary refill, and cyanotic, paralyzed toes. Which of the following is the most appropriate next step in management?

    A. Anticoagulation and emergent embolectomy
    B. Anticoagulation and emergent bypass surgery
    C. Anticoagulation alone
    D. Lumbar sympathectomy
    E. Hyperbaric oxygen therapy

68. Which of the following symptoms or findings best distinguishes patients with serotonin syndrome from patients with other drug- or toxin-related effects?

   A. Tachycardia
   B. Clonus
   C. Shivering
   D. Hyperthermia
   E. Muscular rigidity

69. An 8-year-old male is brought in by his parents after apparently ingesting a pin. He looks well and has a normal physical examination. A flat plate of the abdomen is shown in Figure 7-8. Which of the following is true?

   A. The most common site of perforation is the ileocecal valve.
   B. Perforation occurs in 50% of cases.
   C. Emergent consultation to a pediatric gastroenterologist is required for endoscopic removal.
   D. The patient can be safely discharged home with follow-up with his pediatrician.
   E. The patient's parents should give consent for an emergent laparotomy for surgical removal.

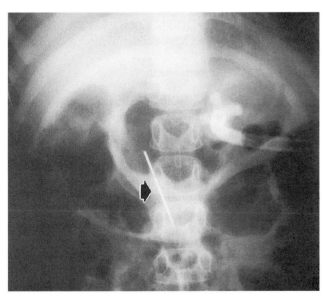

Figure 7-8

70. A 6-month-old male infant is brought in by his mother after 4 days of continuous diarrhea. He appears mildly dehydrated on examination. Which of the following acid–base disturbances is likely to be present?

   A. Elevated anion gap metabolic acidosis
   B. Normal anion gap metabolic acidosis
   C. Metabolic alkalosis
   D. Respiratory acidosis
   E. Respiratory alkalosis

71. A prostaglandin E1 infusion may help with which of the following lesions?

   A. Critical coarctation of the aorta
   B. Hypoplastic left heart syndrome
   C. Critical aortic stenosis
   D. Transposition of the great vessels
   E. All of the above

72. A 43-year-old alcoholic woman presents in coma. A relative states that the patient overdosed on her alprazolam, which she has been taking for many years as an anxiolytic. After initial airway management and IV hydration, which of the following is the most appropriate next step in pharmacologic management?

   A. Fomepizole
   B. Flumazenil
   C. Physostigmine
   D. Glucagon
   E. Thiamine

73. A 44-year-old male with a history of kidney stones presents with progressively worsening left flank pain for several days, dysuria, nausea, vomiting, and fever to 101°F. Urinalysis demonstrates 50 WBC per hpf, positive leukocyte esterase, and positive bacteria. A CT scan of the abdomen and pelvis demonstrates a 7-mm stone at the left ureteropelvic junction. Which of the following is the most appropriate next step in management?

   A. IV antibiotics and admission to the hospitalist
   B. IV antibiotics in the emergency department then discharge home with oral hydrocodone, promethazine, and antibiotics
   C. Discharge home with oral hydrocodone, promethazine, and antibiotics
   D. MRI of the abdomen and pelvis
   E. IV antibiotics and urologic consultation

74. A 34-year-old male overdoses on bupropion. Which of the following serious sequelae is most likely?

   A. Coma
   B. Seizure
   C. Torsades de pointes
   D. Hypotension
   E. Hypertension

75. A 72-year-old female presents by ambulance in pulseless electrical activity. Manual CPR is in progress. Which of the following treatment strategies increases survival to hospital discharge more than this therapy?

   A. Mechanical device CPR
   B. Epinephrine
   C. Vasopressin
   D. Defibrillation
   E. None of these

76. A 32-year-old female G₃P₂ at 39 weeks' gestation presented to your community ED in active labor with a fully dilated cervix. Because your hospital has no obstetrics services, you prepare for delivery. One minute after a successful and apparently uneventful delivery, the patient becomes abruptly hypoxic, severely hypotensive with a BP of 76/palp, and obtunded. The most likely diagnosis is:

    A. Sepsis
    B. Pulmonary embolism
    C. Peripartum cardiomyopathy
    D. Amniotic fluid embolism (AFE)
    E. Eclampsia

77. A 55-year-old male presents with right arm and leg weakness and left-sided facial droop. Which of the following arteries is most likely involved?

    A. Anterior cerebral artery
    B. Anterior communicating artery
    C. Middle cerebral artery
    D. Posterior cerebral artery
    E. Basilar artery

78. Which of the following is true regarding radiographic studies and pregnancy?

    A. The maximum amount of safe fetal radiation exposure is 10 mrad.
    B. Focused assessment of sonography in trauma (FAST) ultrasonography evaluation is approximately 90% sensitive in all trimesters of pregnancy.
    C. The cumulative background radiation exposure to a fetus throughout the 9-month gestation is greater than the exposure due to a single maternal chest x-ray.
    D. Lead shields minimally reduce fetal radiation exposure in the third trimester due to scatter caused by the enlarged uterus.
    E. The highest risk period of radiation exposure is in the first 2 weeks of pregnancy.

79. A 35-year-old male is struck in his leg by the bumper of a car. He is tender just distal to his knee. His knee x-ray is shown in Figure 7-9. Which of the following is true regarding this injury?

    A. Compartment syndrome is a possible complication
    B. Medial collateral ligament injury is seen in most cases
    C. Neurologic injury is seen in most cases
    D. Medial fractures are more common than lateral
    E. Radiographs are over 95% sensitive

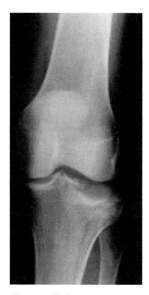

Figure 7-9

80. Which of the following is the most common complication of cirrhosis?

    A. Encephalopathy
    B. Gastrointestinal (GI) bleeding
    C. Spontaneous bacterial peritonitis
    D. Ascites
    E. Hepatocellular carcinoma

81. The parents of a 4-year-old female are referred to the ED by their pediatrician for evaluation of abdominal pain. After arrival, the patient's father refuses to sign the hospital's general consent form which permits the hospital and its providers to treat the patient and bill for their services because he "doesn't want to get gouged." Which of the following is true?

    A. The patient's father should be asked to sign an AMA (against medical advice) form indicating that he has refused care for his daughter
    B. If no emergency medical condition is present after providing a medical screening examination (MSE), the staff can wait for parental consent before proceeding with further examination and treatment
    C. The patient's MSE should be delayed while awaiting parental consent
    D. Child protective services should be called to investigate
    E. Evaluation and treatment of the child should proceed regardless of the father's refusal to sign the form

82. Which of the following is true regarding ischemic stroke and cerebral edema?

 A. Herniation in large strokes resulting from cerebral edema is more common in young patients than in elderly patients.
 B. The effects of hyperventilation on reducing Intracranial pressure (ICP) last for up to 1 week.
 C. Methylprednisolone should be given to all stroke patients with evidence of edema on CT.
 D. Cerebral edema due to ischemic stroke peaks within 2 to 4 hours.
 E. None of the above.

83. You are following up on a positive chlamydia Polymerase chain reaction (PCR) result for a 24-year-old female who presented to the ED 2 days prior. Her gonorrhea result is negative. Chart review indicates that she had no past medical history and lives and works on a Caribbean island as a lifeguard, but is still in town for 1 more day. Which of the following is the best treatment regimen for this patient?

 A. Call in a prescription for azithromycin 1 g PO
 B. Call in a prescription for doxycycline 100 mg PO BID × 7 days
 C. Call in a prescription for albendazole 400 mg PO BID × 10 days
 D. Ask her to return to the ED for ceftriaxone 250 mg IM
 E. Ask her to return to the ED for vancomycin 1 g IV

84. A 42-year-old male is brought into the ED after being thrown from a train during a derailment. He is hypotensive but has no hemothorax, a normal mediastinum, and no pelvic fracture. Focused assessment of sonography in trauma scanning reveals hemoperitoneum. Which of the following is most likely injured?

 A. Spleen
 B. Kidneys
 C. Liver
 D. Diaphragm
 E. Pancreas

85. A 22-year-old female presents with cyanosis. She complains of shortness of breath, headache, and slurred speech. Her friends report that she's been getting high, but they don't know what she's using. SaO_2 is 85% despite aggressive oxygen therapy. Blood drawn from the patient appears extremely dark. Which of the following is the most likely drug ingested?

 A. Lorazepam
 B. Dextromethorphan
 C. Amyl nitrate
 D. Diphenhydramine
 E. Ketamine

86. Which of the following is the most common organism isolated in spontaneous bacterial peritonitis (SBP)?

 A. *Escherichia coli*
 B. *Staphylococcus aureus*
 C. *Streptococcus pneumoniae*
 D. *Klebsiella pneumoniae*
 E. Anaerobic species

87. Which of the following indicates a likely globe injury in a patient with an eyelid laceration?

 A. Vertical laceration through lid margin
 B. Horizontal laceration extending the length of the eyelid
 C. Fat protruding from laceration
 D. Lacerations with a large degree of tissue loss
 E. Stellate lacerations

88. A 35-year-old male presents after a motor vehicle collision with hypotension, tachycardia, and altered mental status. Which of the following is the most appropriate blood product to administer immediately?

 A. Type O negative crossmatched blood
 B. Type O negative uncrossmatched blood
 C. Type O positive crossmatched blood
 D. Type O positive uncrossmatched blood
 E. Fresh frozen plasma

89. The best means of rewarming a frozen or partially thawed extremity is

 A. Direct tissue massage
 B. Direct exposure to dry heat sources such as heat lamps or open fires
 C. Immersion in a water bath maintained between 40°C and 42°C
 D. Slow thaw through immersion in an ice water bath
 E. Forced-air warming device (convection method, e.g., Bair Hugger)

90. A 16-year-old female on day 8 of a 10-day course of trimethoprim–sulfamethoxazole for a urinary tract infection presents for evaluation of a diffuse blanching macular rash over her trunk. She has no airway complaints. In the emergency room, she is noted to be febrile with a temperature of 102.3, but she has no infectious complaints. A repeat urinalysis is negative. Her other vital signs are normal. Which of the following is true?

 A. The best test to determine if the rash and fever are due to the drug is to stop the drug
 B. Nitrofurantoin should be started to complete a 10-day antibiotic course
 C. The erythrocyte sedimentation rate (ESR) is usually low or normal in patients with drug fever
 D. Antibiotics are an infrequent cause of drug fever
 E. Most cases of drug fever present within the first 48 hours after starting the drug

91. Which of the following is the gold standard for diagnosing choledocholithiasis?

    A. CT scan of the abdomen with intravenous and oral contrast
    B. Endoscopic ultrasonography (US)
    C. Cholescintigraphy (e.g., HIDA scan)
    D. Magnetic resonance cholangiopancreatography (MRCP)
    E. CT scan of the abdomen with intravenous contrast only

92. A 23-year-old male with a past medical history of acquired immunodeficiency syndrome (AIDS) presents with fever and headache. Brain CT scan is unremarkable and cerebrospinal fluid (CSF) results from lumbar puncture results are as follows:

    White blood cell (WBC): 35 per μL, lymphocytic predominance

    Red blood cell (RBC): 2 per μL

    Glucose: Normal

    Protein: Normal

    Gram stain: Negative

    India ink: Positive

    Which of the following is the most appropriate medication at this time?

    A. Ceftriaxone
    B. Vancomycin
    C. Acyclovir
    D. Itraconazole
    E. Amphotericin B + flucytosine

93. A 29-year-old male presents to the ED with a 3-week history of diarrhea, crampy intermittent abdominal pain, and a 10-lb weight loss. He denies any bloody stools or vomiting even though his stool guaiac test is positive. He returned from a 1-month trip to India approximately 6 weeks ago and had no problems while he was there. Which of the following is the most likely cause of his symptoms?

    A. *Shigella* spp.
    B. Enterotoxigenic *E. coli*
    C. *Enterobius vermicularis*
    D. *Entamoeba histolytica*
    E. *Campylobacter* spp.

94. Which of the following is the most common presenting symptom of multiple sclerosis (MS)?

    A. Urinary retention
    B. Hemiparesis of the upper extremities
    C. Ataxia
    D. Aphasia
    E. Eye pain and decreased visual acuity

95. Due to its significant morbidity and mortality, early recognition of necrotizing fasciitis is critical. Which of the following is most helpful in making an early diagnosis?

    A. Crepitus on examination
    B. Vesicle and bullae development on the skin surface
    C. Serum C-reactive protein (CRP) ≥150 mg/L
    D. Pain out of proportion to examination findings
    E. Rapidly expanding purplish-red erythema

96. An 8-year-old male presents with right ear pain after a fight. He tells you that he was punched and kicked in the head and ear. On examination, you note the finding visible in the image (see Fig. 7-10). Which of the following is the best step in management?

    A. Incision and drainage followed by application of a pressure dressing
    B. Referral to otolaryngology with follow-up arranged in 2 days
    C. Reassurance and discharge
    D. Application of a pressure dressing only
    E. Aspiration followed by application of a pressure dressing

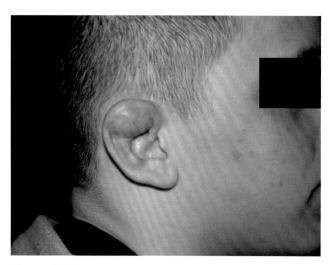

Figure 7-10

97. Which of the following is a known risk factor for subarachnoid hemorrhage?

    A. Hypotension
    B. Smoking
    C. Oral contraceptive use
    D. Hypercholesterolemia
    E. Hypertriglyceridemia

98. A 48-year-old female with a history of menorrhagia is referred to the ED for a blood transfusion after presenting to her primary doctor with mild exertional dyspnea. A CBC reveals a hemoglobin level of 6.8 g/dL. The remainder of her evaluation is unrevealing. She is guaiac negative and reports no active menses. Which of the following is true?

A. She should receive two units of packed red blood cells (PRBCs)
B. She should be admitted for evaluation of a possible concomitant GI bleed
C. A repeat hemoglobin should not be checked until 4 hours after the transfusion is complete
D. A pelvic ultrasound should be emergently performed to evaluate for structural uterine abnormalities
E. She may be a candidate for intravenous iron therapy

99. Which of the following is the most common complication of anterior shoulder dislocation?

A. Axillary nerve injury
B. Brachial artery injury
C. Recurrence
D. Rotator cuff tear
E. Adhesive capsulitis

100. A 42-year-old previously healthy male develops headache, dizziness, decreased responsiveness, right-sided hemiplegia, and aphasia within a minute of emerging from the water after diving to a shipwreck with friends. What is the most likely cause of his symptoms?

A. Arterial gas embolism (AGE)
B. Nitrogen narcosis
C. decompression sickness (DCS)
D. Contaminated air exposure
E. Alternobaric vertigo

1. **Answer A.** Esophageal food impactions usually occur in patients who have pre-existing anatomic abnormality of the esophagus, such as a Schatzki ring, stricture, or cancer. Nitroglycerin IV and glucagon IV are usually attempted but resolve the obstruction less than a quarter of the time. Definitive management usually involves endoscopic removal of the food bolus. Despite the fact that alcohol relaxes the lower esophageal sphincter, alcohol actually puts patients at *higher* risk for esophageal food impaction, probably because of behavioral eating changes. Papain should never be used to facilitate passage of food boluses because it partially digests the already-inflamed esophagus as well as the intended food target.

2. **Answer D.** The skull is a small, fixed space which can't accommodate much more than the brain and its associated neurovascular structures. The majority of epidural hematomas occur in the parietal and temporal regions. When blood accumulates in the epidural space, it compresses the subjacent brain which pushes the brain inferiorly, compressing the oculomotor nerve against the tentorium cerebelli producing pupillary dilation. Brainstem compression may also occur, but is a later, even more serious problem. Traumatic mydriasis is common after a direct blow to the eye, but there is no history suggesting direct eye trauma. A direct injury to the occipital lobe will not produce anisocoria with a dilated pupil but could cause cortical blindness or visual field cuts.

3. **Answer D.** Tube thoracostomy is a procedure that is fraught with potential complications. In a recent series of 47 trauma patients, the complication rate was 30%. Complications that will be evident in the ED are usually related to tube insertion, such as kinked or clotted tubes, intercostal artery lacerations, lung lacerations, diaphragmatic perforation, or insertion of the tube subcutaneously. Infectious complications such as empyema occur well after insertion, requiring at least a few days to develop. REPE is a rare but potentially fatal consequence of tube thoracostomy. However, its incidence is uncertain, because early studies did not report this complication whereas more recent studies have reported an incidence as high as 14%. Patients with pneumothoraces >30% are at greatest risk for developing REPE. Some studies have also shown that the presence of a pneumothorax for a prolonged period (>3 days) before re-expansion is also a risk factor. No controlled studies have demonstrated the best treatment for individuals with such risk factors. However, the consensus of the American College of Chest Physicians is that in patients with a ≥30% pneumothorax, a small bore chest tube (16 to 22 French) should be used and placed to water-seal *only* or to a Heimlich valve device. As some studies have suggested that the rate of re-expansion may also play a role, vacuum suction should not be used. All such patients should be admitted. Because negative pressure is not being applied, lung re-expansion may not occur, and suction may be required especially if the patient is clinically unstable. If REPE develops, treatment is supportive as with other causes of noncardiogenic pulmonary edema.

4. **Answer B.** This patient is presenting with symptoms of idiopathic intracranial hypertension (IIH, also called pseudotumor cerebri). The patient's headaches and sixth nerve palsy (and associated diplopia) are all caused by elevated intracranial pressure. While the exact cause is not known, there is a clear association with obesity and the disease is more common in females. CSF composition is normal in patients with IIH but opening pressure is elevated (≤200 mm H_2O is considered normal pressure while ≥250 mm H_2O is considered clearly abnormal while pressures in between may be considered equivocal). Among cranial nerves, the sixth cranial nerve has the longest intracranial course so it is most impacted by elevations in ICP. Oligoclonal bands are classically found in patients with MS.

5. **Answer D.** Symmetric polyneuropathies produce the classic "stocking and glove" distribution of sensory loss. Many systemic disorders can produce these symptoms, including diabetes, alcoholism, and uremia, from chronic renal insufficiency. However, diabetes is, by far, the most common etiology. Initial symptoms are typically "positive," such as tingling or burning, rather than "negative," such as numbness. The symptoms begin distally and progress more proximally and affect the lower extremities more than the upper extremities. Over time, weakness develops usually involving dorsiflexion of the big toe followed by weakness of foot dorsiflexion, foot drop, loss of ankle jerks, and finally a "steppage gait."

6. **Answer C.** The EKG shows a wide-complex, regular tachycardia, which is almost always ventricular tachycardia (VT). Amiodarone, procainamide, or lidocaine may be used to treat stable VT. Although cardioversion may also be performed, it is painful for awake patients and may not be necessary for patients without hemodynamic instability. Adenosine and diltiazem are both used in patients with narrow-complex tachycardias and have no role in ventricular dysrhythmias. Supraventricular

tachycardia (SVT) with aberrant conduction can also cause a regular, wide-complex tachycardia. VT is far more common, and may be distinguished from SVT with aberrancy by the presence of fusion beats, atrioventricular dissociation, wider QRS complexes (>0.14 second), and concordance of precordial leads. When in doubt, the emergency physician should always treat regular wide-complex tachycardia as VT.

7. **Answer E.** This patient has complete airway obstruction due to foreign body aspiration. The classic triad of foreign body aspiration is coughing, wheezing, and decreased or absent breath sounds. However, approximately 40% of patients may have no significant physical examination findings. Although this patient initially had partial foreign body obstruction, it progressed to complete obstruction and she now requires a definitive airway. Back blows and chest thrusts would be reasonable *initial* approaches in infants with foreign body aspiration. Abdominal thrusts can be used in children older than 12 months, although the Heimlich maneuver is the initial procedure of choice for older children and adults. Blind finger sweeps, which were advocated in the past, are discouraged as they have the potential of converting a partial airway obstruction to complete airway obstruction. In the setting of complete airway obstruction, a definitive airway must be established. The fastest way to accomplish this in this case is by performing a cricothyroidotomy. A needle cricothyroidotomy instead of a surgical cricothyroidotomy should be performed in children younger than 8 years. Surgical cricothyroidotomy is difficult to perform in a small child because of the small size of the cricothyroid membrane, and it places children at risk for subsequent subglottic stenosis. A needle cricothyroidotomy is performed using a 12- to 16-gauge angiocatheter and inserting it through the inferior portion of the cricothyroid membrane into the trachea. The catheter can then be attached to an adapter from a size No. 3.0 endotracheal tube to allow for bag ventilation or to high-flow oxygen tubing for percutaneous transtracheal jet ventilation. In either case, these measures are only temporary until a more definitive airway can be established.

8. **Answer D.** Pericardial tamponade usually results from a penetrating thoracic mechanism causing cardiac or mediastinal injury and accumulation of blood into the pericardium. Pericardial effusion and tamponade are readily seen on the subxiphoid and parasternal views of the FAST scan. Chest x-ray may show a large, water-bottle heart if the effusion is large enough, but tamponade physiology can occur with small, rapidly accumulating effusions which may be invisible on plain radiography. The EKG finding of electrical alternans due to swinging of the heart throughout the cardiac cycle is highly specific for pericardial effusion, but occurs in less than one-third of cases. DPL is highly sensitive for intraperitoneal injury but has no utility in screening for pericardial effusion.

9. **Answer A.** The treatment for aspirin overdose involves gastrointestinal decontamination, hydration, and enhanced excretion of drug. Urinary alkalinization with intravenous bicarbonate increases the amount of ionized salicylate, which is excreted more easily by the kidneys than unionized salicylic acid. A urine pH goal of 7.5 to 8 optimizes this approach. Forced diuresis has been found to increase the risk of cerebral and pulmonary edema and does not result in increased excretion of salicylic acid. Activated charcoal and whole bowel irrigation are recommended in cases of acute intoxications and intoxications with enteric-coated aspirin, respectively. Hemodialysis may be lifesaving for patients who have severe salicylate toxicity, organ failure, or failure of standard, noninvasive management.

10. **Answer E.** The patient has classic alcoholic pancreatitis, the most common cause in men and the second most common cause overall (after gallstones). Autodigestion from pancreatic enzymes due to obstructing gallstones or ethanol damage is the primary pathogenesis. Lipase is the most specific diagnostic test for pancreatitis and is almost as sensitive as amylase. In most cases of acute pancreatitis, emergent abdominal imaging is not necessary. CT abdomen/pelvis may be pursued if a complication such as abscess, necrosis, or pseudocyst is suspected by the presence of fever or systemic toxicity. Ultrasound of the gallbladder should be performed in any patient without a history of alcohol abuse. HIDA scan is used as a more sensitive study (compared to ultrasound) to evaluate gallbladder obstruction. Both MRCP and ERCP are used to evaluate cases of gallstone pancreatitis.

11. **Answer C.** This vignette describes a patient at high risk for a cerebral venous sinus thrombosis (CVT). The factor V Leiden mutation produces a factor V protein that is resistant to inactivation by activated protein C, which usually tempers the activity of factor V (and other coagulation proteins). Unchecked factor V leads to an increased tendency to develop venous thrombosis. Most patients with CVT present with a headache, though the characteristics of the headache are variable and will depend, in part, on the location and extent of the venous thrombosis within the brain. Magnetic resonance venography (MRI with contrast) is the preferred test to demonstrate the absence of flow within the affected sinus. Papilledema is a possible finding due to increased intracranial pressure but its absence doesn't rule out CVT. Negative d-dimer levels also decrease the likelihood of CVT but can't be relied on to exclude it. Seizures are more common in

patients with CVT than in patients with other stroke subtypes.

12. **Answer B.** This patient's x-ray demonstrates the classic "thumb" or "thumbprint" sign signifying a swollen epiglottis. Although nasopharyngoscopy (NP) is an alternative to diagnose epiglottitis through direct visualization, patients with respiratory distress are not candidates for NP until a secure airway is established. Therefore, the lateral soft-tissue neck x-ray will continue to have a role in supporting a diagnosis of epiglottitis. *H. influenzae* is the most common organism causing adult epiglottitis. However, only a minority of throat cultures are positive, suggesting a possibly significant role for viruses as an etiology as well. Patients with epiglottitis may subsequently develop an epiglottis abscess, in which case *Streptococcus* and *Staphylococcus* are the most common isolated species. Although there is no age or seasonal prevalence, men and smokers are most commonly affected. The clinical course is variable, as epiglottitis is frequently preceded by a prodrome resembling a mild upper respiratory infection. In patients who have a brief prodrome with rapid progression of their symptoms, airway complications are more common. Symptoms of epiglottitis include fever, dysphagia, odynophagia, sore throat, and a muffled voice although fever may be absent in up to 50% of patients. Patients frequently have throat pain out of proportion to their physical findings on examination. This can be an important clue in diagnosis, as epiglottitis should be suspected in any patient in whom you expect to find severe tonsillopharyngitis on examination and yet find a relatively benign-appearing oropharynx. Up to one-third of patients with adult epiglottitis were seen within 48 hours before admission with symptoms that were mistaken for another entity, usually pharyngitis. On x-ray, RPA is diagnosed by prominent swelling of the prevertebral tissues. To avoid artifactual effects as a result of redundant tissue, lateral neck films should be taken at full extension with deep inspiration. The retropharyngeal space will appear erroneously enlarged if x-rays are taken in expiration and flexion. RPA should be suspected if the prevertebral soft tissue from the anteroinferior aspect of C2 to the border of the tracheal air column is >7 mm in children and adults or the same space at the level of C6 is >14 mm in children and 22 mm in adults. PTA is a diagnosis that is typically made on physical examination. A CT may be necessary in cases that are unclear, but a lateral neck x-ray generally contributes little to the diagnosis. Bacterial tracheitis is uncommon in adults. Lateral neck films may reveal narrowing of the tracheal air column below the level of the glottis or a ragged posterior tracheal margin. Finally, patients with Ludwig angina are usually diagnosed clinically, although lateral neck films will support the diagnosis and show prominent submandibular soft-tissue swelling.

13. **Answer B.** The causes of painless hematuria vary by age and gender. The most common cause in children is glomerulonephritis, in young adults and older women, UTI, and in older men, bladder cancer. Renal carcinoma is a less common cause of painless hematuria in all age groups. Nephrotic syndrome causes proteinuria without frank hematuria. The combination of urinalysis and appropriate imaging studies (such as helical CT scan) yields the diagnosis in most cases.

14. **Answer E.** A history of a persistent, foul-smelling, bloody vaginal discharge is highly suggestive of a vaginal foreign body. Although the history of a bloody discharge is helpful, few patients remember placing a foreign body in their vagina and few parents witness the act. Therefore, ED physicians should have a high degree of suspicion whenever a patient presents with a foul-smelling bloody discharge. Although many foreign bodies have been documented, small wads of toilet paper are most common. Simple removal followed occasionally by local irrigation, if necessary, is all that is required. Antibiotics are not usually necessary unless a concomitant infectious vulvovaginitis is present. Poor perineal hygiene is the leading cause of vulvovaginitis in the pediatric population. Bacterial pathogens responsible for the infection are typically nonspecific. If the predominant symptom is pruritus, pinworms (*Enterobius*) should be suspected.

15. **Answer D.** This patient is manifesting signs of hepatic encephalopathy (HE). HE is graded on a four-stage scale, and its symptoms range from subtle personality changes and sleep disturbances to confusion, disorientation, stupor, and coma. Although elevated ammonia levels may support the diagnosis, they do not always correlate with the severity of illness and normal levels do not exclude the diagnosis. Roughly 25% of patients will have non-nitrogenous causes of encephalopathy. However, azotemia is the most common precipitant and GI bleeding is a very common cause of azotemia and may frequently trigger or exacerbate HE. The treatment of choice is ammonia-lowering therapy with lactulose, or with neomycin in the case of azotemia-induced causes. Otherwise, treatment should be directed at the underlying precipitant.

16. **Answer E.** The patient is exhibiting a sympathomimetic picture after smoking marijuana, which commonly occurs because of crack cocaine additives. His myocardial ischemia is likely because of a combination of vasospasm and hyperaggregatory platelets. Aspirin is indicated for treatment. His chest pain is resolved and he is not having an ST-segment elevation myocardial infarction, so PTCA, tPA, and GpIIbIIIa inhibitors are not warranted. Metoprolol is relatively contraindicated in cocaine-induced chest pain as there is a theoretical risk of reducing cardiac output by inhibiting β-receptors

in the setting of increased peripheral vascular resistance (due to α-receptor stimulation).

17. **Answer E.** *Compartment syndrome* refers to ischemia that occurs in extremities when pressure in the soft tissues exceeds that of the microcirculation. Such high pressures occur from either increased contents in the compartment or external compression. Normal compartment pressure is zero, and pressures >30 mm Hg are usually enough to predispose to compartment syndrome. Long bone fractures are the usual reason for compartment syndrome, causing extravasated blood and soft tissue edema to accumulate. Tibial fracture is the single most common cause of compartment syndrome, but all the other regions listed can also be involved. The most common symptoms are pain and paresthesias. Diminished pulses generally occur only in extremely advanced cases, as pressure in compartment syndrome is usually well below arterial pressure. Diagnosis is made by directly measuring compartment syndromes with a Stryker needle device. Treatment is with urgent fasciotomy.

18. **Answer A.** The patient has clinical evidence of cavernous sinus thrombosis, with fever, headache, and bilateral ocular paralysis. Among young adults and adolescents, CVT is more common in women than men by 3:1, probably because of oral contraceptives and the increased thromboembolic risk associated with pregnancy. Other causes of CVT include malignancy, infection, and head injury. Magnetic resonance venography (MRV) is the study of choice when CVT is suspected. Symptoms and signs of CVT depend on the location of the thrombosis, but most patients present with a headache. Otherwise, hemiparesis or focal monoparesis is the most predominant finding. Seizures also more commonly occur in patients with a stroke due to CVT than in patients with more common causes of stroke. In cavernous sinus thrombosis, ocular symptoms are paramount with proptosis, eye pain, swelling of the conjunctiva (chemosis), and ocular muscle weakness. Given her fever, this patient's thrombosis is likely caused by an underlying infection, most commonly caused by staphylococci and streptococci. Treatment involves broad-spectrum antibiotics and neurosurgic consultation for possible surgical drainage. Heparin may also be indicated in patients who have extensive thrombosis. Without treatment, mortality is close to 100%, and even with treatment it is close to 30%.

19. **Answer D.** The patient has evidence of acute epididymitis. In men older than 35 years, the most common cause is *E. coli*. In men younger than 35 years, *Chlamydia* is the number one cause, followed by gonococcus. It is crucial for the emergency physician (EP) to distinguish between testicular torsion and epididymitis. Epididymitis is characterized by the gradual progression of symptoms, dysuria,

and the presence of cremasteric reflexes. Focal epididymal swelling is followed by generalized edema and erythema of the scrotum. Low-grade fever is present in most patients. Only half the number of patients with epididymitis have leukocytes in the urine. Treatment involves antibiotics to cover suspected organisms based on age of the patient: Ceftriaxone plus doxycycline for patients younger than 35 years, and trimethoprim–sulfamethoxazole or ciprofloxacin for patients older than 35 years.

20. **Answer C.** One out of every six patients with aortic dissection has a normal chest x-ray—therefore, normal chest x-ray cannot be used to rule out an aortic dissection. CT aortogram is the optimal test to evaluate for aortic dissection. An alternative would be transesophageal echocardiogram, though this may be difficult to obtain in an emergent fashion. The role of D-dimer in the evaluation of aortic dissection is limited to patients who lack high-risk features such as abrupt or severe pain, aortic disease, pulse deficit, shock, or focal neurologic deficit. These lower risk patients may be ruled out with a negative D-dimer test. Emergent coronary angiogram should be reserved only for patients with ST-elevation myocardial infarction or unremitting unstable angina. V-Q scan is important in the evaluation of pulmonary embolism, not aortic dissection. Transthoracic echocardiogram lacks the sensitivity necessary to rule out aortic dissection.

21. **Answer A.** This patient has a partial, pupil-sparing left cranial nerve III palsy. The primary anatomic pathology to exclude is an aneurysm of the posterior communicating artery (called a "PCOM aneurysm"). The best and most consistent test is an MRA though a CT angiogram could also be used to exclude an aneurysm. MRI helps to evaluate nonaneurysmal causes of a CNIII palsy (e.g., brainstem stroke) and is superior to CT. The classic position of the eye in the setting of an oculomotor nerve palsy (cranial nerve III) is "down and out." Superior and inferior rectus muscle weakness cancel each other out while the eye moves outward because of medial rectus weakness and downward because of inferior oblique muscle weakness. In patients with a pupil-sparing but otherwise complete CNIII palsy, the etiology is almost always microvascular ischemia rather than an aneurysm. Such patients typically recover without intervention in 8 to 12 weeks, though most patients are started on aspirin or other antiplatelet medications.

22. **Answer D.** Alcoholic hepatitis is a type of acute ethanol-induced liver disease. Patients usually experience nonspecific symptoms such as fever, myalgias, nausea, and vomiting, in addition to the more specific sign of right upper quadrant tenderness. Laboratory work often shows mild elevations of WBC count, transaminases, and PT. Significant elevations of transaminases are far

more likely to be seen in viral or drug-induced hepatitis. Most patients who have acute alcoholic hepatitis have a chronic history of alcohol abuse and are usually magnesium-deficient. Treatment of alcoholic hepatitis involves symptom control, intravenous fluids, correction of electrolyte abnormalities, and supplementation with thiamine and glucose.

23. **Answer D.** The American Cancer Society estimated that approximately 17,000 people were diagnosed with primary brain tumors in 1999 versus >100,000 people who died with metastatic brain tumors. The most common cause is lung cancer followed by breast carcinoma and colon carcinoma. Malignant melanoma and renal carcinomas metastasize to the brain less commonly. The malignant gliomas, anaplastic astrocytoma, and glioblastoma multiforme are the most common glial tumors, and are typically located in the cerebral hemispheres.

24. **Answer D.** Corneal abrasions should be treated with prophylactic topical antibiotics. Short-term cycloplegics may also be used to reduce the ciliary spasm associated with many abrasions. Eye patching has been shown to increase infection rates. Topical anesthetics have been thought to impede corneal healing if used beyond the acute setting. However, recent studies have contradicted that conventional wisdom. Still, at the time of this writing, topical anesthetics are not available for home use. Topical steroids are indicated only in cases of iritis and are absolutely contraindicated when the possibility of herpetic infection exists. Topical saline solution may be used in corneal abrasions as a remoisturizing medium, but does not reduce superinfection rates or improve healing.

25. **Answer D.** Ciguatera fish poisoning is the most common cause of fish-related food poisoning in the United States. The classic syndrome includes the development of both GI and neurologic manifestations. The relative amount of neurologic or GI symptoms varies by region. GI symptoms occur first and include nausea, vomiting, watery diarrhea, and crampy abdominal pain. Neurologic manifestations are more variable but >90% of patients have distal and perioral paresthesias, cold allodynia, and numbness. Cold allodynia is often incorrectly referred to as *temperature reversal* due to the burning sensation patients experience when coming into contact with cool or cold objects (although it actually represents a painful, burning dysesthesia). Symptoms last for an average of 1 to 2 weeks. There is no effective antidote; therefore treatment is supportive. Rare cases may be associated with bradycardia and hypotension due to anticholinesterase activity. Such cases may require atropine and dopamine.

26. **Answer E.** The patient has acute bacterial prostatitis. Fever, low back pain, and UTI symptoms are common.

A warm, tender prostate is the characteristic physical examination finding. The prostate should never be massaged because of the possibility of bacteremic spread. Etiology is almost always due to gram-negative enteric bacilli, most commonly *E. coli.* Diagnosis is made by physical examination combined with urinalysis, as there is often a concomitant cystitis. Treatment is with either trimethoprim–sulfamethoxazole or a fluoroquinolone. Treatment must be continued for 1 month to assure clinical cure. Ceftriaxone and doxycycline are the drugs of choice for young men with urethritis. Azithromycin is an acceptable alternative for treating chlamydial infections. Three-day and 7-day regimens with a fluoroquinolone are used for treating uncomplicated UTI and complicated UTI, respectively, in women.

27. **Answer B.** Prinzmetal (or variant) angina is characterized by chest pain caused by coronary artery vasospasm, which can result in ST-elevation myocardial infarction, arrhythmia, and sudden death. Prinzmetal angina can occur in concert with atherosclerotic heart disease or may be completely unrelated. A relative reduction in nitric oxide is hypothesized to be the cause. It is often clinically and electrocardiographically indistinguishable from atherosclerotic coronary artery disease (CAD). Patients with Prinzmetal angina can have a decrease, increase, or no change in their pain with exercise—for this reason, history of exertional angina or exercise stress testing is of limited value in diagnosing Prinzmetal angina. Variant angina may be relieved by nitroglycerin. β-blockers, as in atherosclerotic CAD, form part of the cornerstone of management.

28. **Answer E.** *Calcium pyrophosphate dihydrate* crystal deposition disease or pseudogout is most commonly idiopathic. However, it may also be secondary to any of the underlying conditions listed. Attacks are typically not as severe as in gout, although they share the same management.

29. **Answer C.** Sternal fractures are usually caused by blunt thoracic trauma and passengers wearing seat belts are at much higher risk than those who are unrestrained. The belt's position across the chest is thought to put extreme force on the sternum during rapid deceleration. Coexisting mediastinal hematoma or myocardial contusion may occur in <10% of cases, but aortic injury does not occur at appreciably higher rates. Mortality of isolated sternal fractures is <1%. Routine AP views of the chest often miss sternal fractures, but tenderness of the sternum should prompt either a lateral radiograph or CT scan, both of which demonstrate sternal fracture. Concomitant rib fractures are the most common bony injuries associated with sternal fractures, but vertebral fractures do occur at higher rates as well. Treatment involves evaluation for other thoracic injuries and aggressive pain control.

30. Answer B. Of the primary headache syndromes, cluster headaches have the most consistent presentation. The average age of onset is 28 to 30 years. They are strictly unilateral headaches that occur in the ophthalmic division (V1) of the trigeminal nerve. Therefore, the pain is most commonly maximal in the retro-orbital and temporal region, although patients may experience radiating pain to the forehead, temple, cheek, and jaw. The pain is severe and is often described as "boring" or "tearing" in nature. Patients are often very restless or agitated during cluster headaches and characteristically rock or pace back and forth. The headaches last on average from 45 to 90 minutes and occur one to three times daily. The typical cluster period (during which headaches occur) lasts 6 to 12 weeks with typical remissions lasting 12 months. Traditionally, they have been much more common in men, although recent epidemiologic studies have revealed a declining predominance of men. In addition, patients affected by cluster headaches more frequently indulge in cigarette smoking and alcohol abuse. Interestingly, once a cluster period begins, alcohol usually triggers an attack within minutes. There is also a seasonal pattern to the clusters, with exacerbations occurring more often in the spring and fall.

31. Answer D. Given his history of acne, he is very likely taking doxycycline, which is a common cause of pill esophagitis. Other medications that cause pill esophagitis include aspirin and NSAIDs, iron supplements, and bisphosphonates. Symptomatology is the same as that for gastroesophageal reflux disease. Pill esophagitis can be treated supportively or with proton pump inhibitors. Prevention by drinking a full glass of water with the offending medication is useful. Pneumonia is less likely given the lack of dyspnea, fever, cough, crackles, or chest x-ray abnormality. Asthma would be unlikely without cough or shortness of breath. Pericarditis is possible but usually causes some positional changes or EKG abnormalities, sometimes with an antecedent viral syndrome. Psychogenic somatic symptoms should be a diagnosis of exclusion.

32. Answer A. Urethritis in men is commonly caused by *N. gonorrhoeae* and *C. trachomatis.* Symptoms of urethritis are dysuria and penile discharge. Gonococcal urethritis is almost always symptomatic, whereas chlamydial infection can be asymptomatic in one-fourth of cases. Both gonococcus and *Chlamydia* coexist in up to half of the cases of urethritis. Diagnosis is made by urine Gram stain and PCR. Gram-negative intracellular diplococci in the urine are diagnostic for gonococcal infection. Chlamydial infection is much more common in men younger than 20. Treatment of urethritis covers both *N. gonorrhoeae* and *Chlamydia*—ceftriaxone IM with a week of oral doxycycline. Sexual partners should be treated as well.

33. Answer B. The patient's recent diagnosis of schizophrenia and initiation of likely antipsychotic medication strongly suggest neuroleptic malignant syndrome in the setting of his presentation. Hyperthermia, muscle rigidity, altered mental status, and elevated creatine phosphokinase levels are characteristic. Treatment involves aggressive sedation with benzodiazepines, cooling, and paralysis with neuromuscular blockade in severe cases. Acetaminophen is unlikely to be of benefit in patients with hyperthermia because hyperthermia does not exhibit an elevation of the hypothalamic set point as is seen in fever. Amantadine and bromocriptine are dopamine agonists which have not been proven to be beneficial in patients with neuroleptic malignant syndrome. Haloperidol is an antipsychotic which might further exacerbate the pathophysiologic process in this case. Dantrolene, which blocks calcium release in muscle cells may afford some benefit but is unlikely to be more effective than benzodiazepines and paralytics.

34. Answer C. Patients with hypothyroidism who present with significantly altered mental status should be evaluated for myxedema coma. Though lacking precise definition, myxedema coma generally represents the extreme state of hypothyroidism, where the body's metabolic functions are essentially shutting down. Typical findings include bradycardia, hypotension, hypothermia, hypoventilation, hypoglycemia, anemia, etc. Because of decreased ventilatory drive, $Paco_2$ rises. Sodium levels are generally low, usually due to a syndrome of inappropriate diuretic hormone state. Reflexes are described as pseudomyotonic, which refers to the delayed relaxation phase and are one of the most common signs seen in hypothyroidism (though they are seen in other diseases as well). A normocytic normochromic anemia (anemic of chronic disease) is usually observed in hypothyroidism.

35. Answer C. Raynaud phenomenon is nearly universal in patients with scleroderma (also known as *systemic sclerosis*) and is the earliest sign of the disease. Raynaud phenomenon is also common in patients with lupus and RA. The exact mechanism of Raynaud phenomenon in scleroderma (or in other autoimmune diseases) is not known. Raynaud phenomenon may also be a primary problem (in which case it is sometimes referred to as *Raynaud disease*), rather than secondary to an underlying disease. To be considered a primary process, patients need to suffer no ischemic damage in the affected digits (e.g., gangrene, necrosis), have negative serology (e.g., particularly for antinuclear antibodies), have a normal erythrocyte sedimentation rate, have symmetric attacks, and lack physical examination findings which suggest a secondary cause.

36. Answer C. The modified diagnostic criteria for migraine defines migraine headache as a headache lasting 4 to 72 hours, that includes at least two of the following four symptoms:

Unilateral pain

Throbbing

Moderate to severe intensity

Pain aggravated by movement

And one of the following two symptoms:

Nausea or vomiting

Photophobia or phonophobia

Unfortunately, many of these symptoms are similar to those experienced by patients with cluster headaches. However, the pain in cluster headaches is typically described as "boring" or "tearing," despite being of severe intensity. Furthermore, pain associated with cluster headaches is almost always retro-orbital and in the temporal region (due to involvement of the V1 branch of the trigeminal nerve). Cluster headaches are not typically associated with nausea, vomiting, photophobia or phonophobia. The key difference between these two headache syndromes is the cyclic nature of cluster headache exacerbations and the stereotypical presentation of patients with cluster headaches. Sumatriptan is useful for the acute treatment of patients with either headache syndrome.

37. Answer C. The image demonstrates a small bowel obstruction (SBO). Postoperative adhesions account for more than 60% of cases, malignant neoplasms account for approximately 20%, and incarcerated hernias account for roughly 10% of cases. The classic mnemonic for the top three causes of small bowel obstruction is "ABC," representing adhesions, bulges (hernias), and cancer. However, neoplasms are actually the second most common cause. Since this patient has never had abdominal surgery, adhesive disease is not likely. Most tumors are metastatic lesions that cause extrinsic compression of the intestine secondary to peritoneal implants that have spread from an intra-abdominal primary tumor such as from the colon, ovary, or pancreas. The most common hernias to result in obstruction are ventral and inguinal hernias. Flat (or supine) films classically demonstrate multiple dilated loops of small intestine in a "stepladder" pattern without evidence of distal small bowel or colonic distention. Upright films demonstrate multiple air–fluid levels. As a general rule, the larger the number of dilated bowel loops, the more distal the obstruction. The overall sensitivity of plain films for SBO is roughly 60%. (Figure reprinted with permission from Fleisher GR, Baskin MN. *Atlas of Pediatric Emergency Medicine*. Philadelphia: Lippincott Williams & Wilkins; 2003.)

38. Answer A. Tranexamic acid is an antifibrinolytic lysine analogue that inhibits plasminogen activation through competitive inhibition at lysine-binding sites. The CRASH-2 trial was a multinational trauma trial that enrolled over 20,000 trauma patients with significant hemorrhage to study transexamic acid's impact on mortality as well as vascular occlusive events and blood transfusion. It was published in the Lancet in 2010 and revealed a decrease in overall mortality without a significant increase in thrombotic events compared to placebo. The trial showed no significant change in transfusion requirements. While the mortality benefit was relatively small (absolute risk reduction of 1.5%), tranexamic acid's safety profile and low cost make it a very useful adjunct in trauma patients with life-threatening hemorrhage. Though the trial allowed patients to receive the drug up to 8 hours after injury, subgroup analysis revealed that almost all the benefit occurred in patients receiving the drug within 3 hours after the injury.

39. Answer A. Somatization disorder refers to a constellation of physical symptoms that cannot be explained by a known medical condition. Pain, gastrointestinal, sexual, and neurologic symptoms predominate. An integral part of the diagnosis is that the patient is not faking the symptoms—he or she truly is experiencing them and will argue against any evidence that indicates somatization. Somatizing patients have an uncontrollable need to assume the "sick role," which allows them to be cared for. The most common personality disorder associated with somatizing patients is histrionic—well over half the number of patients meet the diagnostic criteria. Management of these patients in the ED involves empathetic recognition and acknowledgment of the patient's symptoms, evaluating for true medical illness as a cause of the symptoms, and referral to psychiatry or primary care for outpatient evaluation. It is crucial for the EP to review old records of patients suspected of somatization disorder, as these patients often undergo repeated unnecessary testing in the ED. Discussions with the patient's primary care physician is mandatory as this will help to tailor emergent workup. Pharmacotherapy is of little benefit in the acute setting.

40. Answer A. The incidence of *B. pertussis* infection is rising, with the number of reported cases in the United States increasing sixfold since 1980. This has occurred despite immunization rates of 80% among young children. Most of the increase is due to an increased number of adolescents and adults diagnosed with the disease. Furthermore, it is widely thought that the true scope of the problem is grossly underestimated because of the failure of physicians to recognize the illness, as well as their failure to report the illness when it is diagnosed. Almost all cases of pertussis in adolescents and adults occur in patients who have been previously *vaccinated* or in patients who have been previously infected with *B. pertussis*. Contrary to popular belief, neither *B. pertussis* infection nor vaccination with either the cellular or acellular vaccine confers lifelong immunity. In fact, natural infection with *B. pertussis* results in approximately 15 years of immunity to reinfection. This is much greater than the 4 to 8 years worth of immunity offered by the vaccines (the acellular vaccine, which is currently used in the United States, offers a shorter duration of immunity than the cellular vaccine, roughly from 4 to 6 years). The recommended vaccination schedule in the United States advises that infants be vaccinated at 2, 4, and 6 months of age, with boosters at 18 months and then again between 4 and 6 years. Therefore, most children born in the United States should carry immunity through the ages of 10 to 12 years. Since the most severe illness occurs in children less than 1 year, adolescents and adults have not been offered booster shots beyond childhood. However, because of the rising incidence of recognized disease in adolescents and adults, as well as the likely enormous asymptomatic disease burden in this population, the CDC and the US Advisory Committee on Immunization Practices (ACIP) now recommends that all adults under 65 receive a single acellular booster along with tetanus and diphtheria in Tdap (Boostrix), which is often given in the ED in the setting of trauma (in place of isolated tetanus toxoid). Patients >65 years old receive Adacel, a different Tdap formulation. *B. pertussis* infection in adults ranges from subclinical infection to a prolonged illness mostly characterized by a nagging, paroxysmal cough, which may interfere with sleep. The mean duration of illness in adults is 36 to 48 days. Erythromycin is the drug of choice for the treatment of *B. pertussis* infection although azithromycin and clarithromycin have been shown to be equally efficacious with fewer side effects. TMP-SMX is an additional alternative. Erythromycin is also recommended for prophylaxis of individuals who have come into contact with patients who are infected. It is thought to be effective in preventing disease as long as it is given before the onset of symptoms. Owing to the decreased infectivity of *B. pertussis* as the disease progresses, prophylaxis is generally unnecessary in individuals who come into contact with a patient who has been symptomatic for >3 weeks.

41. **Answer D.** The patient has scattered human bite marks, which are circular in nature and have a perforated, erythematous border. Human bites are a common sign of child abuse. Management involves tetanus prophylaxis, treatment of associated cellulitis, and notification of appropriate social services. The rash of Henoch–Schönlein purpura presents as palpable purpura on the buttocks and lower extremities. ITP presents as nonpalpable petechiae and purpura with laboratory evidence of low platelets. The rash of Lyme disease, erythema migrans, is an erythematous rash with central clearing, classically on the trunk in a patient with travel to an endemic area. Roseola presents as sudden onset of fever in young

children, followed by a generalized macular rash after the patient has completely defervesced. (Figure from Reece RM, Ludwig S. *Child Abuse: Medical Diagnosis and Management.* 2nd ed. Philadelphia, PA: Lippincott Williams & Wilkins, 2001;150, with permission.)

42. **Answer A.** Initial treatment of thyroid storm consists of beta-blockers (usually propranolol), a thionamide (propylthiouracil or methimazole), glucocorticoids, and cholestyramine. Beta-blockers are critical to blunt the impact of increased adrenergic tone often resulting in significant tachycardia or atrial fibrillation. Sinus tachycardia is the most common dysrhythmia in thyroid storm. Propranolol should be used cautiously in patients with overt CHF. Glucocorticoids are useful because patients with thyroid storm may develop relative adrenal insufficiency as a result of the increased metabolic demands. In addition, high-dose corticosteroids inhibit release of thyroid hormone from the thyroid gland as well as peripheral conversion of T_4 to T_3. Thionamides block new hormone synthesis. Cholestyramine is a bile acid sequestrant that reduces enterohepatic recirculation of thyroid hormone. Iodine-containing preparations such as SSKI or potassium iodide–iodine (Lugol solution) are useful adjuncts in thyroid storm because they decrease T_3 and T_4 release from the thyroid. However, they should not be used until 1 hour after thionamides are given since administration of iodine before thionamides increases thyroid hormone synthesis and could worsen the patient's symptoms and outcome. Most patients with thyroid storm have underlying Graves disease, which is the most common cause of hyperthyroidism. Hashimoto disease is the most common noniatrogenic cause of primary *hypo*thyroidism (although it may cause a transient thyrotoxicosis in its acute phase).

43. **Answer B.** The chief use of EKG in the evaluation of patients with a suspected PE is to rule out the presence of other causes of chest pain such as myocardial ischemia or acute MI and pericarditis. Numerous EKG findings have been reported in the setting of acute PE, although "$S_1Q_3T_3$" is perhaps the most famous. Several papers have reliably refuted the utility of this finding. $S_1Q_3T_3$ was first described in a 1935 study of seven patients who all likely had massive pulmonary embolus. Similar studies have all been plagued by a selection bias for patients with large or massive PE. Several EKG findings are more specific in patients with massive PE, but other clinical signs and symptoms (e.g., hypoxia, dyspnea, tachypnea, and chest pain) are typically more useful than EKG.

44. **Answer A.** The patient has a corneal abrasion, indicated by the fluorescein uptake in the cornea. Management of corneal abrasions is with topical antibiotics to prevent infection and occasionally cycloplegics to help reduce painful iris contraction. Steroids should never be given in

patients with corneal abrasions—use of topical steroids should be contingent on ophthalmologic recommendation. Eye patching was once thought to be effective for corneal abrasions and is now thought to increase the possibility of infection. (Figure From Reece RM, Ludwig S. *Child Abuse: Medical Diagnosis and management.* 2nd Ed. Philadelphia, PA: Lippincott Williams & Wilkins, 2001.)

45. **Answer B.** Etomidate does transiently reduce adrenal function (<24 hours in duration) but this decrease has not been shown to increase mortality. Several studies raised the possibility that the reduced adrenal function could cause increased mortality in septic shock patients but subsequent analyses showed that this was not true. Ketamine, not etomidate, can cause increased intracranial pressure and laryngospasm. Thiopental is a reasonable induction agent for rapid sequence intubation, but attempting to use a new drug for the first time is not a sound strategy for a critically ill patient when other alternatives are available. Etomidate does have side effects such as myoclonus, vomiting, and reduced adrenal function, but none of these is associated with increased mortality. Choice E lies well outside the normal bounds of professionalism and violates basic tenets of patient safety organizations.

46. **Answer E.** Fibromyalgia syndrome is a noninflammatory condition of chronic hypersensitivity of muscles in response to painful stimuli. Patients with fibromyalgia syndrome experience pain at lower thresholds of somatic stimuli. Over 90% of patients with fibromyalgia exhibit fatigue and over 50% carry a concomitant diagnosis of mood disorder. Sleep is frequently affected as well. Elevations in CPK are found in diagnoses such as polymyositis, steroid myopathy, and rhabdomyolysis but are absent in fibromyalgia. ESR and CRP elevations are seen in polymyalgia rheumatica and other inflammatory diseases, not fibromyalgia syndrome. Jaw claudication is frequently seen in temporal arteritis, which can occur concomitantly with polymyalgia rheumatica, not fibromyalgia syndrome.

47. **Answer A.** Patients with tibial shaft fractures usually have concomitant fibular fractures as well, due to the close proximity of the two bones. Mechanism of injury usually involves direct trauma; only rarely do pathologic fractures occur in the tibia. Due to the sparse soft tissue surrounding the anterior surface of the tibia, fractures are often open and require emergent operative repair. The most common site for compartment syndrome is in the leg, due to tibial fracture. The common peroneal nerve is the most common nerve to be injured in tibial fractures, but this does not occur in most patients. Vascular compromise with tibial fractures is rare, but when present, mandates aggressive management.

48. **Answer A.** Hypernatremia is almost always caused by the loss of free water and rarely by sodium gain (which is usually iatrogenic). Regardless of the underlying cause, it almost never occurs in alert patients with an intact thirst mechanism. It is a known complication of multiple doses of activated charcoal, occurring in 6% of patients receiving such therapy. Treatment with saline should only occur in patients who have hemodynamic compromise. Almost all patients, however, require treatment with half-normal saline or more dilute solutions with lower tonicity. The main complication of therapy is cerebral edema, so the rate of correction should be 0.5 to 1.0 mEq/L/hour on average (though it may be more rapid for the initial few hours if the patient is suffering life-threatening complications of hypernatremia). Central pontine myelinolysis is a complication of therapy for hyponatremia.

49. **Answer D.** Posterior hip dislocations account for 90% of all hip dislocations. The most common mechanism of injury is a "dashboard injury," in which a seated patient strikes the dashboard with a flexed knee, driving the femur posteriorly. Owing to the force required to dislocate the well-protected hip joint, posterior hip dislocations are often associated with multisystem trauma. Patients will present with a shortened leg, with the hip internally rotated, adducted, and slightly flexed. Approximately 10% of posterior hip dislocations are associated with sciatic nerve injury, which is usually a neuropraxia. After reduction, this is manifest by hamstring weakness as well as weakness of all lower leg muscles, loss of ankle reflex, and hypoesthesia of the posterior thigh and complete lower leg. Posterior hip dislocations must be reduced emergently because of the high risk of avascular necrosis of the femoral head. Films should be obtained before reduction to determine the presence of associated femur or pelvis fractures, however, unless a pulse deficit is present. Femoral head fractures are much more common in anterior femoral dislocations, occurring in as many as 77% of patients versus only 10% of patients with posterior dislocations. Because the femur is internally rotated and adducted, the shadow of the lesser trochanter is not seen on an AP projection. This is one critical tool to help differentiate posterior dislocations from anterior dislocations. Another is to examine the size of the femoral head. Because the posteriorly dislocated femoral head is closer to the x-ray cassette, it often appears smaller than the unaffected femoral head.

50. **Answer D.** As many as a third of deliveries involve a loop of umbilical cord wrapped around the baby's neck, called a nuchal cord. Most evidence suggests that such cords do not worsen fetal outcome at delivery. However, tightly wrapped cords can impede delivery, or sometimes entangle themselves into a knot which could restrict blood flow to the fetus. If the umbilical cord

can't be slipped over the baby's head while in the birth canal, the cord should be quickly double-clamped and cut before the delivery is completed as rapidly as possible. In cases in which there is enough slack in the cord, delivery could proceed without manipulating the cord further. Crowning is a sign of imminent delivery. Do not attempt to push the baby back into the vaginal canal. While the baby's airway should be suctioned before delivery is completed, delivery takes priority over all else since it is impossible to properly resuscitate a neonate while it remains in the birth canal.

51. **Answer B.** The patient does not have definitive evidence of SBP. Diagnosis of SBP is suspected with an ascitic fluid neutrophil count >250 cells per mm^3. In this case, the neutrophil count is 180 cells per mm^3 (i.e., 60% × 300). Leukocyte esterase testing with urine dipstick on ascitic fluid has a high negative predictive value for SBP and may be used as an earlier marker to exclude the diagnosis. SBP is caused by combination of reduced hepatic phagocytotic activity with a protein-poor (therefore, complement-poor) ascitic fluid environment. The incidence of SBP occurs at about 25% of all cirrhotic patients per year. Gram-negative organisms predominate, most commonly *E. coli* and *Klebsiella*, though streptococci are also well represented. It is crucial to note that up to half of all patients with SBP lack fever and only a minority have significant abdominal tenderness or true rebound tenderness. Treatment with cefotaxime would be the appropriate regimen for SBP. Vancomycin and metronidazole do not adequately cover gram-negative organisms and should not be used alone in the treatment of SBP.

52. **Answer E.** CVT is a rare cause of stroke and is extremely variable in its presentation. The most common presenting symptom is headache. In contrast to arterial stroke, patients with CVT present acutely only 30% of the time, subacutely (more than 2 days after symptom onset) in 50% of cases, and chronically (more than 1 month after symptom onset) in 20% of cases. The area of the sinus involved determines the symptoms. The most common sinuses to be affected are the superior sagittal sinus, the cavernous sinus, and the transverse (or lateral) sinus. Thrombosis of other sinuses is less common but may be underdiagnosed because of the difficulty in recognizing the manifestations of thrombosis. MRI and magnetic resonance venography is the gold standard for diagnosis. Although changes consistent with CVT may be visible on CT, its sensitivity is inadequate to exclude the disorder, as it may be normal in up to 30% of cases. Heparin is the mainstay of therapy, even in patients with evidence of hemorrhage, although some patients may be candidates for catheter-directed thrombolysis. In general, CVT has a better outcome than arterial stroke, although patients with deep cerebral and cerebellar venous thrombosis have poor outcomes. Women with CVT outnumber men by a ratio of 3:1, in part due to the use of oral contraceptives and because of the increased risk of venous thrombosis surrounding pregnancy and the immediate postpartum period. Although either focal or generalized seizures may occur, most seizures are focal due to the focal irritation of the cortex affected by the thrombosis.

53. **Answer C.** A passive leg raise is performed by first having the patient sit semi-upright with their head elevated at about 45 degrees, with their legs flat on the bed. After a few minutes, the head is placed flat, and the legs are elevated to 45 degrees. This results in a transient central fluid bolus of as much as 300 mL, caused by moving fluid that had pooled in the legs to the intrathoracic cavity. Patients who are fluid responsive should experience a rise in blood pressure. In this case, an increase in blood pressure is a surrogate for improved cardiac output. One study showed that patients needed at least a 17% increase in systolic blood pressure to be considered "fluid responsive." An alternative to using blood pressure is to use a noninvasive means of assessing cardiac output such as a NICOM device or by following EtCO$_2$ in mechanically ventilated patients. Since this patient had no improvement after a passive leg raise, he is *not* fluid responsive, so the next step is start vasopressors.

54. **Answer D.** Due to rising resistance rates to trimethoprim–sulfamethoxazole, first-generation cephalosporins, and amoxicillin–clavulanic acid, oral second- or third-generation cephalosporins should be the first choice for treating uncomplicated pediatric cystitis. Cefixime is a highly efficacious third-generation cephalosporin. Other choices include cefdinir, cefpodoxime, ceftibuten. TMP-SMX can be the initial drug of choice if local resistance rates are low. Ciprofloxacin is a first-line agent for treatment of adult UTIs, but concerns about musculoskeletal effects in children have prevented its use in the pediatric population. Doxycycline is not typically used to treat UTIs and has traditionally been contraindicated in children because it is thought to stain tooth enamel although more recent data suggest that this doesn't occur at doses and durations typically used in treating most conventional infections.

55. **Answer E.** Management of bacterial meningitis involves steroid therapy to help reduce inflammation as well as antibiotics that can cross the blood brain barrier. Vancomycin and ceftriaxone are effective against the major pathogens seen in bacterial meningitis (*Streptococcus pneumoniae, Neisseria meningitidis,* and *Haemophilus influenza*). Importantly, in patients at extremes of age, *Listeria monocytogenes* becomes more prevalent and requires specific therapy with ampicillin. In this patient, dexamethasone, vancomycin, ceftriaxone, and ampicillin are all warranted.

56. **Answer B.** Drowning victims can develop serious, delayed pulmonary complications, such as acute respiratory distress syndrome and pneumonia. Observation of symptomatic or hypoxic patients is indicated. Arterial blood gas can be helpful in evaluating for hypercarbia, which is more difficult to assess noninvasively than hypoxia. Corticosteroids and prophylactic antibiotics have not been shown to improve outcomes in drowning victim patients (or other aspiration patients). Endotracheal intubation should be reserved for patients with altered mental status, hypercarbia, or hypoxemia refractory to maximal mask oxygen.

57. **Answer A.** The lateral or fibular collateral ligament complex comprises three ligaments that tend to rupture in an anterior to posterior sequence during ankle sprains. The anterior talofibular ligament is the weakest, and rupture results in a positive anterior ankle drawer test. The calcaneofibular is next and the posterior talofibular is the most posterior portion of the fibular collateral ligament. The deltoid ligament is 20% to 50% stronger than its lateral counterpart and is *infrequently* injured in isolation. The anterior inferior tibiofibular ligament is the weakest ligament of the four syndesmotic ligaments that attach the distal tibia and fibula. The syndesmosis prevents displacement of the tibia and fibula relative to one another, and disruption can contribute to significant instability.

58. **Answer A.** Due to the appearance of the nail, the cause of chronic paronychia has traditionally been attributed to fungal superinfection. However, studies demonstrate a much better response to topical glucocorticoids than to oral antifungals. Thus, it is most likely due to an underlying dermatitis and is most likely a manifestation of eczema. As a result, patients are instructed to keep their hands dry and use gloves for any type of wet work.

59. **Answer E.** The patient's acute gastroenteritis is likely from food poisoning with a preformed toxin. The most common causes are *Clostridium perfringens* and *S. aureus*. Management for both toxin-induced and viral gastroenteritis involves supportive care only. Antibiotics are of no value as the toxin is already preformed. Stool leukocytes are rarely helpful in the management of gastroenteritis as they seldom change management due to poor specificity. Ova and parasite examination is helpful in cases of subacute, watery diarrhea lasting longer than 1 week and is not routinely used in acute diarrheal episodes.

60. **Answer B.** Despite their widespread use, verbal and written "contracts for safety" or "no-harm contracts" have not been shown to reduce suicide rates, are discouraged by the APA, and do not increase liability protection. Instead, their use can actually increase liability risk, and their use risks alienating patients, particularly if they are used as an administrative procedure in place of a thorough evaluation to assess actual risk. Such contracts were initially described in a paper by Drye et al. in 1973, in which the contract was used as a risk assessment tool in outpatients with whom the physician had already established rapport. Patients who responded to the contract's firm statements in a negative manner were thought to be at higher risk of future suicide. While the initial researchers did not advocate widespread use of such contracts in crisis settings, their use rapidly expanded nonetheless. Physicians can effectively use such contracts as a tool to express concern about a suicidal patient, but such contracts should never be used as a means to justify discharge or mitigate liability risk.

61. **Answer C.** The patient is presenting in septic shock from an unclear source. She presents from a nursing home, where rates of methicillin-resistant *S. aureus* (MRSA) and *P. aeruginosa* are extremely high. Treatment involves broad-spectrum antibiotic coverage to cover both these pathogens. Metronidazole and clindamycin afford excellent anaerobic coverage, but piperacillin–tazobactam also kills anaerobes and double coverage of anaerobes is not routinely indicated. Choice B would be a reasonable regimen in a patient with septic shock who is not at risk for nosocomial pathogens.

62. **Answer B.** Signs and symptoms of shock may be misleading in the pregnant trauma patient. Acid–base abnormalities such as decreased bicarbonate or elevated lactate or base deficit are the earliest indicators of maternal shock. Due to an increased intravascular volume, pregnant patients will often not develop hypotension or tachycardia until significantly more blood volume is lost than their nonpregnant peers. Thus, early crystalloid administration is indicated to sustain the patient's increased blood volume and to avoid fetal hypoperfusion. If blood loss occurs more gradually, a pregnant woman can lose as much as 35% of her blood volume before the development of blatantly abnormal vital signs. Additionally, because of the physiologic decrease in peripheral vascular tone during pregnancy, pregnant patients in shock may remain warm and dry even in the setting of shock. Finally, abdominal examination is less sensitive in pregnant patients. As many as 50% of pregnant patients with hemoperitoneum will not have peritoneal signs on physical examination. Therefore, ED physicians need to maintain a high suspicion for injury and a low threshold for further diagnostic testing.

63. **Answer C.** The x-ray demonstrates a Salter–Harris III fracture of the distal radius. The Salter–Harris classification is used to describe pediatric long bone fractures near the growth plate. Type I fractures go through the physis only, type II from the metaphysis into the physis, type III from the epiphysis into the physis, type IV is a

combination of types II and III, and type V is a crush injury to the physis. The most common is type II. Types I and V may be invisible on initial plain films. Type V carries the poorest prognosis. (Figure courtesy of Mark Silverberg, MD. In: Greenberg MI, Hendrickson RG, Silverberg M, et al., eds. *Greenberg's Text-Atlas of Emergency Medicine.* Philadelphia, PA: Lippincott Williams & Wilkins; 2004, with permission.)

64. **Answer A.** Biphasic anaphylactic reactions, in which there is a second episode of anaphylaxis that follows complete resolution of the initial episode, are relatively uncommon. Studies about incidence vary, but only about 10% of patients will suffer a biphasic reaction. The incidence may depend on the allergen but there aren't enough data to answer this question. The biggest risk factors for biphasic reactions appear to be high severity of the initial reaction as well as suboptimal or delayed treatment of the initial reaction. When anaphylaxis occurs a second time, it tends to occur at least 10 hours after the initial episode and tends to be less severe. High-dose steroids have not been shown to benefit patients with anaphylaxis even if they are nearly universally included in patient treatment plans. Some investigators theorize that early steroid administration may decrease the incidence of biphasic reactions but there is no evidence to support the claim.

65. **Answer A.** This patient has Henoch–Schönlein purpura (HSP), a small-vessel vasculitis that primarily affects children who present with palpable purpura, arthralgias, abdominal pain, and glomerulonephritis. Purpura is present in 100% of patients, although 75% of patients have arthralgias, typically of the ankles, 65% have abdominal pain, and 40% have renal involvement. Prognosis depends on the presence and severity of renal involvement. Colicky abdominal pain is the most common gastrointestinal manifestation, though vomiting, bleeding, and more rarely, intussusception, may occur. In contrast to the typical ileocolic intussusception that occurs in the general population, patients with HSP experience ileoileal intussusception 70% of the time. In the absence of renal disease, HSP is self-limited and only supportive care is required. In the setting of hematuria or proteinuria, corticosteroids may be beneficial but renal consultation should be sought. When present in adults, HSP is a much more severe disease due to the increased frequency and severity of nephritis. (Figure reprinted with permission from Fleisher GR, Baskin MN. *Atlas of Pediatric Emergency Medicine.* Philadelphia, PA: Lippincott Williams & Wilkins; 2003.)

66. **Answer B.** Myringitis, which is inflammation of the tympanic membrane, is a rare occurrence in the setting of *Mycoplasma* infections and is not required to establish a diagnosis. Furthermore, the presence of myringitis,

bullous or not, is not pathognomonic for *Mycoplasma* infection as a host of other etiologies are possible. *Mycoplasma* commonly occurs in outbreaks in closed communities such as camps, military bases, hospitals, religious groups, and facilities for the mentally ill. Neurologic complications occur in 6% to 7% of children *hospitalized* with *Mycoplasma* infections, and may include aseptic meningitis, encephalitis, and Guillain–Barré paralysis, among other complications. Cold agglutinins are autoantibodies directed toward RBCs, which have been antigenically altered by *Mycoplasma*. Their titers do not rise to detectable levels until approximately 2 weeks after infection and they may not be present in all patients. *Mycoplasma* is not a common cause of pneumonia in the elderly.

67. **Answer A.** The patient has acute arterial occlusion from arterial embolism, likely due to atrial fibrillation caused by hyperthyroidism. Treatment involves anticoagulation and emergent embolectomy due to the limb-threatening nature of the occlusion. Bypass surgery is usually used in patients who have in situ thrombosis. Anticoagulation alone is used as adjunctive ED therapy for patients with acute arterial occlusion, but it is usually not adequate to treat limb-threatening ischemia due to an embolus. Lumbar sympathectomy and hyperbaric oxygen therapy provide no benefit in these circumstances.

68. **Answer B.** The serotonin syndrome is classically described as a triad of cognitive abnormalities, autonomic hyperactivity, and neuromuscular problems. However, there is considerable variability in the severity of the presentation and considerable overlap of the clinical findings with neuroleptic malignant syndrome as well as the anticholinergic toxidrome. Clonus is the most important clinical finding to help differentiate the serotonin syndrome from similar clinical conditions. Clonus may be spontaneous, inducible, or isolated to the ocular muscles. Thus, physicians must perform a thorough, focused examination to specifically look for this finding.

69. **Answer A.** Eighty percent to 90% of objects that have made it into the stomach will pass through the remainder of the GI tract without difficulty. However, as many as 15% to 35% of sharp or pointed objects may cause perforation if untreated. The ileocecal valve is the most common site of perforation. Objects that are in the stomach are amenable to endoscopic removal, but objects distal to this point generally cannot be retrieved. Because this child is asymptomatic, there is no indication for surgery at this point. Surgery is only indicated in cases of perforation, hemorrhage, fistula formation, or obstruction. Because this child has a relatively high risk of perforation, he cannot be discharged home. Appropriate management includes daily abdominal radiographs

to follow the passage of the object. Surgical management should be individualized but may be considered if the object fails to pass for a number of days. (Figure reprinted with permission from Fleisher GR, Baskin MN. *Atlas of Pediatric Emergency Medicine.* Philadelphia, PA: Lippincott Williams & Wilkins; 2003.)

70. **Answer B.** Diarrhea is the most common cause of a normal anion gap metabolic acidosis. Fluid from the intestine distal to the stomach is bicarbonate-rich, so diarrhea results in bicarbonate loss and subsequent metabolic acidosis. As bicarbonate is lost, chloride is avidly reabsorbed by the kidneys resulting in a hyperchloremic metabolic acidosis.

71. **Answer E.** Prostaglandin E1 can maintain the patency of the ductus arteriosus which allows mixing between the left (aorta) and right (pulmonary artery) sides of the circulation. Thus, a patient with any ductal dependent lesion will benefit from a prostaglandin E1 infusion. These lesions include both cyanotic and noncyanotic lesions. Left-sided lesions include critical aortic stenosis, critical coarctation, hypoplastic left heart syndrome, and interrupted aortic arch. Right-sided lesions include tetralogy of Fallot with pulmonary atresia, tricuspid atresia, and critical pulmonic stenosis. Transposition of the great arteries is also duct-dependent and as it consists of parallel circulations, it exists in a category by itself.

72. **Answer E.** The patient presents after benzodiazepine overdose and may or may not have coingested alcohol. The history of chronic alcohol use and altered mental status dictates the use of thiamine therapy, along with folate, multivitamin, magnesium, and dextrose. Fomepizole is indicated only in cases of toxic alcohol poisoning. Flumazenil, a specific benzodiazepine antagonist, is contraindicated here, as it can precipitate withdrawal seizures in patients who are chronically using benzodiazepines. Physostigmine is an acetylcholinesterase inhibitor used in selected patients with anticholinergic toxicity. Glucagon is used in patients with β-blocker and calcium channel blocker toxicity.

73. **Answer E.** The patient has an infected kidney stone, which, at 7 mm, is very unlikely to pass spontaneously. This represents a true emergency and will likely require specific urologic management. The patient should be admitted to the hospital and given intravenous fluids, analgesics, antiemetics, and antibiotics after urinary culture has been sent. Other indications for emergent urologic consultation in patients with kidney stones are the presence of acute renal failure, high-grade obstruction due to the calculus in a patient with only one kidney, and a stone >5 mm with intractable symptoms of pain and/or nausea. Discharging the patient with an infected kidney stone without urologic approval is contraindicated.

MRI will not add significantly to this patient's diagnosis or management and is an unnecessary waste of time.

74. **Answer B.** Bupropion is an atypical antidepressant with dopamine reuptake inhibitory properties. Seizure is the most likely severe effect in overdose and can occur up to 24 hours after ingestion. Seizures can even occur in patients who are taking therapeutic doses of bupropion. They cannot be predicted by clinical or laboratory data and patients with bupropion overdose should be monitored for 24 hours postingestion. Coma, dysrhythmia, hypotension, and hypertension are not common with bupropion ingestion and suggest coingestion of another drug.

75. **Answer E.** Mechanical device CPR has not been shown to increase survival to hospital discharge over manual CPR. It may increase the ability of first responders to safely carry out other tasks, but no well-designed study has demonstrated an increase in patient survival. Epinephrine does not increase survival to hospital discharge in patients with sudden cardiac arrest—it may increase return of spontaneous circulation. Vasopressin has been removed from the 2015 AHA guidelines for out-of-hospital cardiac arrest management as it is no more effective than epinephrine and it unnecessarily increases complexity of management. Defibrillation is not effective in patients with pulseless electrical activity.

76. **Answer D.** AFE is a rare complication of pregnancy also known as the *anaphylactoid syndrome of pregnancy.* Through a still unclear mechanism, amniotic fluid gains entry into the maternal circulation and triggers as immense inflammatory cascade resulting in pulmonary vasoconstriction, pulmonary capillary leak, and myocardial depression. Clinically, patients develop acute hypoxia, hypotension, and altered mental status. Disseminated intravascular coagulation and seizures may also occur. In patients with eclamptic seizures, however, hypertension will be present instead of the profound shock of AFE. AFE most commonly occurs during labor and delivery or within 30 minutes of delivery. Though there are a variety of experimental treatments, treatment is supportive and the mortality rate is high with most survivors suffering permanent neurologic injury.

77. **Answer E.** "Crossed signs," in which a patient has unilateral cranial nerve deficits but contralateral hemiparesis and hemisensory loss are diagnostic of brainstem infarction. The vertebral arteries, which have their origin from the subclavian arteries, merge to form the basilar artery at the pontomedullary junction. At the junction of the pons and the midbrain, the basilar artery again separates into the two posterior cerebral arteries. The brainstem, from the medulla to the midbrain, is therefore supplied by branches of the vertebrobasilar arterial

system. The facial nucleus, which originates within the pons, may be infarcted when branches of the basilar artery are occluded. As the infarction involves the facial nucleus, the entire face, including the forehead, is affected. As the descending corticospinal tract has not yet reached the medullary decussation, occlusion on one side of the pons affects the descending motor fibers reaching the contralateral body and results in contralateral hemiparesis. When this syndrome includes an ipsilateral rectus palsy, it is known as *Millard–Gubler syndrome* due to infarction of both the facial and abducens nuclei, which are in very close proximity in the pons. Infarction of the basilar artery proper is typically a catastrophic event, resulting in quadriplegia and often respiratory failure and death.

78. **Answer C.** Although there is no consensus, a cumulative dose of 5 rads has been proposed as an acceptable threshold for safe fetal exposure. Intrauterine exposure of 10 rads is associated with a small increase in the number of childhood cancers, but does not result in an increase in fetal malformations, spontaneous abortion, or growth retardation. Maternal plain films of the head, cervical spine, thoracic spine, chest, and extremities each expose the fetus to <5 mrad (i.e., 1,000 times less than the safe threshold). Plain films of the lumbar spine, hip, and pelvis expose the fetus to higher doses, but none of these studies comes close to approaching 5 rads. CT scanning of the abdomen, however, results in approximately 2.6 rads of fetal exposure. In comparison to these films, the cumulative radiation exposure to fetus over a 9-month gestation is between 50 and 100 mrad (far more than a single chest x-ray). Lead shielding of the maternal abdomen can reduce fetal exposure by 50% to 75%. The risk to the fetus during the first 2 weeks of pregnancy is so low that normal radiographic procedure can be used. The period of highest risk is between 2 and 7 weeks (organogenesis). Finally, FAST examination is poorly sensitive in the second and third trimesters. Therefore, CT scanning should be performed in all patients in whom abdominal injury is suspected.

79. **Answer A.** The x-ray reveals a tibial plateau fracture. These injuries usually require operative management. Given the location in the tibia, compartment syndrome is definitely possible and should be guarded against. Lateral collateral ligament injuries are more common than medial collateral ligament injuries, but neither is seen in most cases. Neurologic injuries can certainly occur, but are not seen in the majority of cases. Lateral tibial plateau fractures represent the majority of cases. Radiographs can be negative with tibial plateau fracture up to 20% of the time. (Figure from Bucholz RW, Heckman JD. *Rockwood & Green's Fractures in Adults.* 5th ed. Philadelphia, PA: Lippincott Williams & Wilkins; 2001.)

80. **Answer D.** Ascites is the most common complication of cirrhosis, occurring in roughly 60% of patients with compensated cirrhosis for 10 years. Spontaneous bacterial peritonitis is a complication of ascites and occurs in 8% to 25% of patients with cirrhosis and ascites. Esophageal varices are also common and occur in 25% to 40% of patients with cirrhosis. Of those patients, 30% develop bleeding within 2 years. Hepatic encephalopathy is also a common complication, but its incidence depends on the criteria used to diagnose encephalopathy. It most commonly presents as a sleep disturbance, although patients may have trouble with mood, disorientation, or speech.

81. **Answer B.** Though the parents may not be aware of it, by bringing the child to the ED and requesting an examination, they have triggered EMTALA, the Emergency Medical Treatment and Active Labor Act, that requires hospitals to provide an MSE to any person who comes to the ED and requests examination or treatment; and if an emergency medical condition is determined to exist, provide necessary stabilizing treatment or an appropriate transfer. It is not appropriate to delay the MSE despite the parents' consent. It is appropriate to explain to the patient's parents that by bringing her to the ED, they have triggered a federal law that requires you to screen the child for an emergency medical condition. It may be helpful to add that if no emergency medical condition is found to exist, no treatment or services will be provided to the child without their consent. In cases in which the child has a clear emergency condition (e.g., bleeding profusely, or in respiratory distress), it is appropriate to provide any necessary treatment to prevent the child's death or deterioration of her condition regardless of the parents' wishes.

82. **Answer A.** Owing to cortical atrophy, elderly patients have more intracranial space to accommodate the edema associated with large strokes. Therefore, herniation syndromes are more common in younger patients with less baseline atrophy. Overall, medical treatment of cerebral edema is poor. Patients frequently receive corticosteroids, osmotherapy in the form of mannitol or furosemide, or endotracheal intubation followed by hyperventilation as a means of decreasing elevated ICP due to cerebral edema. None of these methods has been conclusively proved to improve outcome. Corticosteroids, in particular, have only been shown to increase the rate of infections, gastrointestinal bleeding, and hyperglycemia. The effects of hyperventilation last 1 to 24 hours, whereas osmotherapy lasts for 48 to 72 hours. While hyperventilation has been part of the standard approach for the management of elevated ICP in the setting of trauma, the resulting hypocapnia causes cerebral vasoconstriction which limits cerebral blood flow, which in turn, can worsen cerebral ischemia. Thus,

hyperventilation has largely been abandoned as a treatment modality for traumatic elevations of ICP. Cerebral edema following ischemic stroke occurs within 24 to 36 hours but typically does not peak for several days.

83. **Answer A.** One-time azithromycin dosing is the standard of care for chlamydial infection. Doxycycline therapy for 7 days is also reasonable, but it carries with it the risk of significant reaction due to photosensitivity. A lifeguard is likely to be exposed to significant sunlight and doxycycline would not be the best choice for this patient. Albendazole is an antiparasitic used in neurocysticercosis infection and does not have a role in chlamydial infection. Ceftriaxone would be the drug of choice for patients with gonococcal infection. Vancomycin is not considered an appropriate treatment for uncomplicated chlamydial infection.

84. **Answer A.** The spleen is the most common organ injured in blunt abdominal trauma. In order of decreasing frequency, it is followed by the liver, kidney, small bowel, bladder, colon, diaphragm, pancreas, and retroperitoneal duodenum.

85. **Answer C.** The patient has evidence of methemoglobinemia, with cyanosis, unresponsive hypoxemia on pulse oximetry, and dark-colored blood. Oxidation of iron from the ferrous to the ferric state prevents hemoglobin from carrying oxygen. Among the answer choices, amyl nitrate is most likely to cause methemoglobinemia. Co-oximetry must be performed to accurately calculate the oxygen saturation. Treatment is with methylene blue to reduce methemoglobin back to hemoglobin. Lorazepam, like other benzodiazepines, may cause sedation and hypotension. Dextromethorphan may cause an opioid toxidrome with sedation, constricted pupils, and respiratory depression. Diphenhydramine causes an anticholinergic state, with sedation, tachycardia, dry mucous membranes, and mydriasis. Ketamine causes a dissociated state of altered mental status with preserved respiratory reflexes.

86. **Answer A.** *E. coli* is isolated in 47% to 55% of the cases of SBP and gram-negative organisms are the most common etiologic agents as a group. *K. pneumoniae* is the second most commonly isolated organism. This is followed by *S. pneumoniae*, and other *Streptococcus* and *Staphylococcus* species. Although there have been isolated reports of anaerobic and polymicrobial infections in SBP, they are generally not considered to be causes of SBP. Fever or abdominal pain in a patient with ascites should raise the suspicion of infection and prompt a paracentesis. The presentation of SBP may be subtle, however, and include only mental status changes without abdominal pain or tenderness upon examination. All patients with an ascitic fluid neutrophil count

≥250 per mm^3 and a clinical picture consistent with infection should be treated with antibiotic therapy.

87. **Answer C.** Eyelids do not contain subcutaneous fat—the presence of fat indicates likely globe injury. Patients with globe injuries should be seen emergently by the ophthalmologist. ED management involves broad-spectrum antibiotics, eye shielding, avoidance of recumbent position or Valsalva maneuvers, tetanus immunization, and treatment of nausea and vomiting. Choices A, B, D, and E are potential indications for ophthalmologic or plastic surgical repair to prevent significant cosmetic defects.

88. **Answer D.** The patient presents in stage IV hemorrhagic shock, with tachycardia, hypotension, and alteration of mental status. These patients will require both crystalloid and colloid fluid resuscitation during the primary survey. Men in hemorrhagic shock can receive Rh positive or negative blood, but preferably should receive uncrossmatched O positive blood so that O negative stores can be reserve for women. Uncrossmatched blood is easily obtainable in the ED and may be given immediately, without laboratory analysis. The Rh factor may be positive in the donor unit when transfusing men and women beyond childbearing years, as there is no danger of formation of antibodies which might occur in future pregnancies in Rh negative women of childbearing age. Fresh frozen plasma is indicated to keep up with clotting factor losses when patients have received four to five units of packed red blood cell (RBC) transfusions during the course of a resuscitation.

89. **Answer C.** There is some disagreement regarding the optimal temperature for rewarming or thawing frost-bitten tissue. However, all authors agree that optimal rewarming occurs through immersion in a water bath with a closely regulated temperature. Most sources cite 40°C to 42°C as the optimal range, although temperatures as low as 35°C have been recommended as they tend to cause less pain during rewarming. Upon arrival, the affected area should be rapidly rewarmed for 15 to 30 minutes or until thawing is complete. Indicators of successful thawing include increased flexibility, erythema, and hyperemia. Rewarming can be intensely painful, and parenteral analgesics may be required, especially in cases of deep frostbite. Direct tissue massage should never be performed as it may cause increased tissue loss. In addition, field rewarming and rewarming with direct heat sources should never be performed because of the high risk of incomplete thawing and refreezing which results in increased tissue loss.

90. **Answer A.** Antibiotics are the most common cause of drug fever. In particular, penicillins, sulfonamides, and nitrofurantoin are common causes of drug fever,

although this may be due, in part, to their more widespread use since they have been in use for many years. Unfortunately, there is no diagnostic laboratory test. While the erythrocyte sedimentation rate (ESR) is often elevated, an elevated ESR is neither sensitive nor specific for drug fever. The presence of a rash may make drug fever more likely, although most patients don't have a rash at the time of diagnosis. Finally, the median time of onset is 8 days after starting the drug but is highly variable and not diagnostic.

91. **Answer D.** MRCP is the current preferred test for the diagnosis of stones in the common bile duct (CBD) among patients without a contraindication (e.g., pacemaker). While ERCP is effective, MRCP is noninvasive, and easy to perform. Although transabdominal US is the gold standard for the diagnosis of cholelithiasis, only 50% of stones in the CBD can be visualized by US. This is due, in part, to the proximity of the duodenum to the CBD and the interference that occurs due to luminal bowel gas. However, US may detect a dilated CBD in excess of 6 mm (the upper limit of normal) in up to 75% of cases. Therefore, US may suggest but does not confirm the diagnosis. Endoscopic ultrasound (EUS), however, is far superior to transabdominal US and equal to MRCP in sensitivity and specificity for the diagnosis of CBD stones. EUS also provides better resolution than MRCP, and is a dynamic rather than static test making it useful for concomitant stone removal. The primary disadvantage to EUS is that it is an invasive procedure. CT scanning is extremely useful in diagnosing complications of gallstones, such as perforation of the gallbladder, abscess formation, pericholecystic fluid, pancreatitis, and gas in the gallbladder wall. The sensitivity and specificity of CT has been improving with the use of helical scanners, however, and its sensitivity and specificity is now roughly 85%. Likewise, cholescintigraphy has inadequate sensitivity and specificity to be useful for the detection of CBD stones.

92. **Answer E.** With a positive India ink stain of the CSF, the patient has fungal meningitis, most likely due to *Cryptococcus neoformans*, an opportunistic infection common in patients with AIDS. Patients usually present with symptoms typical of aseptic meningitis. The CSF WBC and protein are usually only slightly elevated. India ink staining has approximately 80% sensitivity, so CSF should also be sent for cryptococcal antigen, which has close to 100% sensitivity and specificity. Treatment for cryptococcal meningitis is with amphotericin B plus flucytosine, which is superior to itraconazole monotherapy. Fluconazole monotherapy may be used in very mild cases. Ceftriaxone and vancomycin are used for therapy of bacterial meningitis. Acyclovir is used for herpes simplex encephalitis (HSE), which is suggested by altered mental status and elevated CSF RBC count.

93. **Answer D.** Bloody diarrhea in a traveler or immigrant from an endemic area should always raise the possibility of amebic colitis. While patients with bacterial dysentery can also have bloody stools and crampy abdominal pain, their symptoms do not typically last for longer than 1 week. Enterotoxigenic *E. coli* is the most common cause of traveler's diarrhea but is noninvasive, causes a nonbloody, water diarrhea, and typically resolves within a few days to a week. *Entamoeba* is found worldwide, but it is particularly endemic to the Indian subcontinent, central and South America, and Africa. Extraintestinal manifestations, the most common of which is a liver abscess, only rarely occur.

94. **Answer E.** Optic neuritis is the most common cranial manifestation of MS, and describes a syndrome of monocular eye pain, decreased color perception, and variable visual loss primarily affecting central vision. However, sensory disturbances, diplopia (internuclear ophthalmoplegia), Lhermitte sign (trunk and limb paresthesias evoked by neck flexion), limb weakness, clumsiness, gait ataxia, and neurogenic bladder and bowel symptoms may also be presenting signs and symptoms. Approximately 20% of patients with MS will present with optic neuritis and 50% of patients with MS will experience optic neuritis at some point in the disease course.

95. **Answer D.** There is no single, wholly reliable finding in the setting of early necrotizing fasciitis. However, extreme pain with minimal cutaneous findings is often the first manifestation of a serious underlying problem and may be the only indication of an imminent infectious tsunami. Patients often have relatively unexplained pain (i.e., no history of trauma or prior surgical intervention) that is rapidly progressive in the relative absence of associated skin findings (since it is a fascial infection first, which later extends to the skin and underlying muscle). Once the initial erythema yields to ecchymoses with vesicles and bullae, extensive damage has already taken place in the subcutaneous tissues. Among cases of type II necrotizing fasciitis (primarily caused by Group A streptococci in previously healthy patients), crepitus is only present in 10% of patients. There is a laboratory-based scoring system to help risk-stratify patients in whom the diagnosis is being considered, called LRINEC (Laboratory Risk Indicator for Necrotizing Fasciitis). While an elevated CRP ≥150 mg/L accounts for the largest number of points within this scoring system, it is only useful in patients in whom the diagnosis is already seriously being considered. In such cases, the clinician's suspicion of the disease has likely already triggered surgical consultation.

96. **Answer A.** This patient has an auricular hematoma resulting from bleeding in the potential space between the auricular cartilage and the perichondrium to which it is normally adherent. It is important to incise and

drain these hematomas because failure to do so may lead to necrosis of the cartilage and subsequent cosmetic deformation of the ear such as "cauliflower ear." This is the same principle that guides treatment of nasal septal hematomas (cartilage necrosis). Though aspiration is a reasonable strategy, recurrence is common and aspiration is sometimes incomplete. Incision and drainage is more definitive and simple to perform. After drainage of the hematoma, the ear is packed in a bulky pressure dressing to prevent reaccumulation of the hematoma. Moist cotton is placed within the folds of ear and then covered with bulky dry cotton. Several pieces of trimmed gauze are placed between the ear and the scalp. The ear is then bandaged circumferentially against the supporting gauze. The patient is discharged with follow-up arranged within 48 hours to assess for reaccumulation. (Figure courtesy of Kathleen Cronan, MD. In: Chung EK, Atkinson-McEvoy LR, Julie A Boom JA, et al., eds. *Visual Diagnosis and Treatment in Pediatrics*. 2nd ed. Philadelphia, PA: Lippincott Williams & Wilkins; 2010.)

97. **Answer B.** Smoking appears to be a risk factor for subarachnoid hemorrhage, especially in women. Significant hypertension, not hypotension, has been shown to be a risk factor in some, but not all studies. Oral contraceptive use and cholesterol and lipid abnormalities have not been shown to be risk factors.

98. **Answer E.** Any patient with life-threatening anemia should receive a blood transfusion. However, several anemic patients fall into a gray middle zone, in which it is clear the anemia needs treatment, yet no immediate life threat is present. This patient presents such a scenario. Patients with chronic anemia are almost always iron deficient due to chronic blood loss (e.g., menorrhagia). While oral iron therapy is a potential solution, many patients don't tolerate oral iron therapy due to GI side effects and oral iron therapy may not be able to keep pace with the degree of blood (and iron) loss. In such patients intravenous iron is a potential alternative to a blood transfusion. Common options include low molecular weight iron dextran, which can be given as a single, large infusion over an hour, as well as iron sucrose and ferric gluconate. Each hospital will likely have different options on formulary. However, the infusions are often shorter than intravenous levofloxacin, to which no

one bats an eye. Anaphylaxis is extremely uncommon and premedications are not recommended. If a transfusion is ordered instead, only a single unit should be used and oral iron therapy should be prescribed along with possible hormonal therapy to attenuate further bleeding. The habit of ordering two units for every anemic patient only increases the risk to the patient without benefit. Hemoglobin values drawn 15 to 60 minutes after transfusion accurately reflect the new baseline in stable patients (who are not bleeding).

99. **Answer C.** Patients with anterior shoulder dislocation and subsequent relocation are at extremely high risk of recurrent dislocation. Young patients are the highest risk group, probably because of a combination of associated cartilaginous injury and overly aggressive return to previous activity. Surgical stabilization is recommended in these patients to prevent recurrence. The other answer choices are all complications of anterior shoulder dislocation but occur less commonly than recurrent dislocation.

100. **Answer A.** AGE is the second most common cause of diving-related death and the most severe form of pulmonary barotraumas. As a diver ascends, alveoli expand due to the decreasing atmospheric pressure. If the diver does not continuously expire during ascent, the alveoli will expand and may rupture. Air may then cross the ruptured alveolar–capillary membrane, enter the pulmonary venous circulation, and subsequently embolize to any organ system. Embolization to the coronary or cerebral (usually anterior or middle cerebral) arteries is most catastrophic. The most common presentation of AGE is neurologic, consisting of decreased consciousness, dizziness, confusion, headache, cranial nerve symptoms, hemiplegia, and hemisensory loss. Any diver who surfaces unconscious or who loses consciousness within 10 minutes of surfacing should be presumed to have AGE until proven otherwise. The loss of consciousness (LOC) is a sharp contrast from DCS, in which LOC is rare. Alternobaric vertigo is vertigo that results from a pressure differential between the two middle ears. It results when patients with unilateral Eustachian tube dysfunction or blockage (when one Eustachian tube is more or less patent than the other) are exposed to the ambient pressures associated with diving or flying.

QUESTIONS

1. Which of the following patients should be taken to the operating room (OR) for emergent vascular exploration?

    A. A 24-year-old male with a lower leg gunshot wound and an ankle–brachial index of 0.7

    B. A 32-year-old female who suffered a knee dislocation in a motor vehicle collision (MVC) with normal pedal pulses

    C. A 22-year-old male stabbed in the arm with persistent pulsatile blood loss and an absent distal pulse

    D. A 36-year-old male with steady, slow oozing from a left upper leg gunshot wound and an ankle–brachial index of 1.0

    E. A 62-year-old male whose lower leg was inadvertently impaled on a pitchfork with a large amount of bruising and soft-tissue swelling with a diminished dorsalis pedis pulse

2. Which of the following is adequately absorbed by activated charcoal?

    A. Lithium

    B. Ethanol

    C. Iron

    D. Toluene

    E. Acetaminophen

3. A 28-year-old left-hand–dominant man presents with left-hand pain and swelling for 1 day. His hand is shown in Figure 8-1. He states he hurt his hand after falling down the stairs. An x-ray is negative for fracture. Which of the following is the next best step in management?

    A. Suture repair of wounds

    B. Skin adhesive repair of wounds

    C. Doxycycline PO

    D. Ampicillin–sulbactam IV

    E. Radial gutter splint

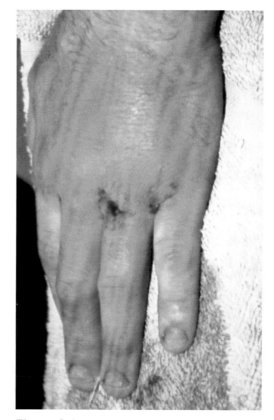

Figure 8-1

4. Which of the following is true regarding elder abuse?

    A. Elder abuse is associated with increased morbidity and mortality.

    B. Men are at higher risk than women.

    C. Sexual abuse is the most common type of elder abuse.

    D. Most elder abuse reporting is performed by physicians.

    E. Most perpetrators are strangers.

5. A 42-year-old male presents in January to your emergency department (ED) with fever, myalgias, cough, sore throat, and malaise for 4 days. He has no past medical history. His vitals are: 100.0, 86, 16, 118/72, 100% RA. His physical examination is unremarkable. Which of the following is the next best step in management?

   A. Prescribe oseltamivir
   B. Prescribe amantadine
   C. Prescribe azithromycin
   D. Give amoxicillin–sulbactam IV in the ED
   E. Supportive care only

6. Which of the following most places women at risk for abruptio placentae?

   A. Preeclampsia
   B. Cigarette smoking
   C. Premature rupture of membranes (PROM)
   D. Cocaine use
   E. Trauma

7. Which of the following is true regarding urinary tract infections in pregnancy?

   A. Pyelonephritis in pregnancy is almost always left sided.
   B. Asymptomatic bacteriuria is less common in pregnant women than in nonpregnant women.
   C. All pregnant women with asymptomatic bacteriuria should receive antimicrobial treatment.
   D. *Candida* spp. is a common cause of urinary tract infections in pregnant women.
   E. All of the above.

8. The Kleihauer–Betke test (KBT):

   A. Should be performed in all pregnant patients in cases of trauma
   B. Determines whether pregnant patients should receive Rh immune globulin
   C. Detects as little as 0.5 mL of fetal blood in the maternal circulation
   D. Is most useful in cases of significant maternal–fetal hemorrhage (MFH)
   E. All of the above

9. Which of the following radiographic views of the knee best identifies longitudinal patellar fractures?

   A. Anteroposterior (AP)
   B. Lateral
   C. Medial oblique
   D. Lateral oblique
   E. Sunrise

10. A 56-year-old unresponsive man with a history of uncontrolled hypertension is brought in to the ED after being found slumped over the steering wheel of his car.

His BP is 245/130, his heart rate (HR) is 62, and he has irregular breathing. On examination, you note that his left pupil is fixed and dilated. What does this physical examination finding likely indicate?

   A. Tonsillar herniation
   B. Uncal herniation
   C. Subfalcine herniation
   D. Sphenoid herniation
   E. None of the above

11. A 24-year-old male with no past medical history presents with intermittent fevers, shortness of breath, cough, and malaise for 1 week. Vital signs are 100.3°F, 85, 20, 145/92, 98% RA. Chest x-ray demonstrates patchy interstitial infiltrates. Which of the following is the most appropriate treatment regimen?

   A. Cefdinir
   B. Vancomycin plus gentamicin
   C. Doxycycline
   D. Amoxicillin–clavulanic acid
   E. Clindamycin

12. A 24-year-old male is brought to the ED for altered mental status. A friend states that they were eating the seeds of a jimson weed plant to get high. Vital signs are 99.6°F, 100, 18, 156/94, 98% RA. The patient is agitated, responds only to name, but has intact airway reflexes. Which of the following is the most appropriate next step in management?

   A. Atropine
   B. Pyridostigmine
   C. Edrophonium
   D. Pralidoxime
   E. Supportive care only

13. Which of the following are the two most common causes of diarrhea in AIDS patients?

   A. *Cryptosporidium* and cytomegalovirus (CMV)
   B. *C. difficile* and *Salmonella*
   C. *Giardia* and *Mycobacterium avium-intracellulare*
   D. *Giardia* and *Isospora*
   E. *Isospora* and *Shigella*

14. Which of the following is true regarding Ludwig angina?

   A. Endotracheal intubation is the preferred method of airway control.
   B. The mortality rate of Ludwig angina is approximately 75%.
   C. Ludwig angina may occur in children without any preceding cause.
   D. Extension to the retropharyngeal space is the most common cause of death.
   E. In patients with an associated oral malignancy, radiation is the therapy of choice.

15. A father and his daughter each present to the ED complaining of elbow pain after falling down ice skating. They were holding hands when they lost their balance and each fell to their outstretched hands. Each of them has limited elbow range of motion on examination but x-rays reveal only a joint effusion. Which of the following is true?

    A. The daughter most likely has a radial head fracture
    B. The father can be placed in a sling
    C. Both the father and the daughter should be placed in a long-arm posterior mold with plaster or fiberglass
    D. The father most likely has an occult olecranon fracture
    E. Compartment syndrome is a common complication of the father's injury

16. Which of the following is true regarding traumatic hemothorax?

    A. Continuous chest tube output of 300 mL/hour for 4 hours is an indication for thoracotomy.
    B. Costophrenic angle blunting occurs on upright chest x-ray with as little as 50 mL of intrapleural blood.
    C. The subclavian artery is the most common source of bleeding.
    D. A 7-French pigtail catheter is adequate for drainage of most hemothoraces.
    E. Pneumothorax almost never occurs concomitantly with hemothorax.

17. A 62-year-old female with a history of chronic atrial fibrillation presents with 2 hours of acute-onset, continuous, excruciating abdominal pain. A few minutes after the onset of pain, she had an urge to defecate and had a large, forceful bowel movement. She denies bloody or melenic stools or a history of postprandial pain. On examination, her abdomen is soft, flat, and only mildly tender. Labs reveal a leukocytosis of 16,000 per mm^3 with a normal chemistry. An initial flat and upright abdominal film is nonspecific and a CT scan is read by the radiologist as having evidence of small bowel thickening. What is the next most important step in management?

    A. Interventional radiology consult for emergent angiography
    B. Surgical consult for emergent laparotomy
    C. Gastroenterology consult for emergent endoscopy
    D. Intravenous antibiotics and admission for presumed infectious colitis
    E. Admission for serial abdominal examinations without specific therapy

18. A 50-year-old male with a history of diabetes and hypertension presents with new-onset vertical diplopia. His examination reveals normal pupils, mild right sided ptosis, and slight inferior deviation of his right eye at rest. At times the right eye appears to "get stuck" after being abducted in downward gaze. Which of the following is most likely affected?

    A. Cranial nerve II
    B. Cranial nerve III
    C. Cranial nerve IV
    D. Cranial nerve VI
    E. Occipital lobe

19. A 71-year-old male with a prosthetic heart valve presents to the ED. Which of the following is an indication for antibiotic prophylaxis?

    A. IV placement
    B. Central line placement
    C. I and D of a forearm abscess
    D. Urethral catheterization
    E. Nasogastric tube insertion

20. Two men are hiking in the mountains of Colorado when one complains of feeling sick. Which of the following is the most sensitive indicator of high-altitude cerebral edema (HACE)?

    A. Cerebellar ataxia
    B. Vomiting
    C. Abducens nerve palsy
    D. Seizures
    E. Slurred speech

21. A 4-week-old male infant is brought in by his parents with progressive, projectile, nonbilious emesis. Labs are drawn and an IV is placed and the patient is sent for an ultrasound. Ultrasonography reveals a hypertrophic pylorus and the surgeon is consulted for pyloric stenosis. What are the labs likely to reveal?

    A. A hypochloremic, eukalemic, metabolic acidosis
    B. A compensatory respiratory alkalosis
    C. A hypochloremic, hypokalemic, metabolic alkalosis
    D. A hyperchloremic, hyperkalemic, metabolic acidosis
    E. A high anion gap metabolic acidosis

22. A 67-year-old male with hypertension presents with acute onset of abdominal pain. The pain is periumbilical and radiates to the left lower quadrant. On physical examination, BP is 140/90 and an abdominal mass is noted near the umbilicus. A bedside ultrasonograph is shown in Figure 8-2. After the ultrasonography, the BP drops to 70/40 and the patient becomes lightheaded and dizzy. Which of the following is the most appropriate next step in management?

    A. CT scan without contrast
    B. CT scan with IV contrast only
    C. CT scan with IV and PO contrast
    D. Emergent surgery
    E. IV crystalloid to normalize BP

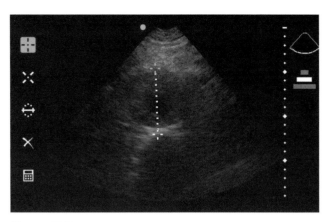

Figure 8-2

23. Which of the following is true regarding post-MI pericarditis?

A. It occurs in a majority of patients with MI.
B. Concave ST elevations are usually seen on EKG.
C. Treatment generally involves nonsteroidal anti-inflammatory drug (NSAID) therapy.
D. A pericardial friction rub is almost never audible.
E. Etiology is likely infectious.

24. In an acute NSTEMI, which of the following advantages does bivalirudin possess over unfractionated and low–molecular-weight heparins?

A. Improved mortality
B. Lower incidence of major bleeding
C. Lower rate of conversion to an ST-elevation myocardial infarction (STEMI)
D. Increased anti-X_a activity
E. Increased anti-XIII activity

25. Which of the following opioids may predispose to serotonin syndrome?

A. Fentanyl
B. Meperidine
C. Propoxyphene
D. Hydrocodone
E. Morphine

26. Among patients who have contraindications to beta-blocker therapy, which of the following calcium channel blockers (CCBs) can be given as a substitute for beta-blockers to patients with a non-ST-elevation MI (NSTEMI)?

A. Nimodipine
B. Diltiazem
C. Amlodipine
D. Nifedipine
E. All of the above

27. Patients with plantar puncture wounds that occurred in the absence of any footwear:

A. Should be given one of the newer fluoroquinolones such as levofloxacin or moxifloxacin instead of ciprofloxacin for better antipseudomonal coverage
B. Infrequently experience wound infection
C. Require high-pressure irrigation to effectively decontaminate the wound
D. Should be given prophylactic antibiotic coverage against *Pseudomonas*
E. Should receive amoxicillin–clavulanate as it is the best oral antipseudomonal option in the setting of fluoroquinolone resistance

28. What is the most common cause of death in patients with hemophilia A?

A. Septic shock
B. Myocardial infarction (MI)
C. Gastrointestinal bleeding
D. Intracranial hemorrhage
E. Congestive heart failure

29. The agent of choice to inactivate coelenterate nematocyst toxin (such as jellyfish) is:

A. 5% acetic acid (vinegar)
B. Ambient temperature fresh water
C. Ambient temperature seawater
D. Ammonia
E. Alcohol

30. What is the most common source of bleeding in a posterior nosebleed?

A. Anterior ethmoidal artery
B. Posterior ethmoidal artery
C. Kiesselbach plexus
D. Nasopalatine branch of sphenopalatine artery
E. Septal branch of superior labial artery

31. A 27-year-old male presents to the ED with pruritus ani, tenesmus, and yellowish mucoid discharge from his rectum. Upon further questioning, he acknowledges recent unprotected anal intercourse. The recommended regimen for treating this patient is:

A. Topical podophyllin b.i.d. × 7 days
B. Ceftriaxone 125 mg IM plus doxycycline 100 mg PO b.i.d. × 7 days
C. Valacyclovir 1 g PO daily × 5 days
D. Benzathine penicillin G 2.4 million units IM × 1 dose
E. Lopinavir

32. A 26-year-old is brought to the ED by emergency medical services (EMS) 3 hours after ingesting an overdose of his mother's digoxin. Which of the following is true?

A. Whole bowel irrigation is an effective means of decontamination.
B. Activated charcoal should be given.

C. A digoxin level may overestimate the amount of digoxin ingested.

D. His underlying heart rhythm is likely sinus tachycardia.

E. Ten vials of Digibind (Fab fragments) should be given to prevent cardiac toxicity.

33. In a human immunodeficiency virus (HIV)-positive patient with pneumocystis pneumonia (PCP) pneumonia who has a sulfa allergy precluding the use of trimethoprim–sulfamethoxazole (TMP-SMX), which of the following is the best outpatient regimen?

A. Primaquine plus clindamycin

B. Levofloxacin

C. Albendazole plus trimethoprim

D. Pentamidine

E. Doxycycline

34. A 17-year-old female with a history of anorexia nervosa is brought to the ED by her parents for evaluation of significant peripheral edema, shortness of breath, and orthopnea. A chest x-ray is consistent with pulmonary edema. The patient had recently begun a refeeding program as part of intensive outpatient treatment. Subsequent blood testing reveals numerous significant abnormalities. Which of the following is most likely present?

A. Hypophosphatemia

B. Hyperkalemia

C. Hyperalbuminemia

D. Hyponatremia

E. Hypermagnesemia

35. A 4-year-old female is brought in by her mother, who is worried that "she swallowed something and it's stuck." The patient was in her usual health until this morning's breakfast, which she could not swallow and rapidly vomited. An anteroposterior (AP) chest x-ray demonstrates a coin positioned *en face* in the upper chest. The patient looks well and is otherwise asymptomatic. What is the next appropriate step?

A. Glucagon 1 mg IV

B. Endoscopy

C. 12 ounces of soda PO

D. Oral papain

E. Heimlich maneuver

36. Which of the following is true regarding topical ophthalmic antibiotics?

A. Ointments have a shorter duration of action than drops.

B. Ointments are absorbed more rapidly than drops.

C. Systemic side effects may occur.

D. Drops are preferred in pediatric patients.

E. Antibiotics should not be prescribed for conjunctivitis without positive cultures.

37. A 44-year-old male is brought to the ED in cardiac arrest due to ventricular fibrillation. He responds to a defibrillation attempt with return of spontaneous circulation, but he is still comatose. You control his airway with endotracheal intubation. You decide to initiate therapeutic hypothermia. Which of the following is thought to be a beneficial mechanism in therapeutic hypothermia?

A. Reduction in postarrest infection

B. Reduction in cerebral oxygen consumption

C. Reduction in pH

D. Increase in cerebral glutamate levels

E. Increase in superoxide levels

38. A 55-year-old female presents with sore throat, runny nose, intermittent low-grade fevers, and generalized malaise. She feels like something is stuck in her throat, causing odynophagia. She is nontoxic appearing, has no respiratory distress, and has normal vital signs. A lateral soft tissue of the neck is shown in Figure 8-3. Which of the following is the most likely etiology?

A. Foreign body

B. Group A *Streptococcus*

C. Anaerobes

D. *H. influenza*

E. Thyromegaly

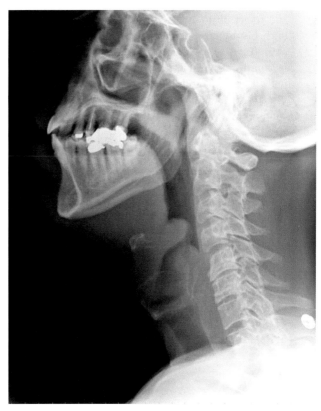

Figure 8-3

39. A 2-year-old male is brought to the ED by his parents for loud breathing for several hours. He had upper respiratory symptoms for several days, followed by a persistent, high-pitched cough. The parents have noticed loud inspiratory noises for the last two evenings. Vital signs are 99.5°F, 112, 24, 93% RA. The patient appears to be in mild respiratory distress, with mild inspiratory stridor and frequent bouts of coughing. Lungs are clear to auscultation. Which of the following is the most appropriate management?

    A. Amoxicillin
    B. Ipratropium
    C. Albuterol
    D. Dexamethasone
    E. Ribavirin

40. Which of the following is the most common complication of otitis media?

    A. Tympanic membrane (TM) perforation
    B. Hearing loss
    C. Labyrinthitis
    D. Meningitis
    E. Brain abscess

41. A 6-month-old infant born at term is brought by her parents for evaluation of cough. The patient has been coughing for 3 days, with rhinorrhea and congestion and fevers up to 101°F. Her past medical history and birth history are unremarkable. Vital signs in the ED are 100.1°F, 133, 42, 90/palp, and 98% RA. The patient is smiling, active, and tachypneic with mild nasal flaring and lungs exhibit moderate expiratory wheezes. Which of the following is true regarding this patient's condition?

    A. Albuterol therapy has been shown to reduce hospitalization rates.
    B. Ribavirin is indicated.
    C. Respiratory syncytial virus (RSV) is the most common cause.
    D. Corticosteroids reduce the duration of illness.
    E. The patient has an 80% chance of developing asthma as a child.

42. A 66-year-old male is brought to the ED after a high-speed motor vehicle collision. He complains of chest pain. Given the extreme deceleration mechanism, you suspect traumatic aortic injury. Which of the following is present in most ED patients with traumatic aortic injury?

    A. BP >140/90
    B. BP <90/50
    C. Intact upper extremity pulses with diminished lower extremity pulses
    D. Systolic murmur
    E. Chest pain radiating to the back

43. What is the most common cause of death in patients with toxic epidermal necrolysis (TEN)?

    A. Electrolyte abnormalities
    B. Respiratory failure
    C. Sepsis
    D. Dehydration
    E. Ventricular dysrhythmias

44. A 6-year-old male presents with diffuse arthralgias, fatigue, and fever for several days. He had a "virus" with fever and sore throat several weeks before, which resolved spontaneously. Physical examination demonstrates a febrile child with significant tenderness and limited range of motion in his left knee with milder findings in his right wrist. Which of the following is the most appropriate next step in management?

    A. Discharge home with azithromycin
    B. Prednisone 1 mg/kg
    C. EKG
    D. Urinalysis
    E. Lumbar puncture

45. The best route and location of epinephrine administration for anaphylaxis is

    A. IM in the deltoid.
    B. Subcutaneous (SQ) in the deltoid.
    C. IM in the lateral thigh.
    D. SQ in the lateral thigh.
    E. There is no preferable route.

46. Which of the following toxins is suggested by the smell of garlic?

    A. Cyanide
    B. Zinc
    C. Toluene
    D. Organophosphate
    E. Hydrogen sulfide

47. A 69-year-old male with a history of hypertension presents with sudden onset of severe chest pain with radiation to the back. His vital signs are: 99.0, 100, 18, 195/90, 99% RA. You diagnose a Stanford Type B aortic dissection on CT aortogram. Which of the following is the next best step in management?

    A. Nitroglycerin IV
    B. Labetalol IV
    C. Nicardipine IV
    D. Nifedipine PO
    E. Clonidine PO

48. A 26-year-old female G2P1 at 25 weeks gestation and a history of placenta previa presents with a chief complaint of lower abdominal pain with vaginal spotting. Which of the following is true?

    A. Most women are diagnosed with placenta previa after an episode of second- or third-trimester vaginal bleeding.
    B. Digital vaginal examination is recommended before ultrasonography for more rapid diagnosis and obstetrician consultation.
    C. Low-lying placentas in early pregnancy tend to migrate toward the cervical os over time.
    D. Disseminated intravascular coagulation is a common complication.
    E. None of the above

49. A father brings in his 8-year-old daughter with a chief complaint of a low-grade fever and a facial rash (see Fig. 8-4). The rash seems to spare the nasolabial fold and perioral area. Which of the following is the cause of this patient's illness?

    A. Rubella
    B. Human herpesvirus 6
    C. Parvovirus B19
    D. Measles virus
    E. Group A *streptococci*

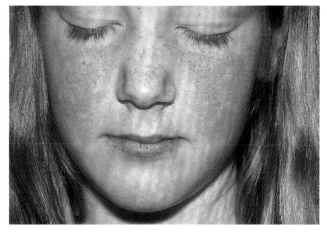

Figure 8-4

50. Which of the following fluids may precipitate a hyperchloremic metabolic acidosis if large volumes are given during trauma resuscitations?

    A. D10 W
    B. Lactated Ringers
    C. D5 0.45 N NaCl
    D. 0.45 N NaCl
    E. 0.9 N NaCl

51. Which of the following is true regarding pediatric EKG analysis?

    A. Left axis deviation is normal in healthy neonates.
    B. Atrial fibrillation is the most common pediatric dysrhythmia.
    C. T-wave inversion in the anterior precordial leads (V1–V3) is a normal finding in school-aged children.
    D. Cardiac dysrhythmias are the most common electrocardiographic manifestation of underlying congenital heart disease.
    E. ST elevation is most commonly associated with myocardial injury.

52. An 18-year-old male presents with fever and left periorbital pain and swelling as shown in Figure 8-5. Which of the following additional tests is indicated at this time?

    A. Brain magnetic resonance imaging (MRI)
    B. Orbital CT scan
    C. Erythrocyte sedimentation rate (ESR)
    D. Cerebrospinal fluid (CSF) analysis
    E. Slit lamp examination

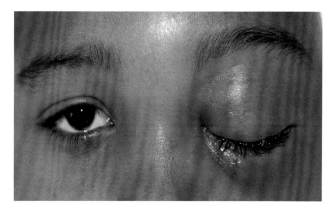

Figure 8-5

53. Which of the following is true regarding hyperkalemia?

    A. Neither calcium chloride nor calcium gluconate should ever be used in the setting of concomitant digoxin use.
    B. The effects of calcium chloride or gluconate last for 3 to 4 hours.
    C. Bicarbonate therapy is more efficacious than either insulin or albuterol.
    D. Sodium polystyrene sulfate (Kayexalate) may exacerbate volume overload.
    E. All of the above

54. An 81-year-old male with no prior medical history presents with acute alteration of mental status with onset 8 hours prior to arrival. His vital signs are 99.0, 100, 22, 185/95, 96% on room air. He is talking, but very confused. He is sent immediately to CT and on return from CT he appears more altered and is unable to answer questions and slips in and out of consciousness. His CT scan is seen on Figure 8-6. After intubation to protect his airway, which of the following is the next best step in management?

A. Hyperventilation to PCO_2 20 mm Hg
B. Blood pressure control to 140 mm Hg systolic
C. Administer a 4-factor Prothrombin Complex Concentrate (PCC) such as factor eight inhibitor bypassing activity (FEIBA)
D. Trendelenburg positioning
E. Administration of IV tPA

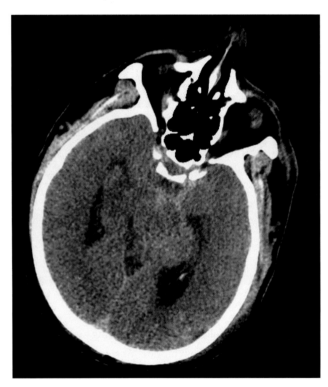

Figure 8-6

55. A 47-year-old female smoker with a history of hypertension presents to the ED with a headache that started 12 hours ago. She looks uncomfortable, prefers to sit in a dark room, and states this headache is more severe than any headache she has had before. Her CT scan is shown in Figure 8-7. Which of the following is true?

A. Seizures may occur in up to one-third of patients.
B. Lumbar puncture should be performed for cerebrospinal fluid (CSF) analysis.
C. Nifedipine 60 mg PO should be given as soon as the CT scan result is obtained.
D. Hypertension should only be treated if her BP exceeds 220/120.
E. All of the above

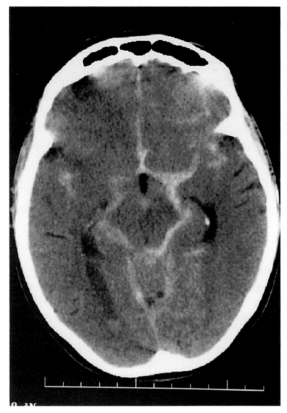

Figure 8-7

56. Which of the following is useful as a sensitive screening test for clinically significant complications of blunt cardiac injury?

A. Creatine kinase, MB isoenzyme (CK-MB)
B. Troponin I
C. Troponin T
D. EKG
E. Exercise stress test

57. A 22-year-old male presents with severe left elbow pain and swelling after being tackled in a football game (Fig. 8-8). His elbow appears to be locked in partial flexion and he guards against any motion. X-rays reveal the image shown. Which of the following is the most common complication of this injury?

A. Median nerve injury
B. Ulnar nerve injury
C. Brachial artery disruption
D. Compartment syndrome
E. Radial nerve injury

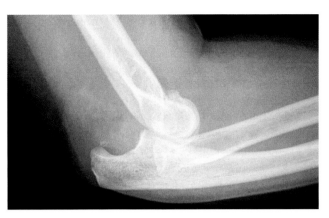

Figure 8-8

58. A 59-year-old male with a history of alcoholic cirrhosis presents with worsening abdominal pain and swelling. He normally receives therapeutic paracenteses every few weeks but has not had one in a month. He has no fever, vomiting, or diarrhea. Vital signs are 98.9°F, 85, 18, 105/65, 99% RA. He has mild cognitive deficits per his baseline with hepatic encephalopathy (HE). He is in no respiratory distress. Abdominal examination demonstrates moderate distention with fluid wave but only mild tenderness and no rebound or guarding. Which of the following is the most appropriate next step in management?

   A. Diagnostic paracentesis
   B. Therapeutic paracentesis
   C. CT of abdomen/pelvis
   D. Ultrasound of right upper quadrant
   E. Discharge home with outpatient follow-up

59. A 62-year-old female with a history of known peptic ulcer disease presents with a chief complaint of hematemesis and black tarry stools. Her vital signs include a pulse of 105 and an SBP of 115 mm Hg. Her initial hemoglobin is 9.6 g/dL. Which of the following is most likely to be useful in this patient?

   A. Continuous famotidine infusion
   B. Sengstaken–Blakemore tube placement
   C. Ewald tube placement
   D. Continuous octreotide infusion
   E. Continuous pantoprazole infusion

60. Which of the following is the most useful treatment modality in patients with heat stroke?

   A. Spraying tepid water on the patient and fanning the patient

B. Intravenous dantrolene
C. Applying ice packs to the axilla, groin, and extremities
D. Delivery of cooled intravenous saline
E. Tylenol or ibuprofen delivered per rectum

61. Which of the following is true regarding the physical examination for patients with abdominal aortic aneurysm (AAA)?

   A. Abdominal bruits are audible in half the number of cases.
   B. Aneurysmal rupture often occurs with deep palpation of the abdomen.
   C. Most aneurysms >5 cm in size are palpable.
   D. Femoral pulses are usually decreased.
   E. Abdominal obesity does not appreciably affect the ability to palpate aortic aneurysm.

62. A 26-year-old male with a history of bipolar disorder is brought in by his mother with a chief complaint of agitation. She states that her son has been very anxious and restless, has not been sleeping, and abruptly stopped taking his lithium medication 2 days ago. His mother has a history of Graves disease but is otherwise healthy. In the ED, the patient's vital signs include a temperature of 104.1°F, pulse of 120, with sinus tachycardia visible on the monitor, and a blood pressure (BP) of 140/70. On examination he is mildly agitated, warm and diaphoretic, tremulous, and has a slight lid lag. Which of the following is the next best step?

   A. Oral lithium administration
   B. Intravenous propranolol administration
   C. Oral administration of Lugol solution
   D. Oral aspirin administration
   E. Intravenous dantrolene administration

63. While watching her grandson's tackle football game, a 72-year-old female presents with right knee and leg pain after being struck by an opposing player. She was knocked over and has had pain on ambulation. She is tender on the lateral aspect of her proximal anterior leg, just distal to her patella. An x-ray of her knee is shown in Figure 8-9. Which of the following is the next best step in management?

   A. Weight-bearing as tolerated
   B. Crutches for 1 week, then weight-bearing as tolerated
   C. X-ray of the ankle
   D. CT without contrast of the leg
   E. CT angiogram of the leg

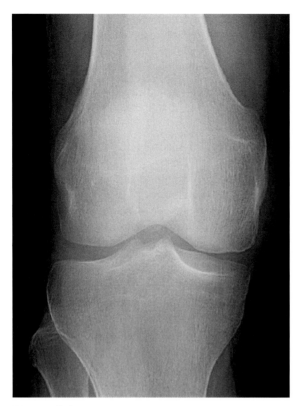

Figure 8-9

64. A group of children are playing outside in the rain when one of them suffers a witnessed lightning strike. The strike did not directly hit the child but it hit the ground very close to where the child was standing. Which of the following is true?

   A. Ventricular fibrillation is the most common cause of death.
   B. He is likely to suffer from severe, deep burns.
   C. Lower extremity paralysis accompanied by mottled, blue, cool, and pulseless extremities typically resolves without treatment.
   D. "Flashover" commonly causes diffuse superficial burns to >50% of the total body surface area.
   E. Myoglobinuric renal failure is the most common complication among survivors.

65. A 29-year-old female presents after going running on the treadmill with cough, shortness of breath, and chest tightness. She has no throat swelling or rash. Her examination is normal except for bilateral wheezes. She has been taking an over-the-counter medication for her intermittent migraine headaches. What medication is the most likely cause?

   A. Acetaminophen
   B. Phenylephrine
   C. Naproxen
   D. Capsaicin
   E. Paracetamol

66. A 27-year-old female presents to the ED with headache and nausea for several days. She is 2 weeks postpartum status post a normal spontaneous special delivery of a healthy infant at term. Her primary care physician instructed her to take Tylenol or ibuprofen for her headache, but she has not had any relief with this. Her vital signs are: 99.6, 85, 16, 165/92, 100% RA. Physical examination is normal, including a normal cranial nerve examination. Which of the following is the next best step in management?

   A. Prescribe tramadol 50 mg PO TID
   B. Prescribe hydrocodone 5 mg PO Q6h
   C. Urinalysis
   D. CT brain with IV contrast
   E. Lumbar puncture

67. Injury to which of the following is the most common cause of traumatic death in children?

   A. Head
   B. Chest
   C. Abdomen
   D. Pelvis
   E. Femur

68. A 46-year-old morbidly obese (BMI >40) male patient is referred to the ED to exclude a deep venous thrombosis (DVT) after he presented to his primary care physician's office with calf swelling and pain for 1 week. His subsequent Doppler study demonstrates a thrombosis limited to the peroneal vein. Which of the following describes the next best steps in management?

   A. Initiate anticoagulation with warfarin or a direct factor Xa or thrombin inhibitor, and refer for primary care follow-up
   B. Treat for superficial thrombophlebitis with pain medicine and anti-inflammatory medicine
   C. Refer the patient for a repeat Doppler study in 1 week but do not initiate treatment
   D. Initiate anticoagulation with warfarin or dabigatran and low–molecular-weight heparin, and refer him to interventional radiology for placement of an inferior vena cava filter
   E. Prescribe furosemide for fluid retention, and counsel the patient to wear support hose and to elevate the legs

69. A 52-year-old diabetic man presents to the ED with fever, crampy abdominal pain, and watery brown diarrhea. He recently completed a 14-day course of clindamycin, which was prescribed by his primary care doctor after she performed an incision and drainage of a small cutaneous abscess on his flank. The patient's symptoms started toward the end of his antibiotic therapy and he has been taking diphenoxylate "around the clock" since then without much benefit. Which of the following is true?

   A. Stool culture is the gold standard.
   B. The patient's diarrhea is an expected side effect of his recent antibiotic therapy.

C. Diphenoxylate is probably contributing to this patient's current illness.

D. Colonoscopy is usually required for effective treatment.

E. Children affected by this illness tend to have milder disease.

70. Which of the following cardiac findings is expected in hypothermic patients?

A. QT interval prolongation

B. Sinus bradycardia

C. Atrial fibrillation

D. J waves

E. All of the above

71. A 56-year-old male with long-standing hypertension and mild renal insufficiency presents to the ED with vague complaints of fatigue and generalized malaise. His EKG is shown in Figure 8-10. Which of the following is the next best step in management of this patient?

A. Nebulized albuterol

B. Insulin

C. Calcium chloride

D. Sodium polystyrene sulfate (Kayexalate)

E. Furosemide

72. In an otherwise normal x-ray, the finding of a "posterior fat pad" on a lateral x-ray of the elbow in adult and pediatric patients is suggestive of which of the following?

A. Normal finding in adults, supracondylar fracture in children

B. Supracondylar fracture in adults and children

C. Radial head fracture in adults, supracondylar fracture in children

D. Olecranon fracture in adults, supracondylar fracture in children

E. Radioulnar dislocation in adults, supracondylar fracture in children

73. A 12-month-old female presents with apparent fussiness with urination. Which of the following is the most appropriate urine collection method for this patient?

A. Diaper collection

B. Bag collection

C. Urethral catheterization

D. Midstream clean catch

E. Suprapubic catheterization

74. A 56-year-old male with chronic hepatitis B presents with mild abdominal pain, weight loss, and weakness. A CT scan of his abdomen revealed a hypodense lesion in the right lobe of his liver suspicious for hepatocellular carcinoma. The consulting oncologist is likely to ask you to add which of the following tests?

A. Beta human chorionic gonadotropin (β-hCG) level

B. Serum total estradiol level

C. Alpha fetoprotein (AFP) level

D. Carcinoembryonic antigen (CEA)

E. Cancer antigen (CA) 19–9

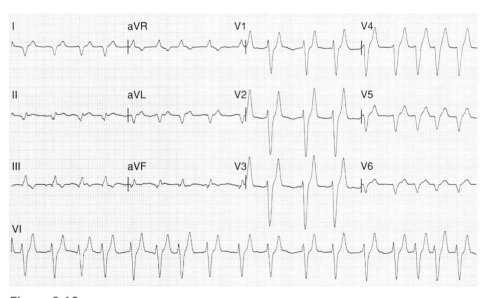

Figure 8-10

75. A mother brings in her 7-year-old daughter to the ED with a chief complaint of painful vaginal lesions and "bumps," burning dysuria, and generalized malaise (Fig. 8-11). On examination, you note tender inguinal lymphadenopathy and the lesions shown. Which of the following is the most likely cause of her symptoms?

    A. Herpes simplex virus type 2 (HSV-2)
    B. Syphilis (*Treponema pallidum*)
    C. Chancroid (*Hemophilus ducreyi*)
    D. Lymphogranuloma venereum (LGV, *Chlamydia trachomatis*)
    E. Granuloma inguinale (*Calymmatobacterium granulomatis*)

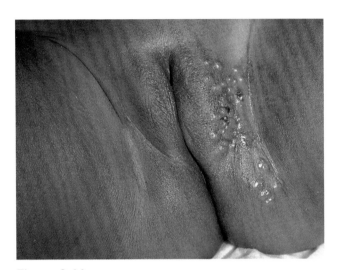

Figure 8-11

76. Which of the following is the most common cause of Ludwig angina?

    A. Pre-existing dental disease
    B. Diabetes mellitus
    C. Mandible fractures
    D. Tongue piercing
    E. Oral malignancy

77. A 4-year-old male is brought by his parents because he swallowed some of his grandmother's antihypertensive medicine. He is sleepy, bradycardic, and hypotensive. Which of the following is the most appropriate treatment?

    A. Atropine
    B. Glucagon
    C. Atropine and glucagon
    D. Atropine, glucagon, and calcium
    E. Atropine, glucagon, calcium, and high-dose insulin with glucose

78. Which of the following is a known property of ketamine?

    A. Analgesia
    B. Anesthesia
    C. Antipsychosis
    D. A and B
    E. A, B, and C

79. Which of the following findings may be present in hypothyroidism?

    A. Nonpitting periorbital edema
    B. Delayed relaxation phase of deep tendon reflexes
    C. Median nerve neuropathy
    D. Hypothermia
    E. All of the above

80. A 30-year-old male presents with right upper quadrant pain and fever. He has just returned from a trip to Brazil. His vital signs are 101.0°F, 105, 22, 155/90, 100% RA. He is exquisitely tender to palpation in the right upper quadrant. You order an ultrasound, which shows a cavitary, fluid-filled lesion in the right hepatic lobe and a normal gallbladder. Which of the following is the most appropriate initial treatment?

    A. Vancomycin
    B. Amikacin
    C. Metronidazole
    D. Methylprednisolone
    E. Surgical drainage

81. A 42-year-old male presents with pain, warmth, and swelling over his posterior elbow (Fig. 8-12). The patient reports frequently having to lean on his elbow while performing electrical work as part of his job. The patient has full range of motion but flexion and extension of the elbow results in increased pain. Fluid is subsequently aspirated from the affected area. Which of the following is true?

    A. Empiric antibiotic therapy should target gram-negative organisms
    B. Olecrnon bursitis is caused by hematogenous spread
    C. Septic bursitis may be present if the bursal white blood cell count is >10,000 per mm^3
    D. Treatment with antibiotics alone is usually successful
    E. The bursa should be incised, drained, and packed

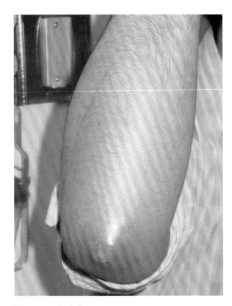

Figure 8-12

82. Which of the following toxins is suggested by a fruity odor to the breath?

   A. Cyanide
   B. Isopropanol
   C. Salicylate
   D. Acetaminophen
   E. Arsenic

83. A 14-year-old male presents with intermittent bilateral hip pain for several weeks. Physical examination demonstrates decreased internal rotation of both hips. Radiographs show slippage of the femoral epiphysis. Which of the following is the most common associated condition?

   A. Hyperthyroidism
   B. Diabetes mellitus
   C. Obesity
   D. Renal failure
   E. Juvenile rheumatoid arthritis

84. Which of the following test results is most concerning in a patient with an acute asthma exacerbation?

   A. Leukocytosis of 14,000
   B. K^+ 3.4
   C. Hyperlactatemia
   D. Eosinophilia
   E. Arterial blood gas (ABG) with pH 7.35, P_{O_2} 60, P_{CO_2} 45

85. A patient in your ED refuses to take penicillin because she is "allergic." The historical feature most suggestive of a true allergy in this patient is:

   A. Paresthesias
   B. Vomiting
   C. Fatigue
   D. Urticaria
   E. Palpitations

86. Which of the following is true regarding aortic dissection?

   A. Dyspnea is the most common symptom.
   B. Syncope often indicates pericardial effusion and tamponade.
   C. Aortic regurgitation occurs in most cases.
   D. Dissection into coronary arteries occurs most often in the left coronary artery.
   E. Interarm differences in SBP of >20 mm Hg occur in most patients.

87. Which of the following is an indication for Fab fragment administration in the setting of a digoxin overdose?

   A. All pediatric ingestions, regardless of the amount ingested
   B. Potassium level >5 mEq/L
   C. Normal sinus rhythm with occasional premature ventricular contractions (PVCs)

   D. Digoxin level >2 ng/mL in the setting of acute toxicity
   E. Digoxin level >2 ng/mL in patients with likely chronic toxicity

88. Which of the following is true regarding anaphylaxis?

   A. Bee stings are the most common cause.
   B. Exercise may trigger anaphylaxis.
   C. Anaphylaxis usually occurs upon first exposure to an allergen.
   D. Anaphylaxis is a type IV hypersensitivity reaction.
   E. The risk of anaphylaxis is greatest in the very young and elderly.

89. Phenytoin most closely resembles which of the following antidysrhythmics?

   A. Procainamide
   B. Amiodarone
   C. Metoprolol
   D. Lidocaine
   E. Verapamil

90. Which of the following is true regarding Guillain–Barré syndrome (GBS)?

   A. The clinical course is more severe in the elderly.
   B. Patients with a rapid onset are more likely to have a benign recovery.
   C. Patients with preceding gastroenteritis caused by *Campylobacter jejuni* have a more benign course.
   D. Autonomic involvement, such as urine retention, ileus, sinus tachycardia, and postural hypotension is uncommon in GBS.
   E. Respiratory failure requiring mechanical ventilation eventually occurs in 75% of patients.

91. Which of the following is the most effective therapy for acute arsenic poisoning?

   A. Activated charcoal
   B. Ipecac
   C. Dimercaprol
   D. Penicillamine
   E. Deferoxamine

92. A 6-year-old female is brought to the emergency room 4 hours after developing a brief choking episode while playing with her toys. Her chest x-ray is shown in Figure 8-13. Where is the foreign body located?

   A. Esophagus
   B. Hypopharynx
   C. Trachea
   D. Anterior mediastinum
   E. Not possible to determine from the information provided

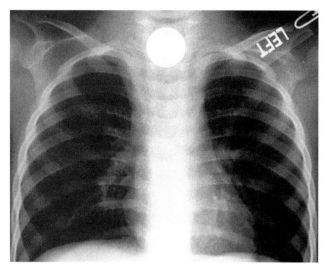

Figure 8-13

93. A 65-year-old female with a history of diabetes and hypertension presents with a 5-hour history of chest pain. Physical examination demonstrates blood pressure of 100/55, jugular venous distension, and hepatomegaly. No crackles are noted. EKG demonstrates inferior ST depressions. You suspect the possibility of right ventricular infarction. You instruct the ED technician to place the rV$_4$ lead at

    A. Right fourth intercostal space, midclavicular line
    B. Right fifth intercostal space, midclavicular line
    C. Right sixth intercostal space, midclavicular line
    D. Right fourth intercostal space, right sternal border
    E. Right fifth intercostal space, right sternal border

94. A 65-year-old male with a history of myasthenia gravis (MG) presents with acute generalized malaise and hypotension. He reports that he ran out of his medicines a week ago but doesn't recall their names. His vital signs are 98.5°F, 85, 18, 90/62, 99% RA. His EKG is normal. Which of the following is the most likely cause of hypotension in this patient?

    A. Addison disease
    B. Glucocorticoid withdrawal
    C. Adrenal hemorrhage
    D. Infection
    E. Myasthenic crisis

95. Which of the following vasculitis syndromes is most likely to present as pulmonary hemorrhage requiring emergent airway management?

    A. Churg–Strauss syndrome
    B. Polyarteritis nodosa
    C. Wegener granulomatosis
    D. Goodpasture syndrome
    E. Mixed cryoglobulinemia

96. A 56-year-old female presents with 1 hour of generalized hives, throat fullness, and cough. She is allergic to certain nuts and just ate a brownie that she thinks had nuts in it. She immediately used the Epi-pen that she carries with her and took 50 mg diphenhydramine orally, but she still feels throat fullness. Vital signs are 99.9°F, 110, 22, 132/75, 94% RA. She appears anxious and has dysphonia. On oropharyngeal examination, you cannot see the inferior border of her moderately edematous uvula and she is spitting her saliva out. She has wheezes bilaterally. Which of the following is the most appropriate next step in management?

    A. Chest x-ray
    B. Arterial blood gas
    C. Fresh frozen plasma (FFP)
    D. Noninvasive positive pressure ventilation
    E. Repeat epinephrine and prepare for endotracheal intubation

97. A 9-year-old male presents with right wrist pain after a fall from playground equipment at school. He has minimal swelling, no ecchymoses, and moderate tenderness over the distal radius, but x-rays demonstrate no fracture. Which of the following is true?

    A. The patient is at high risk for growth restriction affecting the radius
    B. The patient suffered a Salter Harris Type II injury
    C. Splinting the patient in a removal, plastic splint is a good treatment option
    D. The patient should be put in a long-arm posterior mold splint made with plaster or fiberglass
    E. The patient should be placed in a thumb spica splint

98. A 10-year-old presents with findings concerning for orbital cellulitis. CT is most likely to demonstrate which concurrent finding?

    A. Dacryocystitis
    B. Mastoiditis
    C. Orbital blowout fracture
    D. Deviated septum
    E. Ethmoid sinusitis

99. Which of the following is the most common class of psychiatric disorder seen by emergency and primary care physicians?

    A. Thought disorder
    B. Recreational drug use
    C. Anxiety disorder
    D. Somatoform disorder
    E. Factitious disorder

100. A patient with a history of depression on paroxetine presents with acute onset of altered mental status, muscle rigidity, tremor, hyperreflexia, and hyperthermia. Which of the following additional medications is the patient most likely using?

    A. Dextromethorphan
    B. Pseudoephedrine
    C. Diphenhydramine
    D. Acetaminophen
    E. Valproate

ANSWERS AND EXPLANATIONS

1. **Answer C.** There are both "hard" signs and "soft" signs of vascular injury. Hard signs indicate clear vascular injury that will require operative repair while soft signs reflect an increased risk of vascular injury requiring further study. In reality, many surgeons prefer to evaluate stable patients, even in the setting hard signs of vascular injury, with a CT angiogram before proceeding to the OR. However, most examinations stick to the "rule" that patients with hard signs of vascular injury in the setting of extremity trauma are taken emergently to the OR. Hard signs include obvious limb ischemia, absent pulses, compartment syndrome, active hemorrhage, a pulsatile or expanding hematoma, a bruit or thrill in the area of the injury. Soft signs include venous oozing, a nonexpanding hematoma, diminished distal pulses, or an abnormal ankle–brachial index (ABI) or brachial–brachial index (BBI). The ABI is determined by first inflating a blood pressure cuff over the distal lower leg, and, using a Doppler probe, documenting the pressure at which sound is first heard indicating return of flow in artery. This should be done in both the dorsalis pedis and posterior tibial pulses and the highest value should be used. The same test is then performed in both arms while measuring the first pressure at which flow returns to the radial arteries. Both arms should be measured and the higher of the two values should be used. The ratio of the lower extremity to the upper extremity pressure is the ABI. Values <0.9 are abnormal and should prompt CT angiography (CTA) of the affected extremity. In upper extremity injuries, the BBI is used with the same cutoff value of 0.9. In this case, the values obtained from the injured arm are compared to the values from the healthy arm. In the scenarios posed in the question, only the 22-year-old who suffered stab wound has hard signs of vascular injury. All the other victims have either soft signs of injury that warrant CTA.

2. **Answer E.** Activated charcoal prevents absorption of many drugs from all sites in the gastrointestinal (GI) tract. Notable exceptions to the drugs absorbed by activated charcoal are ions, heavy metals, ethanol, and hydrocarbons. Choices A to D all fall into one of these categories, and only acetaminophen is absorbed by activated charcoal.

3. **Answer D.** Injuries to the metacarpals of the ring and little digits commonly occur after punching someone in the face, the so-called fight bite. Metacarpal joint space violation can be serious and the range-of-motion limiting if not treated properly. Optimal management is with broad-spectrum antibiotics and careful wound explora-

tion to ensure that no foreign bodies or tendon injuries are present. Wounds are always left open to heal by secondary intention to avoid the significant possibility of infection if primary closure is performed. Oral antibiotics are inferior to intravenous antibiotics with this injury. Splinting the joint is indicated if x-ray indicates a fracture, but the warm wrapping of the splint could increase the possibility of infection. In this case, an ulnar gutter splint is more appropriate than a radial gutter.

4. **Answer A.** Elder abuse is an under-reported problem that is slowly increasing in incidence with better layperson and health provider education and recognition. Although much data are still lacking, it is clear that elders who undergo abuse are at higher risk for morbidity and mortality than nonabused elders. Women, the extreme elderly, and patients with severe physical and cognitive dysfunction are all at higher risk. The most common type of elder abuse is neglect; sexual abuse occurs but is uncommon. Physicians comprise only a small minority of reporters of elder abuse for a variety of reasons, including lack of awareness or education about the problem. Most perpetrators are family members or direct caregivers. Every ED should have specific protocols for screening for and reporting elder abuse, along with an action plan for confirmed abuse.

5. **Answer E.** The patient has signs and symptoms of influenza virus at the peak time for influenza season. He exhibits no signs of pneumonia or dangerous vital signs warranting further evaluation. Oseltamivir may be useful to reduce duration of illness in the early setting (before 48 hours of symptoms), but is not effective after this in a previously healthy patient. Amantadine and other M2 viral proton channel blockers are no longer indicated for treatment of influenza due to nearly 100% resistance. Azithromycin, while commonly overused in this exact clinical setting, is not indicated in this patient without evidence of pneumonia. Ampicillin–sulbactam, a powerful beta-lactam antibiotic, is similarly not warranted in this patient without evidence of bacterial infection.

6. **Answer A.** Increasing maternal age, cigarette smoking, cocaine use, twin or multiple gestation, pre-existing or pregnancy-induced hypertension (preeclampsia), trauma, chorioamnionitis, oligohydramnios as well as thrombophilias all place women at risk for abruptio placentae. Of these, preeclampsia is the most significant risk factor.

7. **Answer C.** Asymptomatic bacteriuria is a common finding among healthy pregnant and nonpregnant women.

There is a slightly higher incidence of asymptomatic bacteriuria among pregnant women, ranging from 2% to 10% (vs. 1% to 5% in nonpregnant women). However, most of these women have pre-existing bacteriuria, which is detected during routine early pregnancy screening. It is critical to treat all pregnant women with asymptomatic bacteriuria because pregnant women with asymptomatic bacteriuria have a 20- to 30-fold increased rate of pyelonephritis. The development of pyelonephritis in pregnancy increases the risk of preterm delivery and low–birth-weight infants. The increased risk of pyelonephritis in pregnancy is a result of ureteral stasis, which is due in part to the effects of progesterone on ureteral peristalsis and in part to the effects of direct uterine compression of the ureters. The uterus primarily compresses the right ureter such that 75% to 80% of pyelonephritis cases in pregnancy are right sided. As in nonpregnant women, the principle pathogens in pregnant women with urinary tract infection are *E. coli*, *K. pneumoniae*, and *Proteus* spp.

8. **Answer D.** The KBT detects the presence and quantifies the volume of fetal RBCs in the maternal circulation. Unfortunately, it is an insensitive test, requiring a minimum of 5 mL of fetal hemorrhage for detection. Because as little as 0.01 to 0.03 mL of fetal blood may result in maternal Rh sensitization, the KBT is not useful in most pregnant patients. Therefore, all Rh-negative pregnant patients should be given Rh-immune globulin after significant abdominal trauma. The dose is 50 µg in the first 12 weeks and 300 µg after 12 weeks of gestation. However, in cases in which extensive MFH is suspected, the KBT may be useful because it can identify patients in whom >30 mL of MFH has occurred. Such patients should receive a second 300-µg dose of Rh-immune globulin because each 300-µg dose is only enough to prevent sensitization from 30 mL of fetal blood. The only patients in whom this occurs are patients who have suffered catastrophic trauma (<1% of pregnant trauma victims require a second dose). Therefore, the KBT should not be performed in most pregnant ED patients who have suffered trauma.

9. **Answer E.** Patellar fractures usually occur due to direct blows to the patella from falls or motor vehicle collisions. They may be invisible on standard AP and lateral views of the knee, and patellar sunrise views may be necessary for diagnosis. Transverse patellar fractures are the most common type, but longitudinal fractures also occur and are easily seen on the sunrise view.

10. **Answer B.** This patient's symptoms of severe hypertension in concert with a decreased pulse and irregular respirations are consistent with the development of elevated intracranial pressure (ICP). Due to his history of severe hypertension, he likely suffered an acute intracerebral hemorrhage resulting in an acute increase in ICP and transtentorial (or uncal) herniation. The oculomotor nerve (cranial nerve III) is compressed between the uncus and the tentorium cerebelli resulting in parasympathetic paralysis and subsequent mydriasis ("blown pupil"). Tonsillar herniation results from an increase in posterior fossa pressure (e.g., due to a posterior fossa mass). Symptoms may be subtle or may result in acute cardiorespiratory dysfunction (e.g., when a lumbar puncture is performed in the setting of an undiagnosed posterior fossa mass). Subfalcine herniation occurs in association with a cerebral mass lesion, causing the medial surface of the affected hemisphere to be pushed against the rigid falx cerebri and then herniate underneath it. The cingulate gyrus is most commonly affected and it is often clinically silent.

11. **Answer C.** The patient has community-acquired pneumonia (CAP), and while the nature of the infiltrate on chest x-ray can't be used to predict the bacterial etiology of pneumonia, interstitial patterns are most commonly associated with "atypical" organisms, such as Chlamydia and Mycoplasma, especially for the purposes of board testing. Of all the regimens listed, only doxycycline covers both typical and atypical CAP organisms. Cefdinir and amoxicillin–clavulanic acid lack atypical organism coverage and should be supplemented with a macrolide for optimal CAP treatment. Vancomycin plus gentamicin offers excellent nosocomial coverage but is not necessary in this young, healthy patient with no comorbidities or toxic features. Clindamycin lacks appropriate gram-negative coverage for organisms such as *H. influenza* or *Klebsiella*.

12. **Answer E.** Seeds from *Datura stramonium*, commonly referred to as *jimson weed* or *thorn apple*, contain belladonna alkaloids, including atropine and scopolamine, which cause anticholinergic symptoms. Anticholinergic crises are treated supportively, with decontamination, IV hydration, benzodiazepines for agitation or seizures, hyperthermia control, and cardiac monitoring. Physostigmine is an acetylcholinesterase inhibitor that may be used in select anticholinergic poisonings. Physostigmine increases the amount of acetylcholine in the synaptic cleft, allowing it to compete with the anticholinergic agent for the acetylcholine receptor. Physostigmine is contraindicated in patients with tricyclic antidepressant overdoses, as its use may precipitate intractable seizures and asystole. Pyridostigmine is a quaternary amine acetylcholinesterase inhibitor which does not cross the blood–brain barrier, rendering it useless as an agent to reverse agitation in anticholinergic toxicity. Edrophonium is a short-acting acetylcholinesterase inhibitor which is used mainly to diagnose myasthenia gravis (MG) by improving muscle strength in patients with MG and worsening muscle strength in cholinergic crisis patients. Pralidoxime is used in organophosphate

overdoses, where it breaks up the organophosphate–acetylcholinesterase complex and frees acetylcholinesterase—this action would exacerbate the problem in patients with anticholinergic crises.

13. **Answer A.** CMV each causes one-fifth to one-third of all cases of diarrhea in AIDS patients. The other choices do cause diarrheal illness in AIDS patients but far less commonly than choice A.

14. **Answer C.** In children, Ludwig angina may occur without an antecedent cause, although the disease is less common in children than in adults. Asphyxiation is the most common cause of death, and it results due to upper airway obstruction due to the extensive swelling and edema of the floor of the mouth and neck. In patients with impending airway compromise, fiberoptic nasotracheal intubation is the preferred method of airway control. Due to the significant edema, trismus, secretions, and anatomic distortion of the airway, endotracheal intubation may be extremely difficult. Furthermore, although a surgical tray should always be present while fiberoptic intubation is undertaken, cricothyroidotomy is also more difficult to perform in the setting of Ludwig angina. With early antibiotic therapy, the mortality rate of Ludwig angina is <10%. Patients who have an underlying oral malignancy are not treated any differently than other patients with Ludwig angina. All such patients are treated with immediate intravenous antibiotics, with rigorous observation of the airway.

15. **Answer B.** Adults with elbow pain, limited range of motion, and a joint effusion after a fall on an outstretched arm typically have an occult, undisplaced radial head fracture. Such injuries are rarely operative, and treatment with a sling and early mobilization is preferred. However, children with the same symptoms and mechanism of injury typically suffer a supracondylar fracture with a higher rate of morbidity and need for operative repair. Therefore, children should be placed in a long-arm posterior mold with plaster or fiberglass. Compartment syndrome can complicate supracondylar humerus fractures in children but are more common when there is an associated forearm bone fracture.

16. **Answer A.** Traumatic hemothorax may occur after both blunt and penetrating thoracic trauma. Hemorrhage results most often from parenchymal vessel damage, then intercostal and internal mammary artery lacerations, and uncommonly from great vessel injury. At least 200 mL of blood must be present for costophrenic angle blunting to appear on upright chest x-ray. Tube thoracostomy with a large chest tube (36-French or greater) at the fifth intercostal space and midaxillary line is the treatment of choice. Smaller tubes will cause blood to clot and prevent adequate drainage. Pneumothorax

occurs concomitantly in almost a third of hemothoraces and requires suction drainage. Initial chest tube drainage of 1,500 mL, 250 mL/hour of drainage over 4 hours, worsening hemothorax, hemodynamic instability, and cardiac arrest are all indications for thoracotomy.

17. **Answer A.** This patient has mesenteric ischemia, which is a disease that still has a mortality rate of 70%. Therefore, any patient older than 50 years who has risk factors for acute mesenteric ischemia and who presents with acute-onset abdominal pain should be presumed to have mesenteric ischemia until proven otherwise. The key to diagnosis is recognizing patients at risk, which includes any patient older than 50 years who presents with acute abdominal pain and who has known vascular disease, cardiac arrhythmias, recent MI, hypovolemia, hypotension, or sepsis. The most commonly cited clinical finding is patient pain that is out of proportion to tenderness elicited on physical examination. This is a nonspecific finding that needs to be considered carefully in light of the clinical scenario. Unfortunately, there are no laboratory markers or radiologic studies apart from angiography that have sufficient sensitivity and specificity to exclude acute MI early in its course. Lactate levels are elevated in approximately 100% of patients with bowel *infarction*, but this is a late finding and mortality rates are high by the time infarction has occurred. Plain films are most commonly nonspecific, although even minimal findings such as ileus correspond to more severe disease and a higher mortality rate. The sensitivity of CT has been cited to be as high as 82%, but the most common early finding is bowel wall thickening, present in 26% to 96% of cases. Unfortunately, this is also the least specific finding and is often not present in mesenteric ischemia due to arterial embolism or thrombosis, which are the most common causes of acute MI. Pneumatosis intestinalis or gas in the portal venous system is a specific finding but is only present after bowel infarction has occurred. Angiography is the key to diagnosis and allows for therapeutic intra-arterial infusion of papaverine, a potent vasodilator, or thrombolytic drugs.

18. **Answer B.** The vignette describes a partial oculomotor nerve palsy (cranial nerve III). The oculomotor nerve controls the levator palpebrae muscle (which lifts the eyelid), as well as the superior and inferior rectus muscles (which elevate and depress the eye), the medial rectus (which adducts the eye) and inferior oblique muscles (which elevate the eye in adduction and laterally rotate the eye in abduction), and the pupillary constrictor. Most patients presenting to the emergency room with CN III palsies have partial, pupil-sparing palsies brought about by small vessel ischemia due to poorly controlled or long-standing diabetes, hypertension, and hyperlipidemia. The pupillary constrictor muscles are spared because the nerve fibers to the pupillary constrictor

lie in the outer portion of the nerve sheath so they are less affected by inadequate blood flow. Patients with a CN III palsy due to microvascular ischemia tend to have a good prognosis, as the lesions often heal in 8 to 12 weeks without therapy. Antiplatelet medications such as aspirin are typically started after an initial event.

19. **Answer C.** In the ED, antibiotic prophylaxis is needed for surgical procedures of infected skin and soft tissue or urethral catheterization in patients with a known urinary infection. Routine catheterization does not require prophylaxis. Dental procedures are among the highest risk procedures but are not typically performed in the ED. If an I and D of a periapical dental abscess is planned, then prophylaxis is appropriate.

20. **Answer A.** HACE is the most severe form of high-altitude illness and typically follows acute mountain sickness (AMS). Therefore, symptoms of AMS (headache, fatigue, nausea, dizziness, anorexia, and difficulty sleeping) precede the development of HACE. However, AMS may progress to HACE in as a little as 12 hours although 1 to 3 days is more typical. Most cases of severe HACE occur above 12,000 ft. In addition to symptoms of AMS, the cough and dyspnea of high altitude pulmonary edema (HAPE) are also typically present. Specific signs for HACE include generalized seizures, slurred speech, rare neurologic deficits, delirium, and ataxia.

21. **Answer C.** Infants with pyloric stenosis typically present between 2 and 6 weeks of age with progressive, projectile, nonbilious emesis. Persistent emesis results in a loss of hydrogen and chloride ions from the gastric juices (hydrochloric acid) resulting in a hypochloremic alkalosis. With time, cellular exchange mechanisms pump hydrogen ions into the blood in exchange for potassium ions resulting in hypokalemia.

22. **Answer D.** The patient has an AAA seen on ultrasonograph. In association with hypotension and abdominal pain this must be interpreted as an acutely rupturing AAA, and the only management that will save him is surgery. Further confirmatory imaging in this scenario will only prolong definitive management with little yield and high risk for a poor outcome. Administration of intravenous fluids, though important in resuscitation efforts pending operating room and surgeon availability, will not be able to normalize BP or prevent certain death in patients who are hypotensive with a rupturing AAA. (Figure courtesy of Mark Silverberg, MD. In: Greenberg MI, Hendrickson RG, Silverberg M, et al., eds. *Greenberg's Text-Atlas of Emergency Medicine.* Philadelphia, PA: Lippincott Williams & Wilkins; 2004:194, with permission.)

23. **Answer C.** Post-MI pericarditis generally occurs within 4 days of MI and is characterized by a change in the quality of chest pain. It is treated with NSAIDs, in the same manner as idiopathic pericarditis. Less than a quarter of all patients with MI develop pericarditis. EKG changes are usually absent, masked by the MI findings. Pericardial friction rub is characteristic and often audible. The proposed etiology is autoimmune. Dressler syndrome is the term given to pericarditis which occurs 2 to 3 weeks after MI. It is clinically and electrocardiographically indistinguishable from ordinary pericarditis and should be treated in the same way.

24. **Answer B.** Bivalirudin is a direct thrombin inhibitor, which is a synthetic analog of hirudin, a protein originally extracted from leeches. Both drugs are direct thrombin inhibitors that do not require antithrombin III activity. Although bivalirudin also inhibits platelet aggregation, it does not cause thrombocytopenia, which can be associated with both unfractionated heparin and low–molecular-weight heparins. However, in contrast to hirudin, its principal benefit is a decreased rate of major bleeding, particularly among patients who are considered to have an increased risk of major bleeding. Bivalirudin is the recommended drug of choice by the AHA for patients with NSTEMI undergoing an "early-invasive" percutaneous intervention (PCI) and for patients at increased risk for bleeding who are undergoing immediate PCI. Fondaparinux, enoxaparin, and unfractionated heparin are the preferred agents among patients with NSTEMI not undergoing PCI ("conservative" management).

25. **Answer B.** Meperidine may cause serotonin syndrome in patients who are chronically taking selective serotonin reuptake inhibitors (SSRIs) or monoamine oxidase inhibitors (MAOIs). Dextromethorphan also exhibits this effect.

26. **Answer B.** The majority of CCBs used in human pharmacology are dihydropyridines, which are relatively vascular selective with minimal effects on cardiac contractility and conduction. In contrast, verapamil and diltiazem are nondihydropyridines and are less potent vasodilators with more pronounced depressive effects on cardiac contractility and conduction. The use of beta-blockers in patients with NSTEMI is a class I recommendation due to their demonstrated benefit in reducing mortality among patients with acute myocardial infarction. This is primarily based on their ability to limit myocardial oxygen demand by reducing the heart rate as well as the force with which the heart contracts. In patients who are unable to tolerate beta-blockers, nondihydropyridine CCBs, such as verapamil or diltiazem, can be used instead. Each of the other listed CCBs is a dihydropyridine with limited cardiac effects. Nimodipine has a specific affinity for the cerebral vasculature and is used clinically only in patients with subarachnoid hemorrhage to limit vasospasm.

27. Answer B. Infection of plantar wounds suffered in the absence of footwear occurs in roughly 10% of patients, but depends on several factors, including the degree of contamination and the patient's underlying health. When infections do occur, *Streptococcus* and *Staphylococcus* (including MRSA) are the most common causative organisms. *Pseudomonas aeruginosa* does not typically cause infection of plantar wounds unless the patient was wearing a sneaker at the time of the wound puncture. Patients wearing tennis shoes saturated with sweat are at increased risk for *Pseudomonas* infection. Unfortunately, ciprofloxacin resistance is common and rising, and there are no good oral alternatives as newer generation fluoroquinolones have decreased activity against *Pseudomonas*. While gentle cleaning of puncture wounds should always be performed, high-pressure irrigation should be avoided since there is a theoretical risk of introducing bacteria into the deeper tissues.

28. Answer D. Hemophilia A occurs with a genetic deficiency in factor VIII, predisposing the patient to hemorrhagic complications. The most common cause of death is from head trauma causing massive intracranial hemorrhage. Treatment of bleeding episodes in patients with hemophilia A is with factor VIII. Every patient with hemophilia A should receive factor VIII after head trauma (whether or not there is evidence of intracranial bleeding), as the risk of delayed bleeding is high. Sepsis and MI occur with similar incidence to the general population. Gastrointestinal bleeding does occur in hemophiliacs but is not as common a cause of morbidity or mortality as intracranial bleeding. Congestive heart failure may be secondary to high-output failure caused by anemia but is usually a more chronic process and is not primarily responsible for death.

29. Answer A. Many agents have been advocated, but vinegar is the agent of choice. However, some coelenterates have species-specific treatment and most jellyfish stings require no treatment at all. However, in cases in which tentacles and nematocysts remain adherent to skin, vinegar should be liberally poured over the nematocysts before their removal. Tentacles and nematocysts should then be removed by a gloved hand. Fresh water and alcohol may induce further nematocyst discharge and should not be used. Gently rinsing the wound with seawater is advocated as part of general wound care but it does not inactivate the toxin like vinegar.

30. Answer D. Posterior nosebleeds are potentially life-threatening causes of hemorrhage due to the difficulty in management. The most common bleeding vessel is the nasopalatine artery, a branch of the sphenopalatine artery. Posterior nosebleeds are assumed to be present if a nosebleed is unable to be controlled with an adequate anterior nasal pack. Posterior packing devices such as the Epistat may be placed to provide both posterior and anterior tamponade. Patients with posterior packs should be admitted to units that provide telemetry and pulse oximetry monitoring (usually the ICU), given antibiotics to cover gram-positive organisms, and ENT consultation should be sought.

31. Answer B. Any patient with a history of recent unprotected anal intercourse who presents with symptoms of proctitis should be treated empirically for *N. gonorrhoeae* proctitis. Because concurrent infection with *Chlamydia trachomatis* is common in patients infected with gonorrhea, empiric therapy should cover this organism as well. Podophyllin is a treatment for human papillomavirus (condyloma acuminatum). Valacyclovir is a treatment for herpes proctitis, penicillin is a treatment for syphilis, and lopinavir is a protease inhibitor used to treat human immunodeficiency virus (HIV). Owing to this patient's high-risk lifestyle, he should undergo testing for HIV and for syphilis but empiric treatment is not necessary.

32. Answer C. Activated charcoal may be helpful for gastric decontamination when given within 1 to 2 hours of ingestion. Most patients present after this time interval, and patients with significant acute ingestions frequently experience nausea and vomiting which limits oral decontamination. Enhanced elimination by using multidose activated charcoal takes advantage of digoxin's small enterohepatic circulation but has had mixed results. Whole bowel irrigation has not proven to be beneficial in patients with digoxin toxicity. Digoxin has a large volume of distribution, so drug levels drawn before 6 hours overestimate the steady-state plasma concentration. Toxic cardiac effects are correlated to the concentration of digoxin in the heart. However, in the initial hours after ingestion, the drug is located primarily in the plasma. This explains why more significant evidence of toxicity is not seen early in the course of patients who have taken overdoses despite apparently very toxic drug levels (e.g., 16 ng/mL). These patients remain at risk for toxicity, as the drug distributes into the periphery, but drug levels are not useful until at least 6 hours after ingestion. PVCs and bradydysrhythmias are the most common rhythm disturbances. Digibind should be given empirically to patients with evidence of severe cardiac toxicity, such as high-degree AV block, severe bradycardia, with or without hypotension, or for hyperkalemia >5.0 mg/dL. It is not given as a prophylactic measure. The empiric dose of Digibind in patients with acute toxicity is 10 vials, while 5 vials are given in cases of chronic toxicity.

33. Answer A. Both primaquine/clindamycin and pentamidine are alternative regimens for PCP treatment. In addition, trimethoprim–dapsone has equal efficacy to TMP-SMX and can be used in patients who are allergic to sulfa. Pentamidine can only be administered intravenously or by inhalation. In addition, pentamidine use is complicated by significant side effects. Therefore, primaquine and clindamycin comprise the best alternative outpatient regimen. Intravenous pentamidine is the treatment of choice for patients unable to tolerate intravenous TMP-SMX. In addition to allergic responses, TMP-SMX has many side effects including a high incidence of skin rash and bone marrow suppression. In the outpatient regimen of primaquine and clindamycin, the clindamycin is included because primaquine lacks activity against community-acquired pathogens. Because only patients with mild to moderate disease will be discharged from the hospital, it is imperative to include coverage for routine community-acquired pneumonia (CAP) in addition to giving antibiotics which target PCP. In mild cases, or when the patient's CD4$^+$ T-cell count hovers close to 200, it may be difficult to distinguish between PCP and CAP.

34. **Answer A.** This patient is suffering from heart failure which is a common complication of the refeeding syndrome. The refeeding syndrome refers to the effects that result from restoration of normal nutrition in severely malnourished patients such as those with anorexia nervosa or cancer-associated cachexia. Hypophosphatemia is the hallmark of the disorder and is accompanied by hypokalemia, hypomagnesemia, and volume overload. During periods of malnourishment, the phosphate supply is depleted to produce needed ATP and 2,3-DPG (involved in regulating hemoglobin–oxygen binding). Many patients begin refeeding without first receiving electrolyte replacement. While refeeding begins to replenish needed nutrients, it also results in a profound increase in ATP and 2,3-DPG production, which ultimately depletes phosphate levels and curbs further ATP and 2,3-DPG production. This impacts every organ system, though the heart is most profoundly affected. Myocardial contractility is reduced, resulting in heart failure. In addition, patients may experience altered mental status or seizures, rhabdomyolysis, or hemolysis. The treatment is cessation of refeeding and immediate correction of electrolyte abnormalities.

35. **Answer B.** Flexible endoscopy is the procedure of choice for removal of esophageal foreign bodies. A recent trial demonstrated that between 25% and 33% of esophageal coins will spontaneously pass without complications within 8 to 16 hours of ingestion. Spontaneous passage is more likely in older, male children with coins lodged in the distal third of their esophagus. However, this patient has already presented after a tincture of time has passed, and endoscopy remains standard of care. Papain, a proteolytic enzyme that is a common active ingredient in commercially available meat tenderizer, has been used in the past to aid in the passage of

impacted meat boluses. However, its use is associated with an unacceptably high rate of complications including esophageal perforation, aspiration pneumonitis, and hemorrhagic pulmonary edema. Therefore, its use should be avoided in the ED. Glucagon and effervescent agents such as carbonated beverages may both prove useful in alleviating an impacted food bolus. Glucagon is thought to work by relaxing the smooth muscle of the distal esophagus and most markedly, the lower esophageal sphincter. It does not have any appreciable effect on upper esophageal motility. Effervescent agents should be avoided in cases of complete obstruction or obstruction persisting for longer than 24 hours due to the theoretically increased risk of perforation due to ischemia. The Heimlich maneuver is indicated as a life-saving technique for laypersons to help dislodge a foreign body which is obstructing a patient's airway.

36. **Answer C.** Ocular antibiotics may be given by ointment or drops. Either form can cause systemic absorption and side effects. Drops usually require more frequent dosing due to a shorter duration of action. Ointments are easier to apply in pediatric patients for this reason. Antibiotics are indicated in most cases of conjunctivitis, as early presentations of bacterial cases may be clinically indistinguishable from viral ones.

37. **Answer B.** Therapeutic hypothermia is thought to have several beneficial actions, including:

Reduction in cerebral and myocardial oxygen consumption

Reduction in acidosis

Reduction in excitatory neurotransmitter levels (such as glutamate)

Reduction in free radical formation

Certain factors are either unaffected or made slightly worse with therapeutic hypothermia, such as infection and coagulopathy. Therapeutic hypothermia has been shown to be beneficial in cases of cardiac arrest from ventricular fibrillation and pulseless ventricular tachycardia. Cardiac arrests due to asystole and pulseless electrical activity have not shown the same degree of outcome improvement and use of therapeutic hypothermia in these scenarios should be performed on a case-by-case basis.

38. **Answer D.** The patient has epiglottitis. The x-ray shows an enlarged epiglottic shadow—the classic thumbprint sign. The most common cause of epiglottitis in adults is *H. influenzae*. The adoption of the HiB vaccine has drastically reduced pediatric cases of epiglottitis, but adults who have not received HiB are still at risk. Presentation in adults is less dramatic than in children, with less systemic toxicity and airway compromise. Therefore, many cases are missed on initial evaluation and diagnosed as

simple viral pharyngitis. Lateral soft-tissue neck radiography has a sensitivity of about 90%. Management involves confirmation of x-rays with direct nasolaryngoscopy, intravenous antibiotics (usually a third-generation cephalosporin or ampicillin–sulbactam), and admission for airway monitoring. Consider endotracheal intubation (with preparation for backup cricothyrotomy) in patients who have any signs of airway compromise, such as stridor, drooling, or hoarseness. There is no evidence for foreign body on the x-ray. Group A streptococcal infection can cause epiglottitis, less commonly in adults compared to children. Anaerobes are commonly a cause of retropharyngeal abscess or Ludwig angina compared to epiglottitis. Thyromegaly is difficult to appreciate on x-ray but should be palpable on physical examination if large enough to cause odynophagia. (Figure courtesy of Robert Hendrickson, MD. In: Greenberg MI, Hendrickson RG, Silverberg M, et al., eds. *Greenberg's Text-Atlas of Emergency Medicine*. Philadelphia, PA: Lippincott Williams & Wilkins; 2004:51, with permission.)

39. **Answer D.** The patient likely has laryngotracheobronchitis or croup. Croup refers to viral inflammation of the upper airway with possible pulmonary involvement. Parainfluenza type 1 is the most common cause, but other causes include influenza, respiratory syncytial virus, rhinovirus, and adenovirus. Patients are between 6 months and 6 years of age, and croup is the most common cause of stridor in this age-group. Fever, respiratory distress, and a barky cough worse at night are common. Treatment involves humidified oxygen, L-isomer or racemic epinephrine nebulizer, and steroid therapy with oral or intramuscular dexamethasone. Admission is required in some cases due to either respiratory distress or hypoxia. Amoxicillin is not indicated in this viral process. Ipratropium and albuterol are both used for cases of lower respiratory obstructive disease such as asthma or bronchitis but are not necessary in the absence of wheezes on pulmonary examination. Ribavirin can be used in some viral infections but has no proven benefit in croup.

40. **Answer B.** All of the choices are complications of otitis media, but hearing loss is the most common. The primary reason for antibiotic treatment of otitis media is the prevention of these complications. Current treatment guidelines by the American Academy of Pediatrics involve both immediate antibiotic therapy and deferment of therapy with watchful waiting for 48 hours to observe for development of complications.

41. **Answer C.** The patient likely has bronchiolitis, most commonly due to RSV. It usually occurs during the winter months and is more severe in preterm infants. Low-grade fevers, cough, upper respiratory symptoms, and wheezing are seen commonly. Most patients do not appear toxic, but up to 10% of patients with bronchiolitis require hospitalization because of hypoxemia and severe respiratory distress. The only treatment that improves clinical status is oxygen. Bronchodilator therapy with β-agonists is controversial and not clearly proven to be effective. Corticosteroids and antibiotics are not indicated. Ribavirin is used in preterm infants or those with a history of congenital heart/lung disease. Repeated episodes of bronchiolitis as an infant may increase the risk of developing asthma later in life, but the association between the two conditions is still unclear and most patients with bronchiolitis do not go on to develop asthma.

42. **Answer A.** Patients with traumatic aortic rupture who make it to the ED alive usually (over 70% of cases) have *elevated* blood pressures. This is because aortic hematomas tend to stretch sympathetic fibers, causing an increase in systemic vascular resistance. Patients with traumatic aortic injuries tend to have either moderately–severely elevated blood pressures (range 140/90 to 190/120) or no blood pressure at all—the in-between state of normal–low blood pressure is not encountered as often because true rupture of the aorta would lead to almost immediate death if hematoma containment were violated. Positive upper extremity pulses with decreased lower extremity pulses ("pseudocoarctation") occur in about one-third of cases. Systolic murmurs also occur in about one-third of cases. Chest pain radiating to the back is more commonly seen in atraumatic aortic dissection and is present only in a minority of cases of traumatic aortic rupture. This statistic is likely confounded by the fact that many patients with traumatic aortic ruptures have significant distracting injuries or altered mental status preventing accurate assessment of symptomatology.

43. **Answer C.** Fluid loss in patients with TEN is sizable but not as severe as in burn patients. However, the widely denuded skin is an easy access point for a variety of bacteria and sepsis is the most common cause of death.

44. **Answer C.** The patient presents with diffuse arthralgias and fever in the setting of a recent pharyngeal infection. Rheumatic fever is the most important diagnosis to rule out in this setting. A migratory polyarthritis is common and often involves large joints. Major Jones criteria include carditis, polyarthritis, chorea, erythema marginatum, and subcutaneous nodules. Minor criteria include fever, arthralgias, and various study abnormalities. EKG is indicated to assess for the presence of conduction abnormalities, and further evaluation with echocardiogram may be necessary to evaluate for valvular abnormalities. Treatment is with anti-inflammatory agents, antibiotics, and supportive care. Discharging the patient home puts the patient at risk for valvular and

conductive complications of rheumatic fever and is contraindicated. Corticosteroids are controversial. Urinalysis may be conducted in the course of evaluation to assess for the presence of poststreptococcal glomerulonephritis but does not aid the diagnosis of rheumatic fever. Lumbar puncture is not indicated in this case due to the absence of signs and symptoms of meningitis.

45. **Answer C.** Recent studies have demonstrated that serum epinephrine levels are higher and rise faster in patients given epinephrine through IM injection in the lateral thigh instead of through SQ injection. SQ administration results in variable absorption and may be delayed by the vasoconstrictive effect of epinephrine. Patients with epinephrine autoinjectors are taught to inject epinephrine into the lateral thigh musculature (vastus lateralis). Although no trials assessing *outcome* and comparing SQ and IM administration have been performed, the current recommendation is that epinephrine be delivered through the IM route in the lateral thigh.

46. **Answer D.** Patient or toxin odor may provide important clues to the toxic agent. The smell of garlic can be caused by organophosphates, arsenic, or selenium. Cyanide smells like almonds, zinc has a fishy odor, and toluene smells like glue. Hydrogen sulfide has the odor of rotten eggs.

47. **Answer B.** Patients with aortic dissection require aggressive management of both heart rate and blood pressure. The shear forces that contribute to the development and propagation of a false lumen in aortic dissection are worsened by elevated blood pressure as well as the number of times the heart pumps. Labetalol accomplishes reduction of both heart rate and blood pressure and is the optimal first-line agent for management of aortic dissection. Nicardipine is another reasonable choice, but has less effect on the heart rate and, therefore, should be started after labetalol. Nitroglycerin can cause reflex tachycardia and should not be the first-line agent for aortic dissection. Oral medications should not be given in aortic dissection due to unreliable absorption and therapeutic effect.

48. **Answer E.** Placenta previa refers to a placenta that overlies or lies in close proximity to the internal cervical os. The classic presentation of women with placenta previa is painless second- or third-trimester vaginal bleeding. However, most women are asymptomatic and are diagnosed on routine ultrasonography. Digital vaginal examination should never be performed before ultrasonography in the second or third trimester because it can provoke disastrous bleeding in patients with asymptomatic placenta previa. With progression of pregnancy, 90% of low-lying placentas will migrate away from the cervical os. Disseminated intravascular coagulation is a common complication of abruptio placentae but not placenta previa.

49. **Answer C.** This patient has erythema infectiosum (or fifth disease) caused by parvovirus B19. The illness is common and frequently asymptomatic. In symptomatic children, papules develop on the cheeks which promptly coalesce to form a bright, erythematous plaque which spares the perioral area (circumoral pallor) and nasolabial fold. The rash typically lasts for approximately 4 days. Parvovirus B19 is most important in causing aplastic crises in patients with underlying hemolytic anemias. In addition, infection of nonimmune pregnant women rarely results in fetal hydrops and death. No treatment of immunocompetent individuals is required, though practitioners should determine the immune status of exposed pregnant women. (Figure from Harpavat S, Nissim S. *Lippincott Microcards: Microbiology Flash Cards.* 4th ed. Philadelphia, PA: Wolters Kluwer; 2015, with permission.)

50. **Answer E.** The ideal crystalloid solution for trauma resuscitation remains an area of debate. Recently, many experts have begun recommending lactated Ringers (LR) over 0.9 N NaCl in trauma and sepsis resuscitations because LR is a more "balanced" fluid and does not induce the hyperchloremic metabolic acidosis that comes from large volume 0.9 N NaCl infusions. However, at the time of this writing, there remains debate about whether one fluid has substantial clinical advantages over another. However, D10 water, D10 normal saline, and D5 1/2 normal saline are hypertonic solutions containing glucose, which offer no survival advantage and may predispose to hyperglycemia. Half-normal saline alone is hypotonic and would eventually cause electrolyte abnormalities and excessive peripheral edema if given continuously during trauma resuscitation.

51. **Answer C.** T-wave examination has limited utility in pediatric EKG analysis. Upright T waves in the anterior precordial leads (V1–V3) are normal in the neonate, but they invert after the first week of life and remain inverted until early adolescence, at which time they take on the typical adult, upright appearance. In some patients, the "juvenile pattern" of T-wave inversion can persist into a patient's 20s. In contrast, upright T waves in the anterior precordial leads of an otherwise healthy child can be a sign of right ventricular hypertrophy (RVH), which may reflect underlying congenital heart disease. Right axis deviation is a normal finding in healthy neonates due to the large right ventricular mass, but this resolves over time. Left axis deviation is not normally seen. Supraventricular tachycardias are the most common dysrhythmias in pediatric patients. Atrial fibrillation and atrial

flutter are rare and are typically only seen in postsurgical patients after congenital heart disease repair. In general, rhythm disturbances are uncommon presenting manifestations of congenital heart disease. Ventricular hypertrophy and axis deviation are common indications of underlying structural heart disease. ST elevation in otherwise healthy children and adolescents is usually due to benign early repolarization (BER). However, as in adults, ST elevation can indicate myocardial infarction. Since myocardial infarction is exceedingly rare in the pediatric population, other findings supporting a diagnosis of infarction should be sought, such as cardiac enzymes.

52. **Answer B.** Fever and periorbital edema should prompt differentiation between periorbital and orbital cellulitis. Patients with proptosis, oculomotor dysfunction, and pain on oculomotor exercises are more likely to have orbital cellulitis. Staphylococci and streptococci are the most common causes. Diagnosis is confirmed by orbital CT scan. Treatment of orbital cellulitis is with intravenous antibiotics and possibly surgical drainage. Complications include blindness, death, and intracranial extension. Brain MRI may detect complications of orbital cellulitis but provides little advantage in the emergent evaluation. ESR is an extremely nonspecific laboratory test, which is not useful in the diagnosis of most emergent conditions, except temporal arteritis, septic arthritis, and osteomyelitis. Lumbar puncture and CSF analysis are not indicated in this patient in the absence of headache or stiff neck. Slit lamp examination of the affected side is likely to be impossible given the degree of periorbital edema and not useful as a corneal or anterior chamber process is not the primary source of pathology. (Figure from Tasman W, Jaeger EA, eds. *The Wills Eye Hospital Atlas of Clinical Ophthalmology.* 2nd ed. Philadelphia, PA: Lippincott Williams & Wilkins; 2001, with permission.)

53. **Answer D.** Hyperkalemia presumed to be due to digoxin toxicity generally does not require treatment with therapy specifically directed at decreasing the K^+ level. Instead hyperkalemia is a marker of the *severity* of digoxin toxicity rather than a cause of toxicity. Treatment with Fab fragments will result in rapid resolution of hyperkalemia without any adjunctive treatment. If hyperkalemia is presumed to be due to an alternative cause, it may be treated as detailed here. Although calcium may potentiate the effects of digoxin on the cell membrane, it is the first-line agent for the treatment of hyperkalemia resulting in a disturbance of cardiac conduction. In patients taking digoxin, 10 mL calcium gluconate should be diluted in 100 mL of 5% dextrose in water and infused over 20 to 30 minutes. The effects of calcium last for 30 to 60 minutes. Bicarbonate therapy is one of the least effective means of treating hyperkalemia and is less effective than either albuterol or insulin. Furthermore, some authors recommend completely discontinuing its use for the treatment of hyperkalemia. Sodium polystyrene sulfate may exacerbate volume overload due to systemic absorption of sodium in exchange for removed potassium. However, the most serious complication of sodium polystyrene sulfate use is ischemic colitis and colonic necrosis, which are more common with the enema form of therapy.

54. **Answer B.** The patient's CT demonstrates subarachnoid hemorrhage. Moderate blood pressure control (upper limit of 140 mm Hg systolic) is reasonable for the care of this patient. Hyperventilation with accompanying PCO_2 reduction can be employed as a strategy to reduce cerebral blood flow and, consequently, intracranial pressure. However, the lower limit of PCO_2 for hyperventilation should be 30 mm Hg—hyperventilation to a PCO_2 level lower than this can cause worsened outcomes. FEIBA stands for factor eight inhibitory bypass activity, and is used to manage bleeding in hemophilia A and B patients who have developed inhibitors to standard factor therapies. FEIBA contains activated factor VII as well as inactivated factor VII, IX, and X. It does not currently have a role in management of nonhemophiliacs. Trendelenburg positioning increases intracranial pressure and would be contraindicated in patients with subarachnoid hemorrhage. IV tPA is contraindicated in any patient with active bleeding.

55. **Answer A.** The image demonstrates a subarachnoid hemorrhage (SAH). Seizures may occur in up to one-third of patients and may result in rebleeding, a common source of morbidity and mortality in these patients. Although the efficacy of prophylactic anticonvulsant therapy has not been rigorously tested in these patients, most authors recommend prophylactic anticonvulsant therapy in all patients with SAH. As the CT scan demonstrates blood in the subarachnoid space, there is no need for lumbar puncture. Nimodipine 60 mg should be given orally as soon as the diagnosis of SAH is made and every 4 hours thereafter. In obtunded patients, it should be crushed and administered through an orogastric tube. Nimodipine is used to prevent vasospasm, which may result in secondary (or "delayed") cerebral ischemia. No other calcium antagonist has been proven to be as effective, and even the effects of nimodipine are not irrefutably positive. However, because of its safety and ease of use, it is currently recommended in all patients with aneurysmal SAH. Hypertension should be controlled in the ED with intravenous labetalol or nicardipine. Sodium nitroprusside and nitroglycerin should be avoided due to their potential to cause an increase in intracranial pressure. (Figure reprinted with permission from Haines DE. *Neuroanatomy: An Atlas of Structures, Sections, and Systems.* Philadelphia, PA: Lippincott Williams & Wilkins; 2003.)

56. **Answer D.** Blunt cardiac injury results from blunt trauma directed at the sternum, usually from patients striking the steering wheel in a motor vehicle collision. Patients with blunt cardiac injury (formerly known as *cardiac contusion*) may develop myocardial stunning, congestive heart failure (CHF), dysrhythmia, and in rare instances, when a coronary vessel is damaged, MI. The diagnosis should be suspected in any case of blunt thoracic trauma, but physical examination is often not revealing. The best screening tool for the diagnosis is EKG. Patients with any significant abnormal finding on EKG should be admitted for observation, telemetry monitoring, and confirmatory echocardiogram. Cardiac markers have been extensively studied to evaluate for screening or confirming the diagnosis but are not particularly useful in either regard. Stress testing is not indicated in patients with suspected blunt cardiac injury, as the tachycardic response may actually exacerbate the traumatic insult.

57. **Answer B.** The image reveals a posterior elbow dislocation. Brachial artery disruption or injury is the most serious complication of posterior elbow dislocations, but ulnar nerve injuries are the most common complication. Median nerve injuries are the second most common associated injuries and may occur in concert with ulnar nerve injuries. Decreased function in the distribution of either the ulnar, median, or radial nerves *after* reduction is an indication for surgical exploration and decompression. Postreduction functional loss most commonly occurs because of entrapment of the median nerve. Functional loss that exists before reduction is most commonly neurapraxia and spontaneous recovery is the rule. Therefore, such injuries should be well documented and followed by close outpatient observation. The brachial artery is the most commonly injured vascular structure in posterior elbow dislocations. Although the presence of a radial pulse is reassuring, it does not ensure an intact brachial artery, particularly in the setting of a compartment syndrome. Therefore, physicians should have a low threshold to perform angiography on individuals at risk for brachial artery injury. The presence of a distal pulse deficit mandates exploration and repair. A compartment syndrome at the elbow may result in Volkmann ischemic contracture due to ischemia, injury, and fibrosis of forearm structures. In its most severe form, Volkmann ischemic contracture results in elbow flexion, forearm pronation, wrist flexion, thumb adduction, metacarpophalangeal joint extension, and finger flexion. (Figure courtesy of Robert Hendrickson, MD. In: Greenberg MI, Hendrickson RG, Silverberg M, et al., eds. *Greenberg's Text-Atlas of Emergency Medicine.* Philadelphia, PA: Lippincott Williams & Wilkins; 2004:492, with permission.)

58. **Answer A.** Given his history of cirrhosis and resulting ascites, the patient is at risk for SBP. SBP is caused by combination of reduced hepatic phagocytotic activity with a protein-poor (therefore, complement-poor) ascitic fluid environment. The incidence of SBP occurs at about 25% of all cirrhotic patients per year. Gram-negative organisms predominate, most commonly *E. coli* and *Klebsiella*, though streptococci are also well represented. It is crucial to note that up to half of all patients with SBP lack fever and only a minority have significant abdominal tenderness or true rebound tenderness. Diagnostic paracentesis can evaluate for SBP with an ascitic fluid neutrophil count <250 cells per mm^3. Leukocyte esterase testing with urine dipstick on ascitic fluid has a high negative predictive value for SBP and may be used as an earlier marker to exclude the diagnosis. Treatment involves a third-generation cephalosporin, a fluoroquinolone, or ampicillin–sulbactam. Therapeutic (i.e., large volume) paracentesis in the emergent setting should only be performed in cases of significant respiratory distress where the source is suspected to be inadequate tidal volumes due to tense ascites. CT of the abdomen and pelvis has no role in the evaluation of SBP and should instead be pursued in cases of focal abdominal tenderness or suspicion of abscess or other intra-abdominal pathology. Ultrasound of the right upper quadrant may evaluate for further liver disease of biliary pathology, but this is not suspected in the absence of focal abdominal tenderness or jaundice. Patients suspected of having SBP should not be discharged home until SBP and other abdominal emergencies are ruled out.

59. **Answer E.** Patients with severe upper gastrointestinal bleeding (UGIB) require emergent blood transfusion which may be life-saving. In patients with more moderate bleeding, continuous infusions of proton pump inhibitors (PPIs) have been shown to improve the outcome by reducing the need for blood products and reducing the need for reintervention. However, intermittent bolus administration is much less effective than continuous infusion. This is because continuous PPI infusions maintain gastric pH >4 (the threshold for pepsin inactivation). Bolus administration allows gastric pH to fluctuate and episodes of increased gastric acidity may disrupt clot formation. H$_2$ inhibitors do not alter the natural history of UGIB. Sengstaken–Blakemore tubes are rarely used adjuncts to stop hemorrhage from esophageal varices. Though they are effective, they have a high complication rate and should only be used when endoscopy is not immediately available. Ewald tubes are large-bore nasogastric tubes used for gastric lavage. They may be useful to irrigate the stomach before endoscopy or in cases of acute toxic overdose as a means of decontamination. Octreotide is primarily used for acute variceal hemorrhage although it may be useful as an adjunct in cases of nonvariceal UGIB. This question is still being studied.

60. **Answer A.** There are two accepted and commonly used rapid cooling modalities in heat stroke. One involves pouring or spraying tepid water over a patient and using a fan to enhance evaporative cooling through convection. The second is immersion in an ice water bath. Some authors favor ice water immersion because it is thought to result in more rapid cooling. However, ice water immersion presents challenges as patient monitoring and resuscitation is more difficult and immersion containers may not be readily available. The application of ice packs to the axilla and groin should be considered an adjunct only as its use is inferior to tepid water and fanning alone. Antipyretics and dantrolene play no role in the management of heat stroke although dantrolene may be considered in refractory cases, thought to be due to malignant hyperthermia. More invasive cooling means, such as gastric, pleural, or bladder irrigation, as well as intravascular cooling are reserved for only the most severe, refractory cases and have not been studied to support their routine use.

61. **Answer C.** Aneurysms >5 cm in size are usually palpable on physical examination and approximately half the number of aneurysms between 4 and 5 cm are palpable. Audible abdominal bruits due to AAA are rare. Rupture of an aneurysm due to even vigorous palpation almost never occurs. Femoral pulses are usually intact in patients with AAA. Truncal obesity makes detection of AAA on physical examination much more difficult.

62. **Answer B.** This patient is suffering from thyroid storm. There are no specific criteria for establishing the diagnosis of thyroid storm, although scoring systems have been developed to aid in its diagnosis. However, the diagnosis of thyroid storm remains a clinical one, as laboratory abnormalities in thyroid storm are no different than in patients with hyperthyroidism. The clinical manifestations of thyroid storm include fever, tachycardia, and systolic hypertension with a widened pulse pressure, tremor (especially in the hands) as well as dysfunction of the central nervous system (CNS) and GI disturbances. CNS disturbances range from agitation, restlessness, and psychosis to confusion and coma. GI manifestations include vomiting and diarrhea (e.g., hyperdefecation). Most cases of thyroid storm are associated with Graves disease and occur after a precipitating event such as lithium withdrawal. Lithium inhibits thyroid hormone release from the thyroid gland, so abrupt withdrawal may lead to a rapid rise in free thyroid hormone levels. Although lithium can be used for the treatment of thyroid storm, thioamides such as propylthiouracil (PTU) and methimazole are first-line agents as they prevent the production, secretion, and peripheral conversion (in the case of PTU) of thyroid hormone. Lugol solution or other iodine preparations should not be used until at least 1 hour after thioamides are administered. When iodide preparations are given before PTU or methimazole, the intrathyroidal increase in iodine results in increased thyroid hormone synthesis and release. Aspirin should never be given to patients in thyroid storm, because it prevents thyroid hormone from binding to carrier proteins, resulting in an increase in free thyroid hormone levels. Dantrolene is a muscle relaxant that may be useful in neuroleptic malignant syndrome, serotonin syndrome, or malignant hyperthermia. Propranolol is the first-line agent in thyroid storm. It effectively combats the peripheral adrenergic effects in thyroid storm and rapidly improves the clinical scenario.

63. **Answer D.** The x-ray is without significant abnormality, but the patient is at significant risk for occult tibial plateau fracture. Radiographs can be negative with tibial plateau fracture up to 20% of the time. The optimal management for suspected tibial plateau fractures is non–weight-bearing and repeat x-ray imaging in 1 week or CT scan without contrast to evaluate immediately. In a 72-year-old female, non–weight-bearing can be extremely inconvenient and difficult, so immediate CT is preferred. CT angiogram is not needed in this case, and would be more useful with suspected knee dislocation. Delayed weight-bearing recommendations would not be appropriate for this patient with suspected tibial plateau fracture. X-ray of the ankle is not warranted if there is no specific ankle pathology noted. (Figure from Pope TL, Harris JH, eds. *Harris & Harris' The Radiology of Emergency Medicine.* 5th ed. Philadelphia, PA: Wolters Kluwer; 2012.)

64. **Answer C.** Keraunoparalysis typically occurs in the lower extremities and is characterized by transient paralysis associated with mottled, cool, blue, and pulseless extremities. It results from sympathetic nervous system instability and vascular spasm. These changes typically resolve without treatment within minutes to a few hours and are therefore infrequently seen by emergency physicians in the ED. Asystole is the most common cause of death in patients struck by lightning. Although the normal automaticity of the heart may resume spontaneous activity, respiratory arrest may persist, resulting in prolonged hypoxia and the occasional development of secondary cardiac dysrhythmias such as ventricular fibrillation. Burns and myoglobinuric renal failure are uncommon in the setting of lightning strikes. "Flashover" describes the rapid movement of electrical current over the surface of the skin rather than through the patient's body. This usually results in no cardiac or pulmonary effects or cutaneous burns, although a fern-like or "arborescent" skin pattern may result.

65. **Answer C.** The patient likely has aspirin-exacerbated respiratory disease, which is caused by aspirin and other NSAIDs. NSAIDs inhibit cyclo-oxygenase, reducing

the formation of prostaglandin E_2 (PGE_2) from arachidonic acid. PGE_2 normally serves to inhibit formation of inflammatory leukotrienes. With the formation of PGE_2 reduced, leukotrienes are increased, triggering airway inflammation and bronchospasm. Exercise can trigger these bronchospastic attacks. Of the answer choices, only naproxen is an NSAID. Phenylephrine is an alpha-1 adrenergic agent with little effect on airway physiology. Capsaicin is a topical agent that reduces accumulation of substance P in peripheral sensory neurons. Paracetamol is the formulation of acetaminophen that is widely used in the United Kingdom.

66. **Answer C.** With an elevated blood pressure within 6 weeks of delivery, postpartum preeclampsia must be ruled out. Although rare, preeclampsia can occur up to 6 weeks postpartum. Characteristically, blood pressure is elevated above 150/100 in these patients. Diagnosis can be difficult given that gestational hypertension, chronic hypertension, medication-related hypertension, HELLP syndrome, and postpartum preeclampsia all are on the differential. Laboratory evaluation should include urinalysis, complete blood count (CBC), comprehensive metabolic panel, uric acid, coagulation studies, and lactate dehydrogenase (LDH). Neuroimaging can be warranted in the right clinical setting, however in this patient, it should follow laboratory testing. Pain control certainly should occur, aggressive search for the diagnosis should proceed prescriptions for outpatient management. Lumbar puncture may be a step further down on the diagnostic pathway but should not be performed before the urinalysis and evaluation of postpartum preeclampsia.

67. **Answer A.** Head trauma accounts for the large majority of all pediatric traumatic deaths. Falls and MVCs are the most common mechanisms. When compared to adults, children's heads are proportionally larger and heavier relative to the rest of their body resulting in a higher likelihood of serious injury. The possibility of intentional injury should be sought in all cases of pediatric head trauma. Unlike adults, in whom the extent of intracranial bleeding is limited by the fixed bony skull, infants may develop severe hemorrhagic shock from intracranial bleeding into a more flexible skull. Furthermore, intracranial catastrophes such as epidural hematomas may occur due to venous bleeding (rather than arterial bleeding as is more common in the adult) resulting in delayed presentations.

68. **Answer A.** Due to its higher complication rate, proximal (in the thigh) DVT is a more important clinical entity than distal (in the calf) DVT. Proximal DVT is also more commonly associated with persistent rather than transient risk factors. More than 90% of pulmonary emboli originate from a proximal DVT. In low-risk patients diagnosed with a distal DVT who also have transient risk factors (e.g., recent travel, recent prolonged immobilization), a conservative approach involving serial Doppler examinations is reasonable since it limits the significant risks associated with anticoagulation. Many of these patients will experience complete recanalization over time without any extension of the thrombosis to the proximal veins. However, obese patients with a BMI >40 are at significantly increased risk for development of a DVT. Since the patient's obesity is a chronic problem that is not going to be resolved in a short time frame, he is best treated with anticoagulation as for patients with a proximal DVT.

69. **Answer C.** *Clostridium difficile* is a gram-positive rod that is present in approximately 3% of healthy adults. However, antibiotic therapy used to treat unrelated infections increases the carriage rate of *C. difficile* tremendously. It has been implicated in 10% to 25% of patients with antibiotic-associated diarrhea, but in 50% to 75% of patients with antibiotic-associated colitis and nearly all patients with evidence of pseudomembranous colitis. Clindamycin is classically associated with the development of *C. difficile* colitis. However, the use of other antibiotics such as cephalosporins and fluoroquinolones may also result in colitis. The gold standard for diagnosis is considered to be a cell cytotoxicity assay but due to the cost and labor involved, most laboratories use a toxin detection assay. Positive stool cultures are not diagnostic because the bacteria are often present in healthy subjects and are increasingly present in patients who have been on antibiotics. Diphenoxylate (Lomotil) or other antimotility agents may worsen the disease by allowing further overgrowth and increased time for toxin action. Colonoscopy is not required for treatment but may help to rule out other causes or confirm the diagnosis. In mild cases, withdrawal of the offending antibiotic may be all that is necessary. If symptoms do not rapidly resolve, metronidazole is the treatment of choice with vancomycin reserved for refractory cases. Children with *C. difficile* colitis typically have a more severe course, especially in children undergoing chemotherapy.

70. **Answer E.** Though a transient tachycardia may occur, sinus bradycardia develops and the heart progressively slows as the body cools. In fact, the finding of a relative tachycardia in a hypothermic patient should trigger a search for a cause. The PR, QRS, and QT intervals may all become prolonged although this finding is most common in the QT segment and also correlates with the degree of hypothermia. J waves, or Osborn waves, are the most discussed EKG feature in hypothermia. They are additional waves at the junction of the QRS complex and the ST segment and tend to be upright in aV_L, aV_F, and the lateral precordial leads. Any atrial or ventricular dysrhythmia may occur, but atrial fibrillation is the most

common and it usually spontaneously converts to sinus rhythm upon rewarming.

71. Answer C. This EKG reveals changes consistent with hyperkalemia. Cardiac arrhythmias are the most serious consequence of hyperkalemia, and the presence of EKG changes mandates emergent therapy. This patient's EKG demonstrates peaked T waves, which are among the early EKG changes in the setting of hyperkalemia, typically occurring at levels above 6.5 mEq/L. In general, hyperkalemia *decreases* cardiac excitability resulting in flattened P waves, a prolonged PR interval, and a widened QRS interval. Although all the agents listed are beneficial in patients with hyperkalemia, calcium is the agent of choice, as it has a rapid onset of action (1 to 3 minutes) and stabilizes myocardial membranes. Calcium gluconate or calcium chloride may be given, but calcium chloride provides three times the amount of elemental calcium per unit dose. However, calcium chloride may cause tissue necrosis upon extravasation from intravenous lines and is irritating to local veins. Therefore, most authors recommend that calcium chloride is delivered through a large-bore central venous catheter. (Figure reprinted with permission from Wagner G. *Marriott's Practical Electromyography.* 10th ed. Philadelphia, PA: Lippincott Williams & Wilkins; 2001:225.)

72. Answer C. In the setting of trauma, >90% of patients with a "posterior fat pad" sign have an intra-articular elbow injury. The most probable injury in children is a supracondylar fracture, whereas radial head fractures are the most common entity in adults. Although a small anterior fat pad is a common finding in healthy patients, a posterior fat pad is always an abnormal finding.

73. Answer C. Patients with suspected urinary tract infections require either urethral catheterization or a midstream clean catch specimen for adequate sampling and culture. In a 12-month-old child, midstream clean catch would be extremely difficult. Diaper and bag collection methods are notoriously nonspecific and should never be used. Suprapubic catheterization would be necessary only in cases of urethral anatomic abnormalities where direct urethral catheterization would be contraindicated.

74. Answer C. Levels of AFP >500 ng/mL are present in 80% to 90% of patients with hepatocellular carcinoma (in high-incidence populations). This cutoff is used because elevated levels below 500 ng/mL may be present in patients with acute and chronic hepatitis or cirrhosis. Note that although it has been estimated that hepatitis B is responsible for 75% to 90% of hepatocellular carcinoma cases worldwide, metastatic disease is the most common cause of hepatic cancer in the United States.

75. Answer A. HSV-2 is the most common cause of ulcerative vulvar and vaginal lesions, as approximately one in five sexually active adults is infected with the virus. Because it is sexually transmitted, the presence of HSV-2 in a pediatric patient should trigger a meticulous search for other signs of abuse. Patients typically develop multiple scattered lesions in varying types and stages, including vesicles, pustules, and ulcers. The lesions tend to be shallow and painful and frequently coalesce into larger lesions, particularly in women. Primary infections tend to be more severe than recurrent infections and are frequently associated with systemic symptoms, including fever, generalized malaise, headache, and fatigue. Syphilis is initially characterized by a painless chancre, which disappears without treatment. Chancroid is an uncommon infection in the United States and is characterized by multiple genital ulcerations associated with a tender inguinal lymphadenitis called a *bubo*. The lymphadenopathy is typically unilateral and occurs in 50% of patients. LGV is also a rare disease in the United States and is characterized by a painless and often overlooked primary genital lesion. Patients typically present during the second stage of illness, with a tender unilateral lymphadenopathy that may involve the inguinal lymph nodes both above and below the inguinal ligament resulting in a noticeable groove in between ("groove sign"). Granuloma inguinale is another rare disease in the United States characterized by chronic, painless genital ulcerations. (Figure from Burkhart C, Morrell D, Goldsmith LA, Papier A, Green B, Dasher D, Gomathy S. *VisualDx: Essential Pediatric Dermatology.* Philadelphia, PA: Wolters Kluwer, 2009; 2006, with permission.)

76. Answer A. Dental infections are by far the most common cause of Ludwig angina (98% to 99% are odontogenic), and Ludwig angina may follow dental extraction. Other predisposing conditions include diabetes mellitus, malnutrition, alcoholism, immunocompromised states such as AIDS or organ transplantation, mandible fractures, tongue piercing, peritonsillar or parapharyngeal abscesses, submandibular sialoadenitis, and trauma. Ludwig angina describes a rapidly progressive gangrenous cellulitis of the soft tissues of the neck and floor of the mouth that originates in the submandibular space. Patients present with dysphagia, neck swelling, neck pain, and elevation of the tongue. Airway compromise may occur rapidly and without warning, so attention to the airway is the primary task of emergency physicians.

77. Answer E. Overdose with an antihypertensive causing bradycardia, hypotension, and depressed mental status is most likely from a calcium channel blocker (CCB) or β-blocker. These overdoses can be lethal, especially in children. Traditional treatment has focused on atropine, glucagon, and calcium to counteract the effects of both classes of drug. Atropine reverses the effect of vagal stimulation and prevents further bradycardia. Glucagon functions independently of the β-receptor to improve inotropy and chronotropy. Calcium competes for the calcium channel in CCB overdose. Recently, high-dose insulin and glucose has been found to be beneficial in the management of severe overdoses of β-blockers, and probably helps with CCB overdoses as well. Of note, these symptoms could also be due to clonidine, which can cause severe hypotension, bradycardia, respiratory depression, miosis, and somnolence or altered mental status. Such symptoms may be mistaken for acute opiod intoxication or overdose. Naloxone has been advocated by some authors although it may cause severe hypertension and its use is controversial. Generally, the treatment of clonidine overdose is aggressive supportive care (decontamination with charcoal, intravenous crystalloids, pressors).

78. **Answer D.** Ketamine is a dissociative anesthetic and its primary action is to block NMDA-receptors. However, it also has weak opioid-receptor agonist activities which gives it analgesic properties, and is a triple reuptake inhibitor (serotonin, dopamine, and norepinephrine), which is responsible for its antidepressant activity. It *causes*, rather than prevents, psychosis (primarily hallucinations), though this effect is temporary. It has been studied as an effective analgesic that can reduce opioid use in the ED.

79. **Answer E.** Hypothermia is one of the most common manifestations of severe hypothyroidism (e.g., myxedema) although body temperature is rarely <95°F. In the setting of myxedema, a "normal" temperature should trigger a search for a focus of infection. Nonpitting edema is due to hyaluronic acid deposition and is initially found in the periorbital region. Pseudomyotonic or "hung up" reflexes are another common finding (delayed relaxation phase of deep tendon reflexes). Paresthesias are present in >80% of patients and median nerve neuropathy (carpal tunnel syndrome) is the most common manifestation.

80. **Answer C.** The patient has evidence of a liver abscess. Overall, the most common type is pyogenic, which is usually polymicrobial in etiology. However, with the patient's history of foreign travel to an endemic country, amebic liver abscess, caused by the parasite *E. histolytica*, is most likely. Metronidazole therapy is the most appropriate initial choice of treatment. If there is no clinical response to metronidazole, then surgical drainage or drainage by interventional radiolog (IR) is considered. Amebiasis affects about 10% of the world's population, focused specifically in Central and South America and Asia. It usually causes intestinal disease, but hepatic involvement is the most common extraintestinal manifestation. Pulmonary symptoms can occur due to inflammation and frank pulmonary involvement with either right-sided pleural effusions or abscess rupture into the pulmonary airspaces. Vancomycin or gentamicin alone is not adequate therapy for either pyogenic or amebic liver abscess. There is no role for steroid monotherapy in this infectious process.

81. **Answer C.** This patient has olecranon bursitis. Olecranon bursitis most commonly occurs because of repetitive microtrauma caused by leaning or rubbing of the elbow. Hematogenous spread affects deeper bursae. Although most cases of olecranon bursitis are sterile inflammatory reactions, septic bursitis may account for as many as 33% of olecranon bursitis cases. Furthermore, because of the superficial location, septic bursitis is most common in the olecranon and prepatellar bursae, and rarely occurs elsewhere. Predisposing factors to septic bursitis include patients who are immunocompromised because of diabetes, renal insufficiency, and cancer as well as patients with anatomic abnormalities of the joint spaces and surrounding structures such as patients with gouty or rheumatoid arthritis (both of which may involve the bursa). Aspiration of the bursa is the only reliable means available to help differentiate between septic and sterile bursitis. In contrast to the higher number of leukocytes in septic arthritis, septic bursitis may be present when the WBC count is only 10,000 per mm^3 or lower (one study used 2,000 as a threshold). However, the average cell count in septic bursitis exceeds 60,000. Gram stain is positive in only 50% of cases, and *Staphylococcus aureus* is the most common responsible organism. (Figure from Berg D, Worzala K. *Atlas of Adult Physical Diagnosis*. Philadelphia, PA: Lippincott Williams & Wilkins, 2006; with permission.)

82. **Answer B.** Patient or toxin odor may provide important clues to the toxic agent. Isopropanol is metabolized to acetone, which causes a fruity odor to the breath. Ethanol and certain hydrocarbons can also produce this finding. Cyanide smells like almonds, methyl salicylate like wintergreen, and arsenic like garlic. Acetaminophen has no particular odor, but fulminant hepatic failure from acetaminophen toxicity may cause fetor hepaticus.

83. **Answer C.** The patient has evidence of slipped capital femoral epiphysis (SCFE). The most common presenting age is early adolescence, it is more common in boys, and African Americans are the highest risk population. Obesity is the most common associated condition, but hypothyroidism may also be involved. Patients typically present with unilateral or bilateral hip or knee pain, which is intermittent and worse on activity. Physical examination may demonstrate progressive loss of internal rotation, muscle atrophy, and leg length discrepancy. Lateral, AP, and frog-leg radiographs show the femoral epiphysis slipping inferiorly and posteriorly off the femoral neck. Emergency management includes non–weight-bearing and orthopedic consultation.

84. Answer E. The most common acid–base disturbance in the setting of acute asthma exacerbations is a respiratory alkalosis. However, concomitant metabolic acidosis due to lactic acidosis occurs in up to 28% of patients. The etiology of the lactatemia is not known but it has been hypothesized to occur because of fatiguing respiratory muscles. However, recent case reports have demonstrated that lactatemia can occur even in intubated patients who are paralyzed and, therefore, have no respiratory muscle action. Regardless, the clinical relevance of an elevated lactate level accompanying an acute asthma exacerbation is not known, and lactate levels do not predict respiratory failure in critically ill patients. The presence, however, of a respiratory acidosis as indicated by the ABG above is an ominous sign. A normal or elevated P_{CO_2} in a tachypneic asthmatic typically suggests severe obstruction and impending ventilatory failure. Exceptions to this rule occur most commonly in patients with underlying chronic obstructive pulmonary disease who may retain CO_2 at baseline. However, such patients should have a normal pH and an elevated $H_{CO_3}^-$ due to chronic renal compensation. Leukocytosis, mild hypokalemia, and eosinophilia are not useful in the management of acute asthma.

85. Answer D. Adverse drug reactions (ADRs) are serious events that may have fatal consequences. The incidence of ADRs among hospitalized patients is estimated at 15.1%, with half of these events characterized as "serious," whereas the incidence of fatal ADRs is estimated at 0.32%, resulting in >100,000 deaths per year. However, true allergic drug reactions (i.e., through type I IgE-mediated hypersensitivity) represent only 6% to 10% of ADRs (some reports quote as high as 25%). Although 10% of patients claim to be penicillin-allergic, 90% of those patients are subsequently found through skin testing not to have an allergy. Among those mentioned earlier, urticaria is the most likely manifestation of a true allergic response. The remaining symptoms are most likely expected side effects of drug therapy. However, it is very difficult to rely on the patient's history as nearly a third of patients with proven penicillin allergy by skin testing have vague histories.

86. Answer B. Syncope with aortic dissection mandates evaluation of the pericardial space to check for hemopericardium and tamponade. Dissections extending back to the pericardium are ascending and should be taken emergently to surgery. The most common symptom of aortic dissection is chest pain, although dyspnea is often seen as well. Aortic regurgitation is not usually seen in aortic dissection but indicates a valvular disruption when present. Dissection into the coronary arteries occurs rarely, but when it does, the right coronary artery is most frequently affected. Interarm differences in blood pressure due to unilateral extension of the dissection into the subclavian artery occur in the minority of patients with aortic dissection. However, in patients with undifferentiated chest pain, interarm differences of >20 mm Hg indicate a higher likelihood of aortic dissection.

87. Answer B. The use of digoxin-specific Fab fragments to treat digoxin toxicity has dramatically decreased morbidity and mortality from digoxin toxicity. Fab fragments should be given to any patient presenting with hemodynamic instability, malignant or symptomatic rhythm disturbances (*any* ventricular arrhythmia, high-grade AV block [Mobitz type I second-degree block or third-degree heart block, as Mobitz type II almost never occurs in the setting of digoxin toxicity], symptomatic bradycardia), a potassium level >5 mEq/L (an elevated potassium level is a *marker* of toxicity rather than a cause of toxicity), or a digoxin level >10 ng/mL in the acute setting or >4 ng/mL in the chronic setting. The drug level can be used to determine the number of vials needed:

$$[\text{Digoxin ng/mL}] \times \text{patient weight (kg)}/100 = \text{number of vials needed}$$

However, patients who arrive in the ED with a clear indication for Fab administration should be given Fab empirically:

10 vials in acute toxicity.

5 vials in chronic toxicity.

88. Answer B. Foods are the single most common cause of anaphylaxis although up to one-third of causes are unknown. Exercise accounts for 7% of anaphylaxis cases. Anaphylaxis occurs as an immediate type I hypersensitivity reaction mediated by immunoglobulin E (IgE) antibodies. It requires prior sensitization to the allergen in order to develop allergen-specific IgE antibodies. Subsequent exposure to the allergen allows mast cell and basophil degranulation leading to the subsequent anaphylactic response. Anaphylactoid reactions are immediate type I hypersensitivity reactions that do not require prior allergen sensitization and which clinically mimic anaphylaxis. Anaphylactoid reactions (e.g., response to iodinated radiographic contrast material) typically require a larger dose of the offending agent, but the clinical management is identical to anaphylaxis. Patients at the extremes of age are less likely to have anaphylaxis, probably because of less mature immune responses.

89. Answer D. Phenytoin and lidocaine are class IB anti-dysrhythmic agents. Class I agents have their primary effects on fast sodium channels and slow down action potential depolarization and conduction. These effects are greatest in class IC agents (flecainide, propafenone), moderate in class IA agents (procainamide, quinidine), and least in class IB agents. Unlike classes IA and IC, class IB agents shorten repolarization time and action potential duration. Phenytoin is not used in the ED as an antidysrhythmic, because it may cause important cardiac conduction abnormalities in patients who take the drug for its antiepileptic effects. Loading phenytoin intravenously can occur at a rate no greater than 50 mg/minute, as its diluent, propylene glycol, can cause dysrhythmias or hypotension when given too quickly. Fosphenytoin lacks this diluent and may be given more quickly.

90. **Answer A.** The clinical course of GBS is more severe in the elderly. In children with the disease, death is the exception, and rapid recovery is the rule. Overall, the mortality rate is between 4% and 15%, although 20% of survivors have some residual disability. However, rapid-onset GBS predicts a more severe course. Approximately 25% of patients have a preceding *C. jejuni* infection, and these patients typically experience a more severe course and delayed recovery. Autonomic involvement, resulting in urinary retention, ileus, postural hypotension, sinus tachycardia, and cardiac dysrhythmia, is common and respiratory failure is more common in this group of patients. Ultimately, 25% of patients with GBS experience respiratory failure that requires mechanical ventilation.

91. **Answer C.** Acute arsenic poisoning affects multiple organs, including the liver, kidneys, lungs, and heart. It replaces phosphate in high-energy adenosine triphosphate (ATP) bonds and decreases energy production. Management is supportive plus chelation therapy. The first-line therapy for chelation is dimercaprol (or British antilewisite [BAL]). Activated charcoal does not absorb arsenic or heavy metals. Ipecac is almost never indicated for any poisoning. Penicillamine is a less effective alternative to dimercaprol and is only used when the latter's GI side effects are prohibitive. Deferoxamine is used for chelation of iron.

92. **Answer A.** Diagnosis of aspirated foreign bodies relies on plain radiographs. Posteroanterior/lateral chest x-rays and AP and lateral soft-tissue neck films are diagnostic in the case of radiopaque esophageal and tracheal foreign bodies. Esophageal foreign bodies are seen *en face* in AP views and on edge in lateral views, whereas the opposite is true for tracheal foreign bodies. Frequently, both the AP and the lateral views will be needed to determine the exact location of the foreign body. Additionally, the patient may present with ongoing symptoms that provide further clues to the location of the foreign body. Such symptoms include dysphagia, odynophagia, or regurgitation of food in the setting of esophageal obstruction, or stridor, wheezing, or generalized respiratory distress in the case of tracheal foreign bodies. (Figure from Fleisher GR, Ludwig S, Baskin MN, eds. *Atlas of Pediatric Emergency Medicine.* Philadelphia, PA: Lippincott Williams & Wilkins; 2004, with permission.)

93. **Answer B.** Right ventricular infarction can be better assessed with a right-sided EKG, which is the mirror image of a standard 12-lead EKG. The right-sided V_4 lead (rV_4) is placed at the right fifth intercostal space, midclavicular line. Elevation of the ST segment in this lead is most specific for right ventricular infarction. Nitrates should be avoided in patients with right ventricular infarction, as these patients are very dependent upon passive filling of the right heart by the great veins (preload) due to the decreased active contraction of the right ventricle. Reducing the preload with nitroglycerin will reduce the passive filling and cause hypotension.

94. **Answer B.** Most patients with myasthenia gravis (MG) take glucocorticoids. This patient's hypotension is likely caused by adrenal insufficiency precipitated by glucocorticoid withdrawal. The degree of insufficiency depends partly on the dosage, duration, and frequency. Addison disease refers to primary adrenal insufficiency and occurs far less commonly than corticosteroid-induced disease. Adrenal hemorrhage is very rare and most cases do not cause insufficiency. Viral, fungal, and mycobacterial infections can occasionally cause adrenal insufficiency; bacteria are almost never implicated. Myasthenic crises are characterized by generalized or bulbar weakness in most patients and with primary respiratory symptoms in a few patients. Hypotension is not characteristic.

95. **Answer D.** Goodpasture syndrome is characterized by glomerulonephritis and diffuse alveolar hemorrhage (DAH), associated with the presence of a glomerular antibasement membrane antibody. In the past, the 6-month mortality was 80% with half the number of patients succumbing to DAH. A recent study estimated that mortality has improved somewhat, with a 2-year survival rate of 50% in all treated patients. DAH is the most common cause of death.

96. **Answer E.** The patient has a severe allergic reaction with signs of airway compromise. While the patient's presentation does not include a rash, hypotension, or GI symptoms, management is identical to patients with anaphylaxis and should include prompt treatment with epinephrine. Epinephrine can be repeated every 5 minutes if needed, though few patients need more than two epinephrine doses. When more than two doses are needed, an epinephrine infusion should be considered. In addition, antihistamines, beta-agonist nebulizers, and corticosteroids may help. In this case, the patient is at significant risk for airway collapse and requires repeat epinephrine and preparation for immediate airway control. Chest x-ray and arterial blood gas measurements are time consuming and produce unacceptable delays with minimal diagnostic yield. FFP is reported as a possible treatment for angiotensin-converting enzyme (ACE) inhibitor angioedema. FFP does not play a role in allergic

reactions. Noninvasive positive pressure ventilation can provide ventilatory support but is contraindicated in the face of impending airway obstruction due to edema.

97. **Answer C.** This patient's injury is consistent with a Salter Harris Type I fracture, clinically defined as tenderness over the growth plate with no radiographic evidence of fracture. Based on the information provided, there is no clinical evidence a serious injury. There is a lack of evidenced-based data to guide decision making in these patients. However, in the limited data available, patients with Type I Salter Harris fractures achieve equal outcomes whether they are splinted with removable or more permanent fiberglass or plaster splints. Thumb spica splints are reserved for thumb-specific injuries, and Salter Harris Type II injuries reflect a fracture of the distal metaphysis as well as the growth plate but this patient's x-rays were normal.

98. **Answer E.** Though most cases of rhinitis and sinusitis do not result in orbital cellulitis, nearly all cases of orbital cellulitis are preceded by rhinosinusitis. Specifically, ethmoid sinusitis is the most common precursor because the lamina papyracea, which separates the ethmoid sinuses from the orbit, is a paper-thin bone with many natural fenestrations allowing fluid in the sinus to pass easily into the orbit. Dacryocystitis, orbital fractures, orbital foreign bodies, and even dental infections can all lead to orbital cellulitis but ethmoid sinusitis is far and away the leading cause.

99. **Answer C.** The single most common group of psychiatric disorders seen by emergency and primary care physicians is anxiety disorders. This includes simple phobia, generalized anxiety disorder, panic disorder, and obsessive–compulsive disorder. Treatment usually entails long-term SSRIs combined with benzodiazepines, as needed for acute anxiety attacks. Mood disorders are also extremely commonly seen and treated by primary care physicians. Thought disorders such as schizophrenia are usually managed primarily by psychiatrists, as are somatoform disorders and factitious disorders. Most patients who use recreational drugs do not inform their primary care physicians about their drug use and those who do tend to be referred to addiction psychiatry specialists and outpatient rehabilitation centers. Appropriate referral from the ED for anxiety disorders and mood disorders can involve primary care follow-up exclusively. However, patients with thought, somatoform, or factitious disorders should receive dedicated psychiatric follow-up if they do not already have a pre-existing therapeutic relation with a psychiatrist.

100. **Answer A.** The patient has evidence of serotonin syndrome, a constellation of neurologic, GI, and cardiac findings caused by excessive serotonin activity due to medications. The diagnostic criteria include specific symptoms, the presence of two or more serotonergic drugs, and the absence of neuroleptic agents or other cause for the symptoms. Hyper-reflexia, hyperthermia, altered mental status, and diarrhea are characteristic. Medications associated with serotonin syndrome include combinations of the following: Selective serotonin reuptake inhibitors (SSRIs), monamine oxidase inhibitors, catecholamine releasers (cocaine, amphetamines, and dextromethorphan), nonselective serotonin reuptake inhibitors (tricyclic and atypical antidepressants, carbamazepine, meperidine, methadone), and serotonin agonists (buspirone, lithium, LSD, sumatriptan). Treatment of serotonin syndrome is supportive, but cyproheptadine, a serotonin antagonist, may be helpful in some cases. Choices B to E do not contribute to serotonin syndrome.

QUESTIONS

1. Which of the following is true regarding thromboembolic disease in pregnancy?

   A. Ventilation-perfusion (V/Q) scans expose the fetus to less radiation than helical CT chest scans in ruling out pulmonary embolism (PE).
   B. Warfarin is only contraindicated during fetal organogenesis.
   C. Thromboembolic disease is the leading cause of death in pregnancy.
   D. The risk of deep venous thrombosis is highest in the third trimester.
   E. All of the above.

2. A 56-year-old male with a history of alcoholic cirrhosis presents with altered mental status. According to his wife, he reportedly stopped taking his lactulose several days prior to his emergency department (ED) evaluation. He is disoriented and confused and demonstrates asterixis. He has normal vital signs. Laboratory studies are unremarkable except for a chronically elevated prothrombin time (PT). Noncontrast CT of the brain is normal. The ammonia level is only mildly elevated. Which of the following is the next best step in management?

   A. Consult psychiatry
   B. Give lactulose
   C. Perform endotracheal intubation
   D. Perform lumbar puncture
   E. Consult neurology

3. A 26-year-old female G2P1 presents to the ED in labor and delivers her infant onto the stretcher. Upon evaluation, you discover a spontaneously breathing neonate lying relatively still with its arms and legs flexed, with a heart rate of 120, bluish hands and toes with a pink face, who gives s slight whimper when suctioned. Its APGAR score is:

   A. 5
   B. 6
   C. 7
   D. 8
   E. 9

4. A 9-month-old infant is brought to the emergency department (ED) with a bruise on his thigh suffered from falling out of his high chair. Radiographs reveal a midshaft femur fracture. Which of the following is the most likely contributing factor?

   A. Child abuse
   B. Osteogenesis imperfecta
   C. Bone tumor
   D. Bone cyst
   E. Hypocalcemia

5. Which of the following is true regarding ibuprofen overdoses?

   A. Rapid progression to coma and death often occurs within 24 hours.
   B. Significant morbidity and mortality is prevented by timely administration of a specific antidote.
   C. Hemodialysis is required in approximately half the cases.
   D. Urinary alkalinization is effective at reducing toxicity.
   E. Even without treatment, a benign course is characteristic.

6. Which of the following rhythm disturbances is considered pathognomonic for digoxin toxicity?

   A. Atrial flutter with premature ventricular contractions (PVCs)
   B. Sinus bradycardia with PVCs
   C. Bidirectional ventricular tachycardia
   D. Mobitz type II second-degree AV block
   E. Accelerated junctional rhythm

7. A 65-year-old male presents with dyspnea on exertion for several weeks. He does not regularly see physicians and reports no past medical history (Fig. 9-1). Which of the following is the most likely etiology of his symptoms?

   A. Bacterial pneumonia
   B. Viral pneumonia
   C. Congestive heart failure (CHF)
   D. PE
   E. Pancreatitis

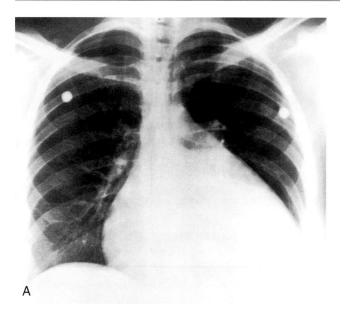

A

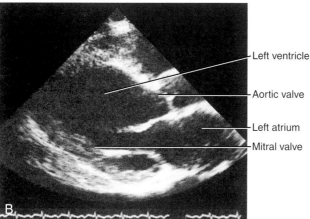

- Left ventricle
- Aortic valve
- Left atrium
- Mitral valve

B

Figure 9-1

8. Which of the following statements is true regarding scarlet fever and acute rheumatic fever?

A. Both occur concomitantly with group A β-hemolytic streptococcal (GAS) pharyngitis.

B. Acute rheumatic fever is a complication of acute GAS pharyngitis that occurs more commonly in adults.

C. Scarlet fever occurs acutely with GAS pharyngitis, but acute rheumatic fever does not typically occur until 2 to 4 weeks after GAS pharyngitis.

D. Scarlet fever is now a rare occurrence due to the *H. influenzae* type B (HiB) vaccine.

E. Both scarlet fever and acute rheumatic fever can be prevented by the use of antibiotics for GAS pharyngitis.

9. Which of the following is characteristic of rotavirus diarrhea?

A. Fecal leukocytes

B. Fecal erythrocytes

C. Peak age is between 3 and 10 years of age

D. Duration of 1 month

E. Vaccination dramatically reduces hospitalization and ED visits

10. A 55-year-old female on long-term steroids for sarcoidosis is brought in by paramedics with generalized weakness and altered mental status. You quickly suspect acute adrenal insufficiency. Which of the following are primarily responsible for the majority of acute morbidity and mortality in acute adrenal insufficiency?

A. Hypernatremia and hypokalemia

B. Hyponatremia and hyperkalemia

C. Hypotension and hypoglycemia

D. Hypothermia and hypercalcemia

E. Anorexia and mucocutaneous hyperpigmentation

11. A 42-year-old female presents with a chief complaint of right-hand numbness. Decreased sensation in the volar aspect of the little finger indicates a problem in which of the following?

A. Radial nerve

B. C5 nerve root

C. Ulnar nerve

D. Median nerve

E. C6 nerve root

12. Which of the following is the most effective method of eliminating symptoms in acquired immune deficiency syndrome (AIDS) patients with *Cryptosporidium* diarrhea?

A. Loperamide

B. Highly active antiretroviral therapy (HAART)

C. Azithromycin

D. Metronidazole

E. Octreotide

13. Intussusception in adults:

A. Most often presents with symptoms of partial intestinal obstruction

B. Most commonly occurs in the large intestine

C. Is most commonly idiopathic, without an identifiable lead point

D. Is the second most common cause of large bowel obstruction

E. Is best diagnosed with barium or water contrast enema

14. A 22-year-old male states that he ingested 20 to 30 condoms containing a total of 1 kg of cocaine 12 hours ago. He subsequently became concerned about rupture of the condoms and now wants to get them out of his body. He is completely asymptomatic. His vital signs are normal and his physical examination is unremarkable. Which of the following is the most appropriate next step in management?

    A. Polyethylene glycol
    B. Activated charcoal
    C. Hemodialysis
    D. Endoscopic removal
    E. Operative removal

15. A 42-year-old female presents with acute onset of abdominal pain. She reports no alcohol use. Her only past medical history is cholecystectomy. Her abdomen is tender in the epigastrium and her lipase returns at 2,500 U/L. Her CBC and her basic metabolic panel return from the lab as unreadable, despite multiple different blood draws. Which of the following is the most likely etiology?

    A. Alcohol
    B. Gallstones
    C. Hypertriglyceridemia
    D. Ibuprofen
    E. Rhinovirus

16. Which of the following is true regarding orbital cellulitis?

    A. Pain with extraocular movements is a characteristic finding.
    B. Hematogenous spread of bacteria commonly occurs.
    C. Sinusitis is an uncommon predisposing factor.
    D. *Aspergillus* is a common cause of acute disease.
    E. Periorbital cellulitis often spontaneously progresses to involve the orbit.

17. A 23-year-old male is brought to the ED by paramedics after a suicide attempt. He had locked himself in the garage and turned on his car for several minutes until his roommates caught him. He is somnolent and barely responsive. You suspect carbon monoxide poisoning. His pulse oximetry is 99%. Which of the following is the most accurate statement regarding this patient?

    A. Because pulse oximetry is 99%, he is unlikely to have had a significant carbon monoxide exposure.
    B. The primary pathophysiologic mechanism of carbon monoxide is hypoventilation.
    C. Pao_2 level is the most accurate test in determining the extent of carbon monoxide poisoning.
    D. Treatment with IV pyridostigmine is indicated.
    E. An emergent blood glucose level should be obtained.

18. Which of the following is true regarding status epilepticus?

    A. Children younger than 16 years have the highest mortality due to status epilepticus.
    B. Treatment with diazepam has better outcomes than with lorazepam.
    C. The most common side effect of benzodiazepines given for status epilepticus is hypoventilation.
    D. Among adults, the most common etiology of status epilepticus is subtherapeutic antiepileptic drug levels.
    E. None of the above is true.

19. Which of the following is true regarding temporomandibular joint (TMJ) syndrome?

    A. It is an extremely rare cause of facial pain.
    B. Young women are at highest risk.
    C. Pain is normally bilateral.
    D. Muscle relaxants are not helpful in management.
    E. Avoidance of hard foods is rarely necessary.

20. Which of the following is true regarding myasthenia gravis (MG) and Lambert–Eaton myasthenic syndrome (LEMS)?

    A. Patients most commonly have worsened muscle weakness in the morning.
    B. Autonomic dysfunction is a common finding.
    C. Colon cancer is the most common associated neoplastic.
    D. Ocular muscle weakness is the most common initial presentation.
    E. Muscle weakness is constant and progressive.

21. A 22-year-old diabetic man presents 1 day after being punctured in his left arm during a hiking accident. Since the accident, he has noted increasingly intense pain in his arm along with mild swelling and redness. On examination, his arm is noted to be mildly swollen and erythematous with an innocuous appearing puncture wound on the volar aspect of his right forearm. His arm is extremely tender, although there is no crepitus. A plain film is obtained which reveals subcutaneous emphysema. Which of the following is the next best step in management?

    A. Irrigation of the wound with sterile saline
    B. Surgical consult
    C. Incision and drainage in the ED
    D. Intravenous antibiotics and admission
    E. MRI of the arm

22. A 27-year-old male presents with a rash (Fig. 9-2). The patient states that his wife first noticed a single spot on his back approximately 10 days ago. He denies fever or pain and complains only of mild pruritus. Over the last few days, many new "spots" have cropped up on

his back and trunk. On examination, you note that the lesions have a fine scale around the border and seem to be arranged along the skin lines of the back. Which of the following is the most likely diagnosis?

A. Secondary syphilis
B. Pityriasis rosea
C. Molluscum contagiosum
D. Tinea corporis
E. Atopic dermatitis

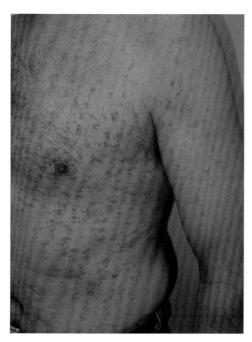

Figure 9-2

23. Which of the following is true regarding orbital wall fractures?

A. The orbital floor is the weakest part of the orbit.
B. Globe injuries occur in almost all orbital floor fractures.
C. The teardrop sign refers to fat extending from the globe into the optic nerve.
D. Antibiotics are indicated in all orbital wall fractures.
E. Patients with orbital wall fractures should be instructed to blow their noses every 6 hours to reduce nasal congestion.

24. Which of the following mechanisms of heat loss can be increased therapeutically to treat heat stroke?

A. Evaporation
B. Conduction
C. Radiation
D. A and B
E. A, B, and C

25. A 63-year-old female is brought to the ED by her children because she is lethargic and has labored breathing. They last saw her 4 days ago when she seemed well. Her vital signs are T 101.8°F, HR 120 per minute, RR 32 per minute, and an SaO_2 of 89% on 100% oxygen by face mask. She is intubated and placed on assist-control ventilation. A subsequent chest x-ray reveals diffuse bilateral infiltrates, and normal heart size. You suspect she has severe pneumonia and acute respiratory distress syndrome (ARDS). Which of the following summarizes the best ventilation strategy?

A. Due to low compliance, patients with ARDS need higher tidal volumes and higher positive end-expiratory pressure (PEEP) to ensure adequate ventilation.
B. Due to significant airway obstruction, such patients require very low or no PEEP similar to asthma patients to avoid air trapping.
C. Due to high compliance, such patients require lower tidal volumes and lower PEEP to improve oxygenation.
D. Due to low compliance, such patients require lower tidal volumes and higher PEEP to avoid barotrauma.
E. Due to high compliance, patients with ARDS do not require PEEP.

26. In a patient with benzodiazepine poisoning, which of the following is an indication for flumazenil use?

A. Accidental pediatric ingestion
B. Coingestion of tricyclic antidepressant
C. Chronic benzodiazepine user
D. Alcoholic patient
E. Seizure activity

27. Which of the following is a manifestation of hypocalcemia?

A. QTc shortening
B. Polyuria
C. Perioral paresthesias
D. Nephrolithiasis
E. None of the above

28. A 65-year-old male presents with sudden, painful loss of vision in his right eye. His visual acuity is markedly decreased in the affected eye. Which of the following is the most likely cause of his symptoms?

A. Acute angle closure glaucoma
B. Central retinal artery occlusion
C. Central retinal vein occlusion
D. Retinal detachment
E. Vitreous hemorrhage

29. A 65-year-old female presents with 2 hours of severe, diffuse, progressively worsening acute abdominal pain. Blood pressure is 150/90, and abdominal examination demonstrates a palpable pulsatile mass. Abdominal CT scan is shown in Figure 9-3. Which of the following is true regarding management of this patient?

    A. Blood pressure should be reduced to systolic 100 mm Hg or below.
    B. The patient should be crossmatched for 10 units of packed red blood cells.
    C. Ultrasound may help better characterize the anatomy.
    D. Angiogram may reduce the need for urgent surgery.
    E. Stable patients may be observed for signs of deterioration.

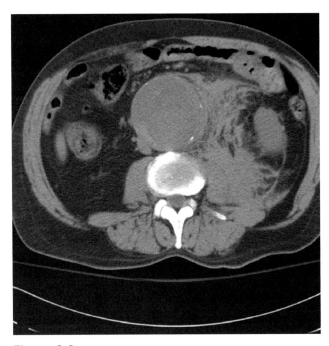

Figure 9-3

30. A 27-year-old female with a history of Wolff-Parkinson-White (WPW) is brought in by EMS with a somewhat irregular, wide-complex tachycardia at roughly 230 beats per minute. Her vitals include a pulse of 230, RR 22, BP 87/58, and SaO$_2$ of 98% on room air. She is mildly diaphoretic and pale. Which of the following is the best treatment?

    A. Procainamide
    B. Electrical DC cardioversion
    C. Adenosine
    D. Amiodarone
    E. Verapamil

31. A 9-year-old female is brought in to the ED with a chief complaint of a palpable, nonblanching rash, achy knee and ankle pain, and colicky abdominal pain (Fig. 9-4). Which of the following is true?

    A. Renal involvement, with progression to renal failure, is common.
    B. Most patients have thrombocytopenia.
    C. Treatment is with high-dose aspirin.
    D. Intussusception complicating this illness is usually ileoileal.
    E. Most patients require inpatient immunosuppressive therapy.

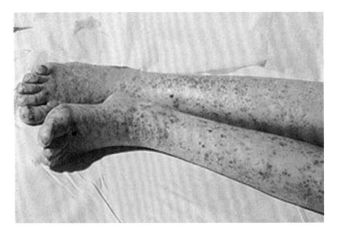

Figure 9-4

32. What is the most common electrocardiographic (EKG) abnormality in patients with heatstroke?

    A. Sinus bradycardia
    B. Atrial fibrillation
    C. QT interval prolongation
    D. Ventricular fibrillation
    E. Supraventricular tachycardia (SVT)

33. A 62-year-old male presents with right eyelid swelling and crusting. He reports no pain or redness in the eye itself. Physical examination of the eyelid is shown in Figure 9-5. Which of the following is the most appropriate therapy?

    A. Topical erythromycin
    B. Topical prednisolone
    C. Topical proparacaine
    D. Intravenous ceftriaxone
    E. Intravenous acetazolamide

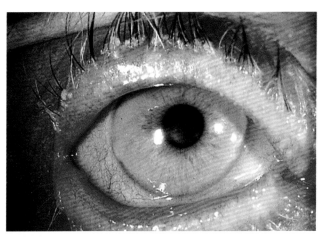

Figure 9-5

34. A 27-year-old nonpregnant woman presents with pelvic pain. Pelvic ultrasonography reveals a 4-cm right adnexal cystic mass. Which of the following is the most likely etiology?

    A. Corpus luteum cyst
    B. Dermoid cyst
    C. Theca lutein cyst
    D. Follicular cyst
    E. Ovarian fibroma

35. A 27-year-old female presents with chronic, intermittent, diffuse, crampy abdominal pain and intermittent nonbloody diarrhea for 10 months. She has seen her primary care physician multiple times for these symptoms and has had a right upper quadrant ultrasound, CT abdomen/pelvis, magnetic resonance imaging (MRI) abdomen/pelvis, HIDA scan, urinalysis, and a comprehensive chemistry lab panel, all of which have been negative. Her vital signs are 98.6°F, 85, 16, 110/65, 99% rheumatoid arthritis (RA). Her examination is unremarkable and her urine pregnancy test is negative. Which of the following is the most appropriate therapy for this patient?

    A. Fiber supplementation
    B. Lithium
    C. Desipramine
    D. Ciprofloxacin and metronidazole
    E. Repeat CT abdomen/pelvis for reassurance

36. A 6-year-old female is brought to the ED by her parents with multiple loose, nonbloody stools for 1 day. She has no vomiting or fever. Many of her classmates in school have similar symptoms. She appears mildly dehydrated, with slightly sunken eyes and dry mucous membranes. Vital signs are 99°F, 115, 22, 95/55, 100% RA. Basic chemistry and complete blood count panels are normal. Which of the following is the most appropriate therapy?

    A. Intravenous fluid therapy
    B. Oral fluid therapy with sugar and salt solution

    C. BRAT diet (bananas, rice, apple sauce, toast)
    D. Metronidazole
    E. Nitazoxanide

37. Which of the following is the most common toxicity associated with cyclosporine?

    A. Hyperuricemia and gout
    B. Hyperlipidemia
    C. Nephrotoxicity
    D. Hepatotoxicity
    E. Hypertension

38. A 25-year-old male with a history of acute myelogenous leukemia presents with acute onset of generalized weakness. He received his first dose of chemotherapy 3 days before presenting for evaluation. Which of the following is the most likely abnormality on laboratory analysis?

    A. Hyperkalemia
    B. Hypercalcemia
    C. Hypophosphatemia
    D. Hyponatremia
    E. Hypomagnesemia

39. Which of the following is the most common cause of nongonococcal urethritis?

    A. *Ureaplasma*
    B. *Trichomonas*
    C. *Hemophilus ducreyi*
    D. *C. trachomatis*
    E. Herpes simplex virus

40. Which of the following is true regarding rust rings?

    A. Removal should be undertaken immediately by the emergency physician (EP).
    B. They are usually caused by copper-containing foreign bodies.
    C. Topical steroids should be used for treatment.
    D. MRI is indicated to evaluate for intraocular foreign bodies.
    E. Ophthalmology follow-up should occur within 48 hours.

41. Which of the following is true regarding avulsed and subluxed teeth?

    A. Avulsed teeth can almost always be successfully reimplanted if returned to their sockets within 3 hours.
    B. Avulsed primary teeth are never reimplanted.
    C. The best known transport medium for avulsed teeth is milk.
    D. Teeth can be temporarily secured for up to 1 week with a periodontal pack made from resin and catalyst paste.
    E. Avulsed teeth should be scrubbed with a povidone–iodine sponge to kill microbes before reimplantation.

42. An 11-month-old male infant is brought in by his parents to the ED with a rash (Fig. 9-6). They state that he appeared to have some discharge from his eyes and then developed a diffuse, tender "redness" to his skin, which had a "rough" feel to it. Their pediatrician diagnosed him with a viral syndrome and prescribed oral antipyretics as needed. Since then, his skin appears to have wrinkled, formed blisters, and is now peeling in large sheets. Which of the following is the treatment of choice?

    A. Amoxicillin
    B. Vancomycin
    C. Valacyclovir
    D. Corticosteroids
    E. Continue with supportive care only

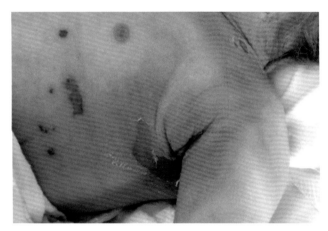

Figure 9-6

43. A 22-year-old primigravida presents to the ED with crampy low abdominal pain. She is 11 weeks by dates and denies vaginal bleeding. Her physical examination reveals a normal vaginal vault and a closed internal cervical os. Ultrasound examination reveals a single intrauterine gestation at 9 weeks, with no fetal heart tones. Persistent failure to expel the fetal and maternal uterine contents would result in a:

    A. Threatened abortion
    B. Incomplete abortion
    C. Complete abortion
    D. Missed abortion
    E. Inevitable abortion

44. A 42-year-old female with a history of migraines presents for evaluation of a throbbing, left-sided parietal headache associated with nausea and refractory to serial doses of sumatriptan at home. Which of the following treatments may be most helpful in treating the patient's acute headache?

    A. A bolus of intravenous fluids
    B. Intravenous dexamethasone

C. Oxygen therapy delivered by nasal cannula ≥2 L/minute
D. Intravenous hydromorphone
E. Intravenous prochlorperazine

45. Which of the following is the most common cause of death in patients with sickle cell disease?

    A. Myocardial infarction (MI)
    B. Stroke
    C. Sepsis
    D. Aplastic crisis
    E. Splenic sequestration

46. The "discriminatory zone" is the quantitative serum β-hCG level at which a normal intrauterine gestation should be seen on ultrasonography. The discriminatory zone for transvaginal ultrasonography is:

    A. <500 mIU/mL β-hCG
    B. 500 to 1,000 mIU/mL β-hCG
    C. 1,000 to 2,000 mIU/mL β-hCG
    D. 2,000 to 3,000 mIU/mL β-hCG
    E. >3,000 mIU/mL β-hCG

47. The joints most commonly affected by decompression sickness (DCS) are:

    A. Ankles and feet
    B. Knees
    C. Hips and axial skeleton
    D. Shoulders and elbows
    E. Wrists and hands

48. Security is called to help restrain an agitated patient in the ED. In helping to restrain the patient, one of the officers is inadvertently stuck by a contaminated needle that the nurse was using to obtain an IV. The patient is known to have chronic active hepatitis B (HepB) and the officer says he was immunized once against HepB but is a "nonresponder." Which of the following is true?

    A. Passive immunization with hepatitis B immune globulin (HBIG) but not active immunization with the HepB vaccine should be given.
    B. The HepB vaccine is incompatible with typical prophylactic drug therapy for human immunodeficiency virus (HIV).
    C. The HepB vaccine should still be given since many initial nonresponders will respond to a second HepB vaccine series.
    D. The patient's wound should be washed with a dilute bleach solution to denature the protein coat of the virus.
    E. HepB is transmitted much less effectively than hepatitis C through needlestick injuries.

49. A 22-year-old male presents with cough, fever, and shortness of breath for 3 days. He has no past medical history. His vital signs are 100.5°F, 92, 22, 122/72, 98% RA. Examination reveals left lower lung field crackles that do not clear on coughing. Which of the following is the most appropriate therapy?

    A. Doxycycline PO
    B. Linezolid PO
    C. Cephalexin PO
    D. Clindamycin PO
    E. Piperacillin–tazobactam IV

50. A 45-year-old female presents with a red eye on waking. She is otherwise completely asymptomatic. She denies any past medical history and takes no medications. The eye is shown in Figure 9-7. Physical examination is otherwise normal. Which of the following is the most appropriate next step in management?

    A. Emergent ophthalmologic consultation
    B. Platelet function assay
    C. Topical antihistamines
    D. Topical antibiotics
    E. No specific therapy

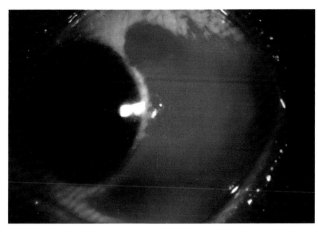

Figure 9-7

51. Which of the following medications or medication classes may exacerbate symptoms in patients with hypercalcemia?

    A. Thiazide diuretics
    B. Bisphosphonates
    C. Calcitonin
    D. Loop diuretics
    E. Glucocorticoids

52. An 87-year-old female is brought to the ED by her caretaker with dehydration and excessive somnolence. Her initial blood work reveals a sodium level of 119 mEq/L and a glucose level of 900. Which of the following represents her actual sodium level?

    A. ~109 mEq/L
    B. ~119 mEq/L
    C. ~125 mEq/L
    D. ~130 mEq/L
    E. ~138 mEq/L

53. The normal anion gap (AG) is primarily due to which of the following?

    A. Phosphate
    B. Albumin
    C. Sulfate
    D. Citrate
    E. Acetone

54. Which of the following Salter–Harris fractures carries the poorest prognosis?

    A. Type I
    B. Type II
    C. Type III
    D. Type IV
    E. Type V

55. Which of the following effects does digitalis exhibit at therapeutic levels?

    A. Decreases intracellular calcium
    B. Decreases intracellular sodium
    C. Increases intracellular potassium
    D. Increases heart rate
    E. T-wave inversion

56. A 36-year-old primigravida presents to the ED at 32 weeks' gestation with epigastric pain. Her BP is 150/100, but other vital signs are normal. While the nurse is performing his assessment in the room, the patient begins to seize. The next best step in management is:

    A. Hydralazine 10 mg IV push
    B. Lorazepam 2 mg/minute IV push
    C. Phenytoin 20 mg/kg IV
    D. Magnesium 6 g slow IV push
    E. Labetalol 20 mg slow IV push

57. Which of the following neurologic findings is characteristic of tick paralysis?

    A. Cranial nerve palsy
    B. Descending flaccid paralysis
    C. Ascending flaccid paralysis
    D. Decreased pain and temperature sensation
    E. Decreased vibratory and position sensation

58. A 23-year-old male with a history of human immuno-deficiency virus (HIV) presents with shortness of breath, fever, and malaise. A chest x-ray is shown in Figure 9-8. Arterial blood gas shows a Pao_2 of 60 mm Hg. Which of the following, in addition to antibiotics, is the most appropriate therapy?

A. Albuterol
B. Prednisone
C. Aspirin
D. Vasopressin
E. Hyperbaric oxygen

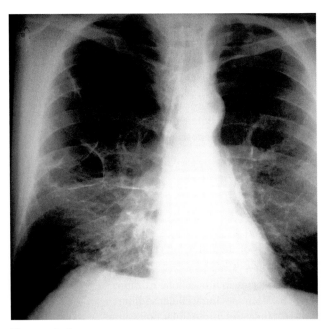

Figure 9-8

59. A 55-year-old male with a history of myasthenia gravis (MG) presents with extreme fatigue and somnolence. He is barely responsive to painful stimuli. His blood glucose level is 95 mg/dL. His pulse oximetry is 96% on room air. Which of the following is the most important next step in management?

A. Chest x-ray
B. Central venous access
C. Endotracheal intubation
D. Noninvasive positive pressure ventilation
E. CT brain

60. A 41-year-old female is referred from her dentist because her blood pressure was 212/105 when she presented for her root canal. She complains of dental pain in the area of the affected tooth, but she denies headache, blurry vision, nausea, or extremity weakness or numbness. The remainder of her review of systems is negative. Her physical examination is unrevealing except for carious teeth. She has never been diagnosed with hypertension, but admits that she had not seen a physician "in years."

She has no drug allergies or known contraindications to any specific drug therapy. Which of the following is the next best step?

A. Administer clonidine 0.1 mg PO every hour until her blood pressure is less than 185/110 and then discharge.
B. Obtain a chest x-ray, EKG, head CT, CBC, basic metabolic panel, and cardiac enzymes to help determine her disposition.
C. Start the patient on hydrochlorothiazide 25 mg PO daily, and discharge her to follow-up with her primary care physician.
D. Administer one dose of IV hydralazine until the patient's BP is lower than 185/110, then switch to oral therapy, and discharge if asymptomatic.
E. Initiate an IV labetalol infusion and admit the patient with a diagnosis of hypertensive urgency.

61. A 64-year-old female is brought in by emergency services (EMS) with a chief complaint of "anaphylaxis." The patient has a known peanut allergy and inadvertently ingested some ground nuts in a dish prepared by a friend. She has a known history of coronary artery disease and is taking metoprolol. Her symptoms do not respond to epinephrine, corticosteroids, or antihistamines. She is intubated but remains hypotensive and unstable. Which of the following may be of benefit?

A. Calcium chloride
B. Atropine
C. Glucagon
D. Nebulized albuterol
E. Terbutaline

62. A 34-year-old female presents with an infection. You decide to prescribe penicillin. She states that she is allergic to penicillin but cannot recall the reaction and has never been skin tested. You consider switching to a cephalosporin. Which of the following is the best estimate for cross-reactivity in this patient?

A. <1%
B. 10%
C. 25%
D. 33%
E. 50%

63. A 32-year-old female presents with cough for 1 week following several days of upper respiratory symptoms. Her vital signs are: 99.2, 75, 16, 119/68, 100% on RA. Her physical examination is normal. You strongly suspect acute bronchitis. Which of the following about this diagnosis is true?

A. Over 50% of cases are caused by bacteria
B. Yellow sputum color is very specific for bacterial illness

C. Procalcitonin levels may be helpful in determining need for antibiotics

D. Nonsteroidal anti-inflammatory drugs (NSAIDs) should be avoided in the acute phase of illness

E. Admission to the hospital for observation is indicated

64. Which of the following signs has over 90% sensitivity for acute appendicitis?

A. Obturator sign
B. Rovsing sign
C. Psoas sign
D. Kehr sign
E. None of the above

65. A mother brings her 4-year-old daughter to the ED, who is complaining of persistent perianal pruritus. The symptoms are worse at night and the mother has had to cut her daughter's nails short because she was scratching and irritating her skin. Which of the following is true?

A. The most sensitive test is a stool sample for ova and parasites.

B. The organism responsible for these symptoms can occasionally cause urinary tract infections and even vulvovaginitis.

C. The infection is most commonly acquired by ingestion of contaminated food or water.

D. Metronidazole is the antibiotic of choice.

E. Eosinophilia is commonly associated with her condition.

66. A 22-year-old primigravida presents to your community ED at 34 weeks of gestation with a chief complaint of headache and mild crampy abdominal pain. Her blood pressure is 160/100. Suspecting preeclampsia, you start a magnesium drip. While the patient is awaiting transfer 2 hours later, the nurse alerts you that she believes the patient is magnesium toxic. Which of the following is a sign of magnesium toxicity?

A. Atrial fibrillation
B. Increased deep tendon reflexes
C. Somnolence
D. Hyperventilation
E. Diarrhea

67. Compared to adults, children with diabetic ketoacidosis (DKA):

A. Are more likely to develop cerebral edema
B. Benefit from sodium bicarbonate as a part of routine therapy
C. Are less likely to have a potassium deficit
D. Should always receive a bolus of intravenous insulin after hydration
E. All of the above

68. A 28-year-old male presents with a chief complaint of abrupt-onset right-sided chest pain and shortness of breath. His vitals are P 105, RR 22, BP 142/90, SaO$_2$ 97% on room air. His x-ray is shown in Figure 9-9. Which of the following is true?

A. Aspiration of air with a 16-gauge catheter is as effective as tube thoracostomy

B. Surgery should be consulted

C. Tube thoracostomy should be performed with a 32-French tube or larger

D. Supplemental oxygen is unnecessary

E. Re-expansion pulmonary edema usually occurs more than 24 hours after re-expansion

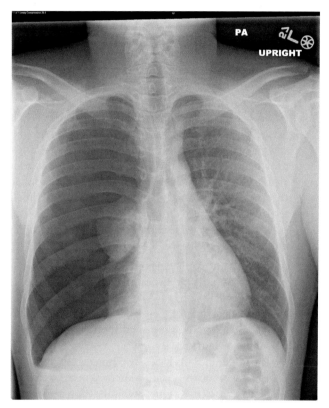

Figure 9-9

69. Traumatic hyphema

A. Is usually associated with an afferent pupillary defect
B. Is treated with supine position and oculomotor exercises
C. May require analgesic treatment with aspirin
D. Can be complicated by rebleeding
E. Rarely requires specific management

70. Which of the following is characteristic of gout but not pseudogout?

    A. NSAIDs are effective in treatment.
    B. Crystal formation is the primary pathophysiology.
    C. Dietary modifications can prevent acute attacks.
    D. The knee and the ankle can be involved.
    E. Erythrocyte sedimentation rate (ESR) is usually elevated in acute attacks.

71. A woman presents to the ED with bilateral pelvic pain. You consider the diagnosis of pelvic inflammatory disease (PID). Which of the following is a risk factor for PID?

    A. Menses within the prior week
    B. Age >30
    C. Diabetes insipidus
    D. Pregnancy
    E. History of ovarian cyst

72. A 57-year-old female with a history of tobacco abuse, hypertension, and end-stage renal disease on hemodialysis through a left upper extremity arteriovenous fistula presents from her dialysis clinic with a chief complaint of chest pain. The pain began 3 hours after the start of her session, and enough fluid was removed to bring her close to her dry weight. She has no associated shortness of breath. Her vitals are stable. The initial EKG demonstrates nonspecific changes. Her chest x-ray is normal. Her subsequent blood tests reveal an elevated cTnI of 0.83 g/μL (reference normal <0.49). She was given four chewable 81-mg aspirin upon arrival to the ED. Which of the following is true?

    A. A cardiac troponin T should be ordered because it is more specific for myocardial infarction in patients on hemodialysis.
    B. The patient has had an non-ST-elevation myocardial infarction (NSTEMI) and appropriate treatment should be initiated.
    C. The troponin is likely falsely elevated.
    D. The MB fraction of creatine kinase should be ordered because it is the most specific test for myocardial infarction in patients on hemodialysis.
    E. Specific treatment for an NSTEMI should be withheld since only serial, repeated enzyme elevations are diagnostic for a myocardial infarction.

73. A 63-year-old male with a history of coronary artery disease, diabetes, chronic obstructive pulmonary disease (COPD), and congestive heart failure (CHF) presents with increased cough and shortness of breath. His vital signs are: 99.5, 102, 24, 185/100, 92% on RA. He has bibasilar crackles and wheezes as well as 2+ lower extremity pitting edema. You order a CBC, basic metabolic panel, chest x-ray, EKG, and troponin. Which of the following additional tests will be helpful in determining the most likely diagnosis?

    A. Lactate
    B. Blood culture
    C. Arterial blood gas
    D. Brain natriuretic peptide
    E. Prothrombin time

74. A 14-year-old male comes to the ED for a diffuse rash. He was in his primary care doctor's office 4 days prior for a sore throat and fatigue and was told he had a viral throat infection. The patient's mother insisted that the patient be given an antibiotic, which he has been taking regularly since then. What antibiotic has this patient most likely been taking?

    A. Penicillin V
    B. Doxycycline
    C. Ciprofloxacin
    D. Amoxicillin
    E. Clindamycin

75. Which of the following toxin–antidote pairings is most correct?

    A. Phosgene–sodium nitrite monotherapy
    B. Sulfur mustard–topical dimercaprol (British anti-Lewisite) and IV ketorolac
    C. Cyanide–hydroxycobalamin (vitamin B12) and sodium thiosulfate
    D. VX–PM monotherapy
    E. Hydrogen sulfide–sodium thiosulfate monotherapy

76. A 17-year-old female presents with bilateral lower quadrant abdominal pain and vaginal discharge for 3 days. She reports having been sexually active with multiple partners in the last month. Her last menstrual period just finished 3 days ago. She denies fever, vomiting, dysuria, and diarrhea. Her urine pregnancy test is negative. Which of the following is most likely to yield the correct diagnosis?

    A. Physical examination
    B. CBC
    C. Urinalysis
    D. Liver function tests
    E. CT scan of the abdomen/pelvis

77. A 33-year-old female presents with acute weakness in her lower extremities that is progressively moving up her body. Along with Guillain–Barré syndrome (GBS), which of the following usually causes a clinical picture of acute ascending paralysis?

    A. Tick paralysis
    B. Botulism
    C. MG
    D. Diphtheria
    E. Paralytic shellfish poisoning

78. A 4-day-old neonate is brought in by her mother for irritability, excessive shaking and tremulousness, and an abnormal cry. The infant's glucose level is 20. Which of the following is the best initial treatment of this infant?

A. 0.03 mg/kg of glucagon delivered IV
B. 5 mL/kg of D10
C. 0.5 mL/kg of D25
D. 1 amp of D50 given IV
E. Continuous IV octreotide infusion

79. Which of the following is most useful in differentiating a patient with acute cholangitis from a patient with acute cholecystitis?

A. Jaundice
B. Fever
C. Abdominal tenderness
D. Leukocytosis
E. Murphy sign

80. The most specific finding for carpal tunnel syndrome (CTS) is:

A. Normal sensation on the medial side but abnormal sensation on the lateral side of the ring finger
B. Weakness of thumb opposition
C. Abnormal sensation of the distal palmar tip of the index finger
D. The presence of a positive Tinel sign
E. Lumbrical weakness

81. A 56-year-old male presents after a high-speed motor vehicle collision. He complains of severe chest pain and chest x-ray demonstrates a widened mediastinum. Chest CT scan shows a traumatic aortic injury (TAI). The patient's heart rate is 95 and blood pressure is 175/77. Operative repair is scheduled in 30 minutes. Which of the following is the most appropriate therapy at this time?

A. No therapy, observe for deterioration
B. Clonidine
C. Hydralazine
D. Labetalol
E. Enalaprilat

82. A 67-year-old female with a history of hypertension and diabetes presents to the ED with a complaint of double vision. On examination you find that she has mild left-sided ptosis and the inability to move her left eye superiorly and medially. The remainder of her eye movements and her pupils are normal. A noncontrast CT scan of the brain is normal. Which of the following is the next step?

A. Cerebral angiogram
B. Lumbar puncture (LP)
C. MRI/MRA of the brain with contrast
D. Administer oral aspirin and admit with a diagnosis of "stroke"
E. Discharge with referral to an ophthalmologist

83. A 22-year-old male presents with forearm pain after being assaulted. Radiographs demonstrate a proximal ulnar fracture with dislocation of the radial head. Which of the following is the most likely nerve injury?

A. Median
B. Radial
C. Ulnar
D. Axillary
E. Brachial

84. Which of the following is true regarding osmotic demyelination syndrome (or ODS, also known as *central pontine myelinolysis*)?

A. Partial recovery occurs after induction of hyponatremia through infusion of 5% dextrose in water.
B. It is more common after correction of acute rather than chronic hyponatremia.
C. It is more common in diabetic patients with pseudo-hyponatremia due to hyperglycemia.
D. Most common initial symptom is burning paresthesias in the hands and feet.
E. Patients do not typically present until a few days after treatment of hyponatremia.

85. You are working in the ED when a 74-year-old female with chronic obstructive pulmonary disease (COPD) presents with an acute COPD exacerbation. You start her on bilevel positive airway pressure (BiPAP) at a rate of 10, an inspiratory positive airway pressure (IPAP) of 10 mm Hg, and an expiratory positive airway pressure (EPAP) of 4 mm Hg. Twenty minutes later, the patient's oxygenation has not improved. Which of the following changes would most likely increase this patient's oxygenation?

A. Increase the patient's IPAP from 10 to 15
B. Increase the patient's rate from 10 to 12
C. Decrease the patient's EPAP from 4 to 2
D. Increase the patient's EPAP from 4 to 7, and the IPAP from 10 to 15
E. Decrease the patient's EPAP from 4 to 2, and decrease the IPAP from 10 to 5

86. A 25-year-old female presents with diffuse myalgias and dark urine after running a marathon. Which of the following treatments is likely to be most effective?

A. Normal saline
B. Potassium
C. Bicarbonate
D. Calcium
E. Furosemide

87. A 63-year-old female presents with an acute, severe headache after an MVC and is diagnosed with a subarachnoid hemorrhage (SAH). Her vital signs are normal. Which of the following should be part of her treatment regimen?

    A. Labetalol
    B. Lorazepam
    C. Isoproterenol
    D. Verapamil
    E. Nimodipine

88. A 33-year-old male presents with severe agitation, psychosis, and violent behavior. Physical examination demonstrates vertical nystagmus. Which of the following is the most likely drug ingested?

    A. Cocaine
    B. Phencyclidine (PCP)
    C. Lysergic acid diethylamine (LSD)
    D. Heroin
    E. Methylenedioxymethamphetamine (MDMA)

89. A 50-year-old male presents after a motor vehicle collision. His primary survey is intact. The pericardial view of his FAST scan is shown in Figure 9-10. Which of the following is the next best step in management?

    A. Emergent pericardiocentesis
    B. Surgical pericardial window
    C. Completion of FAST scan
    D. Needle thoracostomy
    E. Cardiology consultation

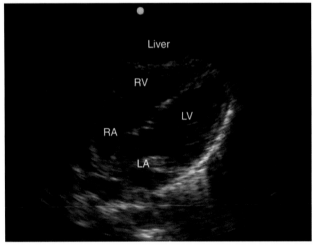

Figure 9-10

90. Which of the following is true regarding adult epiglottitis?

    A. Airway obstruction is usually caused by inflammation of the infraglottic tissues.
    B. Drooling and stridor are infrequent presenting signs.

    C. The disease is more common in winter.
    D. Nebulized racemic epinephrine has been shown to decrease the need for intubation.
    E. Normal lateral neck x-rays can safely exclude epiglottitis.

91. A 65-year-old male with multiple myeloma presents with generalized weakness and fatigue. His physical examination is unremarkable except for severe lethargy. Serum calcium level is 14 mg/dL. Which of the following is the most appropriate next step in management?

    A. Magnesium sulfate
    B. Potassium phosphate
    C. Normal saline
    D. Vitamin D
    E. Hydrochlorothiazide

92. Which of the following is the strongest risk factor for developing an abdominal aortic aneurysm (AAA)?

    A. Hypertension
    B. Obesity
    C. Male gender
    D. Hypertriglyceridemia
    E. First-degree relative with AAA

93. What is the most common source of bleeding in an anterior nosebleed?

    A. Anterior ethmoidal artery
    B. Posterior ethmoidal artery
    C. Kiesselbach plexus
    D. Nasopalatine branch of sphenopalatine artery
    E. Septal branch of superior labial artery

94. Which of the following is true regarding herpes simplex encephalitis?

    A. Bilateral frontal lobe involvement is characteristic.
    B. Herpes simplex virus (HSV)-2 is the most common cause in adults.
    C. Acyclovir reduces mortality.
    D. Most patients recover without neurologic sequelae.
    E. The sensitivity of cerebrospinal fluid (CSF) culture is 90%.

95. What is the most common ultrasonographic finding in women with ovarian torsion?

    A. Intraovarian hemorrhage
    B. Ovarian enlargement
    C. Lack of blood flow through color Doppler imaging
    D. Pelvic-free fluid
    E. All of the above are common findings

96. A 69-year-old female with a history of end-stage renal disease on hemodialysis 3 days per week presents to the ED with severe dyspnea. The patient missed her last dialysis session due to a transportation problem and subsequently became short of breath. On the day of presentation, she felt progressively worse, such that she was breathing "hard and heavy." In the ED, her vitals are T 97.1°F, P 110, BP 172/102, RR 28, SaO_2 84% on RA. Her lung examination reveals diffuse rales, with diminished breath sounds. Though she is on dialysis, she continues to make small volumes of urine. Which of the following is the best initial treatment?

    A. A large bolus of intravenous furosemide (e.g., 200 mg)
    B. Noninvasive ventilation with bilevel positive airway pressure
    C. Continuous positive airway pressure (CPAP)
    D. Continuous intravenous infusion of nitroglycerin
    E. Intravenous enalaprilat

97. A 65-year-old male with a left ventricular assist device presents with fatigue, dizziness, and lightheadedness. His device has alarmed several times. You have a page out to the patient's cardiologist. Which of the following tests can you anticipate the cardiologist will recommend?

    A. CT chest without IV contrast
    B. CT coronary angiography
    C. Echocardiogram
    D. Cardiac MRI
    E. Ventilation–perfusion scan

98. Among patients presenting to the ED with chest pain, which of the following physical examination findings is the biggest risk factor for aortic dissection?

    A. Severe obesity (BMI >40)
    B. Crescendo–decrescendo systolic ejection murmur at the right upper sternal border
    C. Long, slender fingers
    D. A systolic blood pressure difference of 15 mm Hg between the upper extremities
    E. A very muscular physique

99. Possible complications of acute asthma exacerbations include all of the following except:

    A. Pneumothorax
    B. Subconjunctival hemorrhage
    C. Subcutaneous emphysema
    D. Pulmonary embolus
    E. MI

100. Which of the following is the most common cause of hypercalcemia?

    A. Malignancy
    B. Paget disease
    C. Hyperparathyroidism
    D. Adrenal insufficiency
    E. Thiazide therapy

TEST 9

ANSWERS AND EXPLANATIONS

1. **Answer C.** Thromboembolic disease is the leading cause of death in pregnancy. The risk of deep venous thrombosis is highest in the postpartum period (puerpium), although the risk is elevated throughout pregnancy. Warfarin is contraindicated throughout pregnancy due to its strong association with fetal malformations even when given after the period of organogenesis (days 21 through 56 of fetal life). V/Q scans actually expose the fetus to more radiation than helical CT scans when looking for PE.

2. **Answer B.** The patient has clinical evidence of hepatic encephalopathy (HE), likely grade II. Grade I is marked by mild personality changes and cognitive dysfunction; grade II by disorientation, confusion, lethargy, and asterixis; grade III by somnolence and inability to follow commands; and grade IV by coma. Ammonia levels are usually, but not always, elevated in HE and do not correlate accurately with the degree of encephalopathy, which should be clinically assessed. Lactulose should be used to reduce hyperammonemia even when ammonia levels are only mildly elevated. Colonic bacteria convert lactulose into lactic acid, which then acidifies ammonia into ammonium in the gut, inhibiting its resorption and promoting its stool passage. Lactulose may be given by nasogastric tube in patients with altered mental status. Patients with cirrhosis and altered mental status in the ED should never be presumed to have a psychogenic cause of their symptoms. Endotracheal intubation is usually used for patients in grades III or IV HE, where loss of airway protection is more likely. Lumbar puncture is not routinely indicated in afebrile cirrhotic patients with altered mental status; additionally, fresh frozen plasma would be indicated beforehand to avoid epidural bleeding in these coagulopathic patients. Emergent neurology consultation is rarely necessary in these patients.

3. **Answer C.** The APGAR score is a five-category scoring system in which each category is assigned 0, 1, or 2 points to give a general assessment of neonatal well-being at birth. It is typically scored at 1 and 5 minutes postdelivery. The test is named for Virginia Apgar, MD, but her last name is also used as a mnemonic for its categories: Activity (2 for active movement, 1 for flexed limps and arms, and 0 for being limp), Pulse (2 for pulse >100, 1 for pulse <100, and 0 for no pulse), Grimace (in response to stimulation with a suction bulb, for example, also called reflex irritability, scoring 2 points for a strong cry, coughing, sneezing, or pulling away, scoring 1 point for a whimper or grimace without much responsiveness, and 0 for no response), Appearance (scoring

2 for being all pink, 1 for peripheral cyanosis, and 0 for central cyanosis or more diffuse pallor or cyanosis), and Respiratory effort (2 for a strong cry or normal breathing, 1 for irregular or slow breathing, and 0 for apnea). A score of 7 to 10 is considered normal. This baby receives 1 point for activity (flexed legs), 2 points for pulse (>100), 1 point for grimace (whimper), 1 point for appearance (peripheral cyanosis), and 2 points for respiration (normal breathing).

4. **Answer A.** Fractures are found in most abused children. Although no fracture is 100% specific for child abuse, several types are extremely high risk—any fractures in infants (especially of the femur) and spiral, multiple, rib, metaphyseal, humerus, and scapula fractures. Complete skeletal surveys are indicated for patients younger than 5 years who are suspected of being abused. Osteogenesis imperfecta is a rare disease, which causes problems in bone synthesis due to collagen defects. Frequent fractures are common and physical examination may demonstrate blue sclerae, deafness, and ligamentous laxity. Subclinical cases may be more common than previously recognized. Bone tumors and cysts and hypocalcemia may predispose to fracture but are not as likely to cause femoral fractures in the infant as child abuse.

5. **Answer E.** Nonaspirin NSAIDs, including ibuprofen, produce generally benign and self-limited conditions in overdose. Symptoms will occur within 4 hours of ingestion, are usually mild, and resolve within 24 hours. Patients rarely have life-threatening overdoses and almost never require antidotes, decontamination, augmented renal excretion, or invasive therapies such as hemodialysis. Serum levels of nonaspirin NSAIDs are not clinically useful. Of overdoses with nonaspirin NSAIDs, phenylbutazone and mefenamic acid are more serious, potentially causing multiorgan dysfunction and seizures, respectively.

6. **Answer C.** Digoxin toxicity may result in nearly *any* rhythm disturbance. PVCs are the most common, and typically represent the earliest rhythm disturbance. However, the two rhythms that are considered pathognomonic for digoxin toxicity are bidirectional tachycardia and paroxysmal atrial tachycardia with AV block. Clinically, these rhythms are extremely malignant and frequently precede the onset of nonperfusing rhythms. Thus, many patients are treated before these arrhythmias develop and they are not commonly observed.

7. **Answer C.** Chest x-ray demonstrates cardiomegaly and bilateral pleural effusions. The most common cause of

pleural effusion in Western countries is CHF. Malignancy, pneumonia, and PE are less common causes. Outside of Western countries, tuberculosis is the most common cause. Pancreatitis can cause a solitary left-sided pleural effusion. (Figure courtesy of Robert Hendrickson, MD. In: Greenberg MI, Hendrickson RG, Silverberg M, et al., eds. *Greenberg's Text-Atlas of Emergency Medicine.* Philadelphia, PA: Lippincott Williams & Wilkins; 2004:51, with permission.)

8. **Answer C.** Acute rheumatic failure is a nonsuppurative complication of GAS pharyngitis that typically occurs 2 to 4 weeks after the initial pharyngeal infection. Its onset is characterized by the presence of fever plus one or more of the five "major" manifestations, including pancarditis, migratory arthritis, Sydenham chorea, erythema marginatum, and subcutaneous nodules. A diagnosis of acute rheumatic failure is made in the setting of two of these five major Jones criteria and evidence of recent GAS infection, or one of the major criteria and two of the minor criteria (fever, arthralgias, and a history of prior rheumatic fever or rheumatic heart disease). Rheumatic fever is rare in patients older than 20 years. Treatment of acute GAS pharyngitis reduces the subsequent incidence of acute rheumatic failure. Scarlet fever is a consequence of acute GAS infection. Patients usually present with symptoms of GAS pharyngitis *plus* the presence of a diffuse maculopapular rash that has a fine, sandpaper-like feel (caused by an erythrogenic toxin). The rash typically begins in the inguinal creases before becoming quickly generalized. Shortly after generalization, the rash may become more intense along skin folds (e.g., in the antecubital fossa), producing lines of confluent petechiae known as *Pastia lines.* The rash begins to fade 3 to 4 days after its onset and enters a desquamative phase with flakes first peeling from the face and subsequently from the palms and fingers. The tongue is also involved, developing a white coat through which the tongue's erythematous papillae protrude giving the appearance of a "white strawberry" tongue. Treatment of scarlet fever is the same as for acute GAS pharyngitis. Severe scarlet fever with systemic toxic effects is not common.

9. **Answer E.** Rotavirus is an RNA virus that causes a secretory diarrhea in young children, most often in winter months. The peak age range is between 6 months and 2 years. There are two commercially available rotavirus vaccines, both of which are given orally as early as 6 weeks of age. One is a monovalent vaccine while the other contains five human–bovine reassortants. Both vaccines have demonstrated dramatic benefits in reducing the burden of illness, decreasing hospitalization rates as well as visits to the ED. While adults may get infected with rotavirus, they are generally asymptomatic. Among infected children, symptoms include nausea, vomiting, fever, and severe watery diarrhea. The duration of symptoms is generally <2 weeks. Rotavirus does not cause an inflammatory gastroenteritis, so fecal leukocytes and erythrocytes are usually absent. Treatment involves intravenous hydration and supportive care. Antidiarrheals and antibiotics are not indicated. Patients may require admission for rehydration—stool studies should be sent for rotavirus culture and the patient should be contact isolated to help reduce spread of infection to other patients.

10. **Answer C.** Patients with acute adrenal insufficiency should be aggressively treated for hypotension and hypoglycemia, which are the most immediately life-threatening complications. Hypotension from adrenal insufficiency responds to fluids and glucocorticoid replacement therapy far more readily than vasoactive agents. Most patients have moderate–severe hypoglycemia and should be given dextrose-containing fluids. Hypernatremia and hypokalemia are never seen in adrenal insufficiency. In contrast, hyponatremia and hypokalemia are common. However the severity of these electrolyte abnormalities is generally not significant enough to require aggressive correction. Similarly, hypothermia and hypercalcemia do occur but do not cause immediately serious complications. Anorexia is a problem in chronic adrenal insufficiency and can result in significant weight loss. Mucocutaneous hyperpigmentation (occurring in Addison disease but not in secondary adrenal insufficiency) is not a cause for immediate alarm. Emergent dermatologic consultation is not indicated.

11. **Answer C.** One of the guiding principles of peripheral nerve testing is to evaluate nerves in their "autonomous zone" of innervation (i.e., where there is no overlap of adjacent nerves or nerve roots). In the hand, the standard autonomous zone for testing the median nerve is the volar aspect of the index finger, distal to the distal interphalangeal (DIP) joint (the tip of the index finger); the zone for testing the ulnar nerve is the volar aspect of the little finger, distal to the DIP joint (the tip of the little finger). The radial nerve, however, has a far less well-defined autonomous zone as there is much overlap with cutaneous branches of other nerves. The best area for testing is the dorsal aspect of the webspace between the thumb and the index finger. This area overlies the first dorsal interosseus muscle, which is an ulnar innervated structure. However, cutaneous innervation to this area is primarily served by the radial nerve. The C5 nerve root does not have contributions to the hand and the C6 nerve root contributes to the median and radial nerves but not the ulnar nerve which receives contributions primarily from C8 and T1 and occasionally C7.

12. **Answer B.** *Cryptosporidium parvum* is a parasite, which often causes subacute and chronic diarrhea in patients

with AIDS. HAART is the best treatment for *Cryptosporidium* diarrhea. Symptoms are virtually eliminated if CD4 counts are maintained >100 cells per μL. Antidiarrheal agents and antibiotics work with only varying degrees of success and the symptoms are often recurrent after these drugs are stopped. Octreotide has no role in the management of HIV-associated infectious diarrhea.

13. **Answer A.** Only 5% of intussusception cases occur in adults and almost all of them occur in the small intestine. In contrast to pediatric patients, adults with intussusception almost always have an identifiable lead point, which is a malignancy 75% of the time (other lesions include inflammatory lesions and Meckel diverticulum). In adults, the diagnosis is best made with a CT scan. Although barium or water contrast enemas may diagnose and reduce intussusception, it is not as useful in adults because most lesions are in the small intestine and it is thought that the contrast material may help spread malignant cells. Most patients present with signs of incomplete obstruction (only 20% of patients have complete obstruction) with a chief complaint of abdominal pain. Large bowel obstruction in adults is most commonly due to malignancy, with volvulus and diverticulitis being the next most common causes.

14. **Answer A.** People ingest packets of illicit drugs to evade law enforcement officials by two main methods—packing and stuffing. Body packers ingest large amounts of drug in well-sealed packets in a methodical manner; body stuffers, on the other hand, are under time pressure to ingest a small number of packets quickly to avoid being captured with the drugs in their possession. Body packers are less likely than body stuffers to have packets rupture, but more likely to die from ruptured packets, as they usually contain a large amount of drug. Management of asymptomatic patients involves diagnosis with oral contrast radiographs, followed by bowel irrigation with polyethylene glycol and admission to a monitored bed. Charcoal may be of benefit in symptomatic patients shortly after packet ingestion. Hemodialysis is used only if packets have ruptured and drug has been absorbed, but cannot be set up quickly enough in these patients, as death will be sudden. Endoscopic removal is rarely indicated as rupture may occur during packet withdrawal. Operative removal is emergently indicated in patients with any symptoms suggestive of *cocaine* packet rupture, as uncontrolled sympathomimetic crisis will cause death despite even the most aggressive nonsurgical measures.

15. **Answer C.** Hypertriglyceridemia is a rare but important cause of acute pancreatitis. Triglyceride levels are usually above 1,000 mg/dL if pancreatitis is present. This degree of lipemia can significantly affect the interpretation of basic lab studies and result in multiple error results. Alcohol and gallstones together cause the majority of cases of pancreatitis but do not result in laboratory errors and her history puts her at low risk of these two conditions. While multiple drugs and viruses are known to cause pancreatitis, ibuprofen and rhinovirus are not usually implicated.

16. **Answer A.** Pain with extraocular movements, decrease in visual acuity, proptosis, and ophthalmoplegia more commonly occur in orbital cellulitis than in periorbital cellulitis. The majority of cases of orbital cellulitis result from direct spread of adjacent infections in the paranasal sinuses (such as the ethmoid sinusitis). In contrast, sinusitis precedes a relative minority of periorbital cellulitis cases. Most cases are caused by local inoculation (insect bites, trauma), or by local extension from other sources (dacryocystitis). *Aspergillus* species can cause a chronic orbital cellulitis lasting from weeks to months. Orbital cellulitis may cause blindness, and the infection can extend inside the cranium to involve the dural sinuses and meninges. In the absence of trauma, progression of periorbital cellulitis to orbital cellulitis is rare, even in untreated cases, and it is very rare for either infection to involve the globe.

17. **Answer E.** Carbon monoxide displaces oxygen from hemoglobin due to its far greater affinity for the heme subunit. Pulse oximetry senses only two specific wavelengths of light—oxygenated hemoglobin and deoxygenated hemoglobin—and calculates a percentage based on the ratio of the two. Unfortunately, carbon monoxide is sensed as *oxygenated* hemoglobin and pulse oximetry is falsely normal. Primary pathophysiology in carbon monoxide poisoning is inadequate oxygen delivery to tissues despite a normal to even slightly elevated dissolved oxygen level (Pa_{O_2}). Carboxyhemoglobin to oxyhemoglobin ratio is the test of choice in evaluating carbon monoxide poisoning. A ratio of above 25% is considered serious toxicity, though this is subject to various other clinical features. Pyridostigmine is a cholinesterase inhibitor used to treat MG and has no role in the management of carbon monoxide poisoning. Patients with carbon monoxide poisoning should get maximal possible oxygen therapy to compete with carbon monoxide for hemoglobin binding. This can be performed noninvasively with a 100% nonrebreather mask or using endotracheal intubation and mechanical ventilation. Any patient with altered mental status or somnolence should have emergent blood glucose level checked. Additionally, patients with suicidal attempts often ingest large quantities of alcohol, which can cause hypoglycemia.

18. **Answer D.** Children have the lowest mortality from status epilepticus, whereas elderly adults have the highest mortality. In the most widely cited study of status

epilepticus to date (the "Richmond" study), overall mortality was 3% in children younger than 16 years and 38% in elderly adults older than 60. Although lorazepam is favored by many physicians, there is no clear evidenced-based drug of choice. In the Veterans Affairs Cooperative Study, there was no statistically significant difference when lorazepam was compared with phenobarbital, diazepam plus phenytoin, or phenytoin alone as front-line agents. There was only a statistically insignificant trend in favor of lorazepam. The most common side effect of benzodiazepines given for status epilepticus is hypotension. Hypoventilation is the second most common side effect. Subtherapeutic drug levels are the most common trigger of status epilepticus and status epilepticus due to subtherapeutic drug levels has a low mortality. The next most common cause of status epilepticus among adults is cerebrovascular accidents.

19. **Answer B.** TMJ syndrome refers to a vague set of disorders involving the TMJ, such as pain, joint locking, and dislocation. It is considered the most common cause of facial pain after dentalgia. Young women comprise the highest risk category, and many patients have concomitant psychiatric conditions. The pain is normally unilateral. Evaluation involves imaging to assess for structural abnormalities and laboratory tests to check for associated systemic diseases such as RA, degenerative joint disease, and ankylosis. Treatment is with nonsteroidal anti-inflammatory drugs (NSAIDs), muscle relaxants, and a soft-food diet during acute episodes to prevent further exercise of the muscles of mastication.

20. **Answer D.** MG is an autoimmune disorder, which targets postsynaptic acetylcholine receptors. Fluctuating muscle weakness is the most predominant clinical feature. In most patients, the weakness is worse later in the day, and after exercise. Ocular symptoms and findings, such as ptosis or diplopia are the most common initial symptoms. Autonomic dysfunction is not a common finding. Approximately 10% to 15% of patients have an associated thymoma (and improve after thymectomy). Deep tendon reflex in patients with MG tend to be preserved while the disease is progressive, symptoms are often very transient during the early stages of the illness.

21. **Answer B.** This patient has necrotizing fasciitis caused by *Clostridium* spp., which gained entry when his arm was punctured while hiking. *Clostridium perfringens* is the most common species and is prevalent in soil. Pain is the most common early finding and is generally intense and unremitting. Swelling, pallor, and tenderness rapidly develop. Hemorrhagic bullae and brownish, serosanguineous discharge may develop as the wound progresses. Crepitus may also be present, but it is neither a sensitive nor specific finding. Treatment should be prompt, including aggressive surgical debridement and intravenous antibiotics. Despite this, amputation is frequently necessary. Use of advanced imaging to delineate spread along fascial planes delays definitive therapy and may result in a worse outcome.

22. **Answer B.** This patient has pityriasis rosea, which is a common, self-limited rash that is thought to be of viral etiology. It most commonly occurs between the ages of 10 and 35 with a mean age of 23. Approximately 20% to 50% of patients present with a "herald patch," a single, 2- to 10-cm salmon-pink plaque with a fine silvery scale that rings the border of the lesion. Many patients believe they have ringworm, and the lesion may commonly be mistaken for ringworm before the development of additional lesions (KOH testing can rule this out). Approximately 1 to 2 weeks after the herald patch, multiple additional 1- to 2-cm round and oval lesions develop on the trunk. The longitudinal axis of the oval lesions runs along the skin lines of the back and the overall pattern may resemble the branches of a pine tree. For this reason, pityriasis is often said to have a "Christmas tree" distribution. No treatment is necessary and the lesions resolve within 2 to 3 months, although ultraviolet B (UVB) phototherapy will hasten resolution and decrease pruritus. (Figure reprinted with permission from Barankin B. *Stedman's Illustrated Dictionary of Dermatology Eponyms.* Philadelphia, PA: Lippincott Williams & Wilkins; 2004.)

23. **Answer A.** The thin orbital floor is the most easily damaged part of the orbit in trauma. Globe injuries occur in one-fourth of patients with orbital floor fractures. The teardrop sign seen on plain radiographs or CT scan is soft tissue that extends inferiorly from the orbital floor into the maxillary sinus, indicating a floor fracture. Antibiotics are often given to patients with orbital wall fractures but are recommended only if the fracture extends through an infected sinus. Patients with orbital wall fractures should be instructed not to blow their nose, as it may worsen the degree of herniation of globe contents into the sinuses. Nasal congestion should be treated with a 3-day course of nasal decongestants.

24. **Answer D.** Evaporation is the most significant mechanism of heat loss at most climates (except for very cold areas). It refers to the transfer of heat that occurs to convert a liquid to a gas. For example, in a patient who is sweating from running, liquid sweat evaporates to gas by using up excess body heat. Conduction refers to a colder object taking heat from a warmer object. Fan mist therapy uses both evaporation and conduction in decreasing heat. Radiation refers to constant background emission of heat from all bodies and cannot be increased or decreased therapeutically.

25. **Answer D.** In ARDS, the alveoli are flooded with protein-rich fluid due to leaky pulmonary capillaries. The result is poorly ventilated and poorly compliant alveoli (i.e., fluid-filled alveoli are difficult to distend). Owing to the presence of poorly compliant alveoli, both peak and plateau airway pressures in ARDS are higher than in healthy subjects. Ventilating such patients with "normal" or high tidal volumes further elevates the airway pressure and may result in barotrauma and further injury to the lung. The ARDS Network group of investigators published a study in 2000 describing a "lung protective" strategy in which such patients were ventilated with tidal volumes that were much lower than normal. The idea of this strategy is to reduce ventilator-associated lung injury as a result of alveolar overdistension from high tidal volumes and airway pressures. Owing to the low tidal volumes, however, such patients require higher PEEP levels to recruit alveoli in order to ensure adequate oxygenation. The goal is to use the lowest PEEP required to achieve an Fio_2 ≤0.50. An inadvertent result of this strategy is hypoventilation and a resultant rise in $Paco_2$ levels (hypercapnia). Some studies suggest that the resulting acidosis (respiratory acidosis from high $Paco_2$ levels) may actually be protective, although the ARDS Network investigators treated the acidosis with bicarbonate infusions. An ideal strategy regarding this has not yet been developed.

26. **Answer A.** Flumazenil is a benzodiazepine antagonist that is used only in selected cases to reverse benzodiazepine overdose. The only real indications for flumazenil are to speed recovery in accidental pediatric ingestions and during procedural sedation. Flumazenil can precipitate seizures in patients who are chronic benzodiazepine users, alcoholics, and those who have coingested medicines which lower the seizure threshold. The morbidity and mortality of benzodiazepine overdose is mostly from respiratory depression. Therefore, standard airway management, oxygenation, and ventilation preclude the use of flumazenil in almost all cases.

27. **Answer C.** The most common symptoms of hypocalcemia are neurologic and generalized irritability such as twitching and paresthesias which may progress to frank tetany, perioral paresthesias, as well as Chvostek and Trousseau signs. Chvostek sign is a twitch of the upper lip when the area around the facial nerve is tapped. Trousseau sign is carpopedal spasm when a blood pressure cuff is inflated over the arm at greater than systolic blood pressure for longer than 3 minutes. The other signs and symptoms listed are all manifestations of hypercalcemia.

28. **Answer A.** Of all the choices, acute angle closure glaucoma is most likely to cause painful loss of vision. All the other choices are much more likely to cause painless (rather than painful) loss of vision.

29. **Answer B.** The patient has a ruptured abdominal aortic aneurysm (AAA), as indicated by the adjacent retroperitoneal hematoma. Patients with ruptured AAAs must undergo immediate operative repair unless there is an absolute contraindication to surgery, as loss of complete blood volume can occur within minutes. There is no evidence that aggressive reduction of blood pressure is helpful in AAA, and it increases the unnecessary risk of hypotension and worsened hypoperfusion. Once a ruptured AAA is definitively diagnosed by CT scan, there is little role for further imaging in the ED with angiography or ultrasound. Observation of patients with ruptured AAAs is contraindicated. (Figure courtesy of Robert Hendrickson, MD. In: Greenberg MI, Hendrickson RG, Silverberg M, et al., eds. *Greenberg's Text-Atlas of Emergency Medicine.* Philadelphia, PA: Lippincott Williams & Wilkins; 2004:194, with permission.)

30. **Answer B.** This patient is presenting with an unstable, wide-complex tachycardia. Given that the patient is unstable (hypotensive, pale, diaphoretic), the exact details of her underlying rhythm won't change her need for immediate DC cardioversion. The vignette points to the fact that this patient likely has atrial fibrillation with concomitant WPW (irregular rhythm), but all wide-complex tachycardias should first be considered to be ventricular in origin until proven otherwise. If it's clear that the patient is stable and has atrial fibrillation with WPW, the treatment of choice is procainamide followed by amiodarone or ibutilide. Agents which preferentially block AV node conduction such as adenosine, verapamil, or diltiazem should be avoided because their use may lead to unopposed "shunting" of electrical activity through the unblocked accessory pathway, worsening the dysrrhtyhmia.

31. **Answer D.** This patient has Henoch–Schonlein purpura (HSP), which is a systemic, small vessel vasculitis that most commonly affects children. The classic presentation is a patient with a palpable, purpuric rash in dependent areas such as the buttocks and lower extremities, abdominal pain, hematuria, and joint pain. Renal involvement is common, but typically manifests as microscopic hematuria and resolves without sequelae. However, more severe presentations from nephritis to nephritic syndrome rarely occur. Long-term prognosis in HSP is determined primarily by the degree of renal involvement. Patients with HSP do not have thrombocytopenia. High-dose aspirin is a therapy reserved for patients with Kawasaki disease. HSP is commonly associated with intussusception. However, in contrast to most patients with intussusception in which the obstruction occurs in the ileocolic region, patients with HSP experience

ileoileal intussusception. In the great majority of cases, HSP is a benign, self-limited disease that requires only supportive therapy. Steroids remain controversial and are only used for patients with severe symptoms. (Figure from Van Hale HM, Gibson LE, Schroeter AL. Henoch-Schönlein vasculitis: direct immunofluorescence study of uninvolved skin. *J Am Acad Dermatol* 1986;15:665–670, with permission.)

32. **Answer C.** QT interval prolongation is the most common EKG abnormality in patients with heat-related illness. Interestingly, QT interval prolongation is also very common in patients with hypothermia. Other common EKG findings include sinus tachycardia, atrial fibrillation, SVT, right bundle branch block, and occasional ST segment changes. Sinus bradycardia and ventricular fibrillation do not commonly occur.

33. **Answer A.** The patient has blepharitis, as seen by the crusting and edema of the upper eyelid. Staphylococcal infection has been implicated but the complete pathophysiology is not known. The condition is chronic and there are multiple components to treatment. Eyelid hygiene is very important, as patients should clean the lids with a gentle soap, apply warm compresses, gently massage the lids, and apply topical erythromycin ointment. Topical steroids should never be prescribed by the emergency physician (EP) without ophthalmologic consultation. Topical anesthetics (such as proparacaine) should never be prescribed to patients, as they will retard corneal healing. Intravenous ceftriaxone is used in patients with hyperacute bacterial conjunctivitis due to gonococcus. This patient has no evidence of conjunctival involvement on physical examination. Acetazolamide is used in patients with acute angle closure glaucoma, but the absence of eye pain, headache, and corneal or conjunctival abnormality effectively rules this out. (Figure From Tasman W, Jaeger E. *The Wills Eye Hospital Atlas of Clinical Ophthalmology,* 2nd ed. Philadelphia, PA: Lippincott Williams & Wilkins, 2001.)

34. **Answer D.** Follicular cysts are the most frequent adnexal cystic structures in women with normal ovaries. Follicular cysts represent remnants of previously normal follicles that grew in response to follicle-stimulating hormone and then failed to involute. They are typically clinically silent but they may cause pelvic pain or heaviness, as well as urinary frequency and constipation if they are large enough. They are self-limited and involute over a period of weeks to months. Corpus luteum cysts are less common but more clinically relevant. They also represent remnants of formerly normal physiologic structures; in this case, the corpus luteum. Unlike follicular cysts, they have a propensity to be complicated by intracavitary hemorrhage. If the hemorrhage is brisk, the intracystic pressure may rise very quickly resulting in

rupture. Such an event may result in acute onset, severe pelvic pain, and may be associated with significant hemorrhage depending on the size of the cyst. Theca lutein cysts are uncommon, typically bilateral, and associated with prolonged or excessive ovarian stimulation. Dermoid cysts are benign ovarian teratomas that contain tissue from all three germ cell layers. They do not pose an immediate danger, but patients should be referred for further management because they may undergo malignant transformation, particularly in women older than 40. Finally, ovarian fibromas are the most common, benign, solid neoplasms of the ovary. They are extremely slow growing but may grow to very large sizes.

35. **Answer C.** The patient likely has diarrhea-predominant irritable bowel syndrome (IBS). A hypersensitivity to bowel wall peristalsis resulting in altered gut motility and pain perception is the proposed pathophysiology. While few treatments have undergone rigorous randomized-controlled trials, low-dose tricyclic antidepressant therapy (such as desipramine or amitriptyline) has been found to be effective in many cases. The emergency physician should never prescribe tricyclics without consulting the primary care provider and ensuring adequate follow-up. Fiber supplementation is used primarily for constipation-type (IBS). Lithium is used to treat bipolar disorder but has no current role in the management of IBS. Empiric use of antibiotics in IBS or any other cause of chronic intermittent diarrhea is not recommended. Due to radiation exposure and high cost, repeat CT scanning in a patient without focal abdominal findings (especially when one has already been performed for the symptoms) is not recommended.

36. **Answer B.** The patient likely has viral gastroenteritis with evidence of mild to moderate dehydration. She lacks toxic features and does not have signs of severe dehydration. In the vast majority of cases of pediatric patients with viral gastroenteritis and mild–moderate dehydration, oral fluid supplementation with a sugar and salt solution is preferred over intravenous hydration because of lack of complications, reduced cost, and similar clinical outcomes. Normal diet should be resumed as soon as tolerated by the patient. The BRAT diet has never been shown to improve outcomes in acute gastroenteritis and is not recommended over a normal diet. Metronidazole is used for suspected or confirmed cases of *C. difficile* diarrhea, but the absence of antibiotic use makes this unlikely. Nitazoxanide is an antiparasitic agent used to treat *Giardia* infection, which is usually a subacute watery diarrhea occurring over the course of 1 to 2 weeks.

37. **Answer C.** Cyclosporine exhibits all the listed toxicities, and may also cause tremor, hyperkalemia, hirsutism, and gingival hyperplasia. However, the most common

toxicity associated with its use is dose-dependent nephrotoxicity, which occurs in one-third of patients.

38. **Answer A.** The most likely diagnosis is tumor lysis syndrome, a constellation of events that results from rapid cellular death due to chemotherapy. Rapidly growing and hematologic malignancies highly responsive to chemotherapy are at highest risk for development of tumor lysis syndrome. Hyperkalemia, hyperuricemia, and hyperphosphatemia are the most common laboratory abnormalities. Hypocalcemia is more common than hypercalcemia. Severe fluctuations in magnesium levels are rare. Renal insufficiency and dysrhythmias are the most serious complications. Management involves normalization of electrolyte abnormalities (especially hyperkalemia), intravenous fluids, and treatment of renal insufficiency. Alkalinization therapy to counteract hyperuricemia is not universally recommended, as it may exacerbate electrolyte abnormalities. Renal failure requiring dialysis is a poor prognostic indicator.

39. **Answer D.** *Chlamydia* is the most common cause of non-gonococcal urethritis, accounting for over half of all cases. Symptoms are very similar to a urinary tract infection—however, urethral discharge worse in the morning is more characteristic of urethritis. Screening for other sexually transmitted diseases should be pursued. Therapy is with doxycycline or azithromycin and sexual partners should also be treated. Choices A, B, and E all cause urethritis, but are less common than *Chlamydia.* Choice C causes chancroid, a syndrome of a painful, ulcerated lesion on the genitalia in association with inguinal lymphadenopathy.

40. **Answer E.** Rust rings are the result of iron-containing foreign bodies leaving a residue on the cornea. Patients should see the ophthalmologist within 48 hours, as the ring will migrate to more superficial corneal layers over time, allowing for easier removal. Topical steroids have no role in the management of rust rings or ocular foreign bodies. Metallic foreign body evaluation of the eye with MRI is absolutely contraindicated.

41. **Answer B.** Avulsed primary teeth should never be reimplanted, as they may fuse with underlying secondary teeth and cause considerable cosmetic deformity. Avulsed secondary teeth should be reimplanted as soon as possible. If teeth are reimplanted within 30 minutes, approximately 100% will be viable, but if 2 hours have elapsed since avulsion, the chance of successful reimplantation is essentially zero. The best known medium for transporting an avulsed tooth is its own socket, followed by Hank solution; cold milk is the best alternative if either of these is not available. Teeth may be secured for up to 48 hours by reimplanting the avulsed tooth and securing it to two neighboring teeth on either side with a periodontal pack. Before reimplantation, avulsed

teeth should be gently rinsed with saline. Teeth should never be scrubbed or treated with any cleaning solution as this will destroy the periodontal ligament fibers which are essential for successful reimplantation.

42. **Answer B.** The patient has staphylococcal scalded skin syndrome, also known as *Ritter disease.* The disease is caused by an epidermolytic toxin expressed by *S. aureus,* phage group II, and typically occurs in otherwise healthy children. Infection typically begins as an innocuous infection of the pharynx or conjunctiva until a diffuse erythroderma develops that has a sandpaper-like feel, resembling scarlet fever. The skin ultimately wrinkles, develops transient blisters, and then peels in large sheets revealing glossy, moist red skin underneath. Treatment is directed at *S. aureus,* and given the prevalence of methicillin-resistant *S. aureus,* vancomycin is the best choice. (Figure courtesy of Gary Marshall, MD. In: Chung EK. *Visual Diagnosis in Pediatrics.* Philadelphia, PA: Lippincott Williams & Wilkins; 2006.)

43. **Answer D.** The absence of fetal heart tones in an intrauterine gestation with a crown-rump length >5 mm (correlates roughly to 6.2 weeks of gestation) is convincing evidence of fetal demise. Missed abortion refers to the continued presence of a nonviable fetus aged <20 weeks of gestation for at least 8 weeks without the passage of maternal or fetal tissue. The persistent presence of a dead fetus may result in coagulation abnormalities and disseminated intravascular coagulation. However, this is primarily a historical diagnosis due to the prevalence of US. Therefore, most women present to a physician with vague complaints of crampy abdominal pain or vaginal bleeding or they are noted to have a uterus that is too small for their dates. Subsequent US identifies intrauterine fetal demise before coagulation complications occur, and the patient is referred to an obstetrician for definitive management.

44. **Answer E.** Abortive therapy for patients presenting with acute migraine headaches includes nonsteroidal anti-inflammatory drugs (NSAIDs) as intravenous ketorolac, triptans such as sumatriptan, and dopamine receptor antagonists such as prochlorperazine, metoclopramide, or chlorpromazine. Since this patient has already tried failed triptans prior to her presentation, prochlorperazine (Compazine) is a good choice. Intravenous fluid boluses and oxygen therapy have not been shown to help patients with migraine headaches. Intravenous dexamethasone has been shown to decrease the rate of headache recurrence and is recommended as part of ED therapy for migraines but is not helpful in aborting the acute headache.

45. **Answer C.** Sickle cell disease is a hemoglobinopathy causing sickling of RBCs with any systemic stress,

which results in diffuse microinfarctions. Sickle cell trait is present in approximately 10% of all African Americans, and sickle cell disease is primarily a disease of this population. Symptoms involve multiple organ systems and result in specific acute crises—vaso-occlusive, acute chest syndrome, splenic sequestration, and aplastic. The most common cause of death in patients with sickle cell disease is from infection, usually pneumonia. Due to autoinfarction of the spleen, patients are at risk for overwhelming sepsis from encapsulated organisms, such as *Streptococcus pneumoniae, E. coli,* and *Haemophilus influenzae.* Stroke is another common cause. Aplasia and splenic sequestration occur less often. MI is rare in sickle cell patients, as coronary artery disease, although probably accelerated in these patients, does not usually progress far enough to significantly increase the risk of infarction.

46. **Answer C.** The discriminatory zone is the quantitative serum β-hCG level at which a normal pregnancy can be detected by either transvaginal or transabdominal ultrasonography. As ultrasonographic technology improves, the discriminatory zone continues to drop. Furthermore, these levels may vary somewhat between hospitals due to technologic differences. However, the accepted range is 1,000 to 2,000 mIU/mL for transvaginal ultrasonography and 2,400 to 3,600 mIU/mL for transabdominal ultrasonography. Other sources cite a range of 1,500 to 2,500 mIU/mL as the accepted range in transabdominal ultrasonography. Of course, the higher the discriminatory threshold, the higher the specificity for an abnormal pregnancy, including ectopic gestation.

47. **Answer D.** DCS is due to the presence of nitrogen bubbles in the blood and tissues. It is divided into type I DCS and type II DCS. Type I DCS affects the musculoskeletal system, skin, and lymphatic vessels. Type II DCS involves all other organ systems. The shoulder and elbow are the most common joints involved in type I DCS. The arthralgias experienced by patients with type I DCS are known as *the bends.* Joint pain may be reduced by inflating a blood pressure cuff over the affected joint to 150 to 200 mm Hg. This may also be used to aid in diagnosis although it has a poor sensitivity.

48. **Answer C.** HepB is very effectively transmitted through percutaneous needlestick exposure, even though the rate of transmission depends on the presence of the "e" antigen (hepatitis B e antigen [HBeAg]), indicating higher infectivity. Health care providers exposed to HBeAg-positive needlesticks develop clinical evidence of hepatitis in approximately 33% of cases and serologic evidence in up to 62%. In contrast, exposure to HBeAg-negative patients results in clinical hepatitis in only 1%

to 6% of cases and serologic evidence in up to 37%. In contrast, exposure to a hepatitis C-positive source results in an infection rate of roughly 1.8% (0% to 7%). All patients who have not received the HepB vaccine as well as patients who were vaccinated with a single series but who failed to respond should receive both the HBIG and the HepB vaccine series. The HepB vaccine should always be given in the deltoid muscle with a needle 1 to 1.5 in. long (apparently better response rates have resulted from deltoid injection). There is no evidence that using antiseptics for wound care or expressing fluid by squeezing the wound further reduces the risk of blood-borne pathogen transmission.

49. **Answer A.** The patient is a young adult with clinical evidence of community-acquired pneumonia. In a young patient without serious comorbidity or severe distress, outpatient therapy is appropriate. Major pathogens in this age-group include pneumococcus, *Mycoplasma pneumoniae, Chlamydia pneumoniae,* and others. Appropriate therapy could include a macrolide, a second- or third-generation cephalosporin, a fluoroquinolone, or doxycycline. Doxycycline is inexpensive, covers most organisms implicated in community-acquired pneumonia, and has convenient twice-a-day dosing. Linezolid is used to treat vancomycin-resistant organisms, most often seen in the nosocomial setting. Cephalexin is a first-generation cephalosporin with poor coverage of atypical organisms and gram negatives. Clindamycin provides excellent coverage of gram positives and anaerobes but does not cover atypicals or gram negatives. Piperacillin–tazobactam is a potent, broad-spectrum, antipseudomonal antibiotic used only for nosocomial pathogens causing severe illness.

50. **Answer E.** The patient has a large, spontaneous subconjunctival hemorrhage. There is no apparent chemosis or hyphema. Management is purely supportive with avoidance of NSAIDs. Patients with history of frequent subconjunctival hemorrhage may require coagulopathy workup, but most patients with coagulopathies will have other manifestations of bleeding as well. Emergent ophthalmologic consultation is not indicated in patients with subconjunctival hemorrhage, but bloody chemosis or hyphema would necessitate this. Topical antihistamines or antibiotics are not indicated in patients with subconjunctival hemorrhage. (Figure from Rapuano CJ. *Wills Eye Institute – Cornea.* 2nd ed. Philadelphia, PA: Wolters Kluwer, 2011, with permission.)

51. **Answer A.** Thiazide diuretics increase calcium reabsorption, which will exacerbate symptoms of hypercalcemia. Bisphosphonates, calcitonin, and loop diuretics (such as furosemide) all work to decrease calcium levels. Calcitonin is faster acting than bisphosphonates, and is usually combined with intravenous saline to decrease

calcium levels in symptomatic patients. Bisphosphonates are then given for longer term control. Loop diuretics can be given in addition to intravenous fluids, particularly in patients with congestive heart failure, or symptoms of fluid overload.

52. **Answer E.** Since glucose exerts an osmotic pressure on cell membranes, water is extruded from cells into the intravascular space, thereby diluting plasma sodium. The sodium level must therefore be corrected for hyperglycemia by using the following formula:

$$\text{Corrected Na}^+ = [\text{Na}^+] + \{2.4 \times ([\text{glucose}] - 100)/100\}$$

In their 1999 paper, Hiller et al. found that the classically taught 1.6 correction factor was less accurate and determined that the actual correction factor was 2.4.

53. **Answer B.** The AG is used to signify the difference between the concentration of sodium ($[\text{Na}^+]$), and the sum of the concentrations of chloride ($[\text{Cl}^-]$) and bicarbonate ($[\text{HCO}_3^-]$) such that: $\text{AG} = [\text{Na}^+] - [\text{Cl}^-] - [\text{HCO}_3^-]$. However, because of the law of electroneutrality, all aqueous solutions must have an equal number of positive and negative charges such that the entire solution is neutral. Therefore, the AG does not reflect a true "positive" or "negative" charge in the plasma. Instead, it reflects the presence of an anion which the formula is not measuring. In normal patients, albumin accounts for the bulk of these "unmeasured anions." Each 1 g/dL decrease in the concentration of albumin will decrease the expected AG by approximately 2.5 to 3 (the normal albumin concentration is roughly 4 g/dL × ~3 ≈ expected AG of 12). Therefore, patients with hypoalbuminemia (e.g., cirrhosis, malnutrition) will have a smaller, normal AG. Sulfate, phosphate, and citrate make up the bulk of the remaining unmeasured anions.

54. **Answer E.** The Salter–Harris classification is used to describe pediatric long-bone fractures near the growth plate. Type I fractures go through the physis only, type II from the metaphysis into the physis, type III from the epiphysis into the physis, type IV is a combination of types II and III, and type V is a crush injury to the physis. The most common is type II. Types I and V may be invisible on initial plain films. Type V carries the poorest prognosis.

55. **Answer E.** Digitalis inhibits the membrane Na–K ATPase which normally functions to pump sodium out of the cell and potassium into it. Digitalis, therefore, increases intracellular sodium and decreases intracellular potassium. The increased intracellular sodium causes an increase in intracellular calcium, which produces a positive inotropic effect. In therapeutic doses, digitalis reduces the heart rate and can cause slight ST depression and T-wave inversions.

56. **Answer D.** Magnesium remains the drug of choice for the treatment of seizures in eclampsia as well as for the prophylaxis of seizures in patients with preeclampsia. The recommended dose is 6 g given intravenously over 15 to 20 minutes followed by a continuous infusion at 2 g/hour. Hydralazine, labetalol, and nimodipine are all agents that have been used for BP control in patients with eclampsia. Hydralazine is most commonly used and is typically given in 5 to 10 mg doses every 15 to 20 minutes. Lorazepam and phenytoin are second-line agents for seizure control in patients with eclampsia. An obstetrician should be involved in the care of all patients with eclampsia and can help direct therapy if the initial magnesium bolus is ineffective. Finally, although recommendations vary, treatment of seizures is the first priority. Once seizures are terminated, BP may be controlled only if the diastolic BP remains elevated above 105 to 110 mm Hg. In the absence of seizures, the same BP guidelines apply, and magnesium is given for prophylaxis against seizures.

57. **Answer C.** Tick paralysis is likely due to an unidentified toxin, which is transmitted to the human host within a week of tick attachment. The classic clinical presentation is that of ascending flaccid paralysis with loss of deep tendon reflexes, similar to Guillain–Barré syndrome (GBS). Tick paralysis is not associated with the autonomic instability that often accompanies GBS. Furthermore, many patients present more vaguely with paresthesias despite a normal sensory examination and an abnormal gait before progressing to frank paralysis. Respiratory failure can occur due to diaphragmatic weakness. Cranial nerve and sensory findings are rare. Treatment is careful removal of the tick, which results in complete resolution of symptoms within 2 days.

58. **Answer B.** This HIV patient has bilateral fluffy infiltrates consistent with PCP.[1] Over three-fourths of all patients with acquired immunodeficiency syndrome (AIDS) will develop PCP at some point in their lifetimes. It is also the most common identifiable cause of death in patients with AIDS. *Pneumocystis* is classified as a protozoan, but it has many characteristics of a fungus. Symptoms of PCP, like all pneumonias, include fever, cough, and shortness of breath, but a subacute or mild course is characteristic. Chest radiography classically demonstrates diffuse, bilateral interstitial infiltrates but can be completely normal up to 20% of the time. First-line therapy is with TMP-SMX. Adjunctive corticosteroid therapy is indicated in patients who have significant

---

[1] PCP, or Pneumocystis pneumonia, has been used to describe *Pneumocystis carinii* pneumonia. The variant of *Pneumocystis* that is now recognized to infect humans is *Pneumocystis jirovecii*.

hypoxia ($Paco_2$ <70 mm Hg). Albuterol may be used in patients with pneumonia or bronchitis who have a large bronchospastic component to their symptoms. Aspirin is not indicated in most infectious processes. Vasopressin may be used in patients with septic shock who are adequately volume resuscitated. Hyperbaric oxygen does not currently have a role in the management of PCP. (Figure courtesy of Mark Silverberg, MD. In: Greenberg MI, Hendrickson RG, Silverberg M, et al., eds. *Greenberg's Text-Atlas of Emergency Medicine*. Philadelphia, PA: Lippincott Williams & Wilkins; 2004:1,006, with permission.)

59. **Answer C.** Patients with MG are at risk for severe respiratory muscle weakness and resulting hypercarbic respiratory failure. Patients with MG who present with somnolence should be assumed to have severe hypercarbia until proven otherwise. Emergent endotracheal intubation should be performed in any case where the airway appears tenuous. The absence of significant hypoxia merely underscores the different type of respiratory failure at play (hypercarbic vs. hypoxemic). Chest x-ray should be performed after the airway is secured—often MG patients have aspiration that is concomitant with or even causing their myasthenic crisis. Central venous access is not necessary as long as good peripheral lines are in place. Noninvasive positive pressure ventilation is contraindicated in patients who have significant alteration of mental status. CT brain can be performed as part of the altered mental status evaluation but should never delay airway and respiratory evaluation.

60. **Answer C.** Asymptomatic hypertension is an enormous, often mismanaged, problem in EDs for which there is little data to guide emergency physicians. Most of the confusion arises from the use of the term "hypertensive urgency." Hypertensive urgency has been variably defined but generally has included any patient with a blood pressure greater than 185/110 regardless of symptoms. There is no evidence that the "urgent" treatment of such patients is helpful. In contrast, many patients have been needlessly treated with an overly aggressive approach that has led to more harm than good. Asymptomatic patients require no screening testing as long as appropriate follow-up can be arranged. Physicians may choose to initiate low-dose, mild therapy, such as hydrochlorothiazide or chlorthalidone, as a bridge to more comprehensive therapy. Clonidine is not a first-, second-, or third-line agent for the treatment of hypertension and has no role in the ED management of hypertension unless it is part of the patient's existing regimen. There is no role for admission, extensive testing, or IV therapy in asymptomatic patients. Symptomatic patients should undergo a workup based on their symptoms, and should only receive IV therapy if there is also an emergent condition necessitating an emergent

reduction in blood pressure. It is reasonable to check renal function if starting antihypertensive therapy, particularly with ACE inhibitors, but it is not mandatory if the patient has close follow-up.

61. **Answer C.** Patients on β-blockers may be difficult to treat in the setting of anaphylaxis. On the one hand, β-blockade may blunt or prevent some of the beneficial effects of epinephrine. However, epinephrine also has the potential to worsen anaphylaxis in the setting of beta-blockade due to subsequent unopposed alpha receptor stimulation. This may result in an increased release of the vasoactive mediators in anaphylaxis. Clinically, this may be manifest in worsened bronchoconstriction, bradycardia, and coronary vasoconstriction. Like epinephrine, glucagon exerts its influence through the formation of intracellular cyclic AMP. However, glucagon bypasses the β-adrenergic receptor by binding to a discrete G protein receptor. Therefore, glucagon may be effective even in the setting of β-blockade. This is also the basis for glucagon's use in β-blocker overdose. Other agents that may be beneficial include vasopressors (dopamine, norepinephrine), nebulized albuterol (specifically for relief of bronchospasm), atropine (for bradycardia), and isoproterenol (as a last resort).

62. **Answer A.** Patients with *reported* penicillin allergies rarely have true immune-mediated allergic reactions. Most simply have one of a variety of adverse medication effects. The historically quoted cross-reactivity rate between cephalosporins and penicillins of 10% is likely flawed. Early studies demonstrating this 10% rate occurred at a time when penicillin impurities were present during cephalosporin production in laboratories. Furthermore, most second-, third-, and fourth-generation cephalosporins have a penicillin cross-reactivity rate no greater than other antibiotics. Current estimates of cross-reactivity in patients with *reported* penicillin allergies are <1%, and some experts argue that it is *far* less than 1%. Patients with confirmed true allergic reactions to penicillin still have a <5% cross-reactivity rate. Patients who report a nonanaphylactic allergy to penicillin can safely receive a cephalosporin if watched briefly in the ED for adverse events.

63. **Answer C.** Procalcitonin is a prohormone released by the lungs in response to bacterial infection. It is extremely useful in distinguishing between bacterial and nonbacterial infections of the lower respiratory tract and can be used to aid in the decision to withhold antibiotics if normal. Only about 5% of cases of bronchitis are due to bacteria such as *Mycoplasma* or pertussis. Sputum color has no proven association with bacterial illness in bronchitis. NSAIDs are perhaps the most important element of supportive care recommended for the vast majority of cases of acute bronchitis (except in geriatric

patients). Admission to the hospital for a patient with this chief complaint and with no comorbidities, normal vital signs, and a normal physical examination is not warranted.

64. **Answer E.** Physical examination findings generally produce only moderate (50% to 80%) sensitivity in the evaluation of acute appendicitis. Of the signs listed, only Rovsing sign approaches this sensitivity. The obturator sign's sensitivity is so low that it is no longer a clinically useful study. The psoas sign is used to detect a retrocecal appendix but sensitivity is reported at under 50%. The Kehr sign (referred pain at the shoulder due to diaphragmatic irritation) is seen more often in the setting of splenic rupture, ectopic pregnancy, and diaphragmatic lesions.

65. **Answer B.** This patient is infected with the common pinworm or *Enterobius vermicularis*. It is probably the most common parasitic infection in the United States. The most common clinical manifestation is pruritus ani. However, most infections are asymptomatic. Adult worms are white colored, are approximately 1 cm in length, and live in the cecum. At night, pregnant female worms containing an average of 10,000 ova migrate to the perianal skin, deposit their eggs, and die. The resulting pruritic sensation induces the patient to scratch and enables further autoinoculation or spread to other persons unless the patient engages in proper hand washing before touching others. The most sensitive test is the "scotch tape" test in which tape attached to a tongue blade is pressed against the perianal skin in an attempt to affix some of the *Enterobius* ova to the tape. The contents of the tape are then spread on a slide and viewed under a microscope in toluene. Stool samples for ova and parasites are not effective because the organism is not shed in the stool. Metronidazole is not effective for treatment. Instead, treatment is with albendazole, mebendazole, or pyrantel pamoate. Eosinophilia generally does not occur. On occasion, *Enterobius* may cause urinary tract infections and vulvovaginitis through retrograde migration into the urethra or vagina. Interestingly, girls with urinary tract infections are twice as likely to have a concomitant pinworm infection.

66. **Answer C.** Magnesium depresses the CNS and slows nerve conduction. It is used in preeclampsia to prevent progression to eclampsia, which is characterized by the presence of seizures. Magnesium slows neuromuscular conduction and decreases CNS irritability. Remembering this provides an easy means of remembering the actions of magnesium. It will decrease the respiratory rate, decrease deep tendon reflexes, and decrease the degree of consciousness. The loss of deep tendon reflexes is generally the first sign of magnesium toxicity.

67. **Answer A.** Though the mechanisms of cerebral edema are unknown, it is clear that children with DKA are susceptible to cerebral edema as a consequence of treatment. Children <5 years old are at highest risk. Initially the rate of fluid administration was tagged as the culprit, though it is not clear that the rate of fluid administration is the cause. Still, most guidelines advise slow fluid resuscitation with an aim to replete the fluid deficit over 48 hours. Furthermore, there appears to be no benefit to fast fluid administration. Most patients have a significant total body potassium deficit but fluid administration should occur before potassium depletion to avoid dangerous, abrupt increases in potassium. Not only should bolus insulin be avoided, but lower insulin infusion rates of 0.05 units/kg/hour may cause less hypokalemia without impacting the time to DKA resolution. Sodium bicarbonate has not been shown to be helpful and is not recommended unless the patient is severely acidotic (pH <6.9) with evidence of problems with cardiac contractility due to acidosis or in the case of life-threatening hyperkalemia.

68. **Answer A.** The patient has a spontaneous large right-sided pneumothorax. Historically, the decision about whether to treat a spontaneous pneumothorax invasively hinges on the size of the pneumothorax. Unfortunately, there is no standard definition about what constitutes a "large" pneumothorax. Some studies define "large" as a rim of air ≥2 cm at the hilum (which roughly correlates to half the lung volume) while others use 3 cm as a threshold. However, in stable patients even a large pneumothorax can be successfully treated with oxygen administration alone. The main benefit of invasive treatment is more rapid resolution and avoidance of hospital admission. Aspiration is a safe, less invasive technique than traditional tube thoracostomy. This is usually performed with a commercial kit using a one-way valve and manual aspiration. If, after 2.5 L of air has been aspirated, there remains a significant pneumothorax, tube thoracostomy should be performed. In patients with a simple pneumothorax, small caliber tubes (≤22 Fr) should be used. Re-expansion pulmonary edema is a frequent complication of pneumothorax treatment, though often asymptomatic. It tends to develop fairly rapidly after re-expansion.

69. **Answer D.** Hyphema refers to the presence of blood in the anterior chamber of the eye. The eye may rebleed after the initial traumatic hyphema, especially in patients with severe myopia or with large hyphemas. General treatment of traumatic hyphema involves analgesia and antiemetics, head elevation, restriction of eye movement, and avoidance of therapies that may cause bleeding. Ophthalmologic consultation should be sought emergently, especially for large hyphemas, as specific management with topical steroids or operative drainage

may be instituted. There is usually no afferent pupillary defect.

70. **Answer C.** Gout occurs due to uric acid crystal accumulation in the joints. Mechanisms include uric acid overproduction and undersecretion as well as exogenous precursor ingestion of dietary purines converted to uric acid by xanthine oxidase. High purine foods include mussels, organ meats, salty fish (sardines, herrings, etc.), alcohol, and poultry. Pseudogout occurs due to synovial deposition of calcium pyrophosphate crystals. There are no dietary modifications that will aid in preventing pseudogout flares. Although the most common joint affected in gout is the first metatarsophalangeal, the knee and the ankle can also be affected. The knee is the number one joint to be affected in pseudogout, followed by the wrist and the ankle. ESR is elevated in most acute attacks of both diseases. NSAID therapy is first-line for acute attacks of both.

71. **Answer A.** Most cases of PID occur within 1 week of menses. One hypothesis for this is that menstrual blood flow provides an optimal culture medium for bacteria. Other risk factors include young age (<20), history of any sexually transmitted infection (especially gonorrhea or chlamydia), and multiple sexual partners. PID is rare during pregnancy, as thickened cervical mucus is thought to prevent bacterial ascension. Diabetes insipidus and ovarian cysts are not risk factors for PID.

72. **Answer B.** Falsely positive and nondiagnostic elevations of serum troponins and creatine kinase are common among dialysis patients. However, cTnI is much more specific for myocardial injury than either cardiac troponin T (cTnT) or the CK-MB. In a large trial of asymptomatic dialysis patients, only 0.4% had cTnI values greater than 0.6 µg/L. In smaller studies of patients with suspected myocardial infarction, there has been no trend in false elevations of cTnI. While it is true that the most specific finding for a myocardial infarction is serial elevation of cTnI, an initial significant elevation in the setting of a history, and findings suggestive of NSTEMI should prompt initiation of appropriate treatment. Delays in treatment and poorer outcomes are common among patients with end-stage renal disease, in part due to the mistaken belief that most increased cTnI values are falsely elevated. Even among patients without chest pain, there is increasing evidence that elevated troponin is correlated with increased short- and long-term mortality due to significant cardiac events. The etiology for this finding is not entirely clear.

73. **Answer D.** Brain natriuretic peptide (BNP) aids in the diagnosis of CHF especially in cases where the signs and symptoms of COPD can mimic those of an acute heart failure exacerbation. If elevated, the BNP level points to CHF as the likely etiology. There are important false positives to an elevated BNP level, including sepsis and pulmonary embolism. Importantly, obesity can falsely depress BNP levels. Lactate is an excellent indicator of prognosis and mortality, but is not specific enough to point to a certain diagnosis. The yield on blood cultures in general is extremely low, especially in cases where infection is not the leading diagnosis. An arterial blood gas is not generally useful in the acute setting except to evaluate for hypercarbia, as hypoxia can be estimated using pulse oximetry and acidosis can be estimated with a venous blood gas if needed. The prothrombin time is not useful in the absence of suspected coagulopathy or known anticoagulation use.

74. **Answer D.** This patient has Epstein Barr virus (EBV) pharyngitis, also known as *mononucleosis*. As it is a viral infection, antibiotics have no role in treatment. Furthermore, the specific use of amoxicillin may result in the development of a morbilliform (i.e., measles-like) rash. Although this does not represent a true allergy, nor is it dangerous to the patient, it is an irritating and unnecessary outcome. The tonsillitis in EBV infections is non-exudative and may be considerably large, rarely resulting in airway obstruction.

75. **Answer C.** Cyanide intoxication is treated with a three-pronged approach. The preferred approach is direct cyanide binding using hydroxycobalamin (vitamin B12), while cyanide detoxification is achieved using sodium thiosulfate (which serves as a sulfur donor to rhodanese which converts cyanide to nontoxic thiocyanate). Amyl or sodium nitrite can also be used to induce methemoglobinemia since methemoglobin binds cyanide more strongly than mitochondrial cytochrome oxidase. However, methemoglobin also more tightly binds oxygen (shifts the dissociation curve to the left), resulting in decreased tissue oxygen delivery which may have important negative effects in critically ill patients. Phosgene is a common industrial chemical that smells like freshly mown hay when aerosolized. It is a direct pulmonary irritant, like chlorine or ammonia, and causes pulmonary edema. Treatment is supportive. Sulfur mustard is a vesicant which causes redness, pain, itching, and blistering of the skin, as well as gastrointestinal, pulmonary, and ocular damage. Vesicants are slow to act and are rarely fatal, but there is no specific antidote. VX is a "nerve agent" which inhibits acetylcholinesterase resulting in a cholinergic toxidrome. PM is used along with atropine to treat victims. PM should *never* be used as monotherapy because of transient PM-mediated acetylcholinesterase inhibition. Hydrogen sulfide is a toxic gas that smells like rotten eggs and that decouples mitochondrial respiration like cyanide. Unlike cyanide, however, only induced methemoglobinemia is effective as an antidote, so sodium nitrite is the treatment of choice.

76. **Answer A.** PID is an infection of the fallopian tubes. Risk factors include young age (15 to 25 is the highest risk group), multiple sexual partners, smoking, and bacterial vaginosis. It is caused by *Chlamydia*, gonococcus, and organisms, which cause bacterial vaginosis. The peak time of onset is within 1 week of menses, as menstrual flow is thought to provide an optimal culture medium for bacterial ascension. Symptoms include diffuse pelvic pain, fever, nausea, vomiting, vaginal discharge, and dyspareunia. Patients usually exhibit bilateral adnexal tenderness with significant cervical motion tenderness and cervical discharge. PID is a clinical diagnosis with laboratory and imaging studies useful only to rule out other causes of symptoms. Treatment involves antibiotics to cover *Chlamydia* and gonococcus—the most common regimen is IM ceftriaxone plus doxycycline/ azithromycin. Sequelae of untreated PID are extremely serious, including tubal scarring causing infertility and ectopic pregnancy, chronic pelvic pain, and tubo-ovarian abscess.

77. **Answer A.** Tick paralysis causes an ascending paralysis clinically similar to most variants of GBS (the rare Miller–Fischer variant of GBS causes a descending paralysis that starts with cranial nerve involvement). Signs of tick paralysis start as early as 1 day after the tick has attached. Removal of the tick is curative. Botulism causes a descending paralysis that usually starts with cranial nerve involvement. MG causes gradual, chronic, diffuse muscle weakness with repetitive movements, and ptosis is a common sign. Diphtheria causes an upper respiratory pseudomembrane associated with pharyngeal muscle weakness that can lead to airway compromise. Paralytic shellfish poisoning occurs due to toxins in algae ingested by edible mollusks (mussels, clams, oysters). It causes systemic symptoms such as nausea, vomiting, and lightheadedness associated with sensory disturbances and occasionally airway and respiratory muscle weakness.

78. **Answer B.** As with adults, neonatal hypoglycemia is treated with dextrose. Traditionally, D25 and D50 have been discouraged because of rebound hypoglycemia in hyperinsulinemic infants. In addition, D25 and D50 are thought to put the infant at risk for a potentially dangerous rise in plasma osmolarity. In addition, the amount of glucose to deliver to hypoglycemic infants is best determined by following the "rule of 50." This simple rule stipulates that the volume of dextrose given per kg of body weight multiplied by the dextrose concentration should equal 50. For example:

- 5 mL/kg × 10 (as in D10) = 50
- 2 mL/kg × 25 (as in D25) = 50

Then, all that is needed is the weight of the infant. Glucagon is useful as a second-line agent if the infant is refractory to dextrose. Octreotide and diazoxide are useful agents in infants with hyperinsulinemia but are not usually necessary in the ED.

79. **Answer A.** There is considerable overlap in the clinical presentation of patients with acute cholecystitis and acute cholangitis. However, patients with acute cholecystitis rarely exhibit jaundice and tend to be less toxic-appearing. Although the cystic duct is usually blocked in acute cholecystitis, the hepatic and common bile ducts are patent and free of infection and inflammation. Charcot triad (fever, right upper quadrant pain, jaundice) is the hallmark of acute cholangitis. Fever is nearly universal, present in 95% of patients, right upper quadrant tenderness in 90% and jaundice in 80%. Hypotension and altered mental status are present in 15% of patients and suggests gram-negative sepsis. When present in concert with Charcot triad, these findings are known as *Reynold pentad*. Although mildly elevated bilirubin levels may be present in patients with acute cholecystitis, these levels rarely rise above 4 mg/dL.

80. **Answer A.** This is known as *splitting* the fourth digit, and it represents the dividing line between median and ulnar innervation to the ring finger. The median nerve also serves the "LOAF" muscles, which include the **L**umbricals, as well as the muscles, which allow thumb **O**pposition, **A**bduction, and **F**lexion. However, the hallmark of CTS is sensory involvement, with motor abnormalities developing later. The most sensitive finding for CTS is abnormal sensation of the distal palmar tip of the index finger, as this represents the autonomous zone of the median nerve (the area where there is no overlap with other cutaneous nerves). Tinel sign is the presence of distal paresthesias in the setting of median nerve percussion at the wrist. In the absence of sensory or motor symptoms, Tinel sign has inadequate sensitivity and specificity to guide referral for further specialized testing.

81. **Answer D.** TAI occurs most commonly from high-speed motor vehicle collisions causing blunt thoracic trauma. Most traumatic aortic ruptures are immediately fatal, but patients who survive to ED evaluation are usually successfully treated. The descending aorta just distal to the subclavian artery is the most commonly injured site. Chest and back pain are the most common symptoms. Diagnosis is made by a combination of chest x-ray and CT aortography. Management of TAI involves operative repair, but blood pressure and heart rate control with β-blockers is essential to prevent further damage to the aorta from shear forces. Labetalol is an ideal single agent for reduction of blood pressure and heart rate. Clonidine, hydralazine, and enalaprilat all reduce blood pressure, but often cause reflex tachycardia and require a β-blocker in addition to reduce the number of heart

beats and shear forces to the aorta. Observation alone will result in worsening aortic injury and risks immediate death if the aorta ruptures completely.

82. **Answer C.** This patient has a mononeuropathy of cranial nerve III. In addition, the parasympathetic fibers of the oculomotor nerve seem to be spared. The most likely diagnosis is a diabetic mononeuropathy, which results from microvascular ischemia of a nutrient artery feeding the core of the oculomotor nerve. The peripheral aspect of the nerve, which contains the parasympathetic fibers to the pupil, is less affected because of collateral blood supply. However, a more ominous possibility is an aneurysm of the posterior communicating artery ([PCOM] aneurysm). The oculomotor nerve exits the brainstem between the PCOM and the superior cerebellar artery, so a PCOM aneurysm is well positioned to impinge on the nerve as it exits the brain. However, compression of the nerve usually affects the pupils as well, resulting in anisocoria. In addition to a PCOM aneurysm, it is important to evaluate the brainstem for signs of ischemia (vertebrobasilar insufficiency) as well as ischemic or hemorrhagic infarction. These findings may not be picked up on a routine CT scan of the brain. Although a cerebral angiogram would be useful for diagnosing an aneurysm, it is more invasive and provides less information about the brainstem than an MRI.

83. **Answer B.** The patient has evidence of a Monteggia fracture. Proximal ulnar fracture along with dislocation of the radial head from the capitellum (which may be subtle) is the specific finding. The typical mechanism is a blow to the forearm or fall on outstretched hand. Significant displacement of the radial head can put the patient at risk for radial nerve injury, exhibited by wrist drop. Treatment is surgical in most cases.

84. **Answer E.** ODS is a complication of hyponatremia treatment that most commonly affects alcoholics and patients with chronic malnutrition. It carries a grave prognosis with no known treatment. It does not typically occur after the treatment of patients with acute hyponatremia (<48 hours). Patients with pseudohyponatremia (e.g., diabetic patients with severe hyperglycemia) are not at risk for ODS and have normal sodium body stores. Sensory abnormalities are not common in ODS. The classic presentation is altered mental status (lethargy to coma) with pseudobulbar palsies and spastic quadriplegia after treatment for hyponatremia. Patients most commonly have an initial improvement in their sensorium after treatment of hyponatremia with hypertonic saline, but patients developing ODS then rapidly decline in the ensuing 48 to 72 hours. Most patients present 1 to 6 days after initial treatment of hyponatremia.

85. **Answer D.** BiPAP ventilation emulates pressure support mechanical ventilation with positive end-expiratory pressure (PEEP) in which the machine cycles between two *different* pressure levels during inspiration and expiration. This is in contrast to continuous positive airway pressure in which the pressure is the same throughout inspiration and expiration (i.e., IPAP = EPAP). When a patient's oxygenation status is not improving, the two main adjustments that can be made are to increase the inspired FIo_2 and to increase the PEEP. With BiPAP, there is a limit to the amount of oxygen that can be applied because the oxygen is not being delivered to the lower airways, as is the case with mechanical ventilation. However, the EPAP (i.e., PEEP) can be increased in order to recruit additional alveoli (by stenting them open with increased pressure at the end of expiration), which increases the surface area for gas exchange and hopefully results in improved oxygenation. In order to maintain the PPD during inspiration, the IPAP may be concomitantly increased (to ensure ongoing adequate ventilation). If these measures fail, the patient requires intubation and mechanical ventilation.

86. **Answer A.** The patient likely has rhabdomyolysis, which is due to significant skeletal muscle breakdown from a variety of causes. The most serious complication is acute renal failure from myoglobin accumulation in renal tubules. Treatment involves normal saline hydration in very large quantities (up to 10 to 20 L). No pharmacologic intervention has been shown to improve outcomes in randomized controlled trials. This includes mannitol, bicarbonate, and chelation therapy. These agents may be employed on a case-by-case basis. Potassium should never be supplemented, as myocyte breakdown in rhabdomyolysis releases large amounts of intracellular potassium into the bloodstream. Although hypocalcemia can occur in many cases of rhabdomyolysis, supplementing calcium can actually increase intracellular calcium and worsen myocyte injury. Furosemide and other loop diuretics cause urinary acidosis and should be avoided.

87. **Answer E.** Traumatic SAH results from bleeding in the subarachnoid vessels, causing blood to accumulate in around the brain parenchyma and in the sulci. It is an extremely common cause of traumatic intracranial hemorrhage. Symptoms include headache, vomiting, and photophobia. Focal neurologic deficits are rare due to the diffuse nature of the bleeding and generally low incidence of accompanying increased intracranial pressure. Cerebral vasospasm may occur as a result of the SAH and is associated with worse outcomes. The use of peripheral calcium channel blockers such as nimodipine improves outcomes though it does not actually appear to treat vasospasm. Furthermore, vasospasm is not evident

until about 3 days after hemorrhage, so its role in ED treatment is limited.

88. **Answer B.** PCP causes extreme dissociation, agitation, psychosis, and violent behavior. Superhuman strength often occurs in patients with PCP intoxication, sometimes requiring a dozen people to adequately restrain them. Vertical or rotary nystagmus is a physical examination finding characteristic of PCP intoxication. Cocaine intoxication may cause agitation, psychosis, and mydriasis but not nystagmus. LSD is a typical hallucinogen, and MDMA or ecstasy is similar to a combination of a hallucinogen and an amphetamine. Heroin causes a typical opioid toxidrome, with constricted pupils, sedation, and respiratory depression.

89. **Answer C.** The patient has a normal subxiphoid pericardial view on the FAST scan. There is no hypoechoic stripe indicating pericardial fluid (which is assumed to be blood in trauma) to warrant any further procedure in this patient aside from completion of the remainder of the FAST scan. Cardiology consultation should not be pursued just because the patient has a heart. From Bachur RG, Shaw KN. Fleisher & Ludwig's Textbook of Pediatric Emergency Medicine. 7th edition. Philadelphia, PA: Wolters Kluwer; 2015.

90. **Answer B.** Other than the epiglottis, epiglottitis may involve several supraglottic structures, including the vallecula, aryepiglottic folds, arytenoids, lingual tonsils, and base of the tongue. Inflammation does not extend to the infraglottic tissues because of the robust attachments between the infraglottic mucosa and submucosa. Owing to the variable involvement of several supraglottic structures, epiglottitis is sometimes referred to as *supraglottitis.* Drooling and stridor are unusual presenting signs in patients with epiglottitis. Historically, however, it has been thought that patients presenting with these symptoms, especially if they have developed over a short time period, are at higher risk for subsequent airway obstruction. No large, prospective trials have been conducted to sort this out. Most often, patients with epiglottitis present with a severe sore throat and painful dysphagia. Adult epiglottitis does not demonstrate any seasonal variation, but appears more common in males and smokers. Neither epinephrine nor corticosteroids have been shown to be beneficial, despite their widespread use. Caution is advised regarding the use of epinephrine as a temporizing measure in patients with epiglottis due to possible rebound upper airway constriction after the treatment is completed. Ninety percent of patients with epiglottitis will have abnormal lateral neck films. The classic finding is the "thumb" or "thumbprint" sign, indicating the presence of a swollen, inflamed epiglottis. However, a normal film cannot exclude the disease. Direct nasopharyngoscopy has been the gold standard of diagnosis, as it allows direct visualization of the tissue in question.

Recently, however, the "vallecula" sign has been suggested as another method of screening for the presence of epiglottitis on lateral neck films. This method relies on the physician's ability to locate the base of the tongue and trace it inferiorly toward the hyoid bone to locate the vallecula. If the vallecula is not deep and roughly parallel to the pharyngotracheal air column, then epiglottitis is present. In a small trial, this sign was shown to be 98% sensitive and 100% specific for epiglottitis.

91. **Answer C.** Hypercalcemia is extremely common in cancer patients and is probably the most common type of severe metabolic abnormality in this population. Mechanisms include direct bone destruction with release of calcium into the serum as well as PTH-like hormones secreted by some tumors. Symptoms of hypercalcemia include fatigue, nausea, vomiting, altered mental status, and abdominal pain. Treatment involves urgently lowering the serum calcium level with either oral hydration in mild cases or intravenous saline hydration with optional furosemide therapy. Bisphosphonates may also be used when the calcium level is extremely elevated. Magnesium sulfate may be given in patients with concomitant hypomagnesemia but is not indicated for solitary hypercalcemia. Although hypokalemia commonly accompanies hypercalcemia (and is often exacerbated by therapies which lower calcium levels), phosphate salts should be avoided for hypercalcemia, as they may cause precipitation of calcium phosphate. If potassium levels are borderline or low, potassium chloride should be used for replacement while calcium levels are being lowered. Vitamin D and hydrochlorothiazide both increase serum calcium levels and are contraindicated in patients with hypercalcemia.

92. **Answer E.** Family history in older patients with abdominal or flank pain is an extremely strong risk factor—an affected first-degree relative puts an individual at 20 times higher the risk than the general population. Other risk factors include age older than 50, peripheral vascular disease, hypertension, and patients with other large artery aneurysms.

93. **Answer C.** All of the vessels mentioned provide blood flow to the nose. Kiesselbach plexus is the most anterior and the most easily traumatized. Anterior nosebleeds are usually easily stopped by cautery with silver nitrate or packing with Merocel gauze. Nosebleeds that persist despite adequate packing are posterior in origin until proven otherwise.

94. **Answer C.** Herpes simplex encephalitis is clinically indistinguishable from other types of meningoencephalitis, causing headache, stiff neck, fever, and altered mental status. Temporal lobe involvement is typical and may be visible on neuroimaging. HSV-1 is the usual cause in adults; neonates have a higher incidence of HSV-2 due

to maternal infection. As in other cases of suspected meningoencephalitis, lumbar puncture and CSF studies are indicated, though HSV culture is negative in most cases. Acyclovir reduces mortality and the frequency of residual neurologic sequelae, which occur in the large majority of untreated patients.

95. **Answer B.** Ovarian torsion is relatively uncommon among patients in the ED but it is an important cause of acute pelvic pain. The classic history is the development of severe, acute pelvic pain associated with nausea and vomiting. The patient may note that a sudden change in position precipitated the pain. Interestingly, recent reviews have demonstrated that the onset is often much more subtle, with pain lasting from several hours to several weeks and only rarely associated with nausea or vomiting. Torsion is more common in young women with an average age at onset in the mid 20s. In addition, it is much more prevalent in patients with adnexal masses as ovarian tumors are ultimately revealed in approximately 60% of women. Finally, there is an increased rate of torsion in pregnant women, as roughly 20% of cases occur during pregnancy. Owing to obstructed venous drainage, the ovary enlarges and ovarian enlargement is the most common finding. Doppler ovarian imaging is difficult because of the dual ovarian blood supply, which may lead to the false perception of maintained arterial flow. Furthermore, many patients may experience spontaneous and recurrent torsion and detorsion. Ultrasonographies performed with a normal ovarian lie will not reveal vascular abnormalities. Finally, the presence of a large ovarian mass or hemorrhage within the ovary may make detection of vascular flow exceedingly difficult. Abnormal color Doppler imaging is highly predictive of torsion, but 50% of patients with surgically proven torsion have normal Doppler imaging.

96. **Answer B.** This patient is presenting with symptoms of acute decompensated heart failure (ADHF) due to severe volume overload as a result of missing dialysis. The approach to such patients mirrors the approach to patients with ADHF without concomitant renal failure. Since this patient presents with clear respiratory distress, stabilization of her oxygenation and ventilatory status is the chief concern. While furosemide, nitroglycerin, and CPAP may also be helpful in this setting, noninvasive ventilation with bilevel positive airway pressure will most rapidly and completely address her respiratory distress. CPAP is functionally similar to PEEP, as it is not a ventilatory mode, and patients must initiate all breaths. While CPAP has demonstrated efficacy in patients with ADHF, bilevel positive airway pressure allows clinicians to specify a pressure gradient between inspiration (inspiratory positive airway pressure) and expiration (expiratory positive airway pressure) which allows for true ventilation. Intravenous

enalaprilat is not recommended for the treatment of ADHF, since its effects on blood pressure are unpredictable and its use may be associated with worsened outcomes in patients with ADHF in the setting of acute myocardial infarction.

97. **Answer C.** In patients with left ventricular assist devices (LVADs), echocardiogram is extremely helpful for routine outpatient monitoring of ventricular function as well as evaluating for symptoms suggesting malfunction, including fatigue, lightheadedness, and dizziness. Although not all LVAD patients who present to the ED should receive an echocardiogram, the symptoms in the case do warrant this. CT of the chest or coronary vessels is not indicated routinely in this case. Cardiac MRI is contraindicated in patients with LVADs. A ventilation–perfusion scan is used to evaluate pulmonary embolism, and is not routinely ordered in patients without explicit chest pain, shortness of breath, or other symptoms of venous thromboembolic disease.

98. **Answer C.** Hypertension is the most common risk factor for aortic dissection though it is present in <75% of patients with diagnosed aortic dissection. Young patients with aortic dissection are much less likely to have hypertension (only approximately one-third of patients under 40 have hypertension). Marfan syndrome is a connective tissue disorder characterized by several skeletal, cardiovascular, and ocular manifestations. Arachnodactyly (long, slender fingers) is one of the major diagnostic criteria and one of the most easily recognized manifestations of the disease. Other major manifestations include a short trunk with long legs, pectus carinatum or excavatum, reduced elbow extension, and significant scoliosis. While an upper extremity blood pressure disparity is a classically described finding in patients with aortic dissection, it is unreliable and should be at least 20 mm Hg. A pulse deficit between the upper extremities is a more reliable sign of underlying dissection but is present in only 15% of patients. The classic heart murmur in aortic dissection is the murmur of aortic regurgitation, which is present in up to one-third of patients and more than 40% of patients with type A dissections. Obesity is not a risk factor for aortic dissection. Power lifting, or very intense weightlifting, can cause transient elevations of intra-aortic pressure to more than 300 mm Hg and is thought to be a risk factor for dissection. Other risk factors include cocaine use, third-trimester pregnancy, and other connective tissue disorders such as that found in Turner syndrome or Ehlers–Danlos syndrome.

99. **Answer D.** Pneumothorax, pneumomediastinum, subcutaneous emphysema, and subconjunctival hemorrhage are all complications related to the acute elevations in intrathoracic pressure during an asthma exacerbation. Pressures may be further exaggerated by

fits of coughing which may accompany an asthma exacerbation. MIs may occur in patients who have underlying cardiac disease, as severe asthma exacerbations place an extensive demand on the heart. Furthermore, patients with severe asthma attacks may be hypoxic for a period of time resulting in cardiac ischemia as oxygen supply is outstripped by demand. Pulmonary emboli are not related to asthma exacerbations.

100. **Answer C.** More than 90% of cases of hypercalcemia are caused by primary hyperparathyroidism or malignancy. Most cases of primary hyperparathyroidism are caused by benign parathyroid adenomas. Malignant causes of hypercalcemia occur either through osteolytic metastatic lesions as in breast cancer or melanoma or through secretion of parathyroid hormone-related peptide as in squamous cell carcinoma or renal cell carcinoma.

TEST 10

QUESTIONS

1. A 26-year-old female presents with intermittent nausea and vomiting, orthostatic lightheadedness, and mild diffuse abdominal pain. She also notes that her skin has darkened over the last month although she has been indoors. Which of the following laboratory abnormalities are you most likely to find?

    A. Hyponatremia
    B. Hyperglycemia
    C. Low thyroid-stimulating hormone levels
    D. Hypokalemia
    E. Elevated urinary metanephrines

2. Which of the following leads to the most severe acute ocular injury?

    A. Acid
    B. Alkali
    C. Ultraviolet light
    D. Hand soap
    E. Cigarette ashes

3. A 38-year-old female with a history of asthma presents to the emergency department (ED) with a chief complaint of wheezing and chest tightness typical of her asthma. She had recently run out of her medicines and complains of upper respiratory symptoms for the last week. Accompanying her is her 6-year-old son and 72-year-old mother, both of whom have asthma. Which of the following summarizes the treatment differences of acute asthma exacerbations between these groups?

    A. Corticosteroids are avoided in pediatric populations because of concerns about their effects on growth.
    B. The treatment of children with acute asthma exacerbations is similar to the treatment of adults and includes β-agonists, anticholinergics, and corticosteroids.
    C. Cromolyn sodium has a prominent role in the treatment of acute exacerbations of pediatric but not adult asthma.

    D. The first-line agent in treating elderly patients with acute asthma is ipratropium due to the high likelihood of underlying coronary artery disease and subsequent risk with β-agonist–induced tachycardia.
    E. Leukotriene modifiers have recently been shown to be useful in acute asthma exacerbations in elderly but not in pediatric or young adult patients.

4. A 71-year-old female without any past medical history presents with acute onset of shortness of breath and cough. She denies fever or productivity to her cough. Her vital signs are: 99.5, 110, 22, 122/72, 91% on RA. Her physical examination is unremarkable except for the tachycardia. Her complete blood count (CBC), chemistry, troponin, EKG, and chest x-ray are all normal. Which of the following is the most appropriate next step in management?

    A. Check D-dimer level
    B. Check brain natriuretic peptide (BNP) level
    C. Administer piperacillin–tazobactam
    D. Give dexamethasone
    E. Give albuterol nebulizer treatment

5. Which of the following is the most common form of botulism?

    A. Food-borne
    B. Infant
    C. Wound
    D. Respiratory
    E. Cardiac

6. A 35-year-old male presents with a severe head injury after being struck in the head with a baseball bat. His vital signs are HR 135, BP 82/45, RR 20. Which of the following is the most likely cause of his hypotension?

    A. Epidural hematoma
    B. Subdural hematoma
    C. Subarachnoid hemorrhage (SAH)
    D. Cerebral contusion
    E. Extracranial cause

7. Patients stricken with viral-induced myocarditis will most likely present with symptoms and findings consistent with:

    A. Acute coronary syndrome
    B. Variable degrees of heart block
    C. Congestive heart failure (CHF)
    D. Pericarditis
    E. Cardiogenic syncope

8. A 66-year-old female with a history of atrial fibrillation presents with acute onset of low back pain for 1 day. The pain is severe, diffuse, constant, and radiates down both legs. She reports having difficulty urinating over the last 12 hours. Her medications are metoprolol and coumadin. Vital signs are 98.6°F, 110, 18, 122/68, 98% RA. Her examination is unrevealing except for tenderness to palpation in the midline of the lumbar spine. Which of the following is the next best step in management?

    A. Discharge home with PO hydrocodone/acetaminophen
    B. CT myelogram
    C. CT lumbar spine
    D. MRI lumbar spine
    E. CT brain

9. A 32-year-old female who wears contact lenses presents with eye pain and redness (Fig. 10-1). Which of the following is the correct diagnosis?

    A. Acute angle closure glaucoma
    B. Central retinal vein occlusion
    C. Corneal ulcer
    D. Pterygium
    E. Central retinal artery occlusion

10. A 23-year-old male presents after being assaulted by several men. Per eyewitness report, the patient was kicked and struck with a baseball bat several times. The patient is brought in on a backboard wearing a cervical collar. He is extremely agitated and combative, punching and kicking staff and climbing off the bed. He is yelling, "I want to get out of here!" when any question is asked of him. He appears to be moving every extremity except his left arm. You complete the primary survey, which is intact except for the paralyzed left arm. His vital signs are 98.0, 95, 22, 166/94, and 98% RA. Which of the following is the most appropriate next step in management?

    A. CT brain
    B. MRI brain
    C. CT cervical spine
    D. Rapid-sequence intubation
    E. Sedation with haldol and lorazepam

11. A 24-year-old male with no past medical history presents with sudden onset of shortness of breath and chest pain. He appears uncomfortable. Vital signs are 98.6°F, 100, 24, 150/92, 96% RA. He has significantly decreased breath sounds on his right side. Chest x-ray is shown in Figure 10-2. Which of the following is the most appropriate next step in management?

    A. 100% oxygen by nonrebreather mask
    B. Thoracostomy with 36-French tube
    C. Pleurodesis
    D. Noninvasive positive pressure ventilation
    E. Albuterol nebulizer

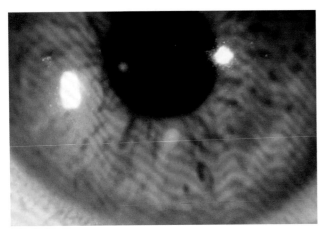

Figure 10-1

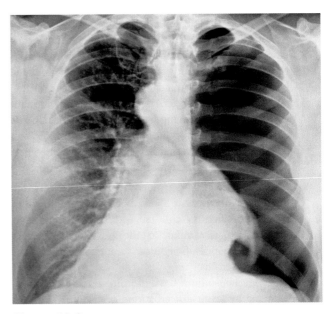

Figure 10-2

12. A 68-year-old male with multiple medical problems including diabetes, coronary artery disease, and hypertension is brought to the ED with a chief complaint of hypoglycemia. His wife called emergency medical services (EMS) after she could not arouse the patient from what she thought was a nap. She subsequently found a suicide note next to his empty bottle of glipizide. His initial blood sugar was 24. EMS administered an ampule of D50 which brought his sugar to 115, but upon arrival to the ED, his sugar has dropped back to 76. What other adjuncts should be given in addition to dextrose?

   A. Continuous intravenous low-dose epinephrine infusion
   B. High-dose intravenous solumedrol bolus
   C. Continuous intravenous glucagon infusion
   D. Activated charcoal with sorbitol
   E. Continuous intravenous octreotide infusion

13. A 67-year-old female with a history of severe heart failure s/p left ventricular assist device placement presents by EMS to the emergency department (ED) after a witnessed collapse in the hospital cafeteria. The patient was brought to the ED emergently after a "Code Blue" was called. Which of the following is true?

   A. Cardiopulmonary resuscitation (CPR) should be started immediately
   B. The patient may not have a palpable pulse even when awake and alert
   C. Ventricular arrhythmias do not impact heart function because patients are dependent on a machine for circulation
   D. Defibrillation is contraindicated in patients with left ventricular assist devices (LVADs)
   E. All of the above

14. Which of the following is the most common valve affected in rheumatic heart disease?

   A. Tricuspid
   B. Pulmonic
   C. Mitral
   D. Aortic
   E. All are equally affected.

15. A 25-year-old G_1P_0 presents at 18 weeks of gestation with a chief complaint of painless vaginal discharge (Fig. 10-3). Her pregnancy has progressed normally to date. Speculum examination reveals an adherent whitish discharge with a pH of 6.0. The wet prep is shown. Which of the following is true?

   A. Metronidazole is the treatment of choice.
   B. Amoxicillin should be used due to the patient's pregnancy.
   C. No treatment is required until the third trimester, after organogenesis has occurred.
   D. Treatment is elective, as the infection poses no health risks to the mother or fetus.
   E. None of the above

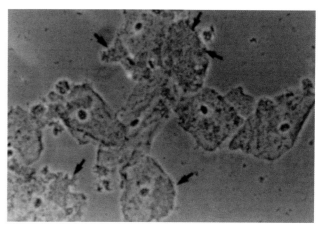

Figure 10-3

16. A 4-year-old male presents with fever, upper respiratory symptoms, and mild conjunctival injection. His mother states that he is unvaccinated due to personal beliefs of harm due to vaccines. Physical examination of the oral cavity reveals the image shown (Fig. 10-4). Which of the following is the likely diagnosis?

   A. Mumps
   B. Rubella
   C. Measles
   D. Chickenpox
   E. *Haemophilus influenzae* type B

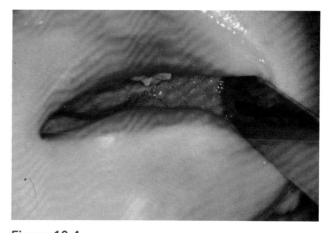

Figure 10-4

17. A patient presents for evaluation 2 weeks after recovering from a sore throat. Which of the following findings is most suggestive of rheumatic fever?

   A. Fever
   B. Sore throat
   C. Increased C-reactive protein (CRP)
   D. Sinus tachycardia
   E. Choreiform movements

18. An 85-year-old female presents with a painless mass in the right side of her neck. She first noticed the mass while brushing her teeth 3 days ago, but waited to see if it would go away before seeking medical attention. She has had pain in her right ear for the last week. She denies fevers, weight loss, foreign travel, night sweats, or a history of smoking. She also denies dysphagia, odynophagia, stridor, or globus. On examination, the patient has a 4 × 2 cm firm, immobile, nontender mass just lateral to her right sternocleidomastoid muscle at the level of her thyroid cartilage. Her right tympanic membrane is retracted with a serous effusion. What is the most likely diagnosis?

   A. Viral lymphadenitis

   B. Bacterial lymphadenitis

   C. Acute otitis media with reactive lymphadenitis

   D. Benign neoplasia

   E. Malignancy

19. An 82-year-old female taking digoxin for congestive heart failure (CHF) is brought to the ED with confusion and an arrhythmia. Her blood tests subsequently reveal a supratherapeutic digoxin level. At baseline, the patient is not known to have any rhythm disturbance or block. Which of the following rhythm disturbances is most likely present?

   A. Sinus bradycardia with multiple premature ventricular contractions (PVCs)

   B. Atrial fibrillation with rapid ventricular response

   C. AV nodal reentrant tachycardia

   D. Sinus tachycardia

   E. Mobitz type II second-degree heart block

20. Which cardiac chamber is most commonly injured in penetrating thoracic injury?

   A. Right atrium

   B. Left atrium

   C. Right ventricle

   D. Left ventricle

   E. All chambers are injured equally as often.

21. An 18-year-old depressed male is brought to the ED after a suicide attempt by ingestion of some sort of powdered poison. The patient called EMS almost immediately after ingesting "about a teaspoon" of the poison, stating he had "second thoughts" and "didn't want to die." En route to the hospital, the patient appears to have a seizure but remains awake throughout the event, and has an awkward, persistent "smile" per EMS providers. They administered 5 mg of midazolam IV which seemed to

have a small beneficial effect. Which of the following is likely responsible for the patient's symptoms?

   A. Superwarfarin

   B. Thallium

   C. Arsenic

   D. Strychnine

   E. Ergocalciferol

22. A 44-year-old male 2 years s/p laparoscopic roux-en-y gastric bypass presents for evaluation of generalized abdominal pain and food intolerance. The patient reports mild bloating and a fullness sensation that he hasn't had before. CT reveals a mesenteric swirl sign. Which of the following is the most likely diagnosis?

   A. Marginal ulcer

   B. Dilation of the gastric remnant

   C. Biliary colic

   D. Internal hernia

   E. Intussusception

23. Which of the following is indicated for treatment of acute angle closure glaucoma?

   A. Topical cycloplegics

   B. Topical antivirals

   C. Aspirin

   D. Acetazolamide

   E. Lateral canthotomy

24. A 45-year-old male presents after a high-speed motor vehicle crash. He was the unrestrained driver of a vehicle traveling 70 mph when he rear-ended a car stopped in front of him. He remembers that he struck his chest on airbag and he complains of severe chest pain. His primary survey is intact and his vital signs are normal. A chest x-ray is performed and is normal. Pelvic x-ray and focused assessment with sonography in trauma (FAST) scans are negative. Secondary survey reveals no additional injuries and the cervical spine is cleared clinically. Which of the following is the most important next step in management?

   A. Angiogram

   B. Check troponin levels

   C. CT chest with IV contrast

   D. Admit for observation

   E. Discharge home

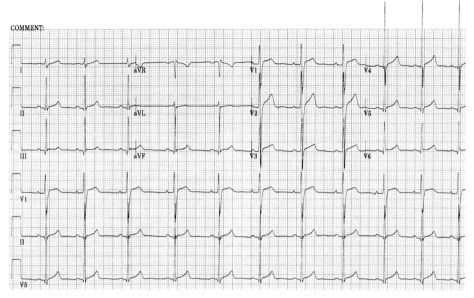

Figure 10-5

25. A 24-year-old male presents with nonexertional, atypical chest pain. His EKG is shown in Figure 10-5. Which of the following is true?

   A. The EKG reveals an acute ST-elevation MI.
   B. The patient likely has congenital heart disease.
   C. The ST-segment elevation is due to early repolarization.
   D. The patient is at risk for sudden cardiac death.
   E. All of the above are true.

26. A 37-year-old previously healthy woman is brought to the ED by her family with a complaint of fever, headache, and delirium with a depressed level consciousness. Empiric antibiotics for community-acquired meningitis were started and a CT scan was performed, which was negative. Her lumbar puncture revealed the following: WBC 412 per mm^3 with a differential of 98% lymphocytes, elevated protein, and normal glucose. Which of the following should be added to her regimen?

   A. Acyclovir
   B. Ampicillin
   C. Dexamethasone
   D. Amphotericin B
   E. None of the above

27. Which of the following is one of Kanavel cardinal signs of flexor tenosynovitis?

   A. Symmetrical swelling of the digit
   B. Tenderness to palpation of the volar aspect of the digit
   C. Pain upon passive extension of the digit
   D. Maintenance of the digit in a flexed posture
   E. All of the above

28. A 46-year-old male presents with a chief complaint of a painful penile erection that has persisted for 6 hours after using sildenafil. Which of the following is true?

   A. Sildenafil causes high-flow priapism
   B. Norepinephrine should be injected into the corpora spongiosum
   C. Due to high blood flow, future erectile dysfunction doesn't occur until an erection persists for 18 hours
   D. Saline irrigation should always be part of priapism treatment
   E. At least 5 to 10 mL of blood should first be aspirated from the corpora cavernosa prior to injection of a sympathomimetic agent

29. A 34-year-old male with a history of leukemia undergoing induction chemotherapy presents with fever of 101.5°F. He denies any symptoms except for fever and chills. Physical examination is normal except for fever. Basic laboratory work is normal except for a total WBC count of 1,400 cells per mm^3 with 5% neutrophils. Which of the following is the most appropriate next step in management?

   A. Discharge home with oncology follow-up
   B. Discharge home with oral ciprofloxacin and amoxicillin–clavulanate and oncology follow-up
   C. IV cefepime and admission to the hospital
   D. Lumbar puncture, dexamethasone, ceftriaxone, vancomycin, ampicillin, admission to the hospital
   E. IV ceftriaxone, G-CSF (Neupogen), then discharge home with cefpodoxime

TEST 10

30. A 44-year-old female presents with right leg pain. She has noticed increasing pain in the middle of her tibia over the last few weeks since she started training for a marathon. Physical examination of the entire lower extremity is normal except for mild tenderness to palpation in the area of pain. Radiographs of the tibia are normal. Which of the following is true regarding this patient's condition?

   A. Most cases require surgery for definitive management.
   B. The patient may only engage in nonimpact exercise.
   C. Magnetic resonance imaging (MRI) is the test of choice to differentiate shin splints from stress fractures.
   D. Men are at higher risk than women.
   E. The metatarsals are the most common bones involved.

31. Which important anatomical structure is at risk of injury during aspiration or incision and drainage of a peritonsillar abscess (PTA)?

   A. Vagus nerve
   B. Lingual artery
   C. Carotid artery
   D. Internal jugular vein
   E. Hypoglossal nerve

32. A 72-year-old male presents to the ED with a bump on his nose (Fig. 10-6). He denies any pain associated with the lesion but has noticed that it has been growing over the last several months. Which of the following is the most likely diagnosis?

   A. Basal cell carcinoma (BCC)
   B. Melanoma
   C. Kaposi sarcoma

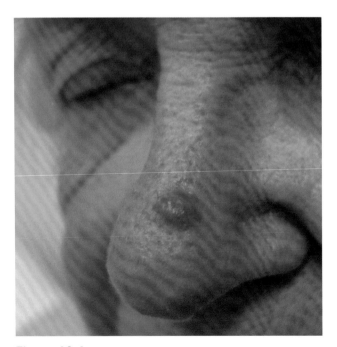

Figure 10-6

   D. Mycosis fungoides
   E. Squamous cell carcinoma (SCC)

33. A 22-year-old gang member is brought to an urban ED with a gunshot wound to his arm. Primary survey of the patient is intact, but a handgun is found in the patient's clothes. Which of the following is the most appropriate action by the physician at this time?

   A. Check to see if the gun is loaded.
   B. Fire the gun into the floor to discharge all the ammunition.
   C. Place the gun away from care providers and notify local law enforcement.
   D. Hold the gun personally so no one can take it.
   E. Use the gun to attack rival gang members in retribution.

34. A 26-year-old male is brought to the ED after being bludgeoned in the head with a baseball bat. His Glasgow Coma Scale is 7. After intubation, a noncontrast CT brain demonstrates a subdural hematoma. Which of the following is a proven benefit of administering seizure prophylaxis to this patient?

   A. Can prevent additional, acute seizures
   B. Can prevent delayed, subacute seizures
   C. Can prevent chronic epilepsy
   D. Can reduce cerebral perfusion pressure
   E. Can reduce mean arterial pressure

35. Which of the following findings on urinalysis is found in pyelonephritis but not cystitis?

   A. White blood cells (WBCs)
   B. WBC casts
   C. Nitrites
   D. Leukocyte esterase
   E. Bacteria

36. Risk factors for decompression sickness (DCS) include which of the following?

   A. Patent foramen ovale
   B. Obesity
   C. Cold ambient temperature after diving
   D. Dehydration
   E. All of the above

37. Which of the following is true regarding genital herpes simplex infection?

   A. The primary attack is usually more severe than recurrent episodes.
   B. Lesions are almost always painless.
   C. The Tzanck smear has >90% sensitivity and specificity.

D. Vesicles should be unroofed to allow drainage of fluid.

E. Antibiotics are indicated during outbreaks to prevent bacterial superinfection.

38. A 75-year-old male is brought to the ED in out-of-hospital cardiac arrest. Which of the following treatments will be most effective at improving the patient's likelihood to be discharged from the hospital in good neurologic condition?

A. Vasopressin

B. Low-dose epinephrine

C. High-dose epinephrine

D. Empiric tissue plasminogen activator

E. High-quality chest compressions

39. A 48-year-old male presents after a motor vehicle collision in which his car was severely rear-ended. He has an intact primary survey, but exhibits significant midline cervical spine tenderness at C7-T1. You decide to order cervical spine imaging. Which of the following is most correct regarding this patient?

A. Cervical spine radiographs have over 95% sensitivity to identify fractures

B. Cervical spine imaging clinical decision rules are of limited utility

C. The most common cervical spine fracture is at the C4–5 junction

D. CT cervical spine is indicated

E. Pain medication should be withheld in trauma to localize tenderness

40. Which of the following is true regarding treatment of otitis media?

A. Few cases will resolve spontaneously without antibiotics.

B. Oral antibiotics are superior to intramuscular (IM) antibiotics in efficacy of treatment.

C. High-dose amoxicillin (80 mg/kg/day) should be reserved for those patients who are older than 2 years of age.

D. Otitis media represents the number one reason for outpatient antimicrobial prescriptions in the United States.

E. Auralgan may be beneficial in patients with tympanic membrane perforations.

41. Which of the following is a common cause of death in patients with acute renal failure?

A. Hypercalcemia

B. Hyperkalemia

C. Hypermagnesemia

D. Hypernatremia

E. Hyperphosphatemia

42. A 44-year-old cancer patient with known chemotherapy-induced neutropenia is sent by her oncologist to the ED with a fever of 101.5°F. Which of the following is the most appropriate initial empiric antibiotic regimen?

A. Doxycycline

B. Cefepime

C. Clindamycin

D. Metronidazole + gentamicin

E. Metronidazole + aztreonam

43. A 45-year-old female presents with headache, fluctuating mild confusion, and fatigue for 1 week. She reports intermittent diffuse headaches, which occur in different locations in her head and do not follow any predictable pattern. She has also noticed that she feels tired easily on her daily activities. Her husband states she is confused at times. Physical examination is normal except for temperature of 100.5°F and pale conjunctivae. She exhibits no meningismus. Laboratory work is as follows:

WBC: 8,000 cells per mm^3

Hemoglobin: 8.5 g/dL

Platelets: 15,000 cells per mm^3

Na: 135 mEq/L

K: 4.4 mEq/L

Cl: 100 mEq/L

HCO$_3$: 24 mEq/L

Blood urea nitrogen: 13 mEq/L

Cr: 1.1 mEq/L

Glucose: 109 mEq/L

Which of the following is the most appropriate next step in management?

A. Platelet transfusion

B. Hemodialysis

C. Splenectomy

D. Plasmapheresis

E. Acyclovir

44. Which of the following is true regarding tinea versicolor?

A. Recurrence of lesions after treatment is common.

B. Sunlight accelerates repigmentation.

C. Griseofulvin is inactive against the disease.

D. The upper trunk is the most commonly affected area.

E. All of the above.

45. A 28-year-old male presents to the ED with an extensive vesicular, weeping, and crusted eruption arranged in a linear pattern on his lower legs. He tells you that he cleaned out the brush from the woods behind his house a couple of days ago. You suspect he has a contact dermatitis due to poison ivy. In addition to cool compresses and antihistamines to help control pruritus, the ideal course of corticosteroids should be:

A. Topical triamcinolone until resolution.

B. Three days of oral prednisone.

C. A commercially available steroid dose pack (e.g., Medrol Dosepak).

D. At least 14 days of oral prednisone.

E. Corticosteroids are unnecessary in most cases of poison-ivy–induced contact dermatitis.

46. A 34-year-old male presents with chest pain and shortness of breath after being struck in the right side of the chest with a baseball bat. Chest x-ray demonstrates a moderate to large pneumothorax on the right. Which of the following is the most appropriate management at this time?

A. Needle thoracostomy at the second intercostal space, midclavicular line

B. Needle thoracostomy at the fifth intercostal space, midclavicular line

C. Tube thoracostomy at the second intercostal space, midaxillary line

D. Tube thoracostomy at the fifth intercostal space, midaxillary line

E. Observation alone

47. Which of the following is true regarding neck trauma?

A. Delayed neurologic deficits after blunt neck trauma suggest carotid artery dissection.

B. All patients suspected to have an esophageal injury should receive a barium contrast esophagram.

C. Zone III injuries are most amenable to surgical exploration.

D. All neck wounds should be probed to determine the depth of the wound and integrity of vital structures.

E. Impaled objects should always be removed in patients with penetrating neck trauma.

48. A 76-year-old female with a history of atrial fibrillation presents with acute, diffuse abdominal pain for 6 hours. The pain has been consistently severe since onset, and she developed chills for the last 2 hours. She reports that she ran out of her coumadin 2 weeks prior. Vital signs are 100.2°F, 115, 18, 168/88, 99% RA. Her abdomen is mildly tender diffusely without focal rebound tenderness. Which of the following is true regarding this patient's most likely diagnosis?

A. A normal WBC count essentially excludes serious sequelae

B. CT angiography is the diagnostic test of choice

C. Lactate has close to 100% sensitivity

D. Mortality is about 15%

E. Venous thrombosis is the most common etiology

49. A 26-year-old female is brought to the ED after she was ejected in a motor vehicle accident. Initial evaluation reveals a confused patient with multiple scalp wounds and vital signs of P 130, BP 85/55. After intubation and fluid resuscitation, initial plain films reveal clear lungs but an obvious pelvic fracture. Focused assessment with sonography in trauma (FAST) examination reveals hemoperitoneum. Which of the following is the next step in management?

A. Abdominal CT to better determine the need for laparotomy

B. Pelvic angiography

C. Thoracotomy with cross clamping of the aorta

D. Exploratory laparotomy

E. Use diagnostic peritoneal lavage (DPL) cell counts to determine the need for laparotomy

50. A 44-year-old alcoholic man presents with nausea and vomiting. He reports drinking alcohol for 2 days straight. Physical examination is normal except for a mildly intoxicated patient with extremely dry mucous membranes. Urine dip is positive for ketones. The chemistry panel is as given:

Na^+, 134 mEq/L

K^+, 4.0 mEq/L

Cl^-, 92 mEq/L

HCO_3^-, 18 mEq/L

BUN, 32 mg/dL

Cr, 1.6 mg/dL

Glu, 114 mg/dL

Which of the following is the most appropriate next step in management?

A. Bicarbonate

B. Insulin

C. Glucose

D. Potassium

E. Magnesium

51. A 24-year-old female presents with a chief complaint of bleeding from her mouth after having her tooth extracted earlier in the day. Which of the following may help stop the bleeding?

A. Tranexamic acid mouth wash
B. Gelfoam
C. Cocaine soaked gauze
D. Thrombin
E. All of the above

52. Aside from the eyes, methanol overdose most commonly has pathologic effects on which of the following sites?

A. Basal ganglia
B. Facial nerve
C. Vagus nerve
D. Olfactory nerve
E. Glossopharyngeal nerve

53. A 15-year-old female is brought to the ED by her parents because they suspect her of drug use. Friends dropped their daughter off after going to a party where she became confused and started grinding her teeth. They noted her heart was beating very fast, and she had trouble focusing her eyes. Her friends report that she took something to "feel closer" to her friends. Which of the following is the most likely drug used?

A. LSD
B. PCP
C. 3, 4-MDMA
D. Sertraline
E. Phenelzine

54. A 45-year-old male presents with abrupt onset of fever, cough, chills, and shortness of breath. One week earlier, he was present in a government office where an explosion thought to be a terrorist attack occurred. He appears toxic and in moderate respiratory distress. Chest x-ray is shown in Figure 10-7. Which of the following is the most appropriate therapy at this time?

A. Ciprofloxacin
B. Aztreonam
C. Tobramycin
D. Ceftriaxone
E. Methylprednisolone

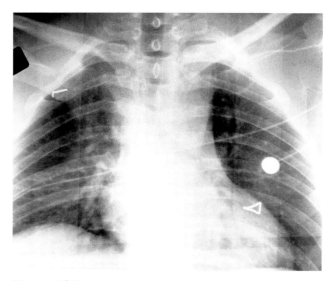

Figure 10-7

55. A 55-year-old female with a history of rheumatoid arthritis presents with progressive swelling and pain in her knee for 6 days. She denies trauma to the area or fever. She is on prednisone for her rheumatoid arthritis, and states that her standard flares involve her ankles and fingers. Vital signs are 99.0°F, 100, 20, 132/65, 98% RA. Physical examination reveals a moderate-sized knee effusion with warmth and tenderness and extreme pain on range of motion of the joint. Which of the following is the most appropriate next step in management?

A. Joint aspiration
B. MRI of the knee
C. Colchicine PO
D. Stress-dose steroids
E. Indomethacin PO

56. A 25-year-old female presents with white vaginal discharge. Physical examination demonstrates grayish-white discharge with no cervical lesions. A wet mount is positive for the presence of clue cells. The patient states she developed a rash after several days of treatment for an identical problem 1 year ago. Which of the following is the best therapy for this patient?

A. Fluconazole 150 mg PO once
B. Metronidazole 2 g PO once
C. Clindamycin 300 mg b.i.d. for 7 days
D. Ceftriaxone 125 mg IM once
E. Azithromycin 1 g PO once

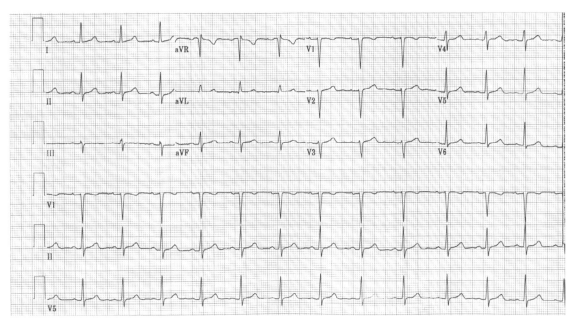

Figure 10-8

57. A 22-year-old male presents with an episode of left-sided chest pain that lasted 4 hours, but resolved an hour before presenting to the ED. The pain was dull and radiated to his left shoulder. The patient states that he used cocaine at a party 12 hours ago. Physical examination is unremarkable and vital signs are normal. The electrocardiogram (EKG) is shown in Figure 10-8. Which of the following is most appropriate at this time?

A. Nitroglycerin
B. Metoprolol
C. Morphine
D. Aspirin
E. Tissue plasminogen activator (tPA)

58. A 27-year-old female at 33 weeks of gestation presenting with liver tenderness and evidence of coagulopathy is most suggestive of:

A. Acute fatty liver of pregnancy (AFLP)
B. Preeclampsia
C. Hepatitis
D. Cholecystitis
E. Intrahepatic cholestasis of pregnancy (ICP)

59. Which of the following can be used to treat hypertrophic cardiomyopathy?

A. Digitalis
B. Isoproterenol
C. Furosemide
D. Phenylephrine
E. Metoprolol

60. Excision of thrombosed hemorrhoids is not recommended or effective after:

A. 12 hours
B. 24 hours
C. 48 hours
D. 96 hours
E. 1 week

61. A 24-year-old previously healthy woman presents with a cutaneous abscess on her left thigh. She is afebrile and her thigh examination reveals a tender, fluctuant area 4 cm × 6 cm in size. There is no surrounding erythema. In addition to incision and drainage, which of the following has been shown to provide the better outcomes in abscess management?

A. Irrigation of abscess cavity
B. Prednisone 40 mg PO q.d. × 5 days
C. Cephalexin 250 mg PO q.i.d. × 10 days
D. Packing of wound with iodoform gauze
E. None of these

62. A pregnant woman at 34 weeks' gestation is undergoing tocographic and fetal monitoring in your small community ED after a motor vehicle accident (Fig. 10-9). While discussing the case with the on-call obstetrician, she asks for your interpretation of the fetal strip. Which of the following is represented in the strips?

A. Head compression
B. Uterine rupture
C. Umbilical cord compression
D. Placenta previa
E. Uteroplacental insufficiency

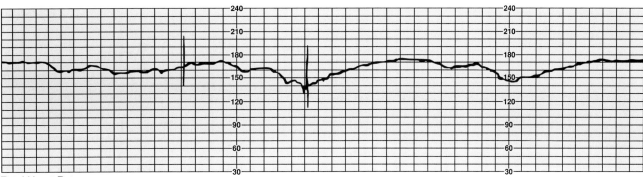

Fetal Heart Rate

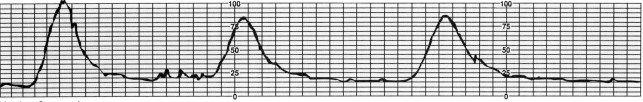

Uterine Contractions

Figure 10-9

63. A 25-year-old male presents with chest pain. The pain lasts for seconds at a time, is not pleuritic, and is nonexertional. He has no past medical history, takes no medications, is a nonsmoker, and does not drink alcohol or use drugs. His vital signs are normal and his physical examination is unremarkable. His EKG reveals a normal sinus rhythm without ST-segment changes. His chest x-ray is normal. Which of the following is the next best step in management?

A. Discharge with outpatient follow-up with his primary care physician.
B. Prescribe 324 mg aspirin every day and discharge
C. Enoxaparin 1 mg/kg IV and discharge
D. Aspirin 324 mg PO and admit to the hospital telemetry floor
E. Tissue plasminogen activator IV and admit to the ICU

64. Which of the following is the most sensitive physical examination test for an anterior cruciate ligament (ACL) tear?

A. Anterior drawer
B. Posterior drawer
C. Lachman
D. McMurray
E. Thompson

65. A 55-year-old male without any past medical history presents with chest pain. Physical examination is normal. The EKG is shown in Figure 10-10. Which of the following represents the likely site of pathology?

A. Pericardium
B. Pulmonary artery

C. Left circumflex artery
D. Left anterior descending (LAD) artery
E. Right coronary artery

66. An otherwise healthy 22-year-old male presents to the ED after a "spider bite." He states that he felt a pinprick sensation on his hand when he lifted the hood of an old car he has been storing in his driveway. He continued working, but soon developed crampy muscle aches that spread up his arm and now seem most severe in his chest and abdomen. In the ED, his abdomen is rigid and the patient is complaining of dizziness, nausea, and severe "stomach cramps." Which of the following is the likely culprit?

A. Tarantula
B. Hobo spider
C. Brown recluse spider
D. Wolf spider
E. Black widow spider

67. A 2-year-old male is brought in by his parents with a rash on his trunk. On examination, you discover a rose-colored maculopapular rash on his chest, neck, and arms. The patient is currently afebrile, but the parents tell you that the patient was seen by one of your colleagues yesterday for a febrile seizure. Which of the following is the most likely diagnosis?

A. Roseola infantum
B. Rubeola
C. Rubella
D. Erythema infectiosum
E. Scarlet fever

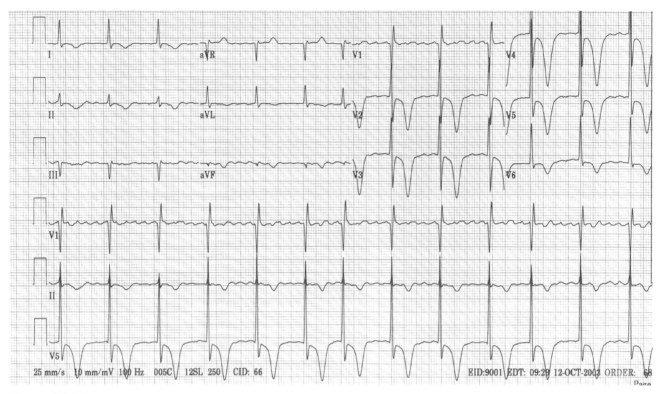

Figure 10-10

68. A 36-year-old female with a history of asthma presents with the following rash (Fig. 10-11). It started out as exquisitely pruritic normal-appearing skin and then progressed to this after she scratched it frequently for several days. Which of the following is the most likely diagnosis?

    A. Group A streptococcal infection
    B. Eczema
    C. Toxic epidermal necrolysis
    D. Toxic shock syndrome
    E. Erysipelas

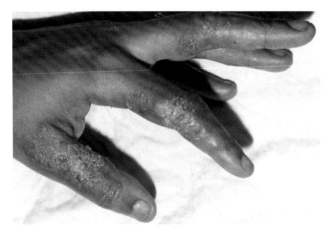

Figure 10-11

69. A 22-year-old female presents with sudden onset of palpitations. She is 10 weeks pregnant with a confirmed intrauterine fetus. Her vital signs are 98.6, 190, 20, 124/67, 98% RA. The EKG shows a regular, narrow-complex tachycardia with absent P waves. Which of the following is the most appropriate next step in management?

    A. Digoxin 0.125 mg IV
    B. Adenosine 6 mg IV
    C. Lidocaine 100 mg IV
    D. Amiodarone 150 mg IV
    E. Procainamide 1 g IV

70. A 24-year-old female presents with a diffuse rash (Fig. 10-12). She had "sores" of her mouth and eyes as well as numerous "spots" on her trunk, but now the rash has spread throughout her body. She is uncomfortable and her skin is warm and tender. Pressure applied to skin adjacent to the lesions seems to extend the lesion into the normal-appearing skin. In exploring her recent history, which of the following is most likely?

    A. She recently had a viral upper respiratory infection (URI).
    B. She was being treated for a urinary tract infection.
    C. She has human immunodeficiency virus (HIV).
    D. She was recently diagnosed with leukemia.
    E. She has gout.

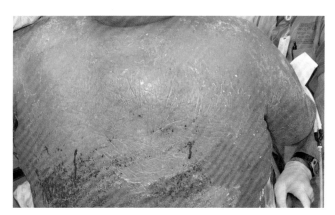

Figure 10-12

71. A 24-year-old healthy female is brought to the ED by EMS after having ingested "a large number" of her mother's digoxin tablets. Her EKG reveals asymptomatic sinus bradycardia with first-degree AV block and occasional PVCs. Her vital signs reveal a pulse of 48 but are otherwise normal. Subsequent laboratory tests demonstrate a potassium level of 6.8 mEq/L. How should the elevated potassium level be treated?

    A. Intravenous Digibind (Fab) administration
    B. Intravenous calcium chloride
    C. Intravenous sodium bicarbonate infusion
    D. Continuous albuterol nebulization
    E. Intravenous insulin and intravenous dextrose

72. A 65-year-old female presents to the emergency room with signs and symptoms of digitalis toxicity, ventricular tachycardia, and a digoxin level of 8.5 ng/mL. She is treated with digitalis antibody fragment therapy and the cardiac rhythm reverts to normal sinus rhythm. However, a repeat digoxin level after the fragments are given is 12 ng/mL. Which of the following is the most appropriate next step in management?

    A. No acute therapy
    B. Cardioversion at 50 J
    C. Procainamide 1 g IV
    D. Calcium chloride 1 g IV
    E. Potassium chloride 40 mEq IV

73. A 47-year-old male smoker with a history of hypertension and hyperlipidemia presents for evaluation of left-sided mid back pain and shortness of breath. He reports he awoke with the pain which has worsened throughout the day. His vitals are: T 98.6°F, RR 22, P 100, BP 124/71, SaO$_2$ 94% on 4 L NC. A CT scan is performed and reveals the image shown in Figure 10-13. An hour after presenting for care, his vital signs are essentially unchanged. Which of the following is true?

    A. Tissue plasminogen activator (tPA) is indicated
    B. An echocardiogram should be performed to guide therapy
    C. Embolectomy is the treatment of choice
    D. An IV heparin infusion should be started to initiate anticoagulation
    E. An inferior vena cava (IVC) filter should be placed

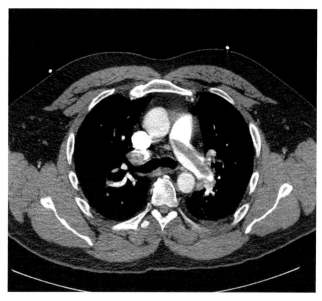

Figure 10-13

74. Which of the following tick-borne illnesses is responsible for the most deaths?

    A. Rocky Mountain spotted fever
    B. Ehrlichiosis
    C. Lyme disease
    D. Colorado tick fever
    E. Babesiosis

75. A 65-year-old male presents with a chief complaint of double vision. On examination, covering either eye causes the diplopia to resolve. Which of the following is the most likely cause?

    A. Multiple sclerosis
    B. Thyroid disease
    C. Isolated cranial nerve palsy
    D. Myasthenia gravis
    E. Orbital abscess

TEST 10

76. Which patients with a transient ischemic attack (TIA) and the following associated signs and symptoms are at lowest risk for recurrent TIA or future stroke?

    A. Isolated monocular blindness (amaurosis fugax)
    B. Aphasia and new-onset atrial flutter
    C. "Crescendo" TIA (more than three ischemic events in 72 hours)
    D. Left arm weakness in a patient who is already taking aspirin therapy
    E. Left arm weakness and facial droop in a diabetic patient that persisted for 45 minutes

77. A 56-year-old male presents with tremor, anxiety, tachycardia, and hypertension. He has a past medical history of chronic renal insufficiency. He reports heavy alcohol use but has not had a drink in the last 2 days. Which of the following is the most appropriate next step in management?

    A. Haloperidol
    B. Lorazepam
    C. Chlordiazepoxide
    D. Diphenhydramine
    E. Droperidol

78. A 42-year-old male with hypertension presents with significant swelling of his lips and tongue. He has been taking lisinopril for the past 8 months. Which of the following is true?

    A. This adverse drug event is most common in the first week after therapy.
    B. This patient's symptoms may be resistant to treatment with epinephrine.
    C. These patients typically do not have urticaria.
    D. Angiotensin-receptor blockers (ARBs) are unsafe to use in this patient.
    E. All of the above.

79. Which of the following is true regarding hyperosmolar hyperglycemic syndrome or state (HHS), also known as *hyperglycemic hyperosmolar nonketotic coma* (HHNC)?

    A. The presence of ketonuria rules out the diagnosis.
    B. The mortality rate is lower than in patients with diabetic ketoacidosis (DKA).
    C. Infection is the most common precipitant.
    D. The degree of mental status change correlates with the plasma pH.
    E. Insulin infusions are the most important component of initial therapy.

80. An 85-year-old male presents with right upper quadrant pain, chills, and nausea. His pain is worse after eating. He is febrile, appears toxic, and has significant right upper quadrant tenderness to palpation. You suspect acute cholecystitis. A right upper quadrant ultrasound reveals pericholecystic fluid and gallbladder wall thickening but no gallstones. Which of the following is the next best step in management?

    A. CT abdomen/pelvis with oral contrast
    B. CT abdomen/pelvis with IV contrast
    C. CT abdomen/pelvis with oral and IV contrast
    D. IV ampicillin–sulbactam
    E. Discharge home with outpatient surgery referral

81. A 56-year-old female is sent immediately to the ED by her primary care provider for a blood pressure of 200/100. She is asymptomatic and has not taken her hydrochlorothiazide and lisinopril for 6 months. Which of the following is the next best step in management?

    A. Nitroglycerin 0.4 mg SL
    B. Labetalol 20 mg IV
    C. Hydralazine 20 mg IV
    D. Nicardipine 5 mg/hour IV drip
    E. Recheck blood pressure in 30 minutes

82. A 30-year-old female presents with painless hematuria and increased urinary frequency. Which of the following is the most likely cause?

    A. Renal carcinoma
    B. Bladder carcinoma
    C. Urinary tract infection (UTI)
    D. Glomerulonephritis
    E. Nephrotic syndrome

83. A 65-year-old female with a history of chronic alcoholism presents with confusion, ataxia, and nystagmus. Which of the following is the most appropriate therapy?

    A. Lorazepam
    B. Haloperidol
    C. Thiamine
    D. Pyridoxine
    E. Potassium

84. Which of the following is true about babesiosis?

    A. Babesiosis is a tick-borne illness
    B. Asplenic patients are at highest risk for severe infection
    C. Infection is often associated with hemolytic anemia
    D. Diagnosis hinges on microscopic evaluation of a thin blood smear
    E. All of the above

85. Which of the following is true regarding osteomyelitis?

    A. Patients usually appear toxic.
    B. The sensitivity of erythrocyte sedimentation rate (ESR) is 50%.
    C. The sensitivity of radiographs is higher early in the illness.
    D. CT is superior to MRI for diagnosis.
    E. *Staphylococcus aureus* is the most common cause.

86. A 20-year-old male who has recently recovered from gastroenteritis due to *Shigella flexneri* is most at risk for developing which of the following?

   A. Ankylosing spondylitis
   B. Systemic lupus erythematosus
   C. Rheumatoid arthritis
   D. Psoriatic arthritis
   E. Reactive arthritis (Reiter syndrome)

87. Which of the following is the most common location of uncomplicated anal fissures?

   A. Anterior midline
   B. Posterior midline
   C. Right lateral
   D. Left lateral
   E. Circumferential

88. An 80-year-old female presents with a distal radius fracture of her nondominant hand after a trip and fall. She did not strike her head and this is her first fall ever. She has no other injuries and takes no other medications. Her only medical history is chronic intermittent constipation. Which of the following is the most appropriate pain management regimen for her?

   A. Ibuprofen 400 mg every 6 hours as needed
   B. Ibuprofen 400 mg every 6 hours scheduled
   C. Acetaminophen 650 mg every 6 hours as needed
   D. Acetaminophen 650 mg every 6 hours scheduled
   E. Oxycodone 10 mg every 6 hours scheduled

89. The use of "triptans" for the treatment of migraine-related headache should be limited to 2 days per week for which of the following reasons?

   A. Prolonged use may result in pulmonary fibrosis
   B. Increased risk of rebound headache
   C. Increased risk of cardiac ischemia
   D. Development of permanent lower extremity paresthesias and numbness
   E. They increase the risk of ischemic stroke

90. While working in the ED, a mass-casualty alert is called in by EMS after a bomb was detonated outside an office building downtown. After the most critically ill patients are successfully managed, a 29-year-old male is brought to the ED by EMS. EMS estimates that he was approximately 100 feet from the detonation site. The patient states he was thrown a few feet and knocked down but did not suffer loss of consciousness. He complains of headache, dizziness, shortness of breath, and decreased hearing with ringing of the ears. Which of the following is true?

   A. Tympanic membrane (TM) rupture is a sensitive indicator of blast lung injury.
   B. Oropharyngeal petechiae are always present in the setting of critical abdominal solid organ trauma.

   C. The primary blast wave predominantly affects solid organs.
   D. Blast lung injury is the most common fatal injury among initial survivors.
   E. High-energy explosives generate blast waves which maintain their pressure and velocity over long distances.

91. A 28-year-old female presents with a low-grade fever, arthralgias, fatigue, and the rash shown (Fig. 10-14). Which of the following is the best therapy?

   A. Acyclovir
   B. Azithromycin
   C. Doxycycline
   D. Amoxicillin–clavulanic acid
   E. Supportive care

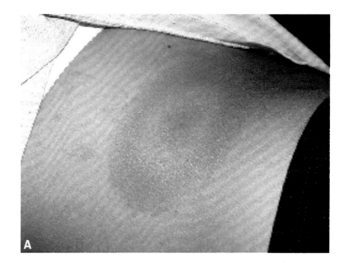

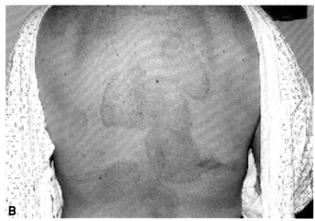

Figure 10-14

92. A 33-year-old male presents with acute onset of bilateral lower extremity weakness several minutes after returning from a deep scuba dive. His physical examination reveals 3/5 strength in both lower extremities and he has patchy loss of sensation throughout the lower half of his body. Which of the following is the most likely cause of his symptoms?

A. Epidural abscess
B. Epidural hematoma
C. Nitrogen bubble formation
D. Guillain–Barré syndrome (GBS)
E. Middle ear barotrauma

93. What is the most common cause of pruritus ani?

A. Inadequate anal hygiene
B. Anal fissure
C. Hemorrhoids
D. Lichen sclerosus
E. Diabetes mellitus

94. Which of the following effects is directly responsible for the QRS prolongation seen in tricyclic antidepressant poisoning?

A. Fast sodium channel blockade
B. Potassium efflux blockade
C. α-1 antagonism
D. Anticholinergic activity
E. Magnesium channel blockade

95. A 67-year-old female presents in septic shock due to pyelonephritis. Her vital signs are: 101.2, 110, 20, 94/59, 99% on RA. Apart from intravenous antibiotic therapy, which of the following is most likely to help reduce her mortality?

A. Corticosteroids
B. Checking a lactate level
C. Placing a central venous catheter
D. Phenylephrine therapy
E. Aggressive intravenous fluids

96. A 62-year-old female with a history of O_2-dependent chronic obstructive pulmonary disease (COPD) presents to the ED with a chief complaint of dyspnea and increased cough productive of yellow phlegm. The patient uses 2 L of O_2 at home. The patient is an ill-appearing, dyspneic woman speaking in sentence fragments. Her SaO_2 reads 85% on 4 L of O_2 by nasal cannula. As you start to increase her O_2, you wonder if you are going to eliminate her respiratory drive. The next best step is to:

A. Immediately intubate the patient using rapid sequence intubation
B. Increase the O_2 to 6 L, because minute ventilation changes little in COPD patients exposed to higher levels of oxygen

C. Decrease the O_2 to 2 L (her baseline) in order to increase the patient's respiratory drive
D. Perform an arterial blood gas (ABG) to assess the patient's exact ventilatory and oxygenation status because you do not know what effect changing the oxygen will have
E. Leave the O_2 at 4 L because the patient is likely hypoxic at baseline and continue treatment hoping the patient will improve

97. Which of the following occurs earliest during hepatitis A infection?

A. Nausea and vomiting
B. Fecal excretion
C. Viremia
D. Transaminitis
E. Jaundice

98. Which of the following is true regarding the afterdrop phenomenon in hypothermic patients?

A. Afterdrop may predispose patients to the development of abnormal heart rhythms.
B. Afterdrop is exacerbated by active external rewarming.
C. Afterdrop is caused by the return of cold peripheral blood to the core upon rewarming.
D. Afterdrop may exacerbate hypotension in moderate and severe hypothermia.
E. All of the above.

99. A 59-year-old female presents with a chief complaint of an acute headache, dizziness, balance problems,

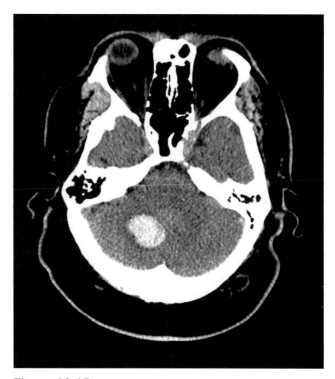

Figure 10-15

and vomiting. A head CT is performed as part of her evaluation and reveals the image shown in Figure 10-15. Which of the following is true?

A. Hydrocephalus rarely occurs as a consequence of this injury

B. She will likely develop left-sided hemiparesis

C. These patients frequently deteriorate and require surgery

D. These patients rarely experience gaze palsies

E. She is likely to have an associated aphasia

100. An 81-year-old female with no reported past medical history except hypertension presents with acute onset of shortness of breath. Her vital signs are: 98.6, 105, 24, 195/92, and 94% on 4 L NC. She has mild respiratory distress and significant wheezing on bilateral lung examination along with peripheral edema. Which of the following is the next best step in management?

A. Albuterol nebulizer therapy

B. Methylprednisolone IV

C. Azithromycin 500 mg IV

D. Labetalol 20 mg IV

E. EKG, chest x-ray, and laboratory studies

TEST 10

ANSWERS AND EXPLANATIONS

1. **Answer A.** This patient has primary adrenal insufficiency. Due to mineralocorticoid deficiency, the most common electrolyte abnormalities are hyponatremia and hyperkalemia. Hypoglycemia due to decreased gluconeogenesis and increased peripheral glucose utilization is also common. The patient's hyperpigmentation is due to increased adrenocorticotropic hormone secretion by the pituitary gland and subsequent stimulation of melanocytes. More than 50% of patients with adrenal insufficiency have intermittent nausea and vomiting and often present with volume depletion.

2. **Answer B.** Alkali causes liquefaction necrosis, which allows the alkali to spread to deeper tissues and cause further necrosis. Acid causes coagulation necrosis, which hardens the tissue and limits spread of the acid to deeper tissues. Chronic exposure to ultraviolet light causes long-term *ocular injury* and eventual blindness but acute symptoms are usually mild. Most commercially available soaps are generally nontoxic and cause only local conjunctival irritation. Cigarette ashes may cause superficial corneal burns, but the duration of exposure is rarely long enough to produce serious injury.

3. **Answer B.** Fortunately for emergency medicine physicians, management of acute asthma exacerbations is consistent across age-groups. The foundation of effective management of acute asthma exacerbations is the concomitant administration of systemic corticosteroids, β-agonists (albuterol), and frequently ipratropium as an adjuvant therapy. Cromolyn sodium has no role in the management of acute asthma exacerbations. It works by inhibiting the release of inflammatory mediators from mast cells through chlorine channel blockade (also known as a *mast cell stabilizing agent*) and is used to prevent inflammation in long-term management. There are limited data that suggest that leukotriene receptor antagonists (e.g., montelukast, zafirlukast) are beneficial in the treatment of patients with acute asthma exacerbations who fail initial β-agonist therapy. Until further studies are done, however, leukotriene modifiers are not currently recommended for acute asthma management.

4. **Answer A.** With shortness of breath, tachycardia, hypoxia, a normal physical examination, and a normal chest x-ray, pulmonary embolism is a very likely diagnosis. Diagnostic evaluation with either a D-dimer or a CT angiogram should be pursued. An argument can be made to do either test, but among the answer choices, D-dimer is the only one present. BNP levels are only helpful in the setting of signs of CHF complicated by possibility of other diagnoses such as COPD. There is no indication for giving piperacillin at this time, given that the patient has no risk factors for nosocomial pathogens. Similarly, without a history of COPD or other obstructive lung disease, neither steroids nor albuterol is indicated.

5. **Answer B.** Botulism is a neurologic syndrome caused by *Clostridium botulinum*, an anaerobic, gram-positive bacillus that produces botulinum toxin. Botulinum toxin is the strongest known biologic toxin, but is heat-labile, and can be inactivated by adequate preparation. Infant botulism, usually spread by honey, is the most common form of botulism, followed by food-borne botulism. Botulinum toxin blocks presynaptic acetylcholine release, causing cranial nerve palsies, parasympathetic inhibition, and descending paralysis. The diagnosis is generally made clinically, with specific toxin assays to aid in confirmation. Management involves aggressive airway evaluation and protection (due to pharyngeal muscle weakness), monitoring of vital capacity and respiratory strength, and equine antitoxin. There is little data regarding the efficacy of antibiotic therapy, and currently antibiotics are not indicated.

6. **Answer E.** Adult trauma patients with head injury are rarely hypotensive because of the intracranial process itself, except in the end stages of herniation or severe scalp injuries. The fixed bony skull limits the degree of hemorrhage in adult patients. In infants, the flexibility and larger proportional size of the skull may allow enough bleeding to cause hypotension. In adult trauma patients, an extracranial cause of hypotension should aggressively be sought, such as bleeding in the chest, abdomen, retroperitoneum, pelvis, or femurs. Treatment of hypotension in the head-injured patient should be undertaken quickly because cerebral blood flow is dependent on mean arterial pressure (MAP) and limited by intracranial pressure (ICP).

7. **Answer C.** Viral and postviral myocarditis are the most common causes of myocarditis. The most common manifestation of acute and chronic myocarditis is dilated cardiomyopathy with a decreased ejection fraction leading to symptoms of CHF. Patients with acute lymphocytic myocarditis can occasionally present with findings that are confused with an acute coronary syndrome. However, the coronary arteries are normal upon subsequent catheterization. While CHF is the most common presentation, patients can present with variable degrees of heart block, pericarditis, syncope, malignant ventricular arrhythmias, or sudden cardiac death.

8. Answer D. The patient has evidence of spinal epidural hematoma. Anticoagulation is a common causative mechanism. The absence of true neurologic weakness or sensory deficits does not exclude the diagnosis, as these signs can lag the pain by days. MRI is the gold standard for diagnosis of spinal epidural processes. Discharging the patient home with oral opioids is not appropriate in patients with back pain in the setting of anticoagulation and early urinary retention. CT myelogram can be pursued if MRI is contraindicated (such as in cases with metallic foreign bodies) but has lower specificity for the diagnosis. CT lumbar spine does not adequately image the spinal canal and is used more for bony disease. CT brain in this case is less useful because of the bilateral lower extremity symptoms and absence of headache.

9. Answer C. The patient has a small whitish patch in the cornea consistent with a corneal ulcer. Management includes topical antibiotics and emergent ophthalmologic consultation. Acute angle closure glaucoma would not be likely in a 32-year-old female without any prior history or in the absence of characteristic ocular findings such as cloudy cornea, fixed and mid-dilated pupil, or loss of vision. Central retinal vessel occlusion is signified more by acute painless loss of vision rather than eye pain and redness. Pterygium is a chronic, benign growth in the conjunctiva of little clinical significance except cosmesis. Pterygia can invade the line of vision and needs to be corrected in those cases. (Figure from Rapuano CJ. *Wills Eye Institute—Cornea.* 2nd ed. Philadelphia, PA: Wolters Kluwer; 2011.)

10. Answer E. Although the patient has clear evidence of brain or spinal injury from blunt trauma, no radiographic evaluation can take place until the patient is cooperative. In cases where patients put themselves or caregivers at risk of physical harm, the trauma team leader's first responsibility is to control the patient's behavior to prevent this occurrence. Sedating the patient with lorazepam or haloperidol is the ideal first-line management, but if this is not an option, sedation and paralysis with rapid-sequence intubation should be performed. This will allow the trauma evaluation to take place expediently and reduce the risk of harm to the patient and caregivers. Once the patient's combative behavior is controlled, CT of the brain and spinal cord, along with the rest of the secondary survey may be initiated.

11. Answer A. The patient has a 100% spontaneous right-sided pneumothorax. Treatment involves supplemental oxygen and tube thoracostomy. Pneumothoraces generally resorb at a rate of 2% per day, and this rate is quadrupled by 100% oxygen. The presence of 100% oxygen causes intra-alveolar nitrogen washout and creates a nitrogen gradient that draws nitrogen-rich room air from the pleural space into the alveolar space. However,

patients with a large pneumothorax require thoracostomy with tubes ranging from 7- to 14-Fr pigtail catheters to 28-Fr tubes. Size 36 Fr tubes are usually reserved for fluid-containing pneumothoraces, such as hemopneumothorax in trauma. Pleurodesis is usually performed in patients who have had multiple pneumothoraces due to a secondary cause. Positive pressure ventilation of any form can only exacerbate the pneumothorax as the positive intra-alveolar pressure will serve to worsen intrapleural air accumulation. Albuterol nebulizer treatment is helpful in bronchospasm but has little benefit in pneumothorax management. (Figure courtesy of Harris JH, Harris WH, eds. *Radiology of Emergency Medicine.* 4th ed. Philadelphia, PA: Lippincott Williams & Wilkins; 1999, with permission.)

12. Answer E. Glipizide is a sulfonylurea with a fairly long half-life (7 hours) and prolonged duration of action (12 to 24 hours). Like other sulfonylureas, the duration of action is increased further when taken in overdose. As a result, patients frequently experience prolonged and severe hypoglycemia after sulfonylurea overdose. While dextrose therapy is a critical part of treatment, its use often results in transient hyperglycemia which further increases insulin secretion causing rebound hypoglycemia. This is particularly true when it is used as a bolus injection. Octreotide works by decreasing calcium influx in pancreatic beta islet cells, which results in decreased calcium-mediated insulin release. Octreotide is continued for 24 hours, after which the patient is observed for a prolonged period for recurrent episodes of hypoglycemia. While glucagon and corticosteroids may increase blood glucose, their use does not affect insulin secretion, in contrast to octreotide. Epinephrine has no role in management.

13. Answer B. Left ventricular assist devices (LVADs) are reserved for patients with end-stage heart failure refractory to conventional treatments. They are typically used as a bridge to transplant but have recently been increasingly used as definitive treatment, so-called "destination therapy." LVADs are continuous flow rather than pulsatile devices so patients most often do not have palpable pulses. As a result, blood pressure measurements with either an automated or manual cuff are unreliable. Instead of conventional blood pressure measures, LVAD patients are managed based on mean arterial pressure (MAP). The goal MAP is typically 60 to 90 and is most easily approximated by listening with a Doppler over the brachial artery as a blood pressure cuff is slowly deflated. The pressure at which the first audible sounds occur is the MAP and is used to guide management. When a patient with an LVAD presents with a depressed level of consciousness, the best approach remains to focus on the ABCs. In the case of circulation, providers should auscultate over the chest wall to listen for the "hum" of the LVAD motor, indicating that it is working. If it is, the MAP can be assessed as above. CPR should be avoided unless there are no signs of life (apneic, MAP of 0) because CPR may dislodge the LVAD cannula resulting in uncontrolled hemorrhage. Ventricular fibrillation and tachycardia are frequent in patients with LVADs and defibrillation is needed to restore normal rhythm, especially since the right ventricle is unassisted and depends on normal conduction to pump normally.

14. **Answer C.** The mitral valve is affected about two-third of the time in rheumatic heart disease, followed by the aortic valve in a quarter of cases and then the tricuspid and pulmonic valves. Rheumatic heart disease is the most common cause of mitral regurgitation in non-Western countries (in Western countries, mitral valve prolapse is the most common cause of mitral regurgitation). The murmur of mitral regurgitation is best heard at the apex of the heart and lasts throughout the systolic phase.

15. **Answer A.** This patient has bacterial vaginosis (BV), which is the most common lower genital tract infection among women of reproductive age. Clue cells, which are squamous vaginal epithelial cells coated with bacteria, are evident on the wet mount. Classically, the disease has been diagnosed when three of the four Amsel criteria are present:

   • An adherent and homogenous vaginal discharge
   • Vaginal pH >4.5
   • Detection of clue cells on saline wet mount
   • An amine odor after the addition of potassium hydroxide (whiff test)

   Though these criteria remain widely used, they have been criticized for their subjectivity. New assays are in development. Though *Gardnerella vaginalis* is present in approximately 95% of cases, BV is a polymicrobial infection with poorly understood origins. Furthermore, although it was originally considered a relatively benign illness, recent research has shown a clear correlation with preterm labor and delivery, preterm premature rupture of membranes, spontaneous abortion, chorioamnionitis, and postpartum infections such as endometritis. Therefore, all symptomatic pregnant and nonpregnant women with BV should be treated. As in nonpregnant women, metronidazole is the treatment of choice (250 mg orally three times daily for 7 days) although clindamycin is an acceptable alternative (300 mg orally twice daily for 7 days). (Figure from Mandell GL, ed. *Essential Atlas of Infectious Diseases.* 2nd ed. Philadelphia, PA: Current Medicine Inc; 2001, with permission.)

16. **Answer C.** The picture indicates small whitish spots on the buccal mucosa consistent with Koplik spots. Koplik spots, though uncommonly seen, are pathognomonic

for measles. They tend to occur just before the onset of the classic measles rash (intensely red, diffuse, and maculopapular), about 3 days after onset of symptoms. Vaccines can prevent the illness. Mumps causes a nonspecific viral syndrome combined with parotid enlargement. Rubella causes a viral syndrome with a rash that is less intensely red than measles. Chickenpox occurs from the varicella zoster virus and causes discrete maculopapular lesions with vesicles. *Haemophilus influenza* is a bacterium that causes a variety of illnesses such as otitis media and meningitis. (Figure from Goodheart H, Gonzalez M, eds. *Goodheart's Photoguide to Common Pediatric and Adult Skin Disorders.* 4th ed. Philadelphia, PA: Wolters Kluwer; 2015.)

17. **Answer E.** Rheumatic fever occurs several weeks after untreated streptococcal pharyngitis. The diagnosis is made by the Jones criteria: either two major (polyarthritis, erythema marginatum, chorea, carditis, subcutaneous nodules) or one major and two minor (arthralgias, fever, increased erythrocyte sedimentation rate or C-reactive protein, prolonged PR interval). Migratory arthritis of major joints is the most common symptom, followed by carditis. Chorea and erythema marginatum are uncommon but fairly specific given a history of antecedent pharyngitis. Despite its name, fever is not common in patients with rheumatic fever.

18. **Answer E.** This case demonstrates the "80% rule" of neck masses. Eighty percent of neck masses in children are benign, 80% of nonthyroid neck masses in adults are neoplastic, and 80% of those are malignant. Therefore, most nonthyroid neck masses in adults are malignant. Referred ear pain and signs of otitis media with effusion increase the likelihood of cancer. Any degree of stridor, dysphagia, or severe hoarseness mandates immediate ENT consultation, as airway obstruction may be imminent.

19. **Answer A.** Digoxin toxicity may result in nearly *any* rhythm disturbance. However, PVCs are the most common and typically represent the earliest rhythm disturbance. The key point is to recall that digoxin toxicity exerts its effects in two ways: Increased vagal tone leads to bradyarrhythmias and AV block, while increased automaticity leads to frequent ectopic rhythms. The hallmark of digoxin toxicity is when these two conditions are combined, as in the often cited paroxysmal atrial tachycardia (PAT) (increased automaticity) with AV block (increased vagal tone). However, sinus bradycardia (increased vagal tone) combined with PVCs (increased automaticity) is much more common. Rapidly conducted atrial dysrhythmias (e.g., atrial fibrillation with rapid ventricular response, or SVT) are not observed because of the high degree of AV block associated with digoxin toxicity. However, since digoxin continues to be used as a

second-line agent in patients with atrial fibrillation, many patients with digoxin toxicity present with atrial fibrillation (which is their baseline rhythm, as opposed to a result of drug toxicity). Other common findings include bradydysrhythmias, junctional tachycardia, and bidirectional ventricular tachycardia which along with PAT with block, are frequently considered pathognomonic. While digoxin toxicity results in AV block, Mobitz type II second-degree AV block is among the least common rhythm disturbances caused by digoxin toxicity.

20. **Answer C.** Due to its anterior position and size, the right ventricle is the most commonly affected cardiac chamber from penetrating thoracic injury. The left ventricle is affected next, followed by both atria equally. Multiple chambers are injured in almost one-third of cases. Death occurs from either exsanguination or pericardial tamponade, the latter of which is treated by ED thoracotomy and pericardial incision.

21. **Answer D.** The "awake seizure" is the hallmark of strychnine poisoning. Strychnine is a glycine antagonist and its use results in disinhibition of glycine-mediated inhibitory tone at the level of the spinal motor neurons. This causes significant unopposed motor neuron activity resulting in distinctive muscle spasms called opisthotonus (arched back with a rigid trunk) as well as a unique facial appearance called risus sardonicus (sardonic smile), which is a tetanic contraction of facial muscles resulting in a persistent grimace or smile. The muscle contractions wax and wane without intervention and may be followed by flaccid periods. Ultimately, a rigid chest wall results in respiratory failure, hypoxia, and death if aggressive supportive care is not initiated (ventilation). There are no antidotes. Benzodiazepines are the class of drugs most often recommended, while barbiturates may be necessary in refractory cases. Super-warfarins are the most common agents used in rodenticides and the most common toxic exposure due to rodent poison overdose. Thallium is a heavy metal that causes hair loss and a painful neuropathy. Arsenic causes severe gastrointestinal symptoms, and patients classically present with breath that smells like garlic. In severe poisonings, the initial symptoms lead to shock, acute respiratory distress syndrome, cardiac irritability, and death. Some rodent poisons contain vitamin D (ergocalciferol) which causes hypercalcemia, but such poisons are rarely significantly toxic in humans.

22. **Answer D.** This patient is presenting with symptoms of a small bowel obstruction (SBO) due to an internal hernia. The mesenteric swirl sign is pathognomonic for an internal hernia although it is often missed or absent. Furthermore, internal hernias often present with vague symptoms without clear obstruction and can be missed by radiology. Therefore, it is imperative to discuss these patients with their surgeons and to maintain a high degree of suspicion in patients with symptoms suggestive of a possible bowel obstruction in the setting of abdominal pain and a past history of laparoscopic roux-en-y gastric bypass. Marginal ulcers and dilation of the gastric remnant are other possible postoperative complications, but gastric dilatation will be clear on CT scan, and neither condition produces the noted swirl sign.

23. **Answer D.** Acute angle closure glaucoma is caused by increased pressure in the anterior chamber due to decreased outflow of aqueous humor. Acetazolamide can increase the excretion of aqueous humor and is indicated as one of the medical therapies, along with pilocarpine, timolol, and antiemetics. Cycloplegics inhibit ciliary muscle contraction (which limits miosis), and are contraindicated in glaucoma, as they further inhibit aqueous humor outflow from the anterior chamber. Aspirin and antivirals play no role in the management of glaucoma. Lateral canthotomy is used to treat retrobulbar hematoma. Definitive therapy for acute angle closure glaucoma is surgical and emergent ophthalmologic consultation is necessary.

24. **Answer C.** The patient is at risk for traumatic aortic injury (TAI), which is a common cause of immediate death in motor vehicle crashes. TAI may result in sudden hemodynamic instability and death in patients who initially appear to be stable after blunt trauma. Lateral- and front-impact motor vehicle crashes at high speed, steering wheel impact to chest, and sudden deceleration injuries each constitutes a high-risk mechanism for TAI. Although a normal chest x-ray has good sensitivity (~90%), patients who have a high-risk mechanism and symptoms consistent with the diagnosis of TAI should undergo CT angiography (negative predictive value of close to 100%). Diagnostic peritoneal lavage is usually indicated in patients who are hemodynamically unstable to evaluate for presence of intraperitoneal injury. Pericardiocentesis is only indicated in patients with pericardial tamponade in whom a pericardial window may not be performed at the bedside. Admission to the hospital could eventually be indicated, but a delay in the diagnosis of TAI could cause immediate death, and observation alone would be unhelpful in prevention of this occurrence. Discharging the patient home without any further workup for either TAI or blunt cardiac injury is contraindicated in a patient with such a high-risk mechanism and suggestive symptoms.

25. **Answer C.** Benign early repolarization (BER) is a common pattern of EKG changes that are not thought to reflect any underlying cardiac disease but which can be confused with cardiac ischemia (see Fig. 10-5). Almost 90% of healthy young men have ST-segment elevation of 1 to 3 mm in at least one precordial lead. BER is more

common among young patients, as well as among men, and African Americans. The pattern of changes seen in BER include ST elevation which is most prominent in the anterior to early lateral precordial leads, i.e., V2–V5, with concave upward morphology of the ST segment (sometimes referred to as the "smiley-face" morphology) and with the amplitude of the ST elevation ≤2 mm in the precordial leads and ≤0.5 mm in the limb leads, symmetric, concordant T waves, notching or slurring of the J point or terminal end of the QRS, and relative stability over time. Identification of the J point is best achieved by looking for the first change in direction as the QRS complex shifts into the ST segment. Isolated ST elevation in the limb leads is rarely benign and should be considered ischemic until proven otherwise.

26. **Answer A.** This patient's pleocytosis with a lymphocytic predominance in concert with a normal glucose and elevated protein level supports the diagnosis of a viral etiology. Herpes simplex encephalitis (HSE) is the most common cause of severe encephalitis in the United States despite the fact that arboviruses such as West Nile virus continue to get significant media coverage. The most common symptoms of HSE are fever, altered mental status, decreased level of consciousness, and focal neurologic findings. Focal seizures may also occur (temporal lobe seizures). Because acyclovir is extremely well tolerated and is very effective for treating HSE, it should be started as soon as the diagnosis of HSE is suspected. Dexamethasone is used as an adjunctive treatment in bacterial meningitis and should be given just before or with the first dose of antibiotics. Amphotericin B is an antifungal agent.

27. **Answer E.** Flexor tenosynovitis is a purulent infection of the flexor tendon sheath that usually results from a penetrating wound of the digital flexor surface. The infection spreads unimpeded throughout the sheath and the patient presents with acute pain and signs of inflammation in the involved digits. Kanavel's four cardinal signs of flexor tenosynovitis include all of the signs listed, although tenderness along the flexor tendon sheath is frequently cited as the most significant of these findings. Although early infections may be treated with intravenous antibiotics directed at *Staphylococcus,* incision and drainage is often required. Due to the limited space in the sheath, purulent infections may cause a rapid increase in compartmental pressure resulting in ischemia to tendons and nerves. A hand specialist should be consulted as soon as the diagnosis is seriously considered.

28. **Answer E.** Technically, priapism is defined as a persistent erection not related to sexual desire. Practically speaking, most studies define it as an erection lasting at least 4 hours. Structural damage can occur as early as 4 to 6 hours and future sexual functional steadily declines the longer priapism persists. Priapism is a compartment syndrome of the two corpora cavernosa within the dorsum of the penis. Sildenafil and other medications cause ischemic priapism (also called vaso-occlusive priapism), the most common subtype, which results because of inadequate venous outflow once the corpora are engorged with blood. High-flow priapism is usually due to arterial–venous fistulas caused by trauma and are uncommon. Aspiration and injection of a sympathomimetic agent is the cornerstone of ischemic priapism treatment. Phenylephrine is the preferred agent because of its favorable side effect profile. After a penile block, at least 5 to 10 mL of blood is aspirated from the corpora cavernosa to decompress the corpora. Irrigation with saline can be used if aspiration is difficult due to blood clotting. Phenylephrine is then injected into the corpora cavernosa and the penis is reassessed frequently. Repeat injections can be given every 3 to 5 minutes for up to an hour to achieve detumescence.

29. **Answer C.** The patient has neutropenic fever. His absolute neutrophil count (ANC) $0.05 \times 1,400 = 70$. Patients with neutropenic fever are at considerable risk for serious bacterial infection and require broad-spectrum antibiotics. These patients are most often admitted to the hospital for observation and bacterial culture monitoring, though carefully selected, low-risk patients may be candidates for outpatient management. However, broad-spectrum antibiotics are always administered. Patients with solid tumors are generally low risk. Patients with hematologic cancers undergoing transplant or induction chemotherapy are high risk, in part because chemotherapy regimens result in longer lasting and more severe neutropenia. While there are many possible drug regimens, inpatients are generally treated with antipseudomonal monotherapy including cefepime, ceftazidime, a carbapenems, or piperacillin–tazobactam. While a fever workup should be performed, lumbar puncture is unnecessary unless the patient complains of a significant headache.

30. **Answer C.** While this patient could have a stress fracture, her presentation is most consistent with shin splints (medial tibial stress syndrome). Like stress fractures, shin splints are due to overuse, and are more common in women than men. While the tibia is the obvious bone involved in shin splints, it is also the most common involved bone in patients with stress fractures (metatarsals are second most common). Radiographs are normal in patients with shin splints, and are most often normal in patients with stress fractures. Subacute radiographs (3 to 4 weeks) of patients with stress fractures are abnormal up to 50% of the time. Bone scan has much higher sensitivity than radiographs, but a much lower specificity. Therefore, MRIs have become the test of choice to differentiate

shin splints from true stress fractures if the diagnosis is unclear. However, advanced imaging is not indicated in the vast majority of cases, as management is rarely affected and the diagnosis is most often clinical. Standard treatment with rest (though patients can continue to run at reduced mileage), ice, and nonsteroidal anti-inflammatory drugs (NSAIDs) results in resolution of almost all cases of shin splints syndrome. Stress fractures require more prolonged rest, participation in nonimpact activities only, and a monitored, more graduated return to running.

31. **Answer C.** In adults, the carotid artery lies approximately 1.5 to 2.5 cm posterolateral to the tonsillar fossa. In pediatric patients, the distance can be as low as 6 mm in small, young children, though it steadily increases with age and weight, up to 2.5 cm. Therefore, aspiration of a PTA in very young children is best performed by an otolaryngologist. In adults, needles used for aspiration should be inserted no more than 1 cm into the abscess cavity in adults. One method to achieve this is to create a "needle guard" by trimming the needle cap such that only 1 cm of the needle itself is exposed beyond the trimmed cap edge. Another is to bend the needle approximately 90 degrees 1 cm from the tip. There are numerous other possibilities. The carotid sheath contains the internal carotid artery, vagus nerve, and internal jugular vein. While all of these structures may be injured during incision and drainage of a PTA, the carotid artery is *usually* the most medial structure and is therefore most at risk. The facial artery, which gives rise to the tonsillar artery, also lies lateral to the tonsil and can be injured. However, the potential consequences of facial artery injury are far less grave than carotid artery injury.

32. **Answer A.** The lesion represents BCC, which classically appears as a pearly white papule with raised borders and telangiectasias over the surface of the lesion. BCC is the most common form of skin cancer and most commonly occurs on the face, with approximately one-third of lesions appearing on the nose alone. However, it also frequently occurs in relatively sun-protected areas such as behind the ears. In contrast, SCC, which also most commonly appears on the head and neck, occurs in areas of maximal sun exposure. (Figure from the Dr. Barankin Dermatology Collection, Philadelphia: Wolters Kluwer, 2016.)

33. **Answer C.** During primary and secondary survey of all victims of violent crime, care must be taken to identify objects that are potentially lethal to caregivers. Handguns are particularly dangerous as they may discharge with only minimal movement during exposure of the patient. Any firearm should preferably not be handled at all—if it is in a potentially dangerous position, it should be placed carefully in a safe location and secured by law enforcement. Care providers should never check to see if the firearm is loaded, fire it, or carry it on their person in case spontaneous discharge occurs. Using the firearm for any reason is obviously contraindicated.

34. **Answer A.** Patients with significant head injury requiring mechanical ventilation and possibly operative care have worse outcomes if exposed to episodes of hypotension, hypercarbia, and hypoxia. Early seizures in the setting of intracranial hemorrhage can cause significant periods of hypercarbia and hypoxia, which may further worsen the ischemic penumbra by increasing intracranial pressure. Seizure prophylaxis in the acute setting does nothing more than to reduce the possibility of early seizures. Delayed seizures and chronic epilepsy are not prevented by acute administration of antiepileptics. The goal of antiepileptic therapy is actually to maintain cerebral perfusion pressure. Reductions in mean arterial pressure will reduce the cerebral perfusion pressure according to the following formula:

$$\text{Cerebral perfusion pressure} = \text{mean arterial pressure} - \text{intracranial pressure}$$

35. **Answer B.** The presence of WBC casts indicates infection from a renal source. Other indices on urinalysis cannot distinguish between upper urinary tract infection (UTI; pyelonephritis) and lower UTI (cystitis or urethritis). Clinically, pyelonephritis usually involves back pain and systemic symptoms of fever, nausea, vomiting, and signs of sepsis. Symptoms of uncomplicated cystitis are generally limited to dysuria, increased urinary frequency, and urgency.

36. **Answer E.** The presence of a patent foramen ovale is probably the most significant risk factor for DCS. In general, the risk of DCS increases with the length and depth of a dive (e.g., violating the no-decompression limits). Other risk factors include increasing age, obesity (nitrogen is lipid soluble), dehydration, fatigue, diving at high altitude, flying soon after diving, performing heavy work while diving, exercise after diving, cold water temperature, and rough seas.

37. **Answer A.** Herpes simplex virus (HSV) type 2 causes most genital herpes infections. Primary HSV infection is almost always more severe than recurrences. Outbreaks can occur with any systemic or local stress. The lesions are usually extremely painful and irritating and should never be drained or unroofed as this will inoculate other sites. The sensitivity and specificity of the Tzanck smear are both <80% and viral culture is the gold standard for diagnosis. Antibiotics should not be used in the absence of clear signs of bacterial superinfection. Treatment of HSV outbreaks is with acyclovir, famciclovir, or valacyclovir. Continuous treatment may be necessary to prevent outbreaks in susceptible individuals.

38. **Answer E.** The only treatments that improve survival with good neurologic outcome in out-of-hospital

cardiac arrest are defibrillation, high-quality chest compressions, and postresuscitation targeted temperature management. Importantly, no medication is able to accomplish this outcome when given on a protocolized basis. Patients with known hyperkalemic cardiac arrests may benefit from emergent calcium and bicarbonate therapy. Epinephrine does improve return of spontaneous circulation in out-of-hospital cardiac arrest, but it has not been shown to improve survival with good neurologic outcome.

39. **Answer D.** CT of the cervical spine is the optimal method of ruling out clinically significant fractures. Plain radiographs have, at best, 85% sensitivity, so high-risk cases should have CT instead. Clinical decision rules such as the NEXUS criteria or the Canadian C-spine rules can be very helpful in avoiding unnecessary spinal imaging. Most cervical spine fractures occur at C2, C6, or C7. Pain medication should never be withheld as localization is not decreased with adequate pain control.

40. **Answer D.** Otitis media is the number one reason for antibiotic prescriptions in the United States, despite the fact that more than 75% of cases will resolve spontaneously without treatment. The 2004 American Academy of Pediatrics (AAP) and American Academy of Family Physicians (AAFP) joint guidelines recommend treatment with antibiotics for patients younger than 2 years old, and consider an observation period for patients older than 2 years old an appropriate management strategy if the patient does not have a high fever and is not systemically ill. A 3-day course of IM ceftriaxone is as effective as a 10-day course of amoxicillin. High-dose amoxicillin is recommended for patients younger than 2 years of age, who are in day care, or those with recent exposure to antibiotics. Auralgan, a mixture of benzocaine and antipyrine, is a local anesthetic that may provide some direct analgesia, but should not be used in patients with tympanic membrane perforation.

41. **Answer B.** The most common causes of death in patients with acute renal failure are volume overload and hyperkalemia. Hyperkalemia can result in fatal dysrhythmias. Treatment involves correction of the renal insufficiency, potassium-binding resin, intravenous calcium for cardioprotection, bicarbonate, and insulin and glucose. Hypocalcemia, not hypercalcemia, occurs with acute renal failure due to decreased levels of activated vitamin D. Hypermagnesemia and hypernatremia may occur in renal failure but are usually clinically inconsequential. Hyperphosphatemia also occurs but is usually adequately managed with correction of the renal failure and calcium antacids to bind excess gastrointestinal phosphate.

42. **Answer B.** Neutropenic fever patients are at considerable risk for serious bacterial infection and require broad-spectrum antibiotics. Either gram-positive (*Streptococcus* or *Staphylococcus* species) or gram-negative (*Pseudomonas, E. coli*, and others) organisms can be responsible for infection. Cefepime monotherapy is an appropriate initial antibiotic choice, covering all organisms except for some strains of methicillin-resistant *Staphylococcus aureus* (MRSA). Vancomycin may be added to any antibiotic regimen to adequately cover MRSA in hospitals with a high incidence of this pathogen. Doxycycline covers some gram-positive organisms and atypicals but does not adequately cover gram negatives. Clindamycin does not cover gram-negative organisms. The combination of metronidazole and either gentamicin or aztreonam leaves out adequate gram-positive coverage.

43. **Answer D.** The patient meets clinical criteria for thrombotic thrombocytopenic purpura (TTP). The classic clinical pentad includes fever, microangiopathic anemia, thrombocytopenia, renal dysfunction, and neurologic symptoms. However, in the modern era, patients are diagnosed earlier in the course of the illness and rarely develop all features of the classic pentad. Hemolytic anemia is the hallmark of the disorder, and when combined with thrombocytopenia and neurologic symptoms is diagnostic for TTP. Pathophysiology involves formation of microthrombi in the systemic vasculature, consuming platelets and causing microinfarctions, usually manifested in the kidneys and brain. Confirmation is made by the presence of schistocytes on peripheral blood smear. Notably, hematologic laboratory studies such as prothrombin time (PT), the activated partial thromboplastin time (aPTT or PTT), and disseminated intravascular coagulation (DIC) panel are almost always normal. Treatment is urgent plasmapheresis with or without corticosteroids. Platelet transfusions are contraindicated, as they exacerbate microthrombi formation. Hemodialysis is not usually required as renal dysfunction is rarely severe. Splenectomy is used as a second-line therapy if plasmapheresis is not successful. Acyclovir may be used for patients with herpes simplex virus encephalitis—although the patient has fever and headache, she lacks altered mental status or meningeal findings as would be seen in encephalomeningitis, and the laboratory findings are more suggestive of TTP.

44. **Answer E.** Tinea versicolor is a fungal infection of the skin caused by *Pityrosporum ovale* (oval form) and *Pityrosporum obiculare* (round form). These organisms were previously called *Malassezia furfur*. Tinea versicolor is a benign and common fungal infection of the skin that most commonly occurs in areas of the skin with increased sebaceous activity. It is most common in the upper trunk but it commonly spreads to the arms, neck, and abdomen. Lesions may be a variety of colors, but are classically hypopigmented white or tan macules and

patches. Griseofulvin is not effective against these fungi, but multiple other agents are effective, including topical ketoconazole, selenium sulfide, and terbinafine as well as oral itraconazole, fluconazole, and ketoconazole. Although such therapy is highly effective, recurrence is common after it is discontinued.

45. **Answer D.** Severe poison ivy requires systemic corticosteroids. Commercially available "dose packs" should be avoided because they provide an inadequate amount and duration of medication. In addition, a prolonged course of prednisone treatment is generally required due to the high chance of rebound dermatitis if prednisone is discontinued abruptly. Therefore, a 14- to 21-day taper generally works best. Not surprisingly, most ED clinicians do not prescribe such a lengthy course of prednisone, perhaps because of their lack of exposure to rebound dermatitis in follow-up.

46. **Answer D.** Patients with moderate traumatic pneumothoraces generally require tube thoracostomy to remove intrapleural air and prevent conversion to a tension pneumothorax. Small pneumothoraces *may* be managed conservatively, with supplemental oxygen and observation, but should be monitored carefully for signs and symptoms of deterioration. Needle thoracostomy is only indicated in patients with tension pneumothorax who are hemodynamically unstable and require immediate decompression. Chest tubes are ideally placed in the fourth or fifth intercostal space at the mid- or anterior axillary lines to minimize cosmetic defects. A large tube (36-French or larger) should be placed in adults with traumatic pneumothoraces in case a hemothorax is also present.

47. **Answer A.** Delayed presentation of neurologic deficits is characteristic of vascular injuries to the neck due to blunt trauma. Only 10% of patients who ultimately develop neurologic deficits due to vascular injury exhibit signs and symptoms of injury within the first hour. Most patients experience stroke symptoms such as hemiparesis, hemiplegia, or aphasia between 1 and 24 hours after injury due to carotid artery dissection or thrombosis. Furthermore, a significant percentage of patients will not develop symptoms until after 24 hours has passed. Vertebral artery injury can also occur, although it is less common. Because the vertebral arteries combine to form a single basilar artery, injuries to the vertebral artery do not produce lateralizing symptoms. Patients may present with nausea, vomiting, central vertigo, and visual changes. Esophageal injuries are relatively uncommon, frequently subtle, and often missed in the setting of neck trauma. Because barium may provoke an inflammatory mediastinitis, patients with suspected esophageal injury should first receive an examination with water-soluble contrast such as gastrografin. If the initial study is negative, a follow-up examination with barium can be performed because of its superior sensitivity for smaller defects. Zone II injuries are most amenable to surgical repair due to the relatively uncomplicated surgical exposure and vascular control. Neck wounds should never be probed outside the operating room. If careful examination fails to determine platysma integrity, a surgeon should be consulted for presumed violation of the platysma. Impaled objects should always be left in place because they may tamponade vascular injuries. They should only be removed in the operating room under direct visualization.

48. **Answer B.** With the combination of atrial fibrillation, inadequate anticoagulant therapy, and acute, diffuse abdominal pain, the patient likely has acute mesenteric ischemia. Diffuse pain out of proportion is characteristic. CT angiography is the diagnostic test of choice. As with most serious causes of abdominal pain in the elderly, WBC count is a poorly sensitive marker for significant disease. An elevated lactate is a sign of advanced ischemia or infarction, but sensitivity for early ischemia is very low. Mortality of acute mesenteric ischemia is around 50% but is considerably higher when infarction has occurred. The most common etiology is thromboembolism (usually from a cardiac etiology), followed by direct arterial thrombosis. Venous thrombosis and low cardiac output each causes around 5% of cases.

49. **Answer D.** Hemodynamically unstable patients with evidence of intra-abdominal hemorrhage should be taken to the operating room (OR) for emergent laparotomy, even in the setting of a pelvic fracture. In an unstable patient with a pelvic fracture, a positive FAST scan is suggestive of intraperitoneal hemorrhage and organ injury and is an indication for emergent laparotomy. If the FAST scan is negative, pelvic angiography and stabilization is indicated. In all patients with suspected hemorrhage from pelvic trauma, temporizing and definitive measures to stabilize pelvic bleeding (angiography, external compression with a bedsheet or fixators) should be undertaken as soon as possible. If the patient achieves stability, a CAT scan could be performed to better define the patient's injuries before further interventions.

50. **Answer C.** The patient has nausea, vomiting, elevated anion gap, ketosis, and normal glucose in the setting of excessive alcohol use with starvation. Alcoholic ketoacidosis (AKA) is the most likely cause. Treatment of AKA is with fluid resuscitation, glucose, and thiamine. Bicarbonate is not indicated in most patients with high anion gap metabolic acidosis except in severe, life-threatening cases. Insulin is indicated in patients with DKA, who rarely present with a normal glucose level. Since alcoholic patients have adequate pancreatic endocrine function, glucose administration induces endogenous insulin release which quickly results in glucose utilization and closure of the anion gap (as the stimulus

for ketogenesis is removed). Alcoholics are frequently thiamine-deficient because of poor nutrition, and thiamine is used during glucose metabolism, so supplementation should be given concurrently or before glucose administration. Potassium repletion may be indicated if hypokalemia is present or expected during the course of therapy. Magnesium supplementation is often indicated in chronic alcoholic patients, but glucose therapy is of more importance as an energy substrate in patients with alcohol ketoacidosis.

51. **Answer E.** Tranexamic acid is an antifibrinolytic lysine analog that acts as a procoagulant by inhibiting plasminogen activation through competitive inhibition at lysine-binding sites. It can be used as a 5% mouthwash or it can be used to saturate gauze which is then stuffed into the affected dental socket. Cocaine and thrombin are also used to soak gauze or cotton tips which are then used to apply pressure directly to the socket. Gelfoam is a hydrocolloid made from hydrolysis of collagen that has procoagulant effects and is also used in gauze form to pack the affected socket. While thrombin or cocaine or other topical agents could be used as a spray, actively bleeding wounds will wash away the topical agent as soon as it's applied which limits its effectiveness.

52. **Answer A.** Methanol is metabolized to formaldehyde by alcohol dehydrogenase, and formaldehyde is converted to formic acid by aldehyde dehydrogenase. Formic acid accumulates preferentially in the ocular tissues and the brain, most commonly the basal ganglia. Long-term morbidity of methanol overdose includes blindness and a parkinsonian syndrome, with bradykinesia and rigidity. Treatment of methanol and ethylene glycol overdoses involves correction of the metabolic acidosis with sodium bicarbonate, inhibition of alcohol dehydrogenase with fomepizole or ethanol, and dialysis of the toxic alcohol.

53. **Answer C.** Choice C is also known as *MDMA* or *ecstasy*. It is in a newly assigned class of drugs known as *entactogens*. These drugs have properties of both hallucinogens and amphetamines, causing mild hallucinations, increased interpersonal emotions, and stimulatory neurotransmitter release. Ecstasy is commonly ingested at raves and other dance parties. Pathophysiology includes sympathomimetic effects, hyperthermia, and hyponatremia (both from a central antidiuretic hormone like effect and increased thirst, causing water consumption). Choice A is LSD, which is not as commonly used currently as it was in the 1960s to 1980s. Choice B is PCP, causing an unpleasant psychosis and violence. Choice D is a selective serotonin reuptake inhibitor, and choice E is a monoamine oxidase inhibitor, neither of which is used recreationally.

54. **Answer A.** The patient likely has pulmonary anthrax due to the gram-positive organism *Bacillus anthracis*. Anthrax is a CDC Category A agent of bioterrorism, with the highest risk of weaponization and transmission. Pulmonary anthrax is caused by the inhalation of anthrax spores, which causes a pneumonia-like picture a week after exposure. Hemorrhagic mediastinitis is the characteristic radiographic manifestation, though CT scan should be ordered if initial chest x-ray is negative. First-line therapy is with ciprofloxacin and second-line is with doxycycline. Aztreonam and tobramycin both cover gram-negative bacteria with minimal gram-positive coverage and should not be used. Anthrax has demonstrated intermediate resistance to ceftriaxone. Corticosteroids such as methylprednisolone are not routinely indicated in the treatment of anthrax. Anthrax spores should be disinfected with bleach solution, as ordinary alcohol solutions have no effect. (Figure courtesy of Harris JH, Harris WH. *Radiology of Emergency Medicine.* 4th ed. Philadelphia, PA: Lippincott Williams & Wilkins; 1999, with permission.)

55. **Answer A.** Although the patient has a history of rheumatoid arthritis, which may be responsible for the symptoms, it is crucial to exclude septic arthritis by aspiration of the joint and synovial fluid analysis. Rheumatoid arthritis, like any process that causes joint destruction, predisposes patients to developing septic arthritis. MRI is not useful in the acute setting and will unnecessarily delay appropriate management. Colchicine and indomethacin are used for acute gouty flares and without a clear diagnosis of crystals in the synovial fluid, neither is indicated. Stress-dose steroids may be reasonable in this patient, but should not precede evaluation for a septic joint.

56. **Answer C.** The patient has evidence of bacterial vaginosis, a bacterial overgrowth process due to polymicrobial infection with *Gardnerella*, *Mycoplasma*, and anaerobes. Clue cells refer to vaginal squamous epithelial cells lined with bacteria. The sniff test (fishy odor of the discharge with addition of potassium hydroxide) may also be positive in bacterial vaginosis. Treatment with an antibiotic to cover anaerobic bacteria must be instituted for at least 1 week, unlike in cases of *Trichomonas* vaginitis, in which one-time therapy with a 2-g dose of metronidazole is adequate. First-line therapy for bacterial vaginosis is with metronidazole 500 mg b.i.d. for 7 days, but clindamycin is an acceptable alternative. The single, 2-g dose of metronidazole is not efficacious and not recommended. Furthermore, the patient's report of a rash after being treated for a similar problem raises the possibility of an allergy to metronidazole, so it should be avoided, even if the prior rash only appeared after several doses. Fluconazole is used to treat candidal vaginitis. Ceftriaxone is used to treat gonorrheal infections. Azithromycin

is used to treat chlamydial infections and a number of other sexually transmitted diseases.

57. **Answer D.** The EKG demonstrates no specific findings consistent with acute myocardial ischemia or infarction. Cocaine-induced myocardial ischemia is due to both vasospasm and hyperaggregatory platelets, which may cause acute thrombosis. Aspirin is indicated in patients with cocaine-induced chest pain until it is known for certain that MI or ischemia is not present. In a patient without current symptoms of chest pain, nitroglycerin and morphine are not indicated. Metoprolol is relatively contraindicated in cocaine-induced chest pain as there is a theoretic risk of reducing cardiac output in the face of increased peripheral vascular resistance. tPA is not emergently indicated in a patient with chest pain without ST-elevation myocardial infarction (STEMI).

58. **Answer B.** The HELLP syndrome is a severe manifestation of preeclampsia characterized by *h*emolysis, *e*levated *l*iver enzymes, and *l*ow *p*latelets. However, liver function tests are abnormal in 20% to 30% of patients overall and is not limited to patients with HELLP syndrome. AFLP is an exceedingly rare disorder (at least 10 times less common than HELLP syndrome) that occurs during the third trimester. It is heralded by the presence of nausea and vomiting in the third trimester with associated epigastric pain and liver dysfunction. In contrast to the HELLP syndrome, coagulation abnormalities, including elevated PT, are present early in the disease course. Hepatitis is the most common cause of liver disease in pregnancy. As in nonpregnant women, however, most patients experience a subclinical illness and do not report any symptoms. Symptomatic patients present with jaundice or scleral icterus, nausea and vomiting, and right upper quadrant tenderness with aminotransferase levels in the thousands. The course in pregnant and nonpregnant women is typically benign and indistinguishable from one another. Cholecystitis is the second most common surgical emergency during pregnancy, and patients typically present with fever, right upper quadrant pain, nausea and vomiting, and leukocytosis (although this can be confused with the leukocytosis of pregnancy). ICP is, like AFLP, a rare disorder that typically complicates the third trimester. Patients present with moderate to severe pruritus that typically begins on the palms and soles and progresses in an ascending manner. Approximately 20% of patients will also be jaundiced on presentation. ICP is associated with increased preterm delivery, increased perinatal mortality, and meconium staining. Fetal mortality approaches 20% in untreated patients. The optimal treatment for preeclampsia, AFLP, and ICP is delivery.

59. **Answer E.** Hypertrophic cardiomyopathy is usually a familial condition, which causes increased left ventricular and septal wall size and resultant diastolic dysfunction. Left ventricular hypertrophy can eventually lead to outflow obstruction. Clinical clues include exertional syncope or chest pain in young patients with a systolic murmur at the left lower sternal border. Any agents which increase systemic afterload (phenylephrine) or cardiac contractility (digitalis, isoproterenol) or decrease preload (furosemide) are contraindicated in patients with hypertrophic cardiomyopathy.

60. **Answer C.** Acutely thrombosed hemorrhoids should be excised within the first 48 hours. Although excision provides rapid relief from pain, the natural history of thrombosed hemorrhoids is spontaneous resolution after several days. Therefore, patients with only mild pain from thrombosis and patients who have already dealt with symptoms for several days should be managed conservatively. Excision in these patients will not provide any added relief.

61. **Answer E.** Simple cutaneous abscesses in patients with immune-compromise can be managed with incision and drainage alone. There is no proven benefit of irrigation, steroids, antibiotics, or packing in these patients. Steroids may, in fact, retard wound healing. NSAID therapy is reasonable pain control for these patients, but many may require opiate pain medications. Antibiotics are indicated in patients with signs of cellulitis. In many communities, methicillin-resistant *Staphylococcus aureus* must be covered by the antibiotics selected—cephalexin alone is not adequate for these patients.

62. **Answer E.** The strips demonstrate "late decelerations" of the fetal heart rate relative to uterine contractile activity. Late decelerations typically begin roughly 30 seconds after the onset of a uterine contraction and their nadir occurs after the peak of the contraction. This most often represents uteroplacental insufficiency, which is an interruption in uteroplacental blood flow. Early decelerations have the same gradual slope and shape as late decelerations, but they occur with different timing relative to uterine contractions. The nadir of early decelerations and the peak of uterine contractions occur simultaneously and the fetal heart rate returns to baseline by the end of the contraction. Early decelerations are thought to result from compression of the fetal head, which causes a vagal reflex. Variable decelerations are the most common type of pattern seen during fetal cardiac monitoring. These decelerations have an inconsistent appearance with respect to shape, width, depth, and timing relative to uterine contractions. They represent umbilical cord compression and are typically benign. However, frequent or particularly deep decelerations (i.e., representing fetal bradycardia) may be an indicator of fetal distress. (Figure reprinted with permission from Pilliterri A. *Maternal and Child Health Nursing.* Philadelphia, PA: Lippincott Williams & Wilkins; 2006.)

63. **Answer A.** Given his lack of risk factors or EKG abnormalities, the patient is at extremely low risk for acute coronary syndrome. He is far more likely to have a gastrointestinal, pulmonary, or idiopathic etiology for his chest pain. It is reasonable to discharge this patient home and have him follow up with his primary care physician at this time. Giving this patient full-dose aspirin therapy for presumed acute coronary syndrome would be more likely to result in aspirin-related side effects than any potential benefit from thrombus prevention or treatment. Enoxaparin would be reasonable in patient where pulmonary embolism was a likely diagnosis—in this case, there is nothing from the history or physical examination to suggest pulmonary embolism. Admission to the hospital for this extremely low risk patient is more likely to result in nosocomial complications than any benefit to the patient's health. IV tPA poses a far greater risk of hemorrhage than any benefit to this patient who lacks any diagnostic criteria for myocardial infarction or pulmonary embolism.

64. **Answer C.** The ACL is the most commonly injured ligament in the knee which requires surgery. Diagnosis is often made on history, with acute knee swelling and audible "pop" after twisting or lateral force to the knee. Lachman test is the most sensitive acute physical examination test to evaluate for an ACL tear in the acute setting. It involves placing the knee in 20 to 30 degrees flexion and pulling anteriorly on the leg while holding the distal thigh stable and observing for laxity relative to the contralateral knee. The anterior drawer test is another test for the ACL which is not nearly as sensitive as the Lachman, especially acutely. It is important for the emergency physician (EP) to remember that the Lachman is not 100% sensitive in the acute setting due to limited range of motion from joint effusion. The posterior drawer test is used to assess the posterior cruciate ligament (PCL), which is rarely injured. The McMurray test assesses the medial meniscus. The Thompson test checks for integrity of the Achilles tendon.

65. **Answer D.** The EKG demonstrates deeply inverted T waves in the anterior leads, which is specific for the LAD distribution. When associated with unstable angina, these T waves indicate stenosis of the proximal LAD, called the *Wellens syndrome*. Electrocardiographic findings of pericarditis include concave ST elevation, sinus tachycardia, and PR depression. Sinus tachycardia and right axis deviation are common EKG findings in patients with pulmonary artery embolism. Lateral (I, L, V5, V6) and posterior (V1, V2) abnormalities are often seen in left circumflex lesions. Right-sided coronary artery disease (CAD) may cause an inferior MI (II, III, aVF) or posterior MI (V1, V2).

66. **Answer E.** Black widow spider bites are characterized by an initial pinprick sensation followed by a mild local inflammatory response. However, within 1 hour, crampy myalgias develop at the bite site and spread up the extremity, eventually involving the entire body. Classically, myalgias are most intense in the chest and abdomen and patients may present with a rigid abdomen that is impossible to differentiate clinically from peritonitis. Patients also frequently have associated hypertension, diaphoresis, nausea, vomiting, headache, dizziness, and weakness. Symptoms typically begin to abate within a few hours with only supportive care. Due to their small size, however, children may suffer from complete cardiovascular collapse with the same degree of envenomation.

67. **Answer A.** Roseola infantum, also known as *exanthem subitum* (*sudden rash*), or sixth disease, is caused by human herpes virus 6. Patients develop a sudden-onset high fever from 103°F to 106°F with hardly any associated symptoms. Owing to the rapid rise in temperature and high fever, however, febrile seizures may occur. The fever lasts for 3 to 4 days and then abruptly subsides, at which point the rash begins. The term *exanthem subitum* or *sudden rash* refers to the startling development of a rash just when the patient appears to be recovering. The rash, as with the illness in general, is benign and self-limited. No treatment is necessary. Rubeola (measles) is characterized by the finding of Koplik spots on the buccal mucosa. The hallmark of rubella is generalized lymphadenopathy. Erythema infectiosum is distinguished by its "slapped cheek" appearance. Scarlet fever is caused by group A *streptococci* and is characterized by its sandpaper rash.

68. **Answer B.** The history of normal-appearing skin with intense pruritus gives eczema the moniker, "the itch that rashes." Patients often complain of significant pruritus with minimal findings. Once they scratch the area, the characteristic maculopapular lesion with scales will appear. Treatment includes topical steroids, which must be of sufficient potency to reduce the inflammation—often over-the-counter 1% hydrocortisone cream is not enough to manage these outbreaks. Prevention with adequate skin moisturization is essential. Group A streptococcal skin infection will cause a cellulitis-like picture, with definite erythema, warmth, tenderness, and generally lacking in scales. An example of Group A streptococcal infection is erysipelas, which is a sharply demarcated, bright red area of skin. Toxic epidermal necrolysis involves significant areas of skin exfoliation along with evidence of dehydration and possibly multiorgan dysfunction. Toxic shock syndrome occurs with the classic "sunburn" rash in a patient with hypotension and multiorgan failure. (Figure courtesy of Robert Hendrickson, MD. In: Greenberg MI, Hendrickson RG, Silverberg M, et al., eds. *Greenberg's Text-Atlas of Emergency Medicine.* Philadelphia, PA: Lippincott Williams & Wilkins; 2004:151, with permission.)

69. **Answer B.** A regular, narrow-complex tachycardia at a rate of close to 200 without P waves is likely due to paroxysmal arteriovenous nodal reentrant tachycardia (AVNRT). The initial treatment for a hemodynamically stable patient with AVNRT is adenosine, which is safe to use in pregnancy. Digoxin, amiodarone, and procainamide are not indicated as first-line therapy for AVNRT. Lidocaine is not indicated for any narrow-complex tachycardias.

70. **Answer B.** The patient has toxic epidermal necrolysis (TEN), which is a vesiculobullous disease that is characterized by diffuse epidermal detachment. It is part of a continuum with Stevens–Johnson syndrome (SJS) and is diagnosed when the degree of epidermal detachment exceeds 30% of the body surface area (whereas SJS is diagnosed when epidermal detachment is <10%). Drug exposure, particularly to sulfonamides, and to a lesser degree, anticonvulsants, is the most common cause of SJS and TEN. A recent urinary tract infection implies that this patient had been taking trimethoprim/sulfamethoxazole or possibly nitrofurantoin when she developed TEN. When normal-appearing skin sloughs or develops ulceration in response to gentle pressure, patients are described as having a positive Nikolsky sign. (Figure from Mulholland MW, Maier RV et al. *Greenfield's Surgery Scientific Principles and Practice*. 4th ed. Philadelphia, PA: Lippincott Williams & Wilkins; 2006; reproduced with permission.)

71. **Answer A.** While hyperkalemia is very common in the setting of digoxin overdose, it is not a cause of digoxin toxicity but rather a manifestation of toxicity. Furthermore, the specific treatment of hyperkalemia in this setting has not been shown to reduce mortality. However, since hyperkalemia is a sign of significant toxicity in the setting of digoxin overdose, its presence is a well-defined indication for digoxin Fab administration (Digibind). Digoxin-specific Fab administration should be given to all patients with a potassium level >5.0 mEq/L. Hyperkalemia will resolve with Fab administration itself. Additional therapy with "conventional" therapies for hyperkalemia is not necessary, and may precipitate hypokalemia once Fab is given. In addition, calcium administration is a "classic" contraindication in the setting of digoxin toxicity because of the risk of "stone heart" or sudden cardiac arrest.

72. **Answer A.** The standard serum digoxin assay measures levels of all digoxin in the body, including drug bound to Fab fragments. It is not useful to measure digoxin levels once Fab has been given. Precedence should be given to dialysis to remove the drug–Fab complexes. Cardioversion may be performed in unstable patients but is unlikely to be curative in patients with digitalis toxicity. Procainamide should be avoided in patients with digitalis toxicity as it may exacerbate dysrhythmias. Calcium chloride should be avoided in patients with digitalis toxicity to prevent theoretical risk of "stone heart," which

occurs from massive calcium influx into cardiac myocytes causing sustained contraction. Potassium chloride should be given with extreme caution in patients with digitalis toxicity, as hyperkalemia is life threatening in this setting.

73. **Answer D.** The patient's CT scan reveals a large "saddle" embolus in both branches of the pulmonary artery. Fortunately, the patient's vital signs indicate relative hemodynamic stability. tPA and surgical or catheter-based embolectomy are reserved for patients with hemodynamic instability who may not respond well to conservative therapy with intravenous anticoagulants. Echocardiograms are often performed to determine the extent of right heart strain as a proxy for the extent of clot. However, this patient's clot burden is easily visible and known to be significant. The prognostic value of right heart strain in this patient is not clear. Despite his significant clot burden, the patient's vital signs have been stable in his brief stay in the emergency department and there is no evidence of hemodynamic compromise. As catheter-based embolectomy techniques improve and more data are gathered, the balance may shift to a more interventional approach.

74. **Answer A.** Rocky Mountain spotted fever (RMSF), caused by *Rickettsia rickettsii* transmitted by the *Dermacentor* tick, is responsible for the most tick-related deaths in the United States. Despite its name, cases are seen most commonly in the southeastern states, but nearly all states have reported cases. The characteristic symptoms are fever, constitutional symptoms, abdominal pain, and a centripetal rash (spreading from extremities to trunk). Antibiotic therapy (specifically with doxycycline) has steadily improved the mortality to about 1%. Doxycycline can even be given to children for optimal treatment of RMSF, as no other antibiotic improves outcomes as well. The other tick-borne diseases mentioned are rarely associated with high mortality and are not as common as RMSF.

75. **Answer C.** The patient has binocular diplopia, which resolves when either eye is covered. Causes include all the answer choices, of which choice C (cranial nerve palsy) is the most common. Monocular diplopia occurs in a specific eye and is usually caused by localized eye pathology.

76. **Answer A.** Interestingly, patients with amaurosis fugax are considered low risk because treatment with antiplatelet agents (e.g., aspirin) is twice as effective in preventing strokes versus patients with hemispheric ischemia. High-risk patients include any patient with new-onset atrial fibrillation or flutter (potential cardioembolic source), patients with crescendo TIA (more than three discrete ischemic episodes within a 72-hour period), patients

who develop a TIA while already on aspirin therapy (considered aspirin failure), and any patient meeting several of the "Johnston" criteria. Johnston et al. studied an ED patient population who had ischemic symptoms for an average of 3.5 hours, which is longer than the typical TIA and longer than the newly revised definition of TIA. However, he found five risk factors (age older than 60 years, diabetes mellitus, duration >10 minutes, weakness with episode, speech impairment with episode) that correlated to the risk of stroke within 90 days of ED discharge. The risk ranged from 0% without any of the risk factors to 34% with all five risk factors. These criteria have yet to be prospectively validated.

77. **Answer B.** Alcohol withdrawal occurs as early as 6 hours after cessation of alcohol consumption and generally peaks after 2 to 3 days of abstinence. Signs and symptoms are similar to a sympathomimetic toxidrome—hyperthermia, tachycardia, hypertension, tremor, anxiety, hallucinations, and seizures. Particularly severe cases are often referred to as *delirium tremens*, which may be life threatening. Management of alcohol withdrawal involves aggressive supportive care with fluids, vitamin and electrolyte supplementation, and benzodiazepine therapy. Diazepam and chlordiazepoxide are preferable because their long half-life is thought to yield a smoother withdrawal with a lower risk of recurrent withdrawal after benzodiazepines are discontinued as well as a lower risk of seizures. However, chlordiazepoxide's long half-life is further prolonged by renal failure so this patient is better served by lorazepam which has a shorter half-life and fewer metabolites. Haloperidol and droperidol are two drugs of the butyrophenone class which are used as adjunctive therapy to manage agitation, but they have no effect in preventing seizures. Chlordiazepoxide is a benzodiazepine that may be used to treat alcohol withdrawal but has a very prolonged half-life in patients with renal insufficiency. Diphenhydramine, an antihistamine and anticholinergic agent, has no role in the management of alcohol withdrawal.

78. **Answer E.** Patients receiving angiotensin-converting enzyme (ACE) inhibitors are at risk for developing angioedema, which is a nonpitting, symmetric edema that typically involves the face, tongue, and supraglottic tissues. Most patients present with lip and tongue swelling and do not have either urticaria or pruritus. The response is most common within the first week of therapy but can occur months or years after starting the drug. It is not safe for patients developing angioedema due to ACEI therapy to take ARBs. ARBs are used when patients can't tolerate the side effects, such as cough, due to ACEI therapy. Finally, patients with angioedema due to ACEI therapy may be resistant to all first-line agents for anaphylaxis including epinephrine, corticosteroids, and antihistamines. Symptoms typically resolve within

24 to 48 hours of discontinuation of the drug, but elective intubation should be performed early in the course if there is any sign of respiratory compromise. Typical "rescue" airways may fail in angioedema due to edema of the glottic structures. Therefore, ENT and anesthesia should be involved in the case, and intubations without the use of paralytics should be considered.

79. **Answer C.** Most authors have abandoned the old terminology of HHNC in favor of HHS. HHS reflects the fact that <20% of these patients present in a coma. HHS is the result of an unremitting osmotic diuresis due to hyperglycemia and is characterized by extreme hyperglycemia (mean glucose is >1,000), hyperosmolarity (at least >320 mOsm/L), and dehydration (average fluid deficit is roughly 10 L). Although a minor ketosis may be present, it is never significant. Infections such as pneumonia or urosepsis are the most common precipitants, accounting for 60% of cases. The mortality rate, which hovers at approximately 15%, is significantly higher than in patients with DKA. The degree of mental status change correlates with the serum osmolarity rather than the degree of hyperglycemia. Insulin is a second-line agent in HHS. It should never be given without prior intravenous fluid administration because insulin delivery will encourage glucose utilization and entry into cells resulting in an acute drop in intravascular fluid volume and possible circulatory collapse.

80. **Answer D.** The patient has clinical evidence of acute cholecystitis. While the large majority of cholecystitis is due to gallstones, acalculous cholecystitis can occur in about 10% of cases. The elderly and immune-compromised are at risk. Patients with acalculous cholecystitis are at higher risk of complications such as gangrene and perforation and require aggressive antibiotic management and early surgical consultation. Computed tomography is not indicated in the evaluation of acute cholecystitis, except in cases of cholangitis, which would be suspected with hyperbilirubinemia. Patients with acute acalculous cholecystitis should never be discharged home.

81. **Answer E.** The patient has asymptomatic hypertension, which should not immediately be treated with intravenous antihypertensives. Instead, a period of observation followed by a blood pressure recheck should be pursued. If blood pressure is still elevated at that time, it is reasonable to restart her on her oral medications while avoiding complete normalization of her blood pressure in the ED. Given her chronic hypertension, her cerebral autoregulation zone for optimal cerebral blood flow is likely higher than in a normotensive individual, and rapidly reducing her blood pressure to 120/70 could cause severe hypoperfusion of the brain. Sublingual nitroglycerin is not an appropriate therapy for

asymptomatic hypertension and should be reserved for reduction in preload in acute heart failure exacerbation and pain control in acute myocardial infarction.

82. **Answer C.** The causes of painless hematuria vary by age and gender. The most common cause in children is glomerulonephritis, in young adults and older women, UTI, and in older men, bladder cancer. Renal carcinoma is a less common cause of painless hematuria in all age-groups. Nephrotic syndrome causes proteinuria without frank hematuria. The combination of urinalysis and appropriate imaging studies (such as helical CT scan) yields the diagnosis in most cases.

83. **Answer C.** Altered mental status, oculomotor dysfunction, and ataxia comprise the clinical trial of Wernicke encephalopathy. Alcoholics develop this emergent condition partly due to thiamine deficiency and supplementation remains the mainstay of management. Wernicke encephalopathy may deteriorate into Wernicke–Korsakoff syndrome, which adds the elements of memory disturbance and confabulation. Magnesium therapy, glucose, and intravenous fluids are important adjunctive therapies for these disorders. Lorazepam is used to treat alcohol withdrawal seizures but has no role in the management of Wernicke encephalopathy. Haloperidol may be used to treat agitation and psychosis in alcohol withdrawal. Pyridoxine therapy may be used as part of a multivitamin that contains thiamine, but it is not essential to treat Wernicke encephalopathy. Potassium repletion may be indicated if hypokalemia is present or expected during the course of therapy.

84. **Answer E.** Babesiosis is a tick-borne protozoan illness that results in hemolytic anemia (after infection, it "lives" inside red blood cells). Clinical infection ranges from mild to severe. Most patients will have a subacute illness consisting of vague constitutional symptoms such as fever, general malaise, and cough, as well as weight loss and night sweats. Immunocompromised patients are at highest risk of severe infection, particularly asplenic patients. Diagnosis is made by pathologist examination of a thin blood smear (like malaria). A combination of atovaquone and azithromycin is the recommended treatment.

85. **Answer E.** Osteomyelitis is a bacterial infection of the bone that generally follows a subacute course. The most common cause is S. *aureus*, but streptococci and gram-negative bacilli are also implicated. Patients usually complain of pain in the affected bone, but do not appear toxic and often lack vital sign abnormalities. The sensitivity of ESR is approximately 90%, and the sensitivity of C-reactive protein may be even higher. Radiographs, although commonly used to evaluate osteomyelitis, have notoriously poor sensitivity in the first week after the onset of symptoms. Bone scintigraphy and MRI are the tests of choice in diagnosing osteomyelitis. MRI is superior to CT scan in characterizing the infection.

86. **Answer E.** Reactive arthritis is the name which is now given to arthritis, urethritis, and conjunctivitis that occurs after an infection (thus, "reactive") and which was formerly called Reiter syndrome. It is a reactive arthritis that occurs following C. *trachomatis* infection of the genitourinary tract or *Shigella, Salmonella, Campylobacter,* or *Yersinia* infection of the gastrointestinal (GI) tract. It is part of a group of arthritides known as the *seronegative spondyloarthropathies.* This group includes ankylosing spondylitis, psoriatic arthritis, reactive arthritis, and the arthropathy of inflammatory bowel disease. They are grouped because of their common involvement of the sacroiliac joint, lack of rheumatoid factor, and presence of the HLA-B27 genetic marker. Reiter syndrome is most common in young men aged 15 to 35 and occurs 2 to 6 weeks after an episode of urethritis or dysentery. The classic triad is arthritis, urethritis, and conjunctivitis. The arthropathy in reactive arthritis is an enthesopathy, which refers to pathology at the site of ligament or tendon insertion to bone. It most commonly involves the lower extremities, particularly the Achilles tendon ("lover's heel").

87. **Answer B.** Ninety percent of anal fissures are located in the posterior midline. The remaining 10% are located in the anterior midline. Fissures located elsewhere should prompt consideration of an underlying disease, such as Crohn disease, leukemia, HIV infection, tuberculosis, or syphilis.

88. **Answer D.** Scheduled acetaminophen is the safest and most effective pain management regimen in the older adult. Scheduled therapy is preferable to as needed therapy because older adults tend to limit use of pain medications unnecessarily when prn prescriptions are written. In addition to age-related decreases in creatinine clearance, NSAID therapy carries a high risk of renal injury as well as atrial fibrillation and cardiovascular ischemia. While opiate therapy is reasonable in specific cases, low-dose hydrocodone is preferred to oxycodone and always should be prescribed with concomitant stool softeners (especially in this chronically constipated patient).

89. **Answer B.** The triptans are serotonin 5-HT$_{1B/1D}$ receptor agonists. Triptans are well tolerated though they have a number of irritating side effects, which include tingling, paresthesias, and sensations of warmth in the head, neck, chest, and limbs. Flushing, dizziness, and neck pain or stiffness occur less frequently. However, their use is limited because more frequent use results in rebound headache. In fact, this may occur with other abortive drugs, particularly butalbital. Triptans can cause

coronary artery constriction and may cause chest symptoms, which mimics angina pectoris. Although these symptoms may be frightening, they are rarely life threatening. However, there have been a few case reports of significant myocardial ischemia or infarction in patients using triptans. Therefore, the use of triptans should be considered contraindicated in the setting of ischemic heart disease, poorly controlled hypertension, and cerebrovascular disease.

90. **Answer D.** High-energy explosives, such as TNT, C-4, dynamite, nitroglycerin, and ammonium nitrate, produce supersonic overpressurization shock waves. However, the pressure and velocity within these waves rapidly decays with distance and time. As a result, injuries due to pressure from the primary blast wave are relatively uncommon as those who are close enough to be injured by the primary blast wave often suffer catastrophic secondary injuries (penetrating trauma due to shrapnel or blunt trauma due to being struck by debris or due to being thrown against solid objects). Blast lung injury is the most common fatal injury among initial survivors. Chest x-ray reveals a classic "batwing" or "butterfly" appearance. Air embolism, due to the creation of microscopic alveolovenous fistulas, may also occur. Historically, the integrity of the TMs has been used as a surrogate marker for more serious internal injury. While the pressure required to induce TM rupture is much less than what is required to affect the lungs, brain, or gastrointestinal system, it is a very unreliable marker of more serious injury since several factors affect the likelihood of TM rupture including orientation to the blast wave (perpendicular is worse than parallel) and presence of occlusive cerumen in the ear canal (protective unless directly adjacent to the TM). However, the presence of TM rupture and oropharyngeal petechiae should indicate a higher likelihood of more serious underlying trauma. Due to blast wave physics, air-containing organs such as the ears, lungs, and intestines are more commonly affected than solid organs.

91. **Answer C.** The rash depicted is erythema chronicum migrans, a sign of early Lyme disease. A nonspecific viral syndrome accompanies this about a week after a tick bite carrying the spirochete *B. burgdorferi*. First-line treatment for Lyme disease is doxycycline; amoxicillin is the second-line treatment. Acyclovir would not be appropriate here given the nonviral etiologic agent. Azithromycin can be used to treat Lyme disease, but is the third-line agent, because it is not as effective as either doxycycline or amoxicillin. Amoxicillin–clavulanic acid would be unnecessarily broad therapy for Lyme disease. Supportive care is not appropriate in the early stage of the illness. (Figure from Kline AM, Haut C, eds. *Lippincott Certification Review: Pediatric Acute Care Nurse Practitioner.* Philadelphia, PA: Wolters Kluwer; 2015.)

92. **Answer C.** The patient likely has type II decompression sickness (DCS). DCS occurs when nitrogen bubbles present in the tissues at high pressures underwater expand to form larger bubbles at the lower pressure of sea level when ascending. Type I DCS is also known as the bends and manifests as severe arthralgias and pruritus. Type II DCS is more serious, causing nitrogen bubble formation in high-fat–containing tissues like white matter. Significant spinal cord damage can occur from nitrogen bubble formation. Paresthesias and weakness can be asymmetric, as nitrogen bubble formation and expansion is irregularly distributed. Spontaneous epidural abscess and hematoma formation would be unlikely in a 33-year-old male without known past medical history. GBS is possible but tends to be symmetric and does not exhibit patchy sensation loss. Middle ear barotrauma refers to the inability to equilibrate the pressure on both sides of the tympanic membrane, resulting in rupture and consequent dizziness, vertigo, and delayed infection.

93. **Answer A.** All of the listed items are potential causes of pruritus ani, but the presence of fecal matter on the perianal skin is the most common.

94. **Answer A.** Tricyclics block fast sodium channels, slowing phase zero myocardial depolarization and causing QRS prolongation. Negative inotropy occurs due to reduced numbers of opened calcium channels. Potassium efflux blockade causes QT prolongation from impaired repolarization, α-1 antagonism causes hypotension, and anticholinergic effects cause tachycardia, hyperthermia, urinary retention, and agitation. Tricyclics have no known effect on magnesium channels.

95. **Answer E.** Septic shock should be treated aggressively with intravenous antibiotics and fluids. Corticosteroids have not been shown in most cases to reduce mortality in patients with pyelonephritis (although they likely help in patients with community-acquired pneumonia and acute respiratory distress syndrome (ARDS)). Merely checking a lactate level does not prevent mortality; a sepsis protocol must contain an effector arm to have a clinician act on the basis of that lactate level. Similarly, placing a central venous catheter by itself does not improve mortality. Norepinephrine would not yet be indicated in a patient with moderate hypotension before aggressive (i.e., 30 mL/kg) hydration is pursued.

96. **Answer B.** Hypoxemia is the most immediate life threat to patients with COPD exacerbations. This patient's pulse oximetry of 85% indicates severe hypoxemia. Although an arterial blood gas (ABG) could be performed to *verify* this patient's hypoxemia and to elucidate the degree of CO_2 retention, it is *clear* that what this patient needs is oxygen. A reasonable goal of oxygen therapy should be to titrate it to a saturation of 90%. Early observational studies demonstrated that some degree of worsening

hypercapnia usually occurs following increased oxygen delivery to patients with COPD. This should not be confused with a decrease in the patient's respiratory drive. Instead, increasing hypercapnia results primarily from worsened ventilation/perfusion ($\dot{V}/\dot{Q}$) mismatching and because of the Haldane effect in which oxygenated erythrocytes have a decreased affinity for CO_2, causing CO_2 offloading and an increase in blood CO_2 concentrations. Although this patient may eventually require intubation, it is prudent to try noninvasive measures, including noninvasive ventilation before endotracheal intubation.

97. **Answer C.** Hepatitis A virus infection is extremely common worldwide, but many cases are asymptomatic. Viremia starts first (2 to 4 weeks postexposure), followed by fecal excretion (4 to 6 weeks), transaminitis and nonspecific symptoms such as nausea and vomiting (5 to 10 weeks), and jaundice (6 to 10 weeks). Jaundice is usually the first symptom that causes patients to seek medical attention. By that time, contagiousness and viremia are minimal.

98. **Answer E.** Core temperature afterdrop refers to the phenomenon of a further decline in core temperature after the initiation of warming. It has been blamed for the development of cardiac dysrhythmias and active external rewarming methods are thought to amplify the drop. This has led to recommendations to heat the core before the extremities to avoid peripheral vasodilation and a brisk return of cool, acidic blood back to the core where it decreases core temperature and pH. In most healthy patients afterdrop has not been shown to be of clinical importance but elderly patients with less cardiopulmonary reserve and patients with volume depletion may be adversely impacted.

99. **Answer C.** The CT image reveals a medial cerebellar hemorrhage. Patients with cerebellar hemorrhage frequently deteriorate because the small space in the posterior fossa can't accommodate the edema associated with the hemorrhage leading to brainstem compression which can be fatal. In addition, cerebellar hemorrhage may compress the fourth ventricle leading to obstructive hydrocephalus, increased intracranial pressure, and decreased cerebral perfusion. Thus, such patients require critical monitoring in an ICU and prompt neurosurgical evaluation. Aphasia and hemiparesis are features of cortical strokes in the middle cerebral artery distribution. They are not associated with cerebellar strokes. However, patients with cerebellar bleeds frequently have gaze palsies because of associated cranial nerve injuries in the adjacent brainstem.

100. **Answer E.** Without a prior history of obstructive lung disease, this patient with wheezing likely has acute heart failure, due possibly to acute coronary syndrome. A diagnostic evaluation should proceed and direct further management, such as with venodilators and diuretics. There is often a temptation to treat all wheezing with albuterol nebulizer therapy, but in patients with cardiogenic causes of wheezing, this can worsen the outcome by increasing heart rate and thus, cardiac workload. Albuterol and methylprednisolone would be reasonable with a past medical history of COPD or asthma. Azithromycin would be reasonable if COPD exacerbation were suspected—as monotherapy, it would not be appropriate for community-acquired pneumonia in this age-group. Labetalol IV should be avoided in the setting of acute heart failure as it may further reduce cardiac output.

TEST 10

QUESTIONS

1. Which of the following traumatic mechanisms is the best candidate for emergency department (ED) thoracotomy?

   A. Blunt trauma to the chest
   B. Blunt trauma to the abdomen
   C. Blunt trauma to the pelvis
   D. Penetrating trauma to the chest
   E. Penetrating trauma to the abdomen

2. A 74-year-old male with hypertension and chronic kidney disease presented to the ED for evaluation after a fall. He reports some recent difficulty walking due to "dizziness." Vitals are P 48, RR 20, BP 105/80, SaO$_2$ 97% on room air. His EKG is shown. Blood tests reveal a hemoglobin of 9.2 g/dL, BUN 30 mg/dL, creatinine 1.6 mg/dL, sodium 141 mEq/L, and potassium of 5.1 mEq/L. Which of the following is the best next step (Fig. 11-1)?

   A. Atropine 1 mg IV
   B. Admission for observation and pacemaker placement
   C. Initiation of temporary cardiac pacing
   D. Amiodarone 150 mg IV bolus followed by an infusion of 1 mg/minute
   E. Kayexalate 15 g PO

3. Patients suffering from a hyperviscosity syndrome (leukostasis) due to severely elevated numbers of WBCs (hyperleukocytosis) most commonly present with symptoms reflecting involvement of which of the following organ systems?

   A. Pulmonary and genitourinary
   B. Cardiac and pulmonary
   C. Brain and pulmonary
   D. Cardiac and genitourinary
   E. Brain and cardiac

4. A 52-year-old homeless male presents for evaluation of frostbite in his hands (Fig. 11-2). In patients suffering severe frostbite, which of the following is a positive prognostic sign?

   A. Violaceous color after rewarming
   B. Lack of edema formation
   C. Woody firmness of the SQ tissue
   D. Early formation of clear blebs in the affected tissue
   E. None of the above

5. A 19-year-old male is brought to the ED after being stabbed in the neck. His primary survey is intact, but his secondary survey reveals a large, oblique laceration over his right lateral neck, starting from just lateral to the sternal notch and extending superolaterally to the posterolateral right neck, below the angle of the mandible. The patient denies odynophagia, dysphagia, dysphonia, or dyspnea. Examination of his wound reveals a small amount of ongoing bleeding, but no evidence of an expanding hematoma, clearly audible bruit or thrill. Which of the following is the next best step?

   A. Barium swallow
   B. CT angiogram of the neck

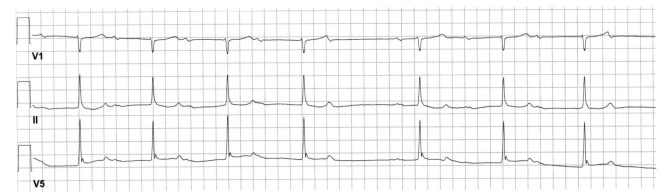

Figure 11-1

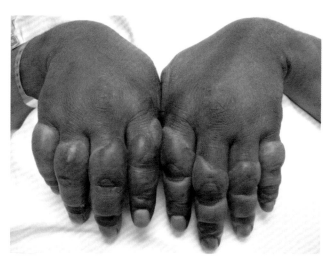

Figure 11-2

C. Closure of the wound and admission for observation
D. Esophagoduodenoscopy (EGD)
E. Bronchoscopy

6. A 20-year-old male presents with fever, sore throat, and fatigue for 1 week. He took a friend's antibiotic after 2 days of illness and developed a red rash all over his body, so he stopped the antibiotic. His oropharynx is mildly red without exudates, and he has cervical lymphadenopathy and splenomegaly. Rapid strep testing and monospot are both negative. Which of the following is the most likely diagnosis?

A. Group A beta-hemolytic streptococcal pharyngitis
B. Infectious mononucleosis
C. Influenza
D. Herpangina
E. Diphtheria pharyngitis

7. A 27-year-old male is brought to the ED after being stabbed in the neck with a knife and robbed. Upon examination, you note a 3-cm wound to zone II of the neck with an intact platysma. Which of the following is the next best step in management?

A. Local wound care, reassurance, and discharge
B. Admission for 23 hours of observation
C. Soft-tissue x-ray of the neck
D. Carotid angiography
E. CT of the neck

8. A 57-year-old male presents in out-of-hospital cardiac arrest with pulseless electrical activity (PEA). Prehospital advanced cardiac life support, including CPR and administration of several doses of epinephrine IV, has been performed for 20 minutes. His monitor still reveals PEA. Which of the following is the next best step in the management of this patient?

A. Synchronized cardioversion at 100 J
B. Defibrillation at 150 J

C. Vasopressin IV
D. CT brain without contrast
E. End-tidal CO_2 level

9. A 15-year-old male presents to the pediatric emergency room with a chief complaint of burning pain to the "tip" of his penis. He is uncircumcised and denies any past history of genitourinary disease. He admits to being sexually active and uses condoms intermittently but denies penile discharge. Physical examination reveals an erythematous, mildly edematous glans without penile discharge. The scrotal examination is unrevealing and there is no inguinal lymphadenopathy. His blood sugar on a finger stick is 96. Which of the following is the most likely cause of his problem?

A. *Chlamydia trachomatis*
B. *Escherichia coli*
C. *Gardnerella vaginalis*
D. Group A *Streptococcus* (GAS)
E. *Candida albicans*

10. A 2-year-old female ingested the leaves of this flowering plant (Fig. 11-3). Which of the following effects can be expected?

A. Dry mouth
B. Renal failure
C. Cardiac dysrhythmias
D. Altered mental status
E. Liver failure

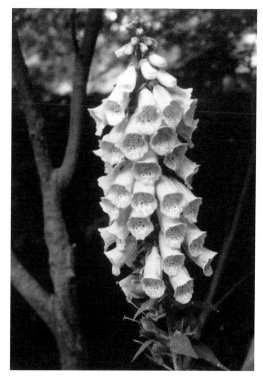

Figure 11-3

11. A complaint that may help differentiate patients with Crohn disease from patients with irritable bowel syndrome is:

    A. Nocturnal diarrhea
    B. Bloating
    C. Weight loss
    D. Colicky abdominal pain
    E. Bilious vomiting

12. Which of the following laboratory abnormalities is most commonly associated with hyperemesis gravidarum?

    A. Hyperkalemia
    B. Elevated liver enzymes
    C. Thrombocytopenia
    D. Hyperglycemia
    E. Elevated erythrocyte sedimentation rate

13. A 65-year-old African-American woman presents with left lower quadrant abdominal pain and slightly loose stools for 3 days. She is afebrile but is tender in the left lower quadrant. You suspect diverticulitis. Which of the following is true regarding diverticulitis?

    A. Diverticulitis most commonly occurs in the ascending colon.
    B. Most patients with uncomplicated diverticulitis do not have recurrences.
    C. Doxycycline is the treatment drug of choice.
    D. High-fiber diet has no proven role in management.
    E. Barium enema is the diagnostic test of choice.

14. An ED thoracotomy is performed on a trauma patient. Which of the following is the structure labeled in Figure 11-4?

    A. Vagus nerve
    B. Phrenic nerve
    C. Sympathetic chain
    D. Spinal accessory nerve
    E. Inferior vena cava

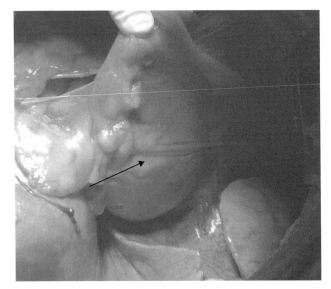

Figure 11-4

15. Which of the following is the most common cranial nerve affected in patients with multiple sclerosis (MS)?

    A. Optic nerve
    B. Oculomotor nerve
    C. Trochlear nerve
    D. Abducens nerve
    E. Facial nerve

16. Which of the following is true regarding the management of epistaxis?

    A. Silver nitrate sticks work best when activated by fresh bleeding.
    B. Silver nitrate sticks should not be used on bilateral surfaces of the septum.
    C. Avoid blowing the nose before placement of packing.
    D. Antibiotics are indicated in patients with posterior packs, but not anterior packs.
    E. Admission is indicated in patients with anterior packs, but not posterior packs.

17. A 34-year-old female with acquired immune deficiency syndrome (AIDS) presents after a first-time seizure. Which of the following is the most likely cause of her seizure?

    A. Mass lesion
    B. Meningitis
    C. Stroke
    D. Electrolyte abnormality
    E. Syphilis

18. Patients with spinal stenosis:

    A. Most commonly present with a radiculopathy that is worse with walking
    B. Typically feel relief when leaning forward
    C. Often have a lumbar radiculopathy at several levels
    D. May be able to walk uphill more easily than downhill
    E. All of the above

19. A 45-year-old male arrives hypotensive after a motor vehicle collision. His physical examination demonstrates clear lungs but an unstable pelvis. The pelvis is secured tightly with a bedsheet, but the patient continues to be hypotensive despite crystalloid and blood replacement. Bedside focused assessment of sonography in trauma scan is negative. Which of the following is the most appropriate next step in management?

    A. CT chest
    B. CT abdomen/pelvis
    C. CT brain
    D. Angiography with embolization
    E. Laparotomy

20. D-dimer levels may be elevated in which of the following?

   A. Elderly patients
   B. Pregnancy
   C. Multiple blunt trauma victims
   D. Postoperative patients
   E. All of the above

21. A 3-year-old male is brought to the ED by his parents with a chief complaint of excessive drowsiness, fever, and decreased oral intake. Examination reveals an ill-appearing child, with tachypnea and increased work of breathing. He is pale, and his extremities are cool and mottled with decreased peripheral pulses. He is not interactive during the examination, and his vitals reveal T 102.7, P 185, BP not measurable, RR 56, SaO$_2$ 93%. An IV is established and the patient is given broad-spectrum antibiotics and three boluses of normal saline at 20 mL/kg per bolus, for a total of 60 mL/kg, with little improvement in his perfusion or clinical status. Which of the following vasopressors is the initial preferred agent?

   A. Epinephrine
   B. Dopamine
   C. Norepinephrine
   D. Milrinone
   E. Dobutamine

22. You diagnose a 68-year-old female with community-acquired pneumonia and decide to admit her to the hospital for inpatient management. Apart from early and appropriate intravenous antibiotic therapy, which of the following would be most likely to improve outcome?

   A. N-acetylcysteine
   B. Oseltamivir
   C. Albumin
   D. Corticosteroids
   E. Lactulose

23. Which of the following patients is at highest risk of developing a lung abscess?

   A. A 28-year-old HIV+ man with a recent CD4$^+$ T-cell count of 301
   B. A 47-year-old female status postlumpectomy for breast cancer
   C. A 68-year-old drunk alcoholic woman with diffuse caries
   D. A 32-year-old male with a history of polypharmacy abuse including IV drug use
   E. A 72-year-old female with Parkinson disease

24. A 22-year-old female presents with a severe sore throat and difficulty swallowing. Her physical examination is consistent with pharyngitis. Which of the following criteria make group A streptococcus (GAS) more likely as a cause of her illness?

   A. Tender anterior cervical lymphadenopathy
   B. Concomitant otitis media

C. Nonexudative tonsillitis
D. The presence of a cough
E. Increased atypical lymphocytes on her peripheral blood smear

25. A 23-year-old male presents with difficulty breathing, altered mental status, and a petechial rash. He suffered a proximal tibia fracture the previous day after being kicked by a horse. Which of the following is the most likely diagnosis?

   A. Meningococcemia
   B. Fat embolism
   C. Pulmonary thromboembolism
   D. Pneumothorax
   E. Pneumonia

26. A 34-year-old female presents with weakness, fatigue, rash, and fever for several days. She was prescribed an antibiotic by her primary care physician for an upper respiratory infection just before the symptoms started. The rash is diffuse, maculopapular, and confluent. Laboratory work demonstrates normal electrolytes, but an elevated creatinine at 3.6 mg/dL. Peripheral blood and urine contain eosinophils. Which of the following is the most likely etiologic agent?

   A. Amoxicillin
   B. Doxycycline
   C. Clindamycin
   D. Azithromycin
   E. Erythromycin

27. Which of the following mushroom toxins is known to cause hepatotoxicity?

   A. Coprine
   B. Ibotenic acid
   C. Amatoxin
   D. Orellanine
   E. Psilocybin

28. Clinically, condyloma acuminatum may be differentiated from condyloma lata by:

   A. Extensive wart-like lesions
   B. Location in the perineum
   C. Drier, keratinized appearance
   D. Foul odor
   E. Bluish superficial telangiectasias

29. A 26-year-old female at 31 weeks' gestation is brought to the ED after a high-speed motor vehicle accident. She was an unrestrained passenger but was not ejected from the vehicle. She is brought in lying on a backboard with a c-collar and is complaining of difficulty breathing. Her room air oxygen saturation reads 82%, although it increases to 93% on a nonbreather. A chest x-ray was taken and is shown in Figure 11-5. Which of the following is true?

   A. Chest tubes should be placed in the fifth intercostal space at the midaxillary line.

B. Chest tubes should be placed over the anterior chest wall.

C. Chest tubes are contraindicated during pregnancy.

D. Chest tubes should be deferred until fetal evaluation is complete.

E. Chest tubes should be placed higher in pregnant than in nonpregnant women.

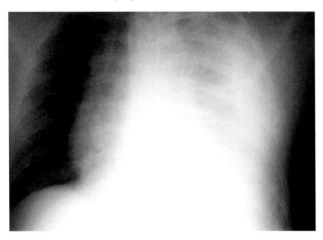

Figure 11-5

30. Which of the following is a biochemical effect of tricyclic antidepressants?

A. α-1 Agonist

B. Dopamine reuptake inhibitor

C. Muscarinic agonist

D. γ-Aminobutyric acid (GABA) agonist

E. Antihistamine

31. A 35-year-old female presents after a fall from a fourth-story window. She was initially moaning, but then became completely unresponsive. Her pupils were initially miotic and equal, but then became dilated and unreactive. She exhibits decorticate posturing in response to pain. Which of the following is the most likely mechanism?

A. Skull fracture

B. Uncal herniation

C. Basilar artery dissection

D. Subarachnoid hemorrhage

E. Brain death

32. Which of the following conditions is the most common cause of lens dislocation?

A. Tertiary syphilis

B. Homocystinuria

C. Marfan syndrome

D. Trauma

E. Ehlers–Danlos syndrome

33. Which of the following is more characteristic of endo-carditis in IV drug users than in nondrug users?

A. Higher mortality from *Staphylococcus aureus*

B. Audible heart murmur

C. Splinter hemorrhages

D. Septic pulmonary emboli

E. Roth spots

34. A 6-year-old male is brought in by his parents for evaluation of dental trauma after a fall. The right maxillary central incisor and left maxillary lateral incisor are loose and somewhat malpositioned. The left maxillary central incisor was completely avulsed (Fig. 11-6). The fall occurred only a few minutes before presentation. Which of the following is true?

A. If the tooth is present, it should be reimplanted after gentle washing.

B. A CT scan should be performed to assess for alveolar bone fracture.

C. The loose teeth will most likely reposition themselves passively.

D. The permanent (secondary) tooth has a better outcome after complete intrusion rather than complete avulsion of the primary tooth.

E. Dental avulsion can result in irreversible problems with speech production.

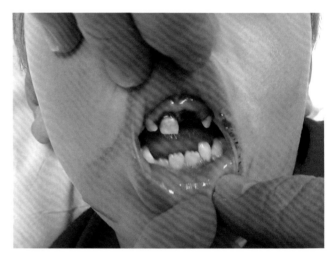

Figure 11-6

35. A 6-month-old infant falls out of her high chair onto the kitchen floor and is brought by her parents for evaluation. The parents note that there was no definite loss of consciousness (LOC), vomiting, or seizure activity. She has not been abnormally sleepy, but her parents note that she should be hungry at this time and has been refusing feeds. Her physical examination, including neurologic examination, is unremarkable. Which of the following is the most appropriate next step in management?

A. Contact Department of Children and Family Services (DCFS)

B. Skull x-rays

C. CT brain

D. MRI brain

E. Discharge home

36. A 20-year-old previously healthy female college student presents to the ED with diarrhea. She went on a camping trip 2 weeks ago but denies any other travel. She notes seven to eight watery, foul-smelling stools per day and generalized abdominal cramping. A test for fecal leukocytes, ordered in triage after the patient had a large diarrheal stool, is negative. Which of the following is the best management?

    A. Azithromycin 500 mg daily for 3 days
    B. Metronidazole 250 mg t.i.d. for 7 days
    C. Ciprofloxacin 500 mg b.i.d. for 3 days
    D. Supportive care with IV hydration and antimotility agents
    E. Vancomycin 125 mg q.i.d. for 10 days

37. A 33-year-old male is bitten by the spider pictured (Fig. 11-7). Which of the following is the next best step in management?

    A. Ibuprofen and lorazepam
    B. Antivenom
    C. Hemodialysis
    D. Plastic surgery consultation
    E. Negative inspiratory force assessment

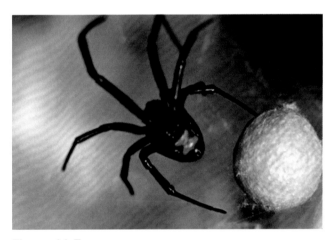

Figure 11-7

38. A 34-year-old male presents with severe left knee pain after a motor vehicle collision. He has a large joint effusion and his knee is unstable in all directions. Plain radiographs demonstrate no fracture. Pulses in the left lower extremity are normal. Which of the following is the most appropriate next step in management?

    A. Discharge with no weight bearing
    B. MRI knee
    C. CT angiography
    D. CT knee
    E. Arthroscopy

39. A 50-year-old male presents with right lower facial swelling for 3 days. He has had right lower molar pain for several weeks but has not seen a dentist. The patient has a history of alcohol abuse. On examination, the patient has a low-grade fever, restricted neck movement, trismus, and firm swelling in the bilateral submandibular and submental regions. Which of the following is true?

    A. The lateral incisors are the most commonly affected teeth.
    B. *Pseudomonas* species are the most common cause.
    C. The most common cause of death is septic shock.
    D. Fiberoptic nasotracheal intubation is the preferred method of airway control.
    E. Corticosteroids are clearly associated with better outcomes.

40. Which of the following is the definition of the shock index (SI)?

    A. Systolic blood pressure (SBP)/heart rate (HR)
    B. (SBP + HR)/respiratory rate (RR)
    C. HR/SBP
    D. HR/mean arterial pressure (MAP)
    E. HR/pulse pressure

41. A 33-year-old male presents by EMS with a chief complaint of palpitations and mild chest pain. Upon EMS arrival, they found the patient awake and normotensive, appearing stable and in a wide-complex tachycardia with a rate of 200. They administered adenosine and the patient converted to a normal sinus rhythm. Which of the following is true?

    A. Adenosine can be used to differentiate supraventricular tachycardia with a block from ventricular tachycardia
    B. The patient has atrial flutter with aberrancy
    C. An echocardiogram will reveal right heart strain
    D. Ventricular tachycardia can convert to sinus rhythm in response to adenosine
    E. The patient should be started on a diltiazem infusion to prevent recurrence.

42. Direct synthesis of which of the following clotting factors is inhibited by coumadin?

    A. Factor XII
    B. Factor X
    C. Factor VIII
    D. Factor V
    E. Factor III

43. The family of a 49-year-old female with a history of hypertension brings her to the emergency department (ED) with a chief complaint of mumbled, incomprehensible speech that started approximately 5 hours ago along with weakness of her right arm, leg, and face. Computed tomography (CT) of her head reveals an area of infarction in her left hemisphere but no evidence of

bleeding. Upon returning from CT, the nurse tells you her blood pressure is 200/105. Which of the following summarizes the best approach to managing this patient's blood pressure?

A. Start a sodium nitroprusside drip and titrate to a systolic blood pressure (SBP) of 160 mm Hg.

B. Give the patient her oral antihypertensive medications at her usual doses.

C. Administer 5 to 10 mg of labetalol IV every 10 to 20 minutes until the patient's SBP is between 140 and 160 mm Hg.

D. Give the patient 60 mg of nimodipine PO because of its dual effects in lowering blood pressure and in preventing vasospasm.

E. Continue to monitor the patient's blood pressure without treatment.

44. A 64-year-old female with small cell lung cancer presents with a chief complaint of fatigue, dizziness, and imbalance. Her blood work is significant for a sodium level of 112 mmol/L. You suspect she has a syndrome of inappropriate secretion of antidiuretic hormone (SIADH) due to her lung cancer. Administering normal saline to this patient will likely:

A. Slowly correct her sodium level.

B. Result in central pontine myelinolysis.

C. Worsen her hyponatremia.

D. Suppress further antidiuretic hormone (ADH) secretion.

E. Make no difference in her sodium level, and cause water retention and edema.

45. A 23-year-old male presents after a stab wound to his right lumbar spinal area. Which of the following is the most likely neurologic deficit?

A. Left leg weakness and left-sided loss of pain sensation

B. Left leg weakness and right-sided loss of pain sensation

C. Right leg weakness and left-sided loss of pain sensation

D. Right leg weakness and right-sided loss of pain sensation

E. Bladder incontinence and bilateral flaccid paralysis

46. Which of the following is a criterion for acute respiratory distress syndrome (ARDS)?

A. Unilateral focal infiltrate

B. Cardiomegaly

C. Pao_2/Fio_2 fraction >200

D. Pulmonary artery wedge pressure >18 mm Hg

E. Acute onset

47. A 55-year-old male with diabetes presents with painful vision loss in his left eye, which occurred when he sat down to watch a movie in the theater. His acuity is markedly reduced in the left eye and his left pupil is poorly reactive to light and measures 4 mm. Which of the following is true regarding this patient's condition?

A. A unilateral shallow anterior chamber is diagnostic.

B. Retinal venules demonstrate a characteristic boxcar appearance.

C. Pilocarpine is typically administered to both eyes.

D. Intravenous therapies are withheld until ophthalmologic evaluation is obtained.

E. Ocular massage is a helpful temporizing measure.

48. Spontaneous intracerebral hemorrhage involving the pons most likely results in which of the following:

A. Seizures and homonymous hemianopsia

B. Gait ataxia, vomiting, headache, gaze palsy

C. Total paralysis, pinpoint pupils

D. Hemiplegia, dysarthria

E. Loss of vertical gaze

49. A 55-year-old female with chronic obstructive pulmonary disease (COPD) presents with acute dyspnea, purulent cough, and fever. Vital signs are 100.4°F, 110, 22, 175/90, 98% on 4 L NC. She has mild neck muscle retractions and bilateral rhonchi. Chest x-ray shows no focal infiltrate. Albuterol nebulizer, methylprednisolone 125 mg IV, and levofloxacin 500 mg IV have only minimally improved respiratory distress. Which of the following is the next best step in management?

A. Azithromycin 500 mg IV

B. Vancomycin 1 g IV

C. Aminophylline 5 mg/kg IV

D. Noninvasive positive pressure ventilation

E. Endotracheal intubation and mechanical ventilation

50. A patient presents with the electrocardiogram (EKG) shown in Figure 11-8. Which of the following is the most likely pathophysiologic mechanism?

A. Reentry

B. Increased automaticity

C. Atrioventricular (AV) blockade

D. Pre-excitation

E. Infarction

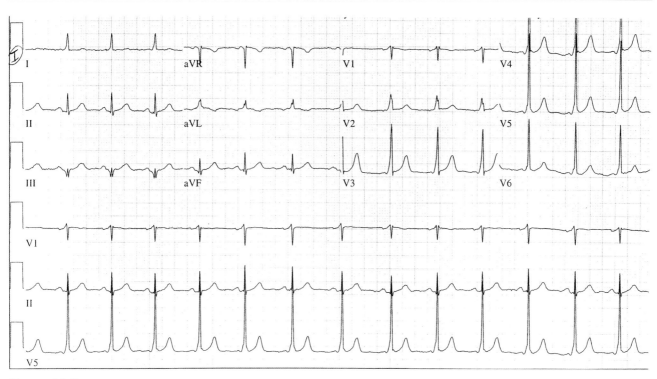

Figure 11-8

51. Among adults, which of the following is the most common cause of acute diarrheal illness in the United States?

A. Viruses
B. *Escherichia coli*
C. *Campylobacter* spp.
D. *Giardia lamblia*
E. *Staphylococcus aureus*

52. The most common cause of acute liver failure is:

A. Acetaminophen toxicity
B. Idiopathic
C. Hepatitis B virus infection
D. *Amanita phalloides* ingestion
E. Reye syndrome

53. Which of the following arteries supplies the atrioventricular (AV) node in most people?

A. Left coronary artery
B. Right coronary artery
C. Left anterior descending artery
D. Left circumflex artery
E. Right posterior descending artery

54. A 60-year-old male presents with acute urinary retention. He has been unable to urinate for the last 10 hours and has extreme discomfort in his lower abdomen. His physical examination is normal except for a distended suprapubic region and nontender prostatic hypertrophy. He appears very uncomfortable. Which of the following is the most appropriate next step in management?

A. Magnetic resonance imaging (MRI) of the abdomen
B. CT scan abdomen with and without IV contrast
C. Renal ultrasonography
D. Complete blood count, chemistry panel
E. Foley catheter placement

55. A 47-year-old female with cirrhosis presents to the ED with mild abdominal pain. Her temperature is 99.1°F and she has a protuberant abdomen with significant ascites. You suspect spontaneous bacterial peritonitis. Aside from antibacterial therapy with IV ceftriaxone, which of the following is most likely to reduce her mortality?

A. Amphotericin
B. Albumin
C. Vancomycin
D. Oseltamivir
E. Midodrine

56. A 67-year-old female presents with acute, severe periumbilical and epigastric abdominal pain. A flat plate and upright is shown in Figure 11-9. Which of the following is true?

A. Cocaine use is a risk factor in younger patients
B. Patients may experience transient paradoxical improvement without treatment.
C. X-ray imaging is only 70% sensitive
D. IV antibiotics, IV fluids, an NG tube, and an intravenous proton pump inhibitor should be started
E. All of the above

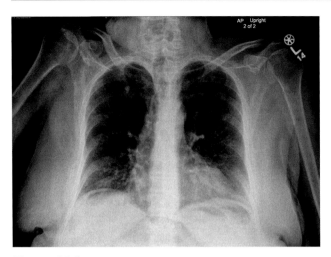

Figure 11-9

57. Which of the following is true regarding patients with temporal (or giant cell) arteritis?

    A. The most specific finding is jaw claudication.

    B. Permanent visual loss occurs in 50% of patients.

    C. Treatment with corticosteroids should be withheld until there is biopsy-proven disease.

    D. Vertigo is the most sensitive clinical finding.

    E. The peak age of onset is 40 years.

58. A 24-year-old female presents with persistent cough for 4 weeks. She had upper respiratory infection (URI)-like symptoms 2 weeks before and then developed a persistent cough for the next month. She states she has had coughing fits many times during the day and "can't stop coughing" for almost a minute once she starts. Which of the following is true regarding this patient?

    A. The disease is caused by a gram-negative coccobacillus.

    B. Antibiotic therapy should eliminate the symptoms within a few days.

    C. Bacterial culture is indicated to confirm the diagnosis.

    D. The disease is not contagious

    E. Mortality is close to 30%.

59. Which of the following is the right remedy for the corresponding bleeding problem?

    A. Desmopressin (dDAVP) for patients with severe uremia and persistent oozing epistaxis

    B. Prothrombin complex concentrate (PCC) for bleeding due to thrombocytopenia

    C. Recombinant factor VIII for a bleeding patient with hemophilia B

    D. Recombinant von Willebrand factor (VWF) for a bleeding patient with hemophilia A

    E. All of the above are appropriate

60. A 47-year-old police officer is brought to the ED after being found unresponsive. The officer was called to respond to an unidentified young female, who was apparently sleeping in a car parked at a shopping center. Bystanders note that after knocking on the windows, the officer opened the door and collapsed to the ground shortly afterward. The bystanders at the scene stated that there was a sharp, foul odor similar to a "rotten egg" that appeared to be coming from the vehicle, so they kept their distance. Which of the following antidotes is most likely beneficial in treating this officer?

    A. Methylene blue

    B. Sodium nitrite

    C. Hydroxycobalamin

    D. Sodium thiosulfate

    E. Succimer

61. A 34-year-old male presents with hypertension. He randomly checked his blood pressure at the drugstore and it was 172/100. His only symptoms are nasal congestion and malaise. He has been told he had borderline hypertension in the past but has not seen a physician in several years. You establish primary care follow-up within 24 hours for him. Which of the following is the next best step in management?

    A. Start metoprolol 50 mg PO b.i.d.

    B. Start amlodipine 10 mg PO q.d.

    C. Refer him to a cardiologist in 2 to 4 days

    D. Instruct him to avoid systemic decongestants

    E. Instruct him to reduce his sugar intake

62. A 35-year-old male presents with acute onset of pleuritic, right-sided chest pain for 2 days associated with mild dyspnea. He has no fever, cough, or chills. He reports no past medical history except smoking. Vital signs are 98.9°F, 105, 20, 120/70, 97% RA. Examination is unremarkable except for tachycardia. Electrocardiogram (EKG) shows sinus tachycardia without any other abnormalities, and chest x-ray reveals a small right-sided pleural effusion with clear lung fields. Which of the following is the next best step in management?

    A. Order blood cultures

    B. Order D-dimer

    C. Give gastrointestinal cocktail and assess response

    D. Give amoxicillin–clavulanic acid

    E. Order right-sided EKG

63. A 3-year-old male had a ventriculoperitoneal shunt (VPS) placed at 22 months due to hydrocephalus. It has not been revised since then and he has had no problems with it. He is now brought to the ED with a history of fever of 38.2°C, headache, and "fussiness." Which of the following is true about this patient?

   A. The risk of VPS infection rises 1 year after insertion.
   B. Urgent lumbar puncture (LP) is indicated.
   C. The mortality of a VPS infection is roughly 75%.
   D. Hydrocephalus on CT scan rules out the presence of VPS infection.
   E. Most patients with a VPS infection have peripheral leukocytosis.

64. A 56-year-old female presents with acute organophosphate overdose, with severe bronchorrhea, bradycardia, and coma. She is intubated for airway protection, and atropine therapy is initiated. After 10 mg of atropine, her heart rate (HR) is 130, blood pressure (BP) is 160/90, and her secretions are still copious. Which of the following is the most appropriate next step in management?

   A. Stop atropine, start epinephrine
   B. Stop atropine, start vasopressin
   C. Stop atropine, start pralidoxime
   D. Continue atropine therapy alone
   E. Continue atropine therapy and add pralidoxime

65. A 25-year-old male ingests the mushroom, which he thought was edible (Fig. 11-10). Which of the following effects can be expected?

   A. Hallucinations
   B. Liver failure
   C. Renal failure
   D. Blindness
   E. Adrenal infarction

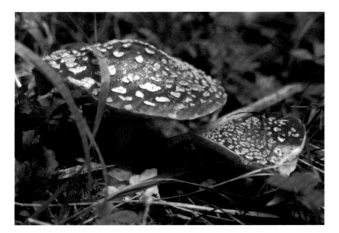

Figure 11-10

66. A 75-year-old female presents to the ED for evaluation of meningitis. She has had 12 hours of acute onset of headache, stiff neck, and fever. Physical examination demonstrates a febrile patient in moderate distress with nuchal rigidity and severe photophobia. A lumbar puncture is performed with the following results:

Cerebrospinal fluid white blood cell (CSF WBC):	700 cells per mL, 80% neutrophils, 20% lymphocytes
CSF glucose:	Decreased
CSF protein:	Elevated
CSF Gram stain:	No organisms seen

On the basis of these results, the presumptive diagnosis of bacterial meningitis is made. Which of the following is the most appropriate therapy?

   A. Dexamethasone and imipenem
   B. Ceftriaxone alone
   C. Ceftriaxone, ampicillin, and vancomycin
   D. Ceftriaxone, vancomycin, and dexamethasone
   E. Ampicillin, ceftriaxone, vancomycin, and dexamethasone

67. A 65-year-old asymptomatic man presents with the EKG as shown in Figure 11-11. Which of the following is the most likely associated condition?

   A. Hypertriglyceridemia
   B. Rheumatic fever
   C. Chronic obstructive pulmonary disease (COPD)
   D. Pulmonary embolism
   E. Hyperkalemia

68. Which of the following is the most common serious complication of the edrophonium (Tensilon) test?

   A. Bradycardia
   B. Atrial fibrillation
   C. Oculogyric crisis
   D. Cough
   E. Seizure

69. A 58-year-old male with a history of hypertension and diabetes presents by EMS with chest pain that developed while he was cutting grass. The patient was normotensive upon EMS arrival. EMS administered two sublingual nitroglycerin tablets en route. Upon arrival, his initial

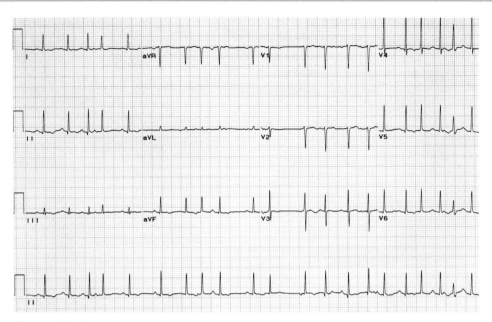

Figure 11-11

vital signs are P 75, RR 18, BP 92/64, SaO$_2$ 98% on room air. His EKG is shown in Figure 11-12. Which of the following is true?

A. Jugular venous distension may be present
B. He is likely to have rales on examination
C. Beta blockers are an important component of therapy
D. Hypotension which develops after nitroglycerin administration suggests left ventricle infarction
E. Intravenous fluids should be avoided due to a concern of heart failure

70. Which of the following is the most common etiology of death from child abuse?

A. Retroperitoneal hemorrhage
B. Hemothorax
C. Intracranial hemorrhage
D. Burns
E. Drowning

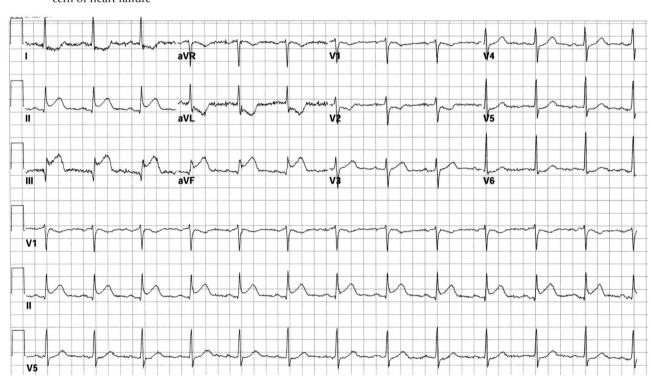

Figure 11-12

71. A 72-year-old male presents with a rash on his right abdomen (Fig. 11-13). He complains of a 1-week history of burning discomfort extending from his low back to his low right abdomen, and a 1-day history of a rash over his abdomen only. The area "tingles" and burns and is "sensitive" to the touch. Which of the following is the most likely etiologic agent?

    A. Herpes simplex virus (HSV)
    B. Varicella zoster virus (VZV)
    C. Human immunodeficiency virus
    D. Epstein–Barr virus (EBV)
    E. Parvovirus

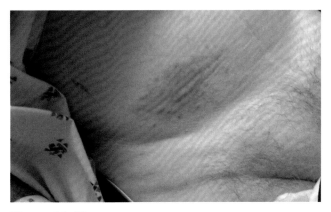

Figure 11-13

72. A 20-year-old male presents with diffuse lower extremity myalgias and dark urine after participating in an adventure race. Which of the following is true?

    A. Hypercalcemia is the most common electrolyte abnormality.
    B. Detection of serum myoglobin is the most sensitive means of diagnosing rhabdomyolysis.
    C. Acute kidney injury is likely if the creatine kinase (CK) is >2,000 Units/L
    D. Loop diuretics are an effective treatment adjunct.
    E. Creatine kinase (CK) has a much longer half-life than myoglobin.

73. Primary chronic adrenal insufficiency is usually due to:

    A. Sarcoidosis
    B. Hemorrhage
    C. Pituitary insufficiency
    D. Idiopathic
    E. Iron deposition

74. Cancer of which of the following organs is the most common cause of superior vena cava (SVC) syndrome?

    A. Breast
    B. Lung
    C. Testicle
    D. Colon
    E. Thyroid

75. Which of the following is true regarding labetalol?

    A. Effect on α-receptors is greater than that on β-receptors.
    B. Reflex tachycardia is a common complication.
    C. Orthostatic changes with IV use are rare.
    D. BP is more easily controlled than with nitroprusside.
    E. It is superior to nitroprusside as monotherapy for aortic dissection.

76. Which of the following is the best adjunct to the physical examination in assessing the severity of an asthma attack?

    A. Arterial blood gas (ABG)
    B. Peak expiratory flow rate (PEFR)
    C. Chest x-ray
    D. Continuous cardiac monitoring
    E. FEV_1 (forced expiratory volume in 1 second, expressed as L/second)

77. A 19-year-old male presents with fevers, chills, malaise, and rash for 5 days. He recently returned from a camping trip. The rash is macular and located on the wrists, ankles, palms, and soles. Routine laboratory work including lumbar puncture is normal. Which of the following is the most appropriate next step?

    A. Watchful waiting
    B. Doxycycline
    C. Acyclovir
    D. Clindamycin
    E. TMP-SMX

78. Which of the following laboratory tests is most likely to be normal in patients with acute disseminated intravascular coagulation (DIC)?

    A. Prothrombin time
    B. Partial thromboplastin time
    C. Platelet count
    D. Hemoglobin
    E. Fibrinogen

79. The development of lethargy, headache, and vomiting in a pediatric patient being treated for diabetic ketoacidosis (DKA) suggests the presence of:

    A. Meningitis
    B. Cerebral edema
    C. Worsening acidosis
    D. Central pontine myelinolysis
    E. Hyponatremia

80. A 27-year-old female with HIV presents for evaluation of a 2-day history of fevers, chills, rigors, cough, and purulent sputum. Which of the following is the most likely cause of infection?

    A. Pneumocystis pneumonia (PCP)
    B. *Streptococcus pneumoniae*

C. Crytptococcus

D. Histoplasmosis

E. Tuberculosis

81. A 64-year-old female with a past history of sick sinus syndrome and recent pacemaker placement presents with neck pain after a low-speed motor vehicle collision. She has midline cervical spine tenderness at C6–7. A cervical spine plain film series is inadequate for visualizing these segments, so a CT scan is performed. The CT scan is normal, but the patient still has pain in her neck. Which of the following is the most appropriate next step in management?

A. Discharge home with soft collar

B. Discharge home with hard collar

C. Flexion–extension cervical spine x-rays

D. Oblique cervical spine x-rays

E. MRI of the cervical spine

82. A 16-year-old male is brought to the ED by his parents after he fell from a bicycle while practicing tricks. He struck the vertex of his helmet as he hit the ground and the fall was witnessed by his brother who said the patient was "out for a second." There was no vomiting, and the patient denies any headache, but he says he cannot remember what happened, and does not remember that he was riding a bike. His mother also states he has been "forgetting new things" since the accident. Which of the following is true?

A. Anterograde amnesia is typically more severe than retrograde amnesia after blunt head trauma.

B. Inability to recall one's birthdate and name in an otherwise alert patient after trauma is most often a sign of malingering.

C. The presence of a skull fracture is a strong predictor of intracranial bleeding.

D. Postconcussion syndrome is more common among young children.

E. There are well-studied, evidenced-based guidelines regarding the optimal time to return to athletic activities.

83. The most common manifestation of barotrauma associated with scuba divers during descent is:

A. Nitrogen narcosis

B. Barosinusitis

C. Temporomandibular joint dysfunction

D. Facial barotrauma

E. Middle ear barotrauma

84. A 34-year-old female has a hemoglobin level of 10.0 g/dL with a low mean corpuscular volume. Which of the following is the most likely cause?

A. α-Thalassemia

B. β-Thalassemia

C. Iron-deficiency anemia

D. Sideroblastic anemia

E. Folate deficiency

85. A 22-year-old male basketball player presents to the ED after developing sudden shortness of breath and a painful sensation on the left side of his chest, which worsens with breathing. Initial chest x-ray reveals a small left apical pneumothorax. The patient's vitals are 128/72, P 95, RR 22 and shallow, and SaO_2 of 97% on RA. The best course of action is:

A. Administer supplemental O_2 and admit the patient to the hospital for 24-hour observation with repeat chest films q6h.

B. Administer supplemental O_2, observe the patient in the ED, and repeat a chest film in 3 to 6 hours.

C. Discharge the patient home with routine follow-up the next day with his *Pneumocystis carinii* pneumonia (PCP).

D. Insert a chest tube and connect it to water-seal

E. Consult cardiothoracic (CT) surgery

86. Which of the following is the most common initial dysrhythmia in symptomatic patients with Wolff–Parkinson–White (WPW) syndrome?

A. Multifocal atrial tachycardia (MAT)

B. Atrioventricular (AV) nodal reentrant tachycardia

C. Mobitz type I second-degree AV block

D. Mobitz type II second-degree AV block

E. Torsade de pointes

87. A 44-year-old female presents with right wrist pain. She fell on her hand the previous day and has pain in her radial wrist. The wrist is tender in the anatomic snuffbox. Plain radiographs of the wrist are completely normal. Which of the following is the most appropriate next step in management?

A. Orthopedics consultation

B. Discharge home with thumb range of motion exercises

C. Discharge home with Velcro wrist splint

D. Discharge home with thumb spica splint

E. Admit for observation of wrist

88. Which of the following is true regarding rheumatoid arthritis (RA)?

A. The distal interphalangeal (DIP) joints are commonly affected.

B. Arthritis is commonly polyarticular and asymmetric.

C. Fifteen percent of patients will have a negative rheumatoid factor (RF).

D. The disease is equally common in women and in men.

E. Arthritic involvement of the spine is uncommon in RA.

89. Which of the following is the number one cause of death in patients with congestive heart failure (CHF)?

    A. Progressive hemodynamic deterioration
    B. Urinary tract infection (UTI)
    C. Pneumonia
    D. Stroke
    E. Pulmonary embolism

90. Which of the following is the most frequent complication during hemodialysis?

    A. Muscle cramps
    B. Headache
    C. Fever and chills
    D. Hypotension
    E. Chest pain

91. A 32-year-old male presents with eye pain and redness. Slit lamp examination is shown in Figure 11-14. Which of the following is the most appropriate next step in management?

    A. Topical prednisolone
    B. Valacyclovir PO
    C. Acetazolamide IV
    D. Erythromycin PO
    E. Ceftriaxone IV

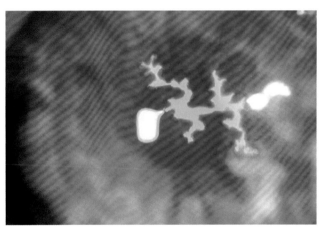

Figure 11-14

92. Which of the following is the most common serious complication of pulmonary contusion?

    A. Acute respiratory distress syndrome (ARDS)
    B. Pneumonia
    C. Pulmonary embolism
    D. Myocardial contusion
    E. Pericardial tamponade

93. A 42-year-old anxious woman presents to the ED with low back pain radiating down her *left* leg. She states that she has a history of a herniated disk but has never had

advanced imaging or surgery. While the patient is lying supine, you lift her *right* leg to approximately 45 degrees, causing the patient to complain of pain radiating down her left leg below the knee. How do you interpret this result?

    A. The patient is malingering.
    B. The patient probably has a vertebral compression fracture.
    C. The patient has cauda equina syndrome.
    D. The patient has a lumbar radiculopathy probably caused by a left-sided herniated disk.
    E. The patient has crossed sensory nerve fibers resulting in paradoxical left-sided pain.

94. A 32-year-old male presents to the ED after an accident while cleaning a paint sprayer. He was trying to dislodge a clog in the nozzle when he inadvertently triggered the sprayer with his index finger over the nozzle. He now comes in with mild pain and a nearly punctate wound at the tip of his left index finger. Which of the following is the next best step in management?

    A. Tetanus prophylaxis, oral antibiotics, splint in the "safe" position, and discharge with orthopedic follow-up in 2 days
    B. Tetanus prophylaxis, irrigate the wound with tap water, oral antibiotics, and discharge with orthopedic follow-up in 2 days
    C. Hand surgeon consultation for immediate operative debridement
    D. Tetanus prophylaxis, oral antibiotics, incision, and drainage of the volar tip of the finger.
    E. Tetanus prophylaxis, oral antibiotics, and digital block with thorough wound exploration to determine the extent of injury

95. A 22-year-old male is brought in for evaluation after drowning. Which of the following is the best predictor of a good neurologic outcome?

    A. Water temperature <40°C
    B. Short submersion time
    C. Patient age <25
    D. Absence of cyanosis
    E. Glasgow coma scale <10

96. Which of the following is true regarding idiopathic thrombocytopenic purpura (ITP)?

    A. Five-year mortality is 50%.
    B. Aspirin is the treatment of choice in adults.
    C. Treatment in children is usually supportive.
    D. There is a male predominance in adults.
    E. Platelet therapy is indicated in patients with <50,000 cells per mm^3.

97. A 4-year-old male presents with penile pain. His physical examination is shown in Figure 11-15. Which of the following is the correct diagnosis?

    A. Phimosis
    B. Paraphimosis
    C. Balanitis
    D. Testicular torsion
    E. Scrotal hernia

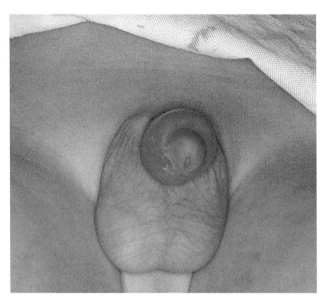

Figure 11-15

98. Which of the following is true regarding acute mesenteric ischemia (AMI)?

    A. Most patients have a lactic acidosis early in the course of their illness.
    B. The mortality rate of AMI is roughly 70%.
    C. In the absence of angiography, intravenous heparin infusion is the standard of management.
    D. Tenderness on physical examination is most often worse than a patient's subjective complaint of pain.
    E. The most common CT finding is gas in the portal venous system.

99. A 13-year-old female is brought to the ED by EMS after a car accident. The patient was the restrained right-sided back-seat passenger within a car that was struck by another vehicle on the same side as her seat. She was extricated by EMS, placed in a cervical collar and on a backboard, and transported to the ED. Upon arrival, her vital signs are HR 164, BP 88/50, T 99.0°F, SaO$_2$ 99% on RA. She is awake and alert but complaining of flank, abdominal, and hip pain. There are abrasions over the right side of her chest and abdomen. A bedside fluid diagnosed by bedside ultrasound (FAST) scan reveals a small amount of fluid in her right upper quadrant. Portable chest x-ray is normal while portable pelvis x-ray reveals a right superior ramus fracture. Which of the following is the next best step?

    A. CT scan
    B. Angiography for pelvic vessel embolization
    C. Take to the operating room (OR)
    D. External fixation of the pelvis
    E. Diagnostic peritoneal lavage (DPL)

100. A 43-year-old male presents with a chief complaint of lower leg pain behind his left ankle. He says he was doing sprints with friends in a morning workout when he felt a sudden "pop" and excruciating pain in the back of the heel. Which of the following examination findings is most sensitive for an Achilles tendon rupture?

    A. Palpation for an Achilles tendon defect
    B. Visualizing ecchymoses and swelling over the Achilles tendon insertion site
    C. Absent passive plantar flexion when the knee is flexed to 90 degrees while the patient is lying prone
    D. Diminished or absent ankle plantar flexion when the calf muscles are squeezed
    E. Tenderness at the Achilles tendon insertion site

ANSWERS AND EXPLANATIONS

1. **Answer D.** Emergency thoracotomy is most useful and successful in patients with penetrating chest wounds who develop traumatic cardiac arrest during or just before the ED resuscitation begins. Patients with pericardial tamponade due to stab wounds have the highest survival rates after ED thoracotomy. In the past, thoracotomies were performed routinely in the ED for traumatic arrest patients. However, concerns about risk to hospital personnel, cost, and low success rates of the procedure have restricted indications for thoracotomy to penetrating chest wounds. Any patient with blunt trauma (even to the chest) is *not* a candidate for ED thoracotomy.

2. **Answer B.** The patient's EKG reveals type I second-degree atrioventricular heart block (Mobitz type I or Wenckebach block). Patients with this type of block experience progressive prolongation of the PR interval before a nonconducted P wave (a P wave that is not followed by a QRS complex). This is usually an asymptomatic, very stable rhythm in young, athletic patients with high vagal tone. However, it may be symptomatic in elderly patients with underlying heart disease who have trouble tolerating the bradycardia that frequently accompanies the rhythm. In such patients, a pacemaker is usually required. This patient suffered a fall, likely as a result of bradycardia and the concomitant relative cerebral hypoperfusion due to type I second-degree atrioventricular heart block. There doesn't appear to be an obvious, reversible cause of his heart block. Given that he has stable vital signs, there is no indication for emergent pacing, or atropine. Amiodarone is not helpful. Kayexalate is not needed to treat the patient's minimal hyperkalemia.

3. **Answer C.** While hyperleukocytosis is a common complication of hematologic malignancies, leukostasis is uncommon except for patients with acute myelogenous leukemia or chronic myelogenous leukemia in blast crisis. When leukostasis occurs, it most commonly affects the lungs and brain. Patients present with shortness of breath and varying degrees of hypoxia (it is important to note that pulse oximetry is a better predictor of arterial O_2 content than blood gases because the large numbers of WBCs remain metabolically active after blood draw and further decrease the O_2, falsely lowering O_2 values during analysis). In addition, patients present with headache, vision and hearing changes, confusion, dizziness, ataxia, and variable degrees of mental status changes. The great majority of patients with hyperleukocytosis and leukostasis also present with fever (~80%), but the fever is only rarely due to an identifiable infectious cause. Since these patients also present with pulmonary infiltrates, it is nearly impossible to differentiate between those with and without infection, so empiric antimicrobial treatment is typically initiated.

4. **Answer D.** Hyperemia and erythema are expected findings upon rewarming frostbitten tissue, but a residual violaceous color is an ominous sign. Positive prognostic signs include a return to normal pliability, early return of normal sensation, and early formation of large clear blebs in the affected area. Persistent firmness of the SQ tissue, lack of edema, or the delayed development of hemorrhagic blebs all portend a worse outcome. (Figure from Sherman SC, Ross C, Nordquist E, et al. *Atlas of Clinical Emergency Medicine.* 1st ed. Philadelphia, PA: Wolters Kluwer; 2015.)

5. **Answer B.** Historically, the evaluation of penetrating neck injuries is based on the zone in which the injury occurs. Zone I is a small area from the sternal notch to the cricoid cartilage. Zone II is the largest and most commonly injured area, extending from the cricoid cartilage to the angle of the mandible. Zone III is another relatively small area which extends above the angle of the mandible to the ear. Traditionally, patients with zone II injuries that are found to violate the platysma upon local exploration are brought to the OR for surgical exploration. However in the absence of other evidence of injury, this leads to a large number of negative surgical explorations and unnecessary added morbidity. Patients with zone I injuries receive a complete workup for tracheal, esophageal, and vascular injury including bronchoscopy, barium swallow, EGD, and a four-vessel angiogram. Though zone III contains the pharynx, the chief concern is a vascular injury, so patients have traditionally received four-vessel angiograms plus additional studies to evaluate the pharynx depending on the extent of the injury. A better approach to evaluating patients with penetrating neck injuries is to evaluate them based on their physical findings and symptoms. There are three broad groups of patients with penetrating neck trauma: Patients with hard signs of vascular or aerodigestive tract injury, patients with soft signs of injury, and asymptomatic patients. Hard signs of vascular injury include significant bleeding, a pulsatile hematoma, an audible bruit or palpable thrill, and hemorrhagic shock or altered mental status secondary to bleeding. Hard signs of aerodigestive tract injury include a gross laceration to the trachea or bubbling in the wound, or blood in the airway or gastrointestinal tract manifested by hemoptysis, or hematemesis. Patients with hard signs of vascular or aerodigestive tract injury are brought to the OR for

further investigation. Most patients, however, have soft signs of injury, that is, a smaller amount of bleeding in the setting of normal blood pressure, no hematoma, mild trouble swallowing or vocal changes, and minimal subcutaneous emphysema. These patients benefit most from CT angiography. CT angiography has replaced the comprehensive workup in most trauma centers because of its speed, the breadth of information obtained, decreased morbidity relative to traditional angiography, and relative ease of patient monitoring. Further evaluation and management is dictated by the findings on CT angiography. Patients who are truly asymptomatic are amenable to primary wound closure and observation. This patient has mild ongoing bleeding. Thus, while there is no pulsatile hematoma or palpable thrill,

there is some risk for an important vascular injury and he should undergo CT angiography (Fig. 11-16). (Figure from Klingensmith M, ed. *The Washington Manual of Surgery.* 7th ed. Philadelphia, PA: Wolters Kluwer; 2015; and adapted from Sperry JL, Moore EE, Coimbra R, et al. Western Trauma Association critical decisions in trauma: penetrating neck trauma. *J Trauma Acute Care Surg.* 2013;75(6):936–940, with permission.)

6. **Answer B.** The patient has clinical signs and symptoms of infectious mononucleosis, usually due to Epstein–Barr virus. The sensitivity of the monospot test is less than 70% during the first week of illness and only about 80% during the second week. Therefore, a negative monospot test in the first 2 weeks of mono does not rule

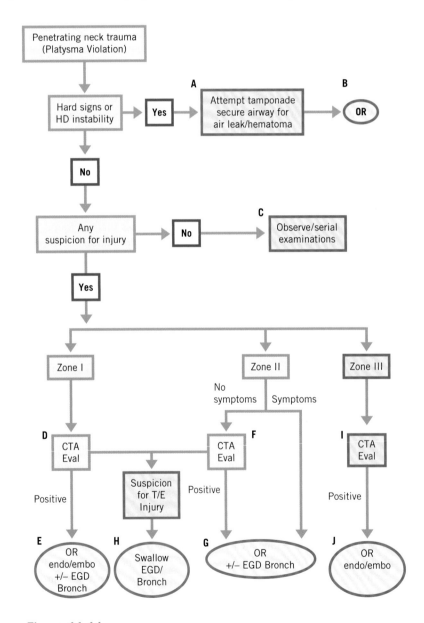

Figure 11-16

out the diagnosis. Group A beta-hemolytic streptococcal pharyngitis usually causes tonsillar exudates and rarely causes splenomegaly. Influenza generally causes a mild pharyngitis without splenomegaly. Herpangina is due to coxsackievirus and causes painful vesicular lesions on the soft palate and tonsils. Diphtheria causes pharyngitis in unvaccinated individuals with a characteristic, grayish-green pseudomembrane that forms when the exudate coalesces. Stridor and frank airway obstruction can form in these cases.

7. **Answer A.** The platysma is the most superficial muscular layer of the neck, as it is sandwiched between the superficial and deep fascia of the neck. There are no vital structures superficial to the platysma. Therefore, patients with penetrating trauma who have an intact platysma can be given local wound care and discharged for routine follow-up. However, although neck wounds may be carefully examined to determine whether the platysma is intact, wounds should never be probed outside of the OR. If, after shallow examination, there is any uncertainty regarding platysma integrity, a surgeon should be consulted for further evaluation and treatment.

8. **Answer E.** The patient has an extremely poor prognosis, given the persistence of PEA despite heroic efforts. An end-tidal CO_2 level of <10 mm Hg at 20 minutes of resuscitation predicted death with 100% accuracy. Cardioversion, either synchronized or unsynchronized (aka defibrillation), has no role in the management of PEA. Vasopressin does not offer any benefit over epinephrine IV and should no longer be used in the management of cardiac arrest. CT brain is not indicated in patients with cardiac arrest—however, if the patient were to have return of spontaneous circulation, then CT brain may be considered to evaluate for the possibility of intracranial hemorrhage.

9. **Answer A.** This patient is presenting with symptoms and findings of balanitis, inflammation of the glans of the penis. When it is accompanied with inflammation of the foreskin, it is called balanoposthitis. In adults, balanitis is frequently a sexually transmitted disease (due primarily to *Chlamydia* and *Neisseria*) or a fungal complication of diabetes (*Candida*). In children, the cause is more often multifactorial but is most commonly associated with poor hygiene among smaller children. In a sexually active adolescent using intermittent protection, the most likely cause is a sexually transmitted disease, and *Chlamydia* is the most common of these. Penile swabs can be obtained for a saline preparation, KOH preparation, group A *Streptococcal* culture, as well as for PCR testing for *Chlamydia* and *Neisseria* to help determine the cause in cases in which it is unclear.

10. **Answer C.** The plant in the picture is the foxglove plant, also known as *Digitalis purpurea*, from which digoxin is derived. Digoxin blocks Na–K ATPase, increasing intracellular sodium, and leading to an increase in intracellular calcium, causing increased cardiac contractility. It is also used as an antidysrhythmic agent, but can cause cardiac dysrhythmias in overdose. Dry mouth is an anticholinergic effect not typically associated with digitalis. Renal and liver failure is seen with other toxins. Altered mental status can occur with digitalis toxicity, but this is less common than cardiac effects. (From Fleisher GR, Ludwig S, Henretig FM, et al., eds. *Textbook of Pediatric Emergency Medicine*. 5th ed. Philadelphia, PA: Lippincott Williams & Wilkins; 2005.)

11. **Answer A.** Nocturnal symptoms point against a diagnosis of irritable bowel syndrome but are common in patients with Crohn disease. Weight loss also points against irritable bowel syndrome but is a less specific complaint. Bilious vomiting is not common in either disease.

12. **Answer B.** There are no clear diagnostic criteria for hyperemesis gravidarum. However, it is generally considered to be nausea and vomiting related to pregnancy that is severe enough to result in weight loss, starvation ketoacidosis, electrolyte imbalance, alkalosis from vomiting, and dehydration. Liver enzymes may be elevated in up to 25% of hospitalized women, although they are not normally increased beyond four times the upper normal limit. This more frequently occurs when hyperthyroidism accompanies hyperemesis. Hyperthyroidism complicating hyperemesis is transient and usually resolves by 14 to 16 weeks of gestation, along with the symptoms of hyperemesis. The elevated levels of thyroid hormone are thought to result from high levels of β-hCG, which is known to stimulate the thyroid-stimulating hormone receptor.

13. **Answer B.** Diverticulitis refers to inflammation and infection of colonic diverticula, which are very common in the Western population (prevalence over 5% in people over 45 and over 75% in people over 85). Uncomplicated diverticulitis refers to disease without frank septic shock, obstruction, abscess, perforation, or necrosis. Most patients with uncomplicated diverticulitis never have a recurrence, though the chance of recurrence increases with younger age at onset of disease. In the Western world, diverticulitis occurs far more commonly in the left (descending) colon; in Japan, right-sided disease is more common. Outpatient antibiotic regimens include ciprofloxacin or trimethoprim–sulfamethoxazole plus metronidazole or amoxicillin–clavulanic acid. High-fiber diets have been shown to reduce both symptoms and chances of recurrence. Barium enema is a

reasonable test to diagnose diverticul*osis* but should never be used in the acute setting of diverticul*itis*.

14. **Answer B.** Emergency thoracotomy is indicated in patients who have traumatic arrest in the ED or shortly before arrival from penetrating thoracic trauma. The initial incision of the chest wall begins in the sternal area and sweeps along the superior border of the rib all the way laterally to the edge of the bed. The rib spreaders are then placed and the left lung is moved out of the way to expose the pericardium. An incision to the pericardium should be made anterior to the prominent phrenic nerve, which is visible in the figure. Damage to the phrenic nerve may cause diaphragmatic weakness and seriously impair respiratory function. (Figure courtesy of Mark Silverberg, MD. In: Greenberg MI, Hendrickson RG, Silverberg M, et al. *Greenberg's Text-Atlas of Emergency Medicine*. Philadelphia, PA: Lippincott Williams & Wilkins; 2004:22.)

15. **Answer A.** Optic (CN II) neuritis is a very common manifestation in patients with MS, and its development often heralds the onset of MS. Oculomotor (CN III) neuropathy causes ptosis, inability to move the eye superiorly or medially, and often pupillary dilation. Trochlear (CN IV) neuropathy causes inability to move the eye inferolaterally. Abducens (CN VI) neuropathy causes inability to move the eye laterally. Facial (CN VII) neuropathy causes facial paralysis and taste and hearing changes.

16. **Answer B.** Silver nitrate sticks should not be applied to both sides of the septum to avoid possible septal perforation. Silver nitrate sticks will *not* work if active bleeding is present. They are best reserved for raw areas of nasal mucosa to which topical vasoconstrictor agents (such as cocaine or phenylephrine) have already been applied. Blowing the nose is essential before placement of any packing material to remove any clot that would prevent effective packing of a site of continuous bleeding. Cephalexin or amoxicillin–clavulanate is generally used prophylactically in patients with any nasal packing; TMP-SMX or azithromycin may be used in the penicillin-allergic patient. Admission is always indicated in patients with a posterior pack.

17. **Answer A.** The single most common identifiable cause of seizures in human immunodeficiency virus (HIV)/AIDS patients is toxoplasmosis, which causes seizures through mass effect. Other mass lesions such as malignancy and abscess are additional causes. In cases that are not due to any identifiable cause, HIV-encephalopathy is postulated to be the etiology. Meningitis, usually cryptococcal, is the second most common identifiable cause. Electrolyte abnormalities, stroke, and neurosyphilis are less commonly implicated.

18. **Answer E.** Patients with spinal stenosis are often elderly and constitute a small minority of patients with low back pain. Most patients present with subacute or chronic pain that frequently mimics symptoms of vascular claudication (often termed *neurogenic intermittent claudication*). This is problematic because vascular claudication strikes the same population. Symptoms of neurogenic intermittent claudication include buttock pain, which frequently radiates to the thighs and lower legs as well as cramping, paresthesias, back pain, and difficulty walking. In contrast to patients with vascular claudication, however, patients with spinal stenosis typically maintain a forward-leaning posture to reduce symptoms. In addition, patients are better able to walk uphill than downhill. Sitting also improves symptoms, which helps to differentiate patients with spinal stenosis from patients with disk herniation. Although patients may have involvement at several lumbar levels, L5 is most commonly involved (75%) followed by L4, L3, and L2.

19. **Answer D.** Patients with a combination of hypotension and pelvic fracture have extremely high mortality and should be managed aggressively. Initial stabilization involves securing the pelvis with a bedsheet or tightening device to reduce the volume into which hemorrhage can occur and copious crystalloid and blood resuscitation. If the patient stabilizes, further evaluation with CT scan may be performed to better delineate the injuries. However, if the patient remains unstable, angiography with embolization should be performed to limit the extent of hemorrhage. As a general rule, hemodynamically unstable trauma patients should *never* have CT scans performed.

20. **Answer E.** Nearly all patients with venous thromboembolism have elevated D-dimer levels. Therefore, assays measuring D-dimer levels have proliferated as they are a highly sensitive but poorly specific screening test for pulmonary embolism (PE). Due to its elevation in numerous other scenarios, an elevated D-dimer level can never be used as proof of the presence of a pulmonary embolus. However, because of the high sensitivity of most D-dimer assays (sensitivity varies depending on the assay used), normal D-dimer levels can safely rule out the presence of a pulmonary embolus in very low-risk patients.

21. **Answer A.** This patient is in severe septic shock. Pediatric patients with shock should first receive aggressive IV fluid resuscitation with three boluses of normal saline at 20 mL/kg per bolus, for a total of 60 mL/kg of fluid. Patients who do not respond to this fluid infusion are said to be "fluid refractory" and require vasopressors. However, vasopressors can be considered and used before 60 mL/kg fluid is infused. The choice of agent depends

on the patient's circulatory status. Patients in "warm shock" have high cardiac output (CO) and low systemic vascular resistance (SVR), which results in bounding peripheral pulses, and warm extremities (hypotensive, vasodilated). Such patients need to increase their SVR, so norepinephrine is used. Patients with cold shock, such as *this* patient, have low CO and high SVR, leading to diminished peripheral pulses and cool, cyanotic, or mottled extremities (hypotensive, vasoconstricted). These patients are in a more advanced stage of shock relative to patients with warm shock. The priority in such patients is to increase CO without affecting SVR, so epinephrine is used. It is often impossible to differentiate the "stage" of shock, and dopamine is often used as the first-line agent, though it is best used in patients who are normotensive with evidence of poor peripheral perfusion. The phosphodiesterase inhibitors, such as milrinone, provide increased inotropic support and may be used as adjuncts but should not be used as monotherapy.

22. **Answer D.** A 2015 meta-analysis by Siemieniuk et al. found that time to clinical stability, hospital length of stay, and development of ARDS were all reduced when adjunctive corticosteroid therapy was given with antibiotics for hospitalized patients with community-acquired pneumonia. The study did not find a statistically significant reduction in mortality, although the trend was in that direction (relative risk 0.67, 95% CI 0.45 to 1.01). Predictably, corticosteroid use was associated with hyperglycemic episodes. Further study will be needed before corticosteroids are prescribed in protocolized fashion for patients with community-acquired pneumonia. Oseltamivir is used to treat influenza, but is not indicated in patients without relevant signs. N-acetylcysteine is used to manage acetaminophen overdose and may have some promise as a general free radical treatment, but this has yet to be proven. Albumin is useful in patients with spontaneous bacterial peritonitis, but not in pneumonia. Lactulose is used to present hyperammonemia in patients with cirrhosis. (Siemieniuk et al. Ann Int Med, 2015.)

23. **Answer C.** Lung abscesses are usually a consequence of aspiration of contaminated oropharyngeal flora. Therefore, the same population of patients who are at risk for aspiration are also at risk for the development of a lung abscess. Risk factors include any syndrome that results in depressed levels of consciousness and consequently increases the risk of aspiration such as alcoholism, massive stroke, head trauma, seizures, and anesthesia. Patients with poor oral hygiene are particularly susceptible because of the increased numbers of organisms among their oral flora. Still, lung abscesses develop in a scant minority of patients who aspirate contaminated oral flora. Although immunocompromised patients are also at risk, the HIV+ patient with a CD4+ T-cell count >200 is unlikely to develop a lung abscess. Although drug abuse may lead to depressed levels of consciousness, IV drug use puts patients at greater risk for infectious complications related to poor skin sterilization techniques, such as endocarditis, phlebitis, or other local skin infections. It also increases the risk of pneumonia due to *S. Aureus*, which rarely causes necrotizing pneumonia. Patients with Parkinson disease may have significant dementia, but it is primarily a motor disease that should not initially put patients at high risk for aspiration.

24. **Answer A.** The Centor criteria, which have been validated in several trials, are most useful to rule out GAS as the cause of pharyngitis. In several trials, patients with none of the four Centor criteria were found to have had only a 2.5% chance of having a positive throat culture for GAS. In contrast, patients with all four criteria were found to have a 56% chance of having a positive throat culture. Furthermore, as the complications of GAS infection are less common in adults than in children, it seems reasonable that the goal of treating low-risk patients should be symptomatic relief rather than the prevention of adverse sequelae. The four Centor criteria are the presence of fever (before the use of antipyretics), the absence of cough, tender anterior cervical lymphadenopathy, and the presence of exudative tonsillitis. McIsaac et al. modified the score such that patients younger than 15 years old receive an extra point, although a point is subtracted from patients who are older than 45. When these data are applied, patients with a score of 0 to 1 have a 1% chance of having a positive throat culture. In this case (a 22-year-old female), no modification of her Centor score occurs. Properly implemented throat cultures have a sensitivity >90%. Posterior cervical lymphadenopathy, nonexudative tonsillitis, and atypical lymphocytes are all features of Epstein–Barr virus (EBV) infection, also known as *infectious mononucleosis*. The presence of a cough, along with other "viral" symptoms such as rhinorrhea and conjunctivitis, also make GAS less likely.

25. **Answer B.** Fat embolism can occur after fracture of any long bone, usually in the lower extremities. Fat droplets from the bone marrow reach the systemic circulation and can embolize to the lungs, brain, eyes, and extremity microvasculature. Respiratory distress, altered mental status, fever, and petechiae commonly occur. Diagnosis is aimed at ruling out other causes of symptoms, and treatment is primarily supportive. Meningococcemia can occur acutely and cause altered mental status and petechiae, but the history of the leg fracture and the respiratory distress point away from this. PE due to thrombus can occur in the post-trauma patient but usually occurs later in the course of the recovery. Pneumothorax and pneumonia in a previously healthy patient are unlikely to cause altered mental status or petechiae.

26. **Answer A.** The onset of renal insufficiency, serum sickness-like signs and symptoms, and eosinophilia points to allergic interstitial nephritis as the most likely cause. A hypersensitivity reaction to various drugs is the usual cause—penicillins, NSAIDs, sulfa drugs, phenytoin, and diuretics are most commonly implicated. Macrolides and tetracyclines are less often involved. Interstitial nephritis may also be due to infectious and immunologic causes. Urinalysis generally demonstrates sterile pyuria with possible hematuria and mild proteinuria. Eosinophilia occurs in approximately half the number of patients. Definitive diagnosis is by kidney biopsy. Renal insufficiency due to allergic interstitial nephritis is usually reversible, and treatment always involves removal of the offending drug.

27. **Answer C.** Mushroom poisonings are divided into the seven major toxins responsible for the pathologic effects:

Mushroom toxin	Pathologic effect
Amatoxin	Hepatotoxicity
Coprine	Disulfiram like
Gyromitrin	Seizures
Ibotenic acid	Anticholinergic
Muscarine	Cholinergic
Orellanine	Nephrotoxicity
Psilocybin	Hallucinations (drug of abuse)

28. **Answer C.** Condyloma acuminatum is a sexually transmitted disease caused by human papillomavirus (HPV). It is usually found in the genital area but may be found elsewhere. It most commonly occurs in young men. It typically starts as small, pedunculated papules that are 2 to 3 mm in diameter and 10 to 20 mm long. They may occur as single papule or in clusters may develop into large, cauliflower-like masses. The surface is dry and highly keratinized, and they are typically asymptomatic unless they become superinfected. In contrast, condyloma lata, which is caused by *T. pallidum* (syphilis), is a weeping, wart-like lesion that emits a foul odor. The two are easily distinguishable clinically and neither lesion has bluish telangiectasias.

29. **Answer E.** Chest tubes should generally be placed in the third or fourth intercostal space during pregnancy and should never be placed lower than the fourth intercostal space. Since the diaphragm elevates approximately 4 cm during pregnancy, there is an increased risk of abdominal placement of chest tubes if they are placed in the typical fifth intercostal space. As in nonpregnant women, the midaxillary line is the least muscular area of the chest wall, which makes it an ideal location for chest tube insertion. Fetal evaluation should always be delayed until maternal evaluation, treatment, and stabilization, even in the setting of obvious fetal distress. (Figure reprinted with permission from Harwood-Nuss A. *The Clinical Practice of Emergency Medicine.* Philadelphia, PA: Lippincott Williams & Wilkins; 2005.)

30. **Answer E.** Tricyclic antidepressants cause *blockade* of the following: α-1, muscarinic, histamine, GABA, cardiac potassium efflux, fast sodium channel, serotonin reuptake, and norepinephrine reuptake. Because of these effects and the potential for lethality in overdose, they are no longer indicated as first-line therapy for the management of major depression.

31. **Answer B.** Cerebral herniation syndromes are a result of severely increased intracranial pressure (ICP), usually because of trauma. Herniation occurs when the increased ICP causes movement of various parts of the brain across fixed structures, such as the falx cerebri (dividing left from right), tentorium cerebella (dividing the cortex from the brainstem and cerebellum), or foramen magnum (dividing intracranial from extracranial structures). Mortality is virtually 100% in untreated patients. Uncal herniation is the most common type, in which the ipsilateral temporal lobe is compressed against the tentorium cerebella and subsequently puts pressure on the underlying brainstem. The initial clinical manifestation is oculomotor nerve injury, causing ipsilateral ptosis, oculomotor dysfunction, and mydriasis. As herniation progresses, contralateral hemiparesis occurs and the contralateral uncus is compressed, leading to bilateral decorticate posturing. Ultimately, uncal herniation often progresses further until the brainstem herniates, causing respiratory failure and death.

32. **Answer D.** Although A, B, C, and E all confer an increased risk of lenticular dislocation, trauma as a whole is the most common cause. Marfan syndrome is the most common cause of inherited lenticular dislocation. Glaucoma and retinal detachment may complicate lens dislocation and must be managed in concert with an ophthalmologist. Iridectomy or lensectomy may be indicated in some cases.

33. **Answer D.** Endocarditis in intravenous drug users (IVDUs) is different from that in nondrug users in several ways: Patients are generally younger, almost universally have fever, and have more pulmonary symptoms due to right-heart vegetations causing septic emboli to the lungs. Although *S. aureus* is a far more common cause of endocarditis in IVDUs, it has less mortality among this patient population. Heart murmurs are less commonly heard in endocarditis in IVDUs because the tricuspid valve, the most common valve affected, is difficult to hear on physical examination. Splinter

hemorrhages and Roth spots are, if anything, less common in right-heart endocarditis as the lungs will filter most septic emboli.

34. **Answer C.** This patient suffered a complete avulsion of his left maxillary central incisor as well as luxation injuries to his right maxillary central incisor and left maxillary lateral incisor. Luxation injuries, in which the teeth are loose and out of position, are more common than complete avulsion injuries, in which the teeth are removed from their socket. Most subluxed teeth will passively return to their anatomic position but patients should be urgently referred to a dentist for teeth that are substantially angulated or displaced. Completely avulsed primary teeth should not be reimplanted, even if present, because doing so risks injuring the developing secondary teeth. In the absence of a severe intrusion injury, in which the teeth are subluxed toward the developing secondary teeth, a CAT scan is unnecessary. Even in the setting of significant intrusion injuries, often a panoramic x-ray (Panorex) is more than adequate to evaluate the underlying teeth and alveolar bone. When alveolar bone fractures are present in the setting of most dental trauma, they are rarely significant and rarely require operative fixation. However, intrusion injuries are more severe than avulsion injuries because of the risk they pose to the development of the secondary teeth. Dental avulsion injuries do not permanently interfere with speech production.

35. **Answer C.** Head trauma accounts for the large majority of all pediatric traumatic deaths. Children's heads are proportionally larger and heavier relative to the rest of their bodies than adults and are more likely to be seriously injured. The PECARN investigators have established the following criteria as low risk in head injured patients <2 years old:

Normal mental status

Normal behavior per routine caregiver

No LOC

No severe mechanism of injury (fall >3 feet, head struck by high impact object, MVC with ejection, death or rollover, pedestrian vs auto)

No nonfrontal scalp hematoma

No evidence of skull fracture

Since this patient is behaving abnormally and fell >3 feet, a CT scan should be performed to evaluate for intracranial injury. Controversy exists as to whether brief LOC should be considered as a sole indication for CT scan in the older child, but in the infant it is an accepted indication given the difficulty of neurologic examination. The EP should always consider contacting DCFS in cases of suspected child abuse, but a clear, consistent history with a normal physical examination is less likely to have

high potential for abuse. Skull x-rays are almost never indicated in head trauma as they do not often change management and require further testing with CT scan anyway if abnormal. MRI offers little benefit over CT scan in the acute setting and is much more technically difficult in the infant. Discharging the patient home without CT scan or serial neurologic examinations is not recommended.

36. **Answer B.** This patient is infected with *Giardia lamblia*, the most common enteric parasite infection worldwide. It is most commonly acquired through drinking contaminated water. However, food-borne and person-to-person transmissions also occur. Backpackers frequently contract the illness after drinking inadequately treated or untreated stream water that is contaminated by animal or human fecal matter. The diarrheal illness is therefore often known as *backpacker's diarrhea*. Giardiasis is a noninflammatory, noninvasive diarrhea, so leukocytes are not seen in stool samples. Instead, diagnosis relies on the detection of trophozoites or cysts ("ova and parasites") in stool specimens. Detection of ova and parasites varies from 60% to 80% after a single stool to greater than 90% after three stools. However, when the clinical history is consistent with giardiasis, a diagnosis can be made presumptively. To prevent chronic infection as well as person-to-person transmission, both symptomatic and asymptomatic patients should be treated. The treatment of choice is metronidazole 250 mg t.i.d. for 7 days and is generally well tolerated.

37. **Answer A.** The spider shown is the black widow spider, also known as *Latrodectus mactans*. Bites from this spider can cause severe muscle spasms, including in the abdominal wall, leading to the term "pseudo-peritoneal signs." Most bites do not cause such severe muscle spasms and mild to moderate symptoms can be treated symptomatically with analgesics and benzodiazepines. Severe envenomations, heralded by severe spasms and vomiting, can be treated with antivenom. Although very effective at alleviating symptoms, antivenom does carry with it the risks of anaphylaxis, allergic reaction, and serum sickness. Hemodialysis is not usually needed for black widow spider bites. Plastic surgery consultation may be pursued in the outpatient setting for brown recluse spider bites which have caused the characteristic necrotic lesion. A negative inspiratory force (NIF) assessment is used to determine the degree of diaphragmatic weakness and respiratory failure in cases of Guillain–Barre syndrome and elapid snake or scorpion envenomations. A normal NIF is 60 cm water; <20 indicates significant respiratory muscle weakness portending respiratory failure. (Figure from Schalock PC, Hsu JT, Arndt KA, eds. *Lippincott's Primary Care Dermatology*. Philadelphia, PA: Lippincott Williams & Williams; 2010.)

38. Answer C. Patients with complete knee instability after significant trauma are suspicious for having a knee dislocation. The knee can spontaneously relocate and be mistaken for a severe sprain with large effusion. The popliteal artery is at high risk for damage, and angiography should be performed in every patient with knee dislocation. The presence of pulses in the foot does not rule out popliteal artery injury, as up to 10% of patients with popliteal injury will have intact peripheral pulses. The most common nerve injury in knee dislocation is the peroneal nerve, which may be tested with foot dorsiflexion and dorsal foot sensation.

39. Answer D. The patient has evidence of Ludwig angina, a cellulitis of the connective tissues of the mouth and neck. The most commonly affected teeth are the molars—usually lower and posterior. Although odontogenic infection is the most common cause, trauma or oral malignancy may also predispose to the condition. Ludwig angina is usually polymicrobial, and the most common species are *Streptococci*, *Staphylococci*, and *Bacteroides*. Airway obstruction is the number one cause of mortality, which may be as high as 10% even in the presence of adequate therapy. Standard oral endotracheal intubation and cricothyroidotomy may be difficult given the edema, secretions, and friability of tissues. Treatment involves high-dose penicillin, clindamycin, or broader-spectrum agents such as piperacillin–tazobactam or ampicillin–sulbactam. The role of steroids is not clearly defined at this time. Intensive care admission should be initiated and ENT should be consulted to address possible tracheostomy placement.

40. Answer C. The shock index (SI) is a simple tool that can be used to quickly identify patients in shock. A shock index of 0.5 to 0.7 is considered normal while a shock index ≥0.9 is predictive of increased mortality and morbidity. The SI also has value in trauma patients, as an SI ≥0.9 doubles the risk of a massive transfusion and dramatically increases the risk of mortality.

41. Answer D. Approximately 10% of patients with ventricular tachycardia (VT) are responsive to adenosine. Fortunately, adenosine-sensitive VT tends to be more stable than other forms of VT and less commonly leads to sudden cardiac death. Still, it is important to recognize that an undifferentiated wide-complex tachycardia should be treated as VT rather than supraventricular tachycardia (SVT) with aberrancy. The patient's stability does not increase the likelihood of SVT or decrease the likelihood of VT.

42. Answer B. Coumadin directly inhibits vitamin-K–mediated synthesis of the following factors: II, VII, IX, and X. Indirect inhibition of factor I (fibrin) also occurs due to the downstream effects of reduced levels of factor II (prothrombin). The prothrombin time is prolonged in patients who are taking coumadin and is used to track therapeutic anticoagulation.

43. Answer E. Because cerebral perfusion pressure (CPP) = mean arterial pressure (MAP) − intracranial pressure (ICP), acute reductions in the MAP may have drastic and potentially grave effects on a patient's CPP. One of the most common errors in the treatment of patients with ischemic strokes is the overly aggressive treatment of hypertension. Because this patient is not a candidate for tPA (because she presented >3 hours after the onset of her symptoms), the general consensus is that her hypertension does not warrant treatment unless her blood pressure is >220/120 mm Hg or her MAP is >130 mm Hg. If this is the case, then either nitroprusside, labetalol, or IV enalapril may be used to rapidly gain control of the patient's blood pressure. Additionally, in patients who are tPA candidates, these medicines can be used to bring a patient's blood pressure below the 185/105 mm Hg threshold required for the administration of tPA. Exceptions to this approach may also apply in patients with ischemic stroke and concomitant myocardial infarction (MI), aortic dissection, or acute renal failure due to malignant hypertension. Such patients may require emergent interventions to decrease blood pressure due to these concomitant conditions. In all other patients with acute ischemic stroke, moderate hypertension as defined in the preceding text is thought to be neuroprotective by maintaining adequate CPP. Nimodipine is a calcium antagonist that is used in patients with subarachnoid hemorrhage (SAH), and it has been shown to improve outcome in such patients. Whether it exerts its protective effects by reducing vasospasm is still an object of study.

44. Answer C. In the setting of SIADH, hypertonic saline (3%) must be given in order to correct hyponatremia. When isotonic normal saline is given (0.9%), the body "desalinates" it, delivering the salt to the kidneys to make concentrated urine, retaining the free water, and worsening the hyponatremia. Therefore, in symptomatic patients with critical hyponatremia (sodium <120 mmol/L), hypertonic saline must be given. However, fluid restriction is the mainstay of treatment for more mild reductions in plasma sodium. Neoplasms are the most common cause of SIADH and small cell lung carcinoma is the most common neoplasm associated with the disorder.

45. Answer C. Patients with penetrating injuries just lateral to the spine often have incomplete cord injury, usually causing hemisection of the cord, known as *Brown–Sequard syndrome*. Neurologic findings include loss of ipsilateral motor function and vibratory/position

sensation and contralateral pain/temperature sensation distal to the injury. The fibers carrying pain/temperature sensation decussate (cross) a few levels after they enter the cord from the periphery, so contralateral findings are observed. The fibers carrying motor axons and vibratory/position sensation do not decussate until high in the spinal cord, so ipsilateral findings predominate. The functional outcome for patients with cord hemisection is favorable overall with few patients losing bowel, bladder, or ambulatory function.

46. **Answer E.** ARDS is a type of noncardiogenic pulmonary edema caused by a variety of systemic and direct pulmonary stressors, most commonly sepsis, usually pneumonia. It is characterized by bilateral patchy infiltrates, absence of cardiogenic etiology, and decreased response to supplemental oxygen. By definition, ARDS is acute in onset. Cardiomegaly may be concomitant, but ARDS implies that left ventricular failure is not present. In ARDS, PaO_2 to FiO_2 ratio is *less than* 200, indicating that the hypoxemia is poorly responsive to supplemental oxygen. A pulmonary artery wedge pressure >18 mm Hg would imply cardiogenic cause due to left ventricular failure—this is not characteristic of ARDS.

47. **Answer C.** The patient has acute angle closure glaucoma. The history of ambient light suddenly decreasing and forcing rapid pupillary dilatation is classic. Patients with glaucoma may often complain of headache, nausea, vomiting, and abdominal pain without any specific ocular symptoms. Bilateral shallow anterior chambers are the specific anatomic abnormality predisposing to closure of aqueous outflow—pilocarpine is therefore administered to both eyes (either eye has an equal chance of being affected by the acute angle closure). Boxcar retinal venules are characteristically seen in central retinal artery occlusion. Although emergent ophthalmologic consultation is required, all modalities for treatment of a severe glaucoma attack should be initiated early—pilocarpine, timolol, apraclonidine, prednisolone, acetazolamide, and mannitol. Intravenous medications may be withheld if intraocular pressures are not severely elevated. Sedatives and antiemetics are used as needed. Ocular massage is absolutely contraindicated, as this will increase intraocular pressure.

48. **Answer C.** Pontine hemorrhage may result in an initial coma, probably because of disruption of the reticular activating system. Patients who later awake may be "locked in," a state in which they experience total paralysis, pinpoint pupils and speechlessness secondary to severe dysarthria. In patients who survive the insult, locked in syndrome is the most severe outcome. More commonly, patients suffer from total paralysis, miotic pupils, and loss of horizontal gaze.

49. **Answer D.** The patient is not responding to initial therapy for COPD exacerbation. She is in moderate respiratory distress but has a normal mental status. In patients with COPD, noninvasive positive pressure ventilation is an excellent alternative to endotracheal intubation and mechanical ventilation. It reduces the risk of endotracheal intubation, ICU length of stay, and overall hospital length of stay. Azithromycin adds little to fluoroquinolone coverage for common pathogens in COPD exacerbations. Vancomycin is used to treat methicillin-resistant *S. aureus*, but this would not be suspected in a patient without frank pneumonia or nosocomial exposure. Aminophylline is a phosphodiesterase inhibitor that is used in asthma exacerbations but is not as effective in COPD exacerbations.

50. **Answer D.** The EKG demonstrates a pre-excitation pattern. Leads V_1 through V_6 exhibit a gradual sloping of the QRS complex (delta wave) combined with a shortened PR interval. The most common type of pre-excitation is Wolff–Parkinson–White (WPW) syndrome. Patients have an accessory conductive pathway from the atria to the ventricles, which pre-excites the ventricular myocytes before the AV node releases the normal sinoatrial depolarization. As a result, patients with WPW have a shortened PR interval and a delayed QRS upstroke, called the *delta wave*. Patients with WPW syndrome can have reentrant dysrhythmias, in which the accessory pathway can either conduct retrograde (in which the AV node conducts in the normal direction, producing a narrow QRS complex and an "orthodromic" pattern) or anterograde (in which the AV node conducts backward, producing a wide QRS complex and an "antidromic" pattern). A patient with WPW syndrome, tachycardia, and wide QRS complexes suggests the presence of an antidromic conduction pattern (where the accessory pathway conducts anterograde and the AV node conducts retrograde). Selective AV nodal active agents are contraindicated in this circumstance, as inhibition of the AV node will cause faster conduction through the anterograde accessory pathway, which is already at high risk for degeneration into an unstable rhythm. The treatment of choice in stable antidromic or irregular tachycardias in patients with WPW is amiodarone or procainamide. Unstable patients require cardioversion.

51. **Answer A.** Noroviruses, which include Norwalk virus, are responsible for 50% to 80% of all cases of acute infectious diarrhea. However, most patients with acute infectious diarrhea do not seek medical treatment. Patients who seek medical attention are more likely to have a bacterial cause, most commonly *Campylobacter* spp.

52. **Answer A.** Hepatitis B infection is the most common viral cause of acute liver failure. However, worldwide,

acetaminophen toxicity is the most common overall cause. Idiopathic causes are probably the third most frequent cause of liver failure.

53. **Answer B.** The right coronary artery supplies the AV node in >80% of patients, and the left circumflex artery supplies the AV node in the rest.

54. **Answer E.** For any patient with acute urinary retention, the goal is to find the cause of urinary obstruction and correct it as rapidly as possible. In this case, as in the majority of older men, the most likely cause is benign prostatic hypertrophy (BPH). Pain and distension in the suprapubic area indicates bladder distention from a more distal obstruction. The correct management is to urgently place a Foley catheter to temporarily stent open the prostatic urethra and decompress the bladder. Any imaging and blood studies may follow this initial management, but should not delay relief of the obstruction. Further management usually involves a basic chemistry panel to assess kidney function, urinalysis to look for concomitant infection, and outpatient urology follow-up.

55. **Answer B.** Patients with spontaneous bacterial peritonitis (SBP) may benefit from early therapy with IV albumin. This benefit may also extend to prevention of renal impairment. Antifungal therapy may be helpful if patients exhibit signs of infection in the face of aggressive antibacterial therapy. Vancomycin is often used for catheter-associated peritonitis, but is less useful to treat the gram-negative infections usually seen in SBP. Oseltamivir could be used in this patient to treat influenza, but the patient has no signs or symptoms suggestive of this. Midodrine, an alpha-agonist, is often used to maintain blood pressure in hypotensive patients with end-stage cirrhosis, but there was no history suggestive of this in the scenario. (Annals Apr 2016)

56. **Answer E.** Most patients suffering from peptic ulcer perforation are elderly, and NSAID use is involved in roughly 50% of cases. Smoking is the leading risk factor for perforation among young patients. Cocaine use may lead to perforation of ulcers of the juxtapyloric region, possibly because of vasoconstriction or vascular thrombosis. The pain of peptic ulcer perforation is classically described in three stages. Initially, patients present with severe, diffuse abdominal pain and may present with signs of shock. After minutes to hours, this phase tends to resolve and patients begin to look and feel better and may have normal vital signs. However, they will nearly always have signs of peritonitis upon physical examination. Most notably, patients will have a rigid, tender abdomen, and signs of pelvic peritoneal inflammation (assessed by a rectal examination). The final stage is characterized by worsening abdominal pain, abdominal distension, and

signs of sepsis. Only ~2/3 of patients will have evidence of intraperitoneal free air on upright chest or abdominal radiography. Insufflating 50 mL of air through an NG tube before x-ray improves sensitivity. Treatment includes IV antibiotics, IV fluids, IV PPIs, and an NG tube. Endoscopy is contraindicated because the insufflation of air may open a spontaneously closed perforation.

57. **Answer A.** Temporal arteritis (or giant cell arteritis) is a large vessel vasculitis that primarily affects branches of the carotid artery. The disease is rare before the age of 50, and incidence peaks in the seventh decade. The most sensitive finding is a new headache, whereas the most specific finding is jaw claudication. However, the disease often presents vaguely with systemic symptoms such as a fever of unknown origin, fatigue, malaise, and anorexia. The diagnosis should be considered in any older person with fever of unknown origin. Scalp pain is a more specific finding than headache, particularly when localized over the temporal artery. Vertigo is not a manifestation of the disease. Permanent visual loss occurs in only 15% of patients and is usually preceded by the development of blurring, diplopia, or amaurosis fugax. Corticosteroids are the treatment of choice and should never be withheld if the diagnosis is seriously considered. Multiple studies have demonstrated that treatment with steroids does not affect the accuracy of biopsy if performed within a few weeks.

58. **Answer A.** The patient has evidence of whooping cough caused by *B. pertussis*, a gram-negative coccobacillus. According to the CDC's definition, whooping cough should be considered in the absence of a more likely diagnosis when a patient has a "cough illness" lasting >2 weeks with one of the following symptoms: Paroxysms of coughing, or inspiratory "whoop," or posttussive vomiting, or apnea in infants <1 year. The disease occurs in three phases—the catarrhal phase, a nonspecific URI-like syndrome lasting 1 to 2 weeks; the paroxysmal phase lasting up to 1 month, with paroxysms of coughing fits; and the convalescent phase lasting up to several months, with a chronic, intermittent cough. Antibiotic therapy with macrolides is usually only effective in the catarrhal phase, but should be given to patients to reduce the high degree of contagiousness. Cultures are useful only in the catarrhal phase, and have low sensitivity during the paroxysmal phase. Mortality is low and usually due to superinfection, most commonly from pneumonia.

59. **Answer A.** Desmopressin (dDAVP) is thought to work by promoting the release of large factor VIII:von Willebrand factor multimers from endothelial cells to promote platelet function. It is fast acting, easy to administer, and effective. While hemodialysis provides a better long-term solution in uremic patients, dDAVP is a much

more effective short-term solution. Given its mechanism, dDAVP can also be used for patients with hemophilia A or von Willebrand disease with mild bleeding. Prothrombin complex concentrates (either 4-factor or 3-factor) are alternatives to fresh frozen plasma in patients with vitamin-K antagonist (e.g., warfarin) associated bleeding. Thrombocytopenia-associated bleeding should be treated with a platelet transfusion. Recombinant factor VIII is used to treat patients with hemophilia A (who have factor VIII deficiency) as opposed to hemophilia B (who have factor IX deficiency). Recombinant von Willebrand factor (VWF) is not appropriate for hemophilia A patients in the absence of recombinant factor VIII.

60. **Answer B.** The officer's sudden collapse in the setting of a gaseous "rotten egg" smell strongly suggests the presence of hydrogen sulfide. The use of hydrogen sulfide as a relatively easy, painless means to commit suicide has gained popularity in recent years. At low concentrations, hydrogen sulfide may cause only minor irritation, cough, and a sensation of dyspnea. At higher levels, hydrogen sulfide inhibits mitochondrial cytochrome oxidase, which uncouples electron transport and terminates cellular respiration. This has profound, rapid effects on the nervous system and quickly leads to coma. Patients who remain awake will often improve after being moved to an area with uncontaminated air and with supplemental oxygen. More severely affected patients require aggressive supportive care (ventilation) and specific treatment with sodium nitrite, which induces methemoglobinemia. As in patients with cyanide intoxication, induction of methemoglobinemia is helpful by providing an alternative binding site for hydrogen sulfide. The combination of hydroxycobalamin (direct cyanide binding) and sodium thiosulfate (enhanced cyanide detoxification) is the treatment of choice for cyanide poisoning. They are not effective in treating hydrogen sulfide poisoning. Methylene blue is used to treat methemoglobinemia. Succimer (meso-2,3-dimercaptosuccinic acid) is an adjunctive treatment for lead poisoning.

61. **Answer D.** Patients with mild essential hypertension will often exhibit rises in their blood pressure if they use systemic decongestants as symptomatic relief for upper respiratory infections. This patient should be counseled specifically to avoid decongestants for this reason. Starting oral antihypertensive therapy in this patient is not warranted given the lack of severe hypertension, the presence of next-day follow-up, and the possibility of side effects or supratherapeutic effect. Cardiology referral for essential hypertension in an otherwise healthy 34-year-old male is not indicated. Sugar intake reduction, while laudable, will not have a significant immediate effect on the patient's blood

pressure (reduction in salt intake would certainly be recommended).

62. **Answer B.** The patient has pleuritic chest pain, shortness of breath, and sinus tachycardia, indicating that he is at some risk for PE. The presence of pleuritic chest pain in the setting of a pleural effusion in a young patient without signs of CHF, pneumonia, or malignancy is most commonly due to PE. D-dimer can be used as a risk stratification test for PE. Blood cultures are rarely helpful in previously healthy patients with dyspnea even with established diagnosis of pneumonia. Gastrointestinal cocktail is only helpful for therapeutic management of gastroesophageal reflux disease or peptic ulcer disease and should never be used as a diagnostic maneuver. The differential diagnosis in this patient includes atypical pneumonia, such as from *Mycoplasma* species. Amoxicillin–clavulanic acid does not adequately cover atypical organisms and should not be used in this case, due the absence of crackles, fever, or focal infiltrate on chest x-ray. Right-sided EKGs are helpful in evaluation of a right-sided MI to assess for right ventricular involvement.

63. **Answer E.** There is a dearth of data regarding pediatric patients with VPS infections. However, several studies have suggested that as many as one-third of patients may present with nonspecific clinical findings. The risk of infection is highest in the first 6 months after insertion or instrumentation (in the case of revision). In addition, patients younger than 4 years old and older than 61 years old have been shown to be at increased risk of infection. LP should never be performed without first obtaining a CT scan and reviewing the findings with a neurosurgeon. The mortality of VPS infection is roughly 30% to 40%. As many as one-third of patients with VPS infection may present with signs and symptoms of obstruction or VPS failure with or without a fever. These include hydrocephalus, papilledema, hypertension with concomitant bradycardia, and irregular respirations (Cushing response), personality changes, ataxia, and cranial nerve palsies. Over 80% of patients with a VPS infection have peripheral leukocytosis.

64. **Answer E.** Organophosphates bind to and inhibit acetylcholinesterase, causing a cholinergic syndrome of systemic hypersecretion: Bronchorrhea, diarrhea, lacrimation, salivation, emesis, and incontinence. Effects on HR are variable. Mortality from organophosphate overdose is usually due to hypoxia from excessive bronchorrhea. Treatment involves high-dose atropine—the endpoint of atropine therapy is the reduction of bronchial secretions. Tachycardia and hypertension are not indications to stop atropine therapy. Over time, the binding of organophosphates to acetylcholinesterase

becomes irreversible. Pralidoxime acts to break up this complex before this process (known as *aging*) occurs.

65. **Answer A.** The mushroom in the picture is *Amanita muscaria*, which contains muscimol, a hallucinogenic. It is intentionally ingested in parts of the world for the hallucinogenic effect. Despite its name, there is very little muscarine present in *Amanita muscaria* mushrooms and no toxic effect from this substance. Liver failure is seen with *Amanita phalloides* mushrooms, also known as the death cap. Renal failure and blindness are seen with ethylene glycol and methanol poisoning, respectively. Adrenal infarction is not a typical sequela of any common toxicologic agent. (Figure from Engelkirk P, ed. *Burton's Microbiology for the Health Sciences.* 10th ed. Philadelphia, PA: Wolters Kluwer; 2014.)

66. **Answer E.** The treatment of bacterial meningitis varies by age of the patient. All patients should be treated with a third-generation cephalosporin to cover meningococcus, pneumococcus, and gram-negative bacilli. At the extremes of age, *Listeria monocytogenes* is a more common pathogen and should be specifically treated with either ampicillin or trimethoprim–sulfamethoxazole. Vancomycin may be used in addition to these therapies to cover methicillin-resistant *S. aureus* in endemic areas. Dexamethasone should be given before or simultaneously with the first dose of antibiotics.

67. **Answer C.** The EKG demonstrates multifocal atrial tachycardia (MAT), which is associated most commonly with COPD, followed by congestive heart failure, hypokalemia, and hypomagnesemia. There are P waves of at least three different morphologies associated with an irregular tachycardia. Management involves treatment of the underlying condition. Patients with MAT rarely have hemodynamic compromise as a result of their dysrhythmia. (Figure from Fowler NO. *Clinical Electrocardiographic Diagnosis: A Problem-Based Approach.* Philadelphia, PA: Lippincott Williams & Wilkins; 2000, with permission.)

68. **Answer A.** Edrophonium is a cholinesterase inhibitor and may, therefore, produce symptoms of cholinergic toxicity, including bradycardia, excessive airway and oral secretions, tearing, and dyspepsia associated with nausea or vomiting. Of these, bradycardia is the most common serious side effect, even though it occurs very infrequently, having been reported in only 0.16% of patients. However, as excessive airway secretions may also occur, caution is advised in patients with lung diseases such as asthma or chronic obstructive pulmonary disease (COPD). Atropine should be at the bedside in case either of these symptoms occurs. Oculogyric crisis describes a dystonic reaction in which patients experience severe torticollis and extreme upward gaze

that may persist for hours. It is most commonly due to treatment with neuroleptics (antipsychotics) and is terminated with the antimuscarinic drug benztropine (Cogentin) in concert with benzodiazepines. Cough, atrial fibrillation, and seizures are not associated with edrophonium use.

69. **Answer A.** This patient has an inferior ST elevation MI with reciprocal ST depressions anteriorly. While the patient likely has concomitant inferior involvement of the left ventricular wall, the patient's hypotension after nitroglycerin strongly suggests right ventricular involvement. A right-sided EKG demonstrating ST elevation in V4R is considered diagnostic (>90% sensitivity and specificity). Agents that reduce preload such as nitrates, opioids, or beta-blockers should be avoided or used with caution in patients with right ventricular involvement or signs of right ventricular failure (elevated jugular venous pressure, peripheral edema, hepatomegaly, clear lung examination). Instead, such patients should receive small boluses of IV fluid to optimize preload. In patients who remain hypotensive despite preload, dopamine may be a helpful adjunct.

70. **Answer C.** More than 2,000 children per year die of child abuse. The most common mechanism is head injury, followed by intra-abdominal bleeding. Evaluation and treatment of injuries from child abuse are often delayed due to the abuser's status as primary or secondary caretaker. Intracranial injuries commonly include subdural hematoma, SAH, and cerebral contusions. A vigorous shaking mechanism alone in an infant is enough to cause a fatal brain hemorrhage. The other answer choices listed are less common causes of death from child abuse. The most common overall manifestations of child abuse are soft-tissue injuries, followed by long-bone fractures.

71. **Answer B.** The patient has a dermatomal rash consistent with shingles, caused by VZV. Shingles is due to reactivation of dormant VZV—primary VZV is also known as *chickenpox*. Many patients with shingles will have a prodrome of pain before the rash appears, and vesicles are not always present. However, the description of this patient's pain is typical of shingles, and pain is, in general, the most common complaint for which patients seek evaluation and treatment. Immunocompromised patients may have disseminated zoster infection, which spreads beyond the initial dermatome and ultimately results in systemic involvement. Older patients (>50 years of age) with shingles recover faster with antiviral therapy if treatment is started within 72 hours of the onset of symptoms. Otherwise, treatment is supportive with effective analgesia. While glucocorticoids are often used, their use does not reduce postherpetic neuralgia so they are not recommended. Steroids appear to hasten

recovery, but their benefit is modest, and their use is associated with significant undesirable side effects, particularly in older patients. (Figure reprinted with permission from Fleisher GR, Baskin MN. *Atlas of Pediatric Emergency Medicine.* Philadelphia, PA: Lippincott Williams & Wilkins; 2003:214.)

72. **Answer E.** This patient presents with rhabdomyolysis. Hypocalcemia is the most common electrolyte abnormality as calcium floods the intracellular space when myocyte membranes fail. Because hyperphosphatemia may also occur, treatment of hypocalcemia is not recommended unless symptoms are severe or unless severe hyperkalemia develops. Otherwise, calcium phosphate may precipitate and form deposits in tissues. Myoglobin has a plasma half-life of only 1 to 3 hours, making detection sometimes difficult. Although myoglobinuria is pathognomonic for rhabdomyolysis, measurement of creatine kinase (CK) is the most sensitive method to detect muscle cell injury. CK has a half-life of 1.5 days. The classic finding of a urine dipstick that is positive for blood while microscopic urinalysis reveals no red blood cells is present only 50% of the time. In addition to trauma, HMG-CoA reductase inhibitors are a well-known cause of rhabdomyolysis. IV fluids are the mainstay of treatment, and should be started when the CK >5,000 Units/L. Alkalinization may be helpful while loop diuretics offer no benefit.

73. **Answer D.** Increasingly, acute adrenal insufficiency is thought to be a *rare* condition, and most cases of acute adrenal insufficiency probably represent an exacerbation of chronic disease. When acute adrenal insufficiency occurs, it is most commonly due to exogenous glucocorticoid administration. Chronic adrenal insufficiency is idiopathic (thought to be autoimmune-mediated destruction of the adrenal gland) in 66% to 75% of cases.

74. **Answer B.** Historically, the majority of cases of SVC syndrome (obstruction of the SVC) were due to syphilitic aortic aneurysms, tuberculosis, and cancer. Today they are primarily due to deep venous thrombosis of the SVC in patients with an indwelling catheter such as a PICC line or Port-a-Cath. Many of these patients have such devices because of cancer treatment, but their cancers are not the primary cause of SVC obstruction. Among neoplastic causes, lung cancer is the most common. Breast and testicular cancer are less common causes of SVC syndrome. Colon and thyroid neoplasms are uncommon causes. Symptoms include facial and upper extremity edema, shortness of breath, cough, and chest pain. Diagnosis is made by physical examination, chest x-ray, and advanced imaging such as echocardiography, CT, and/or MRI. Management has traditionally involved radiation therapy, but chemotherapy and

surgical evaluation have potential roles in the acute treatment as well.

75. **Answer E.** Labetalol antagonizes α-1, β-1, and β-2 adrenergic receptors. The β-blockade is much greater than the α-blockade, although both function to provide rapid, predictable BP control without causing reflex tachycardia. This blunting of the tachycardic response along with concomitant arteriolar vasodilation makes labetalol ideal as the initial single agent for management of aortic dissection, where reduction of heart rate is as important as reduction of BP. Orthostatic hypotension with oral labetalol is rare, but IV formulations can cause major changes. Nitroprusside and labetalol are roughly equal in their ability to control BP rapidly and predictably.

76. **Answer B.** The PEFR (in L/second) and the FEV_1 (in L) are both valuable adjuncts in assessing the severity of airflow obstruction. Because of its portability and ease of application, however, PEFR is much more easily measured and is more useful for EPs. Although the absolute value of the PEFR may be useful, it is most useful in comparison to a patient's typical best (as a percentage). A patient who generates a PEFR <50% of his or her typical best has severe airflow obstruction. The utilization of ABG determination widely varies in clinical practice. As a general rule, patients in whom oxygenation can't be reliably assessed due to an erratic or absent pulse oximetry waveform should receive an ABG. Repeat ABGs are generally not needed to determine whether a patient is improving or deteriorating. Chest x-rays are not generally useful in patients with asthma exacerbations. They do not reflect the severity of the exacerbation. They are generally useful only for those patients in whom pneumonia, or a complication (e.g., pneumothorax) is suspected, or in those patients who remain refractory despite optimal therapy. Neither continuous cardiac monitoring, nor routine EKGs are useful in routine asthma exacerbations. Both of these may be useful, however, in older patients with coexisting cardiac disease. Most patients have pulse rates between 90 and 120, and only 15% exceed this value.

77. **Answer B.** With the history of a recent camping trip, tick-borne illness should be suspected. In this case, the patient likely has Rocky Mountain spotted fever, caused by the intracellular bacterium, *Rickettsia rickettsii.* The organism causes endothelial cell damage, resulting in diffuse vasculitis and multiple organ microinfarctions and failure. Acute respiratory distress syndrome, DIC, and shock all may occur in serious cases. Rash on the wrists and ankles following a nonspecific viral-like syndrome is characteristic. Laboratory work is usually normal, though thrombocytopenia may occur. Treatment is with doxycycline or chloramphenicol. Choices

A, C, D, and E will not adequately treat the rickettsial infection.

78. **Answer D.** DIC is an acquired consumptive coagulopathy which may occur in patients who are critically ill. Disorder of the clotting cascade causes platelets and clotting factors to be consumed, leading to both hemorrhagic and thrombotic complications. Almost all have decreased levels of clotting factors, leading to prolongation in the prothrombin and partial thromboplastin times. Fibrinolysis occurs commonly, leading to decreased fibrinogen levels and an increase in fibrin split products. Acute anemia may not always occur, as some patients have relatively low hemorrhagic burden and hemoglobin levels may take time to equilibrate and not show subtle, acute decreases.

79. **Answer B.** Cerebral edema is the most feared complication of DKA treatment in children. Although reports vary, cerebral edema complicates roughly 1% of pediatric DKA cases, with a mortality rate of 20% to 90%. Survivors have persistent neurologic sequelae 20% to 40% of the time. The development of cerebral edema is almost exclusively a complication of pediatric DKA. There is still no consensus regarding the etiology of cerebral edema in pediatric DKA. However, early clinical signs include headache, vomiting, decreased arousal, relative bradycardia, and relative hypertension.

80. **Answer B.** Though pneumocystis pneumonia (PCP) is an important consideration in patients with HIV, typical organisms associated with community-acquired pneumonia predominate. This is increasingly true as the majority of patients are taking extremely effective highly active antiretroviral therapy (HAART). Unless the CD4 count is <200, opportunistic infections are uncommon. Furthermore, the abrupt onset of this patient's symptoms along with purulent sputum is typical of patients with community-acquired bacterial pneumonia. In contrast, patients with PCP have a nonproductive cough, dyspnea, and a more gradual onset. Tuberculosis should be considered in all HIV patients presenting with pulmonary symptoms. However, the symptoms are typically gradual and subacute to chronic. Patients with early HIV behave like patients who are HIV negative, with symptoms of fever, cough, night sweats, and weight loss. Chest x-ray may reveal cavitation and patients may present with blood-streaked sputum. Cavitation and hemoptysis are often absent in patients with more advanced HIV, who may present with dissemination (e.g., fever without a source) or extrapulmonary TB (cervical lymphadenopathy).

81. **Answer C.** Modern, multidetector CT scanners, which are ubiquitous in the United States, are nearly 100% sensitive in detecting clinically significant cervical spine injuries. Flexion and extension and oblique views don't add additional information. While MRI is more sensitive for detecting ligamentous injuries, those injuries are almost never clinically relevant in patients without neurologic complaints or findings. Patients with persistent tenderness without neurologic complaints or findings may be discharged home with outpatient follow-up. Some guidelines suggest discharging patients in a rigid collar (such as a Miami-J, Aspen, or Philadelphia collar) with short-term follow-up, ideally in consultation with the trauma or neurosurgical team. As pacemakers are increasingly designed to be MRI-compatible, MRI utilization may increase in this patient population. Additionally, reasons for the motor vehicle collision should be aggressively sought—with a recent pacemaker placement for sick sinus syndrome, pacemaker malfunction and dysrhythmia causing syncope may be the causative process. Discharge, therefore, should not take place before both medical and traumatic issues are completely evaluated.

82. **Answer B.** This patient has suffered a concussion. However, the use of the word "concussion" often causes confusion due to competing and vague definitions. The American Academy of Neurology defines concussion as a trauma-induced alteration of mental status that may or may not be associated with loss of consciousness. In the literature, "concussion" is frequently used in reference to those patients with the mildest form of traumatic brain injury. In patients with head trauma, retrograde amnesia is more common and longer in duration than anterograde amnesia. Furthermore, patients who appear unable to recall their name or birthdate and are otherwise well are likely malingering. In contrast to past beliefs, simple (i.e., not depressed) skull fractures do not strongly predict underlying brain hemorrhage. In fact, the fracture of the skull may well dissipate the majority of the energy delivered from the impact before it is transmitted to the brain. Postconcussion syndrome refers to the constellation of symptoms that occurs after head injury, including headache, dizziness, memory problems, and occasional neuropsychiatric complaints. It rarely occurs in young children. While there are several consensus-based guidelines regarding the optimal time to return to athletic activities, there is a lack of prospective data to guide these decisions.

83. **Answer E.** Middle ear barotrauma or "middle ear squeeze" is the most common barotrauma-related problem during descent. Ear pain during descent is the most common symptom, although transient hearing loss may occur. Additionally, if the diver continues to deeper water, further increases in pressure may result in tympanic membrane (TM) rupture. TM rupture may alleviate

some of the pain but it also exposes the middle ear to cold water, which may result in nystagmus and vertigo. A facial nerve palsy also uncommonly occurs. Nitrogen narcosis occurs during descent as increased levels of nitrogen are "forced" into the tissues. Symptoms typically occur at approximately 100 ft and resemble alcohol intoxication. Barosinusitis presents as facial pain that results from pressure changes in one of the facial sinuses. Facial barotrauma occurs when divers fail to equilibrate the airspace created by a dive mask over the eyes and nose. The relative negative pressure causes petechial hemorrhages on the face, subconjunctival hemorrhage, and conjunctival edema. Temporomandibular joint dysfunction is caused by teeth clenching and malocclusion resulting from a poorly fitting mask. The pain is felt near the ear and can be confused with middle ear barotrauma.

84. Answer C. Iron-deficiency anemia is the most common cause of all anemias in women of childbearing age, likely due to menstrual blood loss. Iron-deficiency anemia is the number one cause of microcytic anemia and is characterized by a rapid response to oral iron therapy. Both α- and β-thalassemia cause microcytic anemia, but are far less common than iron-deficiency anemia. Microcytosis is more severe in patients with thalassemia than with iron-deficiency anemia. Definitive diagnosis is made by hemoglobin electrophoresis. Sideroblastic anemia is usually found in elderly patients, alcoholics, and in those with lead poisoning. Folate deficiency, although common, causes macrocytic anemia.

85. Answer B. Guidelines regarding the management of primary spontaneous pneumothorax continue to evolve. In the past, small pneumothoraces were defined as those pneumothoraces occupying <20% of the hemithorax. However, multiple different systems are used to estimate pneumothorax volume, and analysis of plain posteroanterior (PA) chest films tends to underestimate pneumothorax volume. Recently, the British Thoracic Society published new guidelines dividing pneumothoraces into "small" and "large" categories to avoid estimations of percentages. Patients with a rim of air around the lung ≤2 cm are considered to have a small pneumothorax while those with ≥2 cm of air around the lung are considered to have a large pneumothorax. Most small pneumothoraces have no persistent air leak and recurrence in those managed with observation alone is less than in patients treated with tube thoracostomy. Such patients do not require hospital admission, but most ED physicians observe the patient while applying supplemental O$_2$ (which increases the rate of resorption of the pneumothorax by a factor of 4) over a period of 3 to 6 hours after which a film is repeated to ensure that there is no increase in the size of the pneumothorax. Any patient with hypoxia or a patient with more than minimal symptoms of dyspnea requires treatment with either aspiration and admission for observation, or tube thoracostomy and admission for observation. Patients with small pneumothoraces who fail simple observation often have secondary pneumothoraces.

86. Answer B. Wolff–Parkinson–White (WPW) syndrome is the most frequently occurring accessory pathway syndrome. Patients have an accessory conductive pathway from the atria to the ventricles that pre-excites the ventricular myocytes before the AV node releases the normal sinoatrial depolarization. As a result, patients with WPW often have a shortened PR interval and a delayed QRS upstroke, called the *delta wave*. The accessory pathway can cause reentrant dysrhythmias, of which atrioventricular nodal reentry (AVNRT) is the most common. In reentrant dysrhythmias, the accessory pathway can conduct retrograde (where the AV node conducts in the normal direction, producing a narrow QRS complex and an "orthodromic" pattern) or anterograde (where the AV node conducts backward, producing a wide QRS complex and an "antidromic" pattern). MAT is seen in the setting of chronic pulmonary disease and is not usually seen with WPW syndrome. AV blocks and torsade de pointes are not commonly seen in WPW syndrome.

87. Answer D. Patients with fall on outstretched hand (FOOSH) injuries may have bony or ligamentous damage in any part of their upper extremity. The bones of the wrist are most susceptible to injury. The anatomic snuffbox is demarcated by the extensor pollicis brevis and longus tendons just proximal to the thumb and tenderness in this region indicates possible fracture to the scaphoid. Scaphoid fracture is particularly dangerous because of the high rate of AVN and resulting limitation of thumb function. Almost one-fifth of all scaphoid fractures are invisible on acute radiographs, so appropriate management in suspected cases includes immobilization in a thumb spica cast and repeat radiographs in 1 to 2 weeks. There is no need for emergent orthopedic consultation in patients with negative x-rays. Discharging the patient home without a splint that immobilizes the thumb is contraindicated. Admission for observation is not an appropriate use of resources.

88. Answer C. The DIP joints are never affected in RA, which provides a useful means of differentiating the disease from osteoarthritis. The arthritis of RA is typically polyarticular and symmetric, particularly affecting the hands (metacarpophalangeal and proximal interphalangeal joints), wrists, and elbows. The disease is twice as common in women and peaks in the fourth to sixth decade. Two-thirds of patients with RA develop cervical spine disease, although thoracic and lumbar disease is

uncommon. The disease most commonly involves the occipitoatlantoaxial junction, and anterior atlantoaxial subluxation may occur. RFs are autoantibodies directed at the crystallizable fragment (Fc) of human immunoglobulin molecules. The exact incidence of RF depends on the assay used and the threshold titer used to separate positive from negative results. In general, roughly 15% of patients with RA will be seronegative (RF within the normal range), and those patients tend to have milder disease.

89. **Answer A.** Patients with CHF most commonly die due to hemodynamic decline, followed by dysrhythmia. Mortality from fluid overload has been reduced by β-blockers and angiotensin converting enzyme inhibitors, and short-term mortality from dysrhythmias has been reduced by automated internal cardiac defibrillators (AICDs). Choices B, C, D, and E are all important, but are less common causes of death in patients with CHF.

90. **Answer D.** Hypotension complicates roughly 15% to 50% of hemodialysis sessions and is more common among the elderly and female dialysis patients. It is primarily due to the volume and rate of plasma fluid removal. Patients referred to the ED with asymptomatic hypotension after a dialysis session should receive a small bolus of normal saline and frequent reassessment. Though septicemia is a very common cause of death in dialysis patients (second most common, after cardiovascular disease), most septic patients typically have *some* additional evidence of infection, such as fevers, chills, tachycardia or focal symptoms of illness, in addition to hypotension. Muscle cramps are the second most common complication of dialysis, and are also thought to be due primarily to the rate of volume removal. Thus, they are treated with a small fluid bolus, and diazepam, if needed. The FDA has issued a warning against the use of quinine, which has long been prescribed for muscle cramps, due to its long list of adverse side effects.

91. **Answer B.** The slit lamp examination demonstrates dendritic lesions with fluorescein uptake characteristic of herpes simplex keratitis. The dendritic lesions may scar, and ocular HSV is a common cause of corneal blindness in the United States. Management involves oral and/or topical antivirals and ophthalmologic consultation to assess for surgical management. Topical steroids are absolutely contraindicated as they may cause worsening of the corneal epithelial defect. Acetazolamide is used to increase aqueous humor excretion as part of noninvasive temporizing therapies for acute glaucoma attacks. Erythromycin is used to treat corneal ulcers or prevent infections from occurring in patients with corneal abrasions. Ceftriaxone is used in patients with hyperacute bacterial conjunctivitis, which is usually due to gonococcal infection. (Figure from Rapuano CJ. *Wills Eye Institute—Cornea.* 2nd ed. Philadelphia, PA: Wolters Kluwer; 2011.)

92. **Answer B.** Pulmonary contusion refers to direct parenchymal injury from blunt thoracic trauma. It is often associated with other intrathoracic and chest wall injuries, most commonly multiple rib fractures. Impaired oxygenation and ventilation may cause severe deficits in respiratory function requiring endotracheal intubation and mechanical ventilation. The diagnosis is made by initial chest radiography, although CT scan is more sensitive and able to detect other thoracic injuries as well. Atelectasis and pneumonia are the most common complications of pulmonary contusion but may take several days after the injury to develop. Prophylactic antibiotics before the onset of clinical signs and symptoms of postcontusion pneumonia are not recommended. ARDS may develop in patients with particularly severe pulmonary contusions but is less common than concomitant pneumonia. Pulmonary embolism may also occur in patients who are bedridden after severe traumatic injuries but do not occur at significantly higher rates in patients with pulmonary contusion. Myocardial contusion and pericardial tamponade may occur from the same blunt traumatic forces that caused the pulmonary contusion but do not generally occur as a complication of isolated pulmonary contusion.

93. **Answer D.** The "crossed" straight leg raise (SLR) test is performed by raising the *unaffected* leg of a patient complaining of radicular low back pain while keeping the knee straight. The occurrence of pain radiating below the knee in the *affected* leg is nearly pathognomonic for a herniated disk with nerve root compression. Although the normal SLR test (performed on the affected leg) is more sensitive than the crossed SLR test, it has a low specificity. Therefore, many patients without true disk disease will have a positive SLR test. Pain which worsens when the ankle is dorsiflexed (Lasègue sign) may be a helpful adjunct to the initial examination. Of note, the SLR and crossed SLR tests are considered positive only if the patient complains of radicular pain radiating down the leg past the knee. The mere presence of back pain is considered a negative test.

94. **Answer C.** High-pressure injection injuries to the hand are associated with a very high rate of amputation depending on the injected substance and the rapidity of treatment. Amputation rates as high as 80% have been reported. The index finger of the nondominant hand is the most common digit involved. Entrance wounds from high-pressure injection injuries may look deceptively benign. The jet of liquid is under such high pressure that it easily penetrates the skin and gains access

to the tendon sheaths causing rapid distension and an inflammatory response. Over time, compartment pressures increase, the inflammatory cascade mushrooms, and the tissues become ischemic and necrotic. The flexor sheaths of the thumb and index finger (most commonly involved) extend to the thenar space while the long, ring, and little finger sheaths extend to the midpalmar space. In addition to tetanus prophylaxis and antibiotics, a hand surgeon should be consulted immediately for emergent wide incision and debridement to decompress the hand and eliminate inflammatory debris (e.g., paint or grease). Digital blocks are contraindicated by ED physicians due to the subsequent increase in compartment pressures.

95. **Answer B.** Short submersion time (<5 minutes) has been consistently shown to predict better neurologic outcomes. All other predictive factors have not been as robust in terms of their predictive value. However, predictors of a poorer prognosis include age >14 years old, time to resuscitation >10 minutes, duration of CPR >25 minutes, GCS <5, and initial pH <7.1.

96. **Answer C.** ITP causes immune-mediated destruction of platelets. Acute ITP is more often seen in children and chronic ITP is seen in adults. Bleeding is the most common clinical finding and intracranial bleeding is the most common cause of death. Treatment in children is primarily supportive with a high rate of spontaneous resolution. Mortality in young adults and children is below 5%; in older adults, it jumps to almost 50% because of complications surrounding intracranial hemorrhage. Aspirin is contraindicated because of its irreversible platelet-killing effects. There is a female predominance in adult patients. Platelets are not indicated until levels reach <10,000 to 20,000 cells per mm^3. Treatment in adults is with high-dose corticosteroids and/or IVIG.

97. **Answer B.** The patient has symmetric swelling of his foreskin behind his glans without active retraction indicative of a paraphimosis. This is a urologic emergency that can occur in uncircumcised patients which requires prompt reduction to prevent necrosis of the glans. Reduction is performed by squeezing the glans for several minutes to clear the capillaries of blood and pulling the foreskin over the glans. A dorsal slit procedure may need to be performed if noninvasive reduction is unsuccessful. A *phimosis* refers to inability to retract the foreskin over the glans—it does not require emergent reduction. *Balanitis* refers to bacterial or fungal infection of the glans without concomitant foreskin infection (which would be called *balanoposthitis*). Testicular torsion and scrotal hernia are not often evident on simple inspection and require palpation and ultrasonography to definitively diagnose. (Figure from Fleisher GR, Ludwig S,

Baskin MN. *Atlas of Pediatric Emergency Medicine.* Philadelphia, PA: Lippincott Williams & Wilkins, 2004; with permission.)

98. **Answer B.** Owing to its deceptively innocuous early course, the diagnosis of AMI remains problematic. Therefore, the mortality rate has remained essentially unchanged at roughly 70%. The key to diagnosis is recognizing patients at risk, such as any patient older than 50 years of age who presents with acute abdominal pain and who has known vascular disease, cardiac arrhythmias, recent myocardial infarction, hypovolemia, hypotension, or sepsis. The most commonly cited clinical finding is pain that is out of proportion to tenderness elicited on physical examination. This is a nonspecific finding that needs to be considered carefully in light of the clinical scenario. Unfortunately, there are no laboratory markers or radiologic studies apart from angiography that have sufficient sensitivity and specificity to exclude AMI early in its course. Lactate levels are elevated in approximately 100% of patients with bowel infarction, but this is a late finding and mortality rates are high by the time infarction has occurred. Plain films are most commonly nonspecific, although findings such as ileus correspond to more severe disease and a higher mortality rate. The sensitivity of CT has been cited to be as high as 82%, but the most common early finding is bowel wall thickening, present in 26% to 96% of cases. Unfortunately, this is also the least specific finding and is often not present in mesenteric ischemia due to arterial embolism or thrombosis, which is the most common cause of AMI. Pneumatosis intestinalis or gas in the portal venous system is a specific finding but is only present after bowel infarction has occurred. In the absence of angiography, the treatment is emergent laparotomy.

99. **Answer C.** Hemodynamically unstable (tachycardia, hypotension) trauma patients with intraperitoneal FAST should be taken to the OR for an emergent laparotomy. Given that the patient suffered right-sided abdominal trauma, she bears considerable risk for liver laceration. Taking time to further delineate or evaluate her injuries with additional imaging only exposes her to additional risk without benefit. The role of FAST in stable pediatric trauma patients is less clear as the sensitivity and specificity of a FAST scan in such patients is decreased relative to its use in hypotensive patients. In addition to her abdominal injuries, the patient suffered a minor superior pubic ramus fracture. Such a fracture does not typically cause significant hemorrhage, and lateral compression mechanisms generally result in less severe injuries than anterior–posterior compression. In the setting of concomitant significant pelvic trauma and presumed pelvic hemorrhage, external pelvic compression should

be used as a temporizing measure while laparotomy is performed. External compression can be achieved with a bedsheet wrapped around the pelvis, or with external fixation, if time permits.

100. **Answer D.** The Thompson test, in which ankle plantar flexion is assessed as the calf muscles are squeezed, is the most sensitive test to predict Achilles tendon rupture.

The Matles test, which assesses the degree of passive (i.e., natural) ankle plantar flexion when the patient is lying prone with the knee flexed to 90 degrees is also a sensitive and specific test but it is not as predictive as the Thompson test. Finally, while a definite palpable Achilles tendon defect may be diagnostic, frequently soft tissue swelling will limit the ability to determine if a defect is present and the sensitivity and specificity of this test is low.

QUESTIONS

1. Which of the following is the earliest electrocardiogram (EKG) finding in acute myocardial infarction (MI)?

    A. Hyperacute T waves
    B. ST elevation
    C. ST depression
    D. T-wave inversion
    E. Q waves

2. A 60-year-old female presents with painful facial swelling that started acutely over the course of 1 hour (Fig. 12-1). Which of the following is the best imaging modality for evaluation of this condition?

    A. X-ray
    B. X-ray with contrast
    C. CT
    D. MRI
    E. PET scan

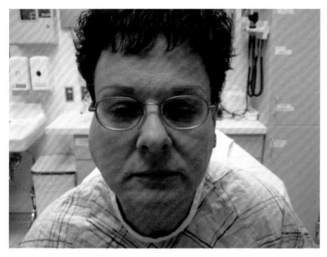

Figure 12-1

3. A 22-year-old male presents with painful oral lesions for 2 days (Fig. 12-2). He has been unable to drink fluids due to significant odynophagia. Which of the following is the most important next step in management?

    A. Nystatin
    B. Incision and drainage
    C. Valacylovir
    D. Methotrexate
    E. Prednisone

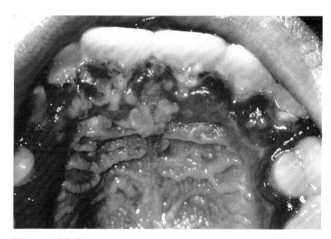

Figure 12-2

4. A 45-year-old male presents with signs and symptoms of bacterial meningitis. Which of the following is the single most likely cause?

    A. Group B streptococcus
    B. *Listeria monocytogenes*
    C. *Streptococcus pneumoniae*
    D. *Neisseria meningitides*
    E. *Hemophilus influenzae*

5. Which of the following is characteristic of the Zika virus?

    A. Fetal macrocephaly
    B. Part of same genus as dengue and West Nile viruses
    C. Absence of rash and myalgias
    D. Outbreak in 2015 starting in Australia
    E. Mortality of 50%

6. Which of the following is true regarding lipase and amylase in the setting of acute pancreatitis?

   A. Lipase is more specific than amylase.
   B. Amylase is more sensitive than lipase.
   C. Amylase peaks earlier and remains elevated for a longer period than lipase.
   D. The degree of elevation of either amylase or lipase correlates with disease severity.
   E. The amylase to lipase ratio may be useful in determining the etiology of pancreatitis.

7. A 23-year-old male presents to the ED with loss of consciousness after being kicked in the head. He is now awake and alert and complains of a headache. Brain computed tomography (CT) is performed and a slice is shown (Fig. 12-3). Right after the CT scan, he becomes unresponsive. Which of the following is the most appropriate next step in management?

   A. Burr hole placement
   B. Endotracheal intubation
   C. Diagnostic peritoneal lavage (DPL)
   D. Emergent thoracotomy
   E. Repeat CT scan

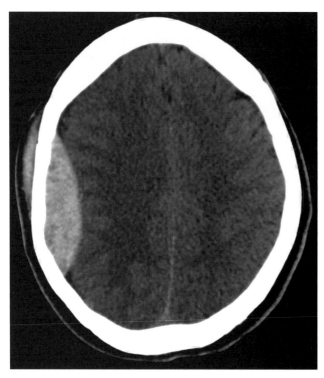

Figure 12-3

8. Which of the following is the most common mode of completed suicide?

   A. Drug ingestion
   B. Firearms
   C. Carbon monoxide
   D. Hanging
   E. Wrist cutting

9. A 25-year-old male ingests an unknown quantity of iron tablets 2 hours before presentation in an overdose attempt. Which of the following is the most appropriate next step in management?

   A. Activated charcoal
   B. Gastric lavage
   C. Ipecac
   D. Polyethylene glycol
   E. Hemodialysis

10. A 42-year-old female presented to the emergency department (ED) with acute-onset epigastric abdominal pain and nausea without vomiting. Her workup revealed acute pancreatitis and she was admitted. After receiving appropriate analgesics and antiemetics, she is now hungry and wants something to eat. Which of the following is true?

    A. She should undergo a period of bowel rest for 48 hours regardless of her laboratory results.
    B. She requires ongoing nasogastric (NG) suctioning until pancreatic enzyme abnormalities resolve.
    C. She should receive total parenteral nutrition for 72 hours.
    D. She should be allowed to eat if abdominal computed tomography (CT) reveals resolution of the signs of pancreatitis.
    E. She may eat a low calorie, carbohydrate-rich diet.

11. Which of the following corresponds to ischemia of the anterior circulation?

    A. Hemiparesis and hemisensory loss of the left leg
    B. Transient monocular blindness
    C. Aphasia and hemiparesis of the right arm, leg, and face
    D. Ataxia, vertigo, nausea, and vomiting
    E. A, B, and C

12. Which of the following is the most common symptom of rheumatic fever?

    A. Chorea
    B. Carditis
    C. Erythema marginatum
    D. Migratory polyarthritis
    E. Fever

13. A 70-year-old female presents with blurry vision in her right eye and a right-sided headache. The patient also complains of malaise, and is tender in her right temporal region. Which of the following is true regarding this patient's illness?

    A. Steroids are ineffective in preventing disease in the contralateral eye.
    B. Patients have a higher risk of arterial aneurysms.
    C. Steroid therapy should be withheld until definitive diagnosis is made.

D. Men are more commonly affected.

E. The disease is very rare in patients older than 50 years of age.

14. An 18-year-old female presents to the emergency department (ED) with acute-onset severe right lower quadrant pain. Initially, she was doubled over with pain and had immediate nausea and vomiting just prior to her ED evaluation. The pain resolved almost completely after 15 minutes, and then she had a second episode while in the ED waiting room. The patient is currently pain-free. Her last menstrual period was 2 weeks ago. She has a family history of kidney stones. Her vital signs are normal. Physical examination is unremarkable except for mild fullness and tenderness in the right adnexa. Her complete blood count (CBC), chemistry, and urinalysis are normal and her urine pregnancy is negative. Which of the following is the most appropriate next step in management?

A. Computed tomography (CT) abdomen/pelvis with oral and IV contrast

B. CT abdomen/pelvis with IV contrast only

C. CT abdomen/pelvis with rectal contrast

D. Pelvic ultrasound

E. Emergent urologic consultation

15. Which of the following wounds will most likely develop a wound infection?

A. A 3-cm face laceration suffered 6 hours before evaluation

B. A fresh, 8-cm lower leg wound in a patient with diabetes

C. A 4-cm hand wound suffered 10 hours prior to evaluation

D. A 2-cm forearm wound that cuts the underlying muscle

E. A 3-cm superficial neck wound suffered 12 hours prior to evaluation

16. A 24-year-old female presents with dysuria and increased frequency of urination for 2 days. She denies fevers, vomiting, or back pain. She is allergic to sulfa drugs and fluoroquinolones. Urinalysis demonstrates 25 WBCs per high-powered field, leukocyte esterase, and nitrites. Which of the following is the most appropriate antibiotic regimen?

A. Ciprofloxacin

B. Trimethoprim–sulfamethoxazole (TMP-SMX)

C. Doxycycline

D. Azithromycin

E. Nitrofurantoin

17. A 20-year-old male presents to the ED with several days of progressive chest pain, fatigue, myalgias, and exertional dyspnea. He states that he had the "flu" 1 week before. He denies illicit drug use or family history of heart disease. Physical examination reveals a temperature of 100.5°F, heart rate of 125, no murmurs on cardiac examination, and scattered bilateral crackles on lung examination. EKG demonstrates sinus tachycardia, chest x-ray reveals cardiomegaly and mild pulmonary edema, and laboratory reports are normal except for troponin I, which is elevated at 10 ng/mL. Which of the following is the most likely etiology?

A. MI

B. Aortic dissection

C. Viral infection

D. Stroke

E. Diabetic ketoacidosis (DKA)

18. Which of the following is associated with carpal tunnel syndrome?

A. Hypertension

B. Diabetes

C. Congestive heart failure

D. Coronary artery disease

E. Osteogenesis imperfecta

19. A healthy 23-year-old female presents with acute bilateral facial weakness. She complains that she "can't taste anything" and that sounds are abnormally loud. She denies any unusual travel and notes only her usual summer camping trip. Which of the following is the most likely cause of her symptoms?

A. Infectious mononucleosis

B. Miller–Fisher variant Guillain–Barré syndrome (GBS)

C. Neurosyphilis

D. Lymphoma

E. Lyme disease

20. The parents of a 12-year-old male bring him to the emergency room after he hit the back of his head while diving for a basketball just prior to arrival. He did not lose consciousness, had no period of confusion, and has not been vomiting, but he has been complaining of a moderate generalized headache and dizziness since the incident. His vitals are stable and his neurologic examination is normal. What guidance should you provide the parents?

A. He hasn't had a concussion and can engage in all activities without restriction

B. He's likely had a concussion but he does not require activity restriction

C. He requires a CT scan before discussing whether he's had a concussion

D. He's had a concussion and he should undergo physical and cognitive rest until his symptoms resolve

E. He hasn't had a concussion, but he should have neurology follow-up to ensure the headache and dizziness resolve.

21. A 50-year-old female with no past medical history presents with acute onset of fever, chills, shortness of breath, and cough. She has crackles in her right middle lung field and chest x-ray shows right middle lobe consolidation. Vital signs in the emergency department (ED) are normal. Which of the following is the most appropriate next step in management?

    A. Blood cultures
    B. Sputum Gram stain
    C. Computed tomography (CT) of chest
    D. Arterial blood gas
    E. Antibiotics

22. A 15-year-old male comes to the ED complaining of shortness of breath and nausea. He admits to "huffing" glue before presentation. Which of the following is the most appropriate therapy at this time?

    A. Supportive care only
    B. Antibiotics
    C. Corticosteroids
    D. Diuretics
    E. Activated charcoal

23. In pediatric patients, osteomyelitis:

    A. Is most commonly from hematogenous spread
    B. Is best diagnosed with magnetic resonance imaging (MRI)
    C. Most frequently occurs in the long bones such as the tibia and femur
    D. Is more common in patients with sickle cell anemia
    E. All of the above

24. A 56-year-old diabetic male presents with a chief complaint of room-spinning dizziness, nausea, and trouble walking. While asking the patient to fixate on a distant object straight ahead while forcibly turning his head to the right (the head impulse test), his eyes are dragged to the right off target before slowly marching back to the midline. This indicates:

    A. He has had a stroke
    B. He has vetebrobasilar insufficiency
    C. He has right vertebral artery dissection
    D. He has a lesion affecting his right vestibular nerve (cranial nerve VIII)
    E. He has an oculomotor nerve palsy

25. A 22-year-old male presents with a painful, red area on his right leg for the last 3 days. It is spreading up his leg and he noted fevers, chills, and lightheadedness today. He also describes a sunburn-like rash on his chest, back, and arms but denies recent sun exposure. Vital signs are 102.5°F, 112, 22, 82/45, 94% RA. Which of the following is true regarding this patient?

    A. *Pseudomonas* is the most likely cause.
    B. A bacterial toxin is responsible for the pathologic effects.

C. Blood cultures are almost always positive.
D. Mortality is <1%.
E. Intravenous fluids usually worsen the clinical outcome.

26. Which of the following is true regarding pemphigus vulgaris?

    A. It is most common in children.
    B. Nikolsky sign is infrequently present.
    C. Antibiotics are the most important part of management.
    D. Oral blisters that spontaneously rupture to form painful erosions are the earliest manifestation.
    E. Outbreaks are commonly triggered by sulfonamides or β-lactam drugs.

27. A 63-year-old female with a history of congestive heart failure (CHF) presents for evaluation of shortness of breath. Her vital signs are P 115, BP 190/100, RR 28, SaO_2 82% RA. Physical examination reveals diffuse rales. Which of the following is true?

    A. Patients in CHF presenting with severe hypertension have a higher mortality rate than normotensive or hypotensive patients
    B. Furosemide is the initial treatment of choice
    C. The patient should undergo rapid sequence intubation and mechanical ventilation
    D. An intravenous nitrate infusion should be started
    E. Noninvasive ventilation is contraindicated in the setting of severe hypertension

28. Which of the following is the most important factor in determining the chance of spontaneous passage of a kidney stone?

    A. Composition of the stone
    B. Size of the stone
    C. Degree of pain
    D. Degree of nausea
    E. Age of the patient

29. A 65-year-old female with hypertension, atrial fibrillation, and type II diabetes presents with acute painless vision loss in her right eye. On examination, visual acuity is markedly decreased and the patient has a striking afferent pupillary defect. She also has a right-sided carotid bruit. Which of the following is the most appropriate next step in management?

    A. Lateral canthotomy
    B. Globe massage
    C. Aspirin
    D. Heparin
    E. Tissue plasminogen activator (tPA)

30. Which of the following is the most common cause of large bowel obstruction?

    A. Malignancy
    B. Sigmoid volvulus
    C. Adhesions
    D. Diverticular disease
    E. Fecal impaction

31. A 1-week-old infant is brought to the ED with central cyanosis. Pulse oximetry is 85% on maximal oxygen therapy, and chest x-ray is shown in Figure 12-4. Which of the following medications may be indicated in the treatment of this patient?

    A. Prostaglandin E₁
    B. Albuterol
    C. Indomethacin
    D. Aspirin
    E. Ribavirin

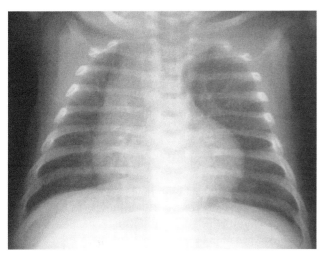

Figure 12-4

32. A term female neonate develops purulent ocular discharge on day 3 of life. Which of the following etiologies carries the greatest morbidity in this patient?

    A. *C. trachomatis*
    B. *N. gonorrhoeae*
    C. *S. aureus*
    D. Nasolacrimal duct obstruction (dacryocystitis)
    E. No organism—chemical conjunctivitis

33. The most common cause of sexually transmitted disease (STD) in the United States is:

    A. *Trichomonas vaginalis*
    B. *Chlamydia trachomatis*
    C. *Treponema pallidum*
    D. *Neisseria gonorrhoeae*
    E. *Candida* spp.

34. Which of the following is the most common cause of acute-onset, nontraumatic hearing loss?

    A. Otitis media with effusion
    B. Tympanic membrane (TM) perforation
    C. Acute foreign body
    D. Cerumen impaction
    E. Idiopathic sensorineural hearing loss

35. A mother brings in her 12-year-old son with a chief complaint of alopecia. The patient denies any complaints and has been well recently. The lesion is shown in Figure 12-5. Which of the following is the treatment of choice?

    A. 2.5% selenium sulfide shampoo
    B. Clotrimazole cream FENa = (urine Na) (plasma Cr)/ (urine Cr) (plasma Na)
    C. High-dose amoxicillin (80 to 90 mg/kg divided b.i.d.)
    D. Terbinafine lotion
    E. Oral griseofulvin

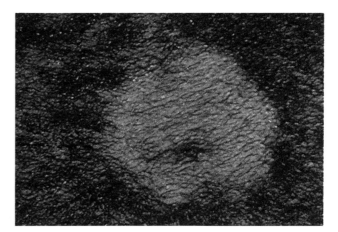

Figure 12-5

36. Among trauma patients, which of the following is the most common incomplete spinal cord syndrome?

    A. Brown–Séquard syndrome
    B. Central cord syndrome
    C. Anterior cord syndrome
    D. Posterior cord syndrome
    E. Conus medullaris syndrome

37. A 22-year-old male presents with left-sided facial and periorbital pain after a fight. A CT scan reveals the image shown in Figure 12-6. Which of the following examination findings may be present?

    A. Decreased sensation of the left cheek
    B. Inability of upward gaze
    C. Enophthalmos
    D. Periorbital emphysema
    E. All of the above

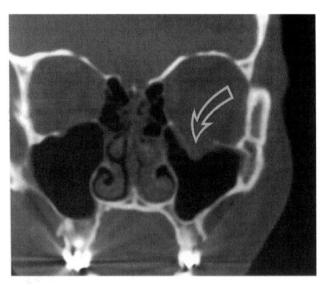

Figure 12-6

38. A 44-year-old female with a history of migraines presents with a 2-day history of her typical migraine symptoms including a frontal, throbbing headache with photophobia and phonophobia. She ran out of her sumatriptan, and acetaminophen has not helped her headache. Which of the following treatments is likely to be most effective?

    A. PO ibuprofen
    B. PO hydrocodone–acetaminophen
    C. IV hydromorphone
    D. IV lorazepam
    E. IV metoclopramide

39. Which of the following is true regarding major depression?

    A. Visual hallucinations have high specificity for the diagnosis.
    B. Paranoid delusions have high sensitivity for the diagnosis.
    C. Either depressed mood or anhedonia is required for the diagnosis.
    D. The prevalence of major depression is the same as bipolar disorder.
    E. In the elderly, depression is easily distinguished from dementia on clinical grounds.

40. A 6-year-old child presents after a seizure. She has had acute gastroenteritis for the past 2 days. Electrolytes are normal. Which of the following is the most likely cause?

    A. *Salmonella*
    B. *Shigella*
    C. *Campylobacter*
    D. *Yersinia*
    E. *Vibrio*

41. An 18-month-old previously healthy child is brought in by his mother with bilateral oral commissure burns after biting an extension cord. He cried immediately after the injury, did not lose consciousness, and he has been acting normally since the injury. On examination, you note a 5-mm burn to both of the patient's oral commissures. Which of the following is true?

    A. He should be transferred to a burn center for immediate debridement and reconstructive repair.
    B. Delayed labial artery bleeding can usually be managed with direct pressure.
    C. All patients with bilateral oral commissure burns should have a CT scan of the face to search for deep tissue injury.
    D. He should be admitted for 24 hours of cardiac monitoring.
    E. Serum creatine kinase and troponin levels should be measured.

42. A 52-year-old previously healthy male presents by EMS for evaluation of a scalp laceration after a fall. His initial CT reveals a small subdural hematoma. However, he later seems more confused and you suspect he will need intubation. Which of the following is the best means of preoxygenation before intubation?

    A. Noninvasive positive pressure ventilation
    B. High-flow nasal cannula set to 15 L/minute
    C. Standard reservoir face mask with oxygen set as high as possible
    D. "Blow by" oxygen over the patient's mouth connected to wall oxygen set as high as possible
    E. A venturi mask set to 50% oxygen at 15 L/minute

43. A 24-year-old female presents with an ankle injury while playing soccer. She inverted her ankle and has pain and tenderness in the lateral malleolar area. She has no tenderness to palpation in the base of the fifth metatarsal, calcaneus, or proximal fibula. An ankle x-ray reveals no fracture. She is able to bear weight, albeit with moderate pain. Which of the following is the most appropriate home care instruction for her?

    A. Non-weight-bearing with crutches until seen by orthopedic surgeon
    B. Toe-touch ambulation with crutches until seen by orthopedic surgeon

C. Stirrup-style ankle brace with weight-bearing as tolerated

D. Lace-up ankle brace with weight-bearing as tolerated

E. Mixed martial arts training with roundhouse kicks on padded dummy

44. A 23-year-old male presents with shoulder pain after falling. A shoulder radiograph is shown in Figure 12-7. Which of the following is the most likely additional injury?

A. Axillary nerve injury

B. Glenoid rim disruption

C. Brachial artery injury

D. Humeral head fracture

E. Biceps muscle tear

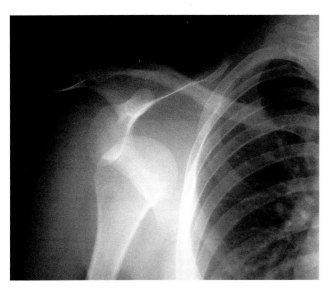

Figure 12-7

45. A 34-year-old female with systemic lupus erythematosus (SLE) is diagnosed with lupus anticoagulant. Which of the following is likely to be seen in this patient?

A. Prolonged PT

B. Venous thrombosis

C. Predisposition to bleeding

D. Most cases occur in lupus patients

E. Most complications are treated with factor VII

46. A 35-year-old marathon runner who is asymptomatic presents from an outside hospital with an "abnormal EKG" (Fig. 12-8). Your advice to the patient is:

A. Telemetry admission for pacemaker

B. Atropine 1 mg IV

C. Amiodarone 300 mg IV

D. Adenosine 6 mg IV

E. No acute therapy, routine follow-up

47. A 45-year-old male presents with acute onset of left flank pain. He is extremely uncomfortable and writhing in pain. After appropriate pain control, he is sent for a CT scan of the abdomen and pelvis, which demonstrates a 2-mm kidney stone in his mid-right ureter. Which of the following is true regarding this patient?

A. He is likely to pass the stone without further medical intervention.

B. Urinalysis is likely to be completely normal.

C. The stone has already traversed the narrowest portion of the ureter.

D. Strict fluid restriction is the management of choice.

E. The stone is most likely composed of cystine.

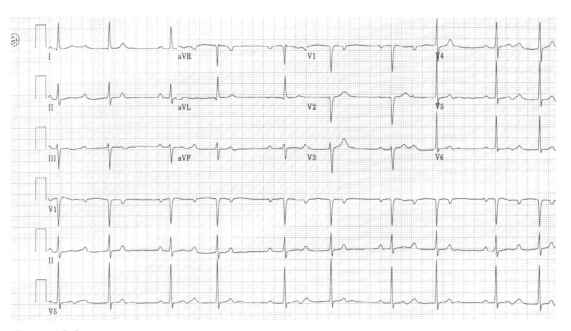

Figure 12-8

48. Which of the following is the most common symptom in patients diagnosed with an abdominal aortic aneurysm (AAA)?

    A. Nausea
    B. Abdominal distention
    C. Constipation
    D. Urinary retention
    E. Asymptomatic

49. Newborns with congenital dislocation of the hip:

    A. Require surgical repair 50% of the time
    B. Most often have an associated connective tissue disorder
    C. Frequently develop a leg-length discrepancy
    D. Most often have normal hips by 2 months of age
    E. Frequently develop the classic Trendelenburg gait pattern

50. A 4-year-old female presents with vomiting and diarrhea. She is diagnosed with acute gastroenteritis. Presence of which of the following findings still allows the patient to be a suitable candidate for oral rehydration therapy (ORT)?

    A. Continued diarrhea
    B. Lethargy
    C. Shock
    D. Abdominal rebound
    E. Bowel obstruction

51. Which of the following occurs in most patients with myocarditis?

    A. Chest pain
    B. Fever
    C. Antecedent viral syndrome
    D. S4 heart sound
    E. Leukocytosis

52. A 3-year-old female swallows a button battery. Plain radiographs demonstrate that the battery is lodged in the esophagus. Which of the following is the most appropriate next step in management?

    A. Expectant management
    B. Endoscopic removal
    C. Ipecac for therapeutic emesis
    D. Activated charcoal
    E. Whole bowel irrigation

53. Which of the following is most characteristic of ethylene glycol overdoses?

    A. Hypocalcemia
    B. Hypokalemia
    C. Microcytic anemia
    D. Thrombocytopenia
    E. Hypermagnesemia

54. Patients with which of the following tumors is at highest likelihood for developing tumor lysis syndrome (TLS) in response to chemotherapy?

    A. Colon cancer
    B. Endometrial cancer
    C. Burkitt lymphoma
    D. Chronic lymphocytic leukemia (CLL)
    E. Prostate cancer

55. A 14-year-old female presents with a blanching, erythematous rash all over her chest and back and arms and legs shortly after starting antibiotics for a sore throat a few days prior to presenting to the ED. The patient's mother reports that the strep swab was negative but antibiotics were started because it "looked like strep." She has posterior cervical lymphadenopathy and bilateral tonsillar exudates on examination. Which of the following is true?

    A. The antibiotic should be changed to clindamycin
    B. The patient has scarlet fever
    C. Amoxicillin is the likely antibiotic given
    D. The patient has an allergic drug reaction
    E. Pastia lines will be present on examination

56. Which of the following may worsen acute renal failure due to rhabdomyolysis?

    A. Mannitol
    B. Saline
    C. Bicarbonate
    D. Furosemide
    E. Deferoxamine

57. A 10-year-old male is brought to the ED after a head injury. Based on his CT scan which of the following physical findings is most likely (Fig. 12-9)?

    A. Left pupillary dilation, coma
    B. Bitemporal hemianopia
    C. Bilateral pupillary constriction, coma
    D. Right pupillary dilation, coma
    E. Left pupillary constriction, left eye deviated inferiorly and laterally, coma

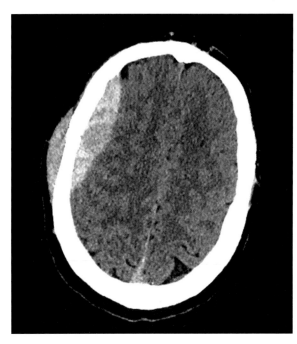

Figure 12-9

58. A 32-year-old pregnant woman in her third trimester presents with dysuria. She has a penicillin allergy. Urinalysis demonstrates bacteria, but no white blood cells, leukocyte esterase, or nitrites. Physical examination is normal. Which of the following is the most appropriate next step in management?

A. Close outpatient observation
B. Trimethoprim–sulfamethoxazole
C. Ciprofloxacin
D. Nitrofurantoin
E. Amoxicillin

59. Diverticular disease:

A. Is more common in the right colon among Japanese-Americans
B. Most commonly affects the sigmoid colon in the Western world
C. Is treated with a high-fiber diet
D. Is the most common cause of massive lower gastrointestinal (GI) bleeding
E. Is all of the above

60. A 3-week-old term male neonate is brought in by EMS in respiratory distress, with minimal wheezes, cyanotic with a room air SaO_2 of 60%. His father reports this began after the baby became fussy while feeding. Applying a 100% nonrebreather results in no improvement. Which of the following is the best next step?

A. Rapid sequence intubation
B. Place the infant in a knee to chest position
C. Infuse intravenous phenylephrine

D. Infuse intravenous esmolol
E. All of the above

61. A 34-year-old female presents with shoulder pain following a fall. Physical examination is normal except for tenderness in the middle of the clavicle. Radiographs demonstrate a nondisplaced clavicle fracture. Which of the following is the most appropriate course of action?

A. Operative repair
B. Figure-of-eight brace
C. Magnetic resonance imaging (MRI) to evaluate rotator cuff injury
D. Shoulder sling
E. Shoulder arthrocentesis

62. A 55-year-old male presents with a "bump" on his upper eyelid (Fig. 12-10). Which of the following is the most appropriate next step in management?

A. Intravenous antibiotics
B. Eyelid culture
C. Warm compresses
D. Needle aspiration of the raised area
E. Topical antivirals

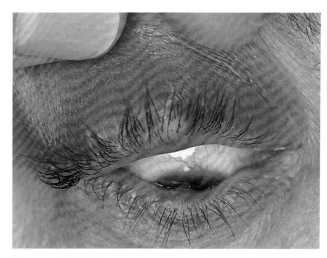

Figure 12-10

63. Which of the following is true regarding pediatric community-acquired pneumonia (CAP)?

A. The most common cause of pneumonia in the neonate is *Mycoplasma pneumoniae.*
B. Toddlers and young children more frequently develop CAP than middle-aged adults.
C. It is easier to differentiate between typical and atypical pneumonia in pediatric patients.
D. *Streptococcus pneumoniae* is the most commonly isolated organism in children aged 5 to 15 years.
E. The presence of rhinorrhea, myalgias, or a concomitant illness in a family member is more common in viral pneumonia.

64. A 42-year-old female presents with sudden onset of acute severe headache. You strongly suspect subarachnoid hemorrhage. Which of the following is the most likely etiology?

    A. Arteriovenous malformation
    B. Neoplasia
    C. Mycotic aneurysm
    D. Moyamoya disease
    E. Amyloid angiopathy

65. A 16-year-old male is brought to the emergency room by his parents after being struck in the face by a baseball while playing for his high school team. He complained of immediate eye pain and vision loss. Which of the following findings is most concerning for an underlying globe rupture?

    A. Hyphema
    B. Subconjunctival hemorrhage
    C. Marked decreased visual acuity
    D. Orbital floor ("blowout") fracture
    E. Bloody chemosis

66. A 46-year-old male presents with chest pain 8 hours after having upper endoscopy for dysphagia (Fig. 12-11). Esophageal perforation is suspected and a screening chest x-ray is ordered. Which of the following is likely to be found on physical examination?

    A. Diffusely diminished heart sounds
    B. Decreased breath sounds at lung bases bilaterally
    C. Shock
    D. A crunching sound upon cardiac auscultation
    E. A rigid, tender abdomen

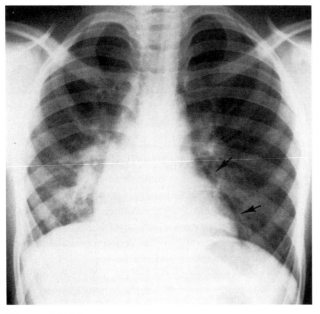

Figure 12-11

67. A 44-year-old female with a history of end-stage renal disease on peritoneal dialysis presents with abdominal pain. You suspect peritonitis as a cause of her pain. Which of the following is the most likely etiologic agent?

    A. *Staphylococcus* species
    B. *Candida* species
    C. *Escherichia coli*
    D. *Klebsiella*
    E. *Pseudomonas*

68. A 24-year-old female presents to the ED with the rash shown in Figure 12-12. She notes that she had a recent "cold sore" and brief febrile illness that resolved on its own. She now complains of general malaise and a rash. The rash is symmetric and is spread over her extremities as well as her palms and soles. The remainder of her examination is unremarkable. Which of the following is true?

    A. Mucosal involvement is common.
    B. A positive Nikolsky sign will be present.
    C. Intravenous immunoglobulin is the only effective treatment.
    D. The rash will resolve on its own
    E. All of the above

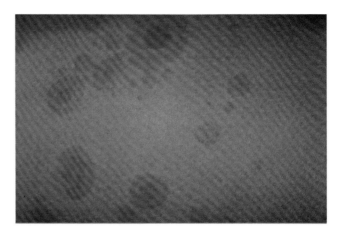

Figure 12-12

69. A 31-year-old G_4P_3 presents to the ED in active labor at 38 weeks of gestation. On examination, the patient is maximally dilated and the umbilical cord is noted at the cervical opening. Which of the following may be helpful?

    A. Place the mother on a stretcher in Trendelenburg position
    B. Place a Foley catheter and instill the bladder with 750 mL of saline
    C. Place the mother's legs in a knee to chest position
    D. Elevate the presenting fetal part to relieve compression on the umbilical cord
    E. All of the above

70. A 5-year-old female presents with the lesion shown in Figure 12-13. It is soft, boggy, and very tender. Which of the following is the most appropriate next step in management?

A. Doxycycline PO
B. Incision and drainage
C. Griseofulvin PO
D. Topical triamcinolone
E. Topical terbinafine

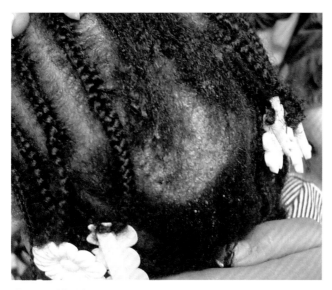

Figure 12-13

71. An institutionalized patient with psychiatric disease presents with abdominal pain, distension, and nausea without vomiting. The image shown in Figure 12-14 suggests which of the following diagnoses?

A. Sigmoid volvulus
B. Small bowel obstruction
C. Intussusception
D. Diabetic gastroparesis
E. Hirschsprung disease

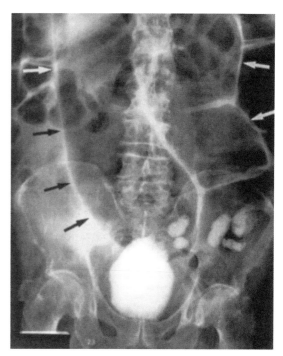

Figure 12-14

72. A 30-year-old, 80-kg male patient presents to the ED with a severe allergic reaction not responding to intravenous diphenhydramine, steroids, and famotidine. You decide to treat him with epinephrine. The appropriate dose is:

A. 0.3 mL 1:1,000 subcutaneously (SQ)
B. 0.5 mL 1:10,000 SQ
C. 0.3 mL 1:1,000 intramuscularly (IM)
D. 0.5 mL 1:1,000 IV
E. 0.3 mL 1:10,000 IM

73. A 52-year-old male with a long-standing history of alcohol abuse presents with a chief complaint of vomiting blood. He was last seen by a doctor 8 months ago because of abdominal swelling and he was told he had "a liver problem." Which of the following is most likely to be useful in this patient?

A. Octreotide
B. Famotidine
C. Pantoprazole
D. Vasopressin
E. Propranolol

74. A 55-year-old male presents with acute, left-sided flank pain. Which of the following increases the likelihood that the patient's pain is due to acute ureterolithiasis as opposed to another etiology?

A. Black race
B. Hypotension
C. Fever
D. Hematuria
E. Abnormal Rovsing sign

75. In most patients diagnosed with community-acquired pneumonia, which of the following contributes most to a patient's Pneumonia Severity Index (PSI) score?

    A. Underlying neoplastic disease
    B. Cirrhosis
    C. Age
    D. Sex
    E. Pulse >125

76. A 72-year-old female presents to the ED with asymptomatic acute kidney injury. Her creatinine is 1.9 mg/dL as measured at her primary care physician's office. She has a past medical history of hypertension, osteoarthritis, and neuropathy. Which of her medications is most likely to blame?

    A. Amlodipine
    B. Metoprolol
    C. Ibuprofen
    D. Hydrocodone
    E. Gabapentin

77. Which of the following is true regarding electrical injury?

    A. Direct current (DC) is more dangerous than alternating current (AC).
    B. In high-voltage injuries, the extent of cutaneous burns is a good predictor of internal tissue damage.
    C. Asystole is the most common dysrhythmia resulting from low-voltage electrical injury.
    D. In contrast to other mass casualty traumatic events, patients without signs of life should be resuscitated first.
    E. All of the above.

78. A 77-year-old male with type 2 diabetes presents with a 4-day history of progressively worsening left ear pain, hearing loss, and discharge. On examination, he has a temperature of 101°F, he appears fatigued, and his tympanic canal is markedly edematous with foul drainage. His glucose level is 400. Which of the following is true regarding this condition?

    A. IV ciprofloxacin and ENT consultation are indicated.
    B. *Streptococcus pneumoniae* is the single most likely pathogen.
    C. Cranial nerve involvement almost always begins with the abducens nerve.
    D. Sinus x-ray may be warranted to evaluate extent of disease.
    E. Antiviral therapy should empirically be started.

79. A 5-year-old male presents with fever and sore throat. Examination reveals exudative tonsillitis and tender cervical lymphadenopathy. You suspect group A streptococcal pharyngitis. Which of the following is true regarding treatment for this condition?

    A. Resistance to penicillin is above 30%
    B. Antibiotic therapy helps to reduce the risk of acute glomerulonephritis
    C. The risk of side effects from antibiotics is higher than the risk of acute rheumatic fever
    D. Macrolides are the drug of choice if penicillins are contraindicated
    E. Oral therapy is more effective than intramuscular therapy

80. A 34-year-old male with a history of schizophrenia is brought to the ED by police with acute agitation. He was reported to be threatening passersby on the street. He now begins to threaten staff, stating that he will kill anyone who comes near him, and starts to swing punches at people standing near him. The patient is physically restrained by security staff and secured to a cart in four-point restraints. He is still yelling at the top of his lungs and struggling against the restraints. Which of the following is the most appropriate next step in management?

    A. Administer medications for agitation and check a CK level to determine if he has neuroleptic malignant syndrome (NMS).
    B. Observe for 1 hour and repeat history and physical examination.
    C. CT scan of the brain without contrast.
    D. Administer haloperidol and lorazepam.
    E. Perform rapid sequence intubation.

81. A 4-year-old male is brought to your office by parents with a fever to 102°F over the last 2 days, malaise, and complaint of right ear pain. Examination reveals an active, febrile child with a bulging right tympanic membrane (TM) minimally mobile on insufflation. Which of the following is the most likely pathogen?

    A. *Mycoplasma pneumoniae*
    B. *Streptococcus pyogenes*
    C. *Moraxella catarrhalis*
    D. *Hemophilus influenza*
    E. Adenovirus

82. A 59-year-old male with a history of diabetes and gout presents for evaluation of a 2-day history of worsening left knee pain and swelling without fever. He is unable to put any weight on it or bend it. Vital signs are 99.4°F, 100, 18, 161/80, 99% RA. Examination reveals a warm, tender knee with a moderate effusion and extreme pain on flexion and extension. Knee radiographs reveal an effusion but no fracture. Which of the following is the next best step in management?

    A. Discharge home with acetaminophen or nonsteroidal anti-inflammatory drugs (NSAIDs)
    B. Discharge home with colchicine
    C. Knee arthrocentesis
    D. MRI knee
    E. Serum uric acid level

83. Which of the following neurologic functions is commonly impaired in patients with anterior cord syndromes?

   A. Vibration sensation
   B. Fine touch sensation
   C. Temperature sensation
   D. Position sensation
   E. Extraocular motor function

84. Which of the following may be a cause of central vertigo?

   A. Basilar artery migraine
   B. Vertebrobasilar artery insufficiency
   C. Multiple sclerosis
   D. Alcoholic cerebellar degeneration
   E. All of the above

85. A 47-year-old female s/p a remote tonsillectomy presents with a chief complaint of a 5-day history of progressive neck pain radiating to her occiput. She does not recall the moment of onset but rather describes gradually worsening neck pain over the past several days. In the day prior to her visit to the ED, she developed a mild sore throat, and more limited range of motion. Specifically, she has difficulty with neck flexion, and turning to the right. She denies any shortness of breath and she has no stridor or wheezing on examination. A CT scan was obtained and is shown in Figure 12-15. The CT image reveals a likely infection in the:

   A. Peritonsillar space
   B. Retropharyngeal space
   C. Submandibular space
   D. Epiglottis
   E. None of the above

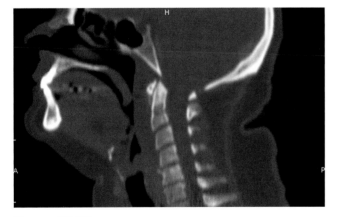

Figure 12-15

86. A 78-year-old male nursing home resident is brought to the ED with fever and hypoxia. He has a history of dysphagia and dysarthria secondary to stroke and receives tube feedings and small spoon feeds. Approximately 1 week before admission, he had an episode of vomiting and appeared to choke on some of the regurgitated contents. His chest x-ray now shows bilateral lower lobe infiltrates. He has a fever of 101.8°F, a WBC of 16,000, and a pulse oximetry of 92% on room air. What is the most likely diagnosis and appropriate initial treatment?

   A. CAP, levofloxacin, and corticosteroids
   B. Aspiration pneumonia, metronidazole
   C. Aspiration pneumonitis, no antibiotics
   D. Aspiration pneumonia, aztreonam
   E. Aspiration pneumonia, piperacillin–tazobactam

87. A 22-year-old male contact-lens wearer presents to the ED with a chief complaint of right eye pain, redness, light sensitivity, and a foreign body sensation. Examination reveals no foreign body but a small, peripheral corneal ulcer and a small amount of yellowish drainage. In addition to removing the contact lenses, which of the following is the best next step?

   A. Patch the eye, erythromycin eye drops
   B. Irrigate the eye with 500 mL of 0.9% normal saline
   C. Ciprofloxacin eye drops
   D. Trimethoprim–polymyxin B ointment
   E. Patch the eye, ophthalmology follow-up in 24 hours

88. A 5-day-old neonate presents for routine follow-up. The child is acting normally. Funduscopic examination demonstrates bilateral retinal hemorrhages. Which of the following is the most likely cause?

   A. Child abuse
   B. Accidental fall
   C. Normal birth trauma
   D. Intracerebral hemorrhage
   E. Congenital finding

89. A 22-year-old male presents with a gunshot wound to the left chest. Chest x-ray is shown in Figure 12-16. Which of the following is the most likely diagnosis?

   A. Pneumothorax
   B. Pericardial tamponade
   C. Hemothorax
   D. Pneumoperitoneum
   E. Diaphragmatic rupture

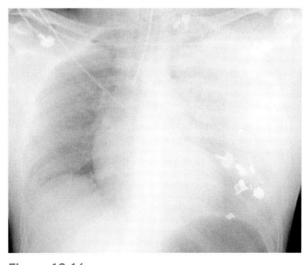

Figure 12-16

90. Which of the following is true regarding West Nile virus (WNV) infections?

    A. It is the most common cause of viral encephalitis.
    B. Following recovery, immunity is likely lifelong.
    C. The most common presentation is "West Nile fever," in which patients present with fever, headache, and malaise, associated with diffuse myalgias.
    D. Neuroinvasive disease may lead to a spastic paralysis.
    E. Valacyclovir is an effective adjunct in treatment.

91. Which of the following is the most common opportunistic infectious agent in AIDS patients?

    A. Tuberculosis
    B. Pneumocystis pneumonia (PCP)
    C. *Cryptococcus neoformans*
    D. *Toxoplasma gondii*
    E. Cytomegalovirus (CMV)

92. Which of the following is a possible complication of left ventricular assist device (LVAD) placement and use?

    A. Gastrointestinal bleeding
    B. Right heart failure
    C. Pump thrombosis
    D. Driveline infection
    E. All of the above

93. Which of the following is the most common symptom seen in pulmonary tuberculosis (TB)?

    A. Weight loss
    B. Night sweats
    C. Shortness of breath
    D. Chest pain
    E. Hemoptysis

94. Comatose patients with bilateral miosis thought to be due to narcotic overdose may sometimes be confused with patients with which of the following?

    A. Lateral medullary syndrome
    B. Locked-in syndrome
    C. Pontine hemorrhage
    D. Pseudobulbar palsy
    E. Retinal detachment

95. Which of the following is true regarding traumatic aortic injury (TAI)?

    A. Dyspnea is the most common symptom.
    B. Normal chest x-ray rules out the diagnosis.
    C. CT aortography has better sensitivity than transthoracic echocardiogram.

    D. Blood pressure control is not useful in the preoperative setting.
    E. The ascending aorta is the site at highest risk for rupture.

96. In patients with measles, where are Koplik spots most likely to be seen?

    A. Hard palate
    B. Soft palate
    C. Tonsils
    D. Tongue
    E. Buccal mucosa

97. Pulmonary infections with which of the following may be transmitted from person to person?

    A. *Coxiella burnetii*
    B. *Y. pestis*
    C. *Histoplasma capsulatum*
    D. *Francisella tularensis*
    E. *Bacillus anthracis*

98. Which of the following is true regarding diaphragmatic injuries?

    A. Left-sided injuries are three times as common as right-sided.
    B. The majority heal spontaneously.
    C. Delayed herniation of abdominal contents into the thorax is extremely rare.
    D. Almost all cases are caused by penetrating trauma to the abdomen.
    E. Ultrasonography is the diagnostic modality of choice.

99. Which of the following EKG changes may be seen in the setting of hypercalcemia?

    A. ST-segment depression
    B. QTc-segment shortening
    C. Widened T wave
    D. Bradycardia
    E. All of the above

100. A 23-year-old female presents with right lower quadrant pain. Which of the following historical features increases the likelihood of acute appendicitis?

    A. Migratory pain from the periumbilical region
    B. Radiation of pain to the right scapula
    C. Pain >48 hours
    D. Unchanged pain with movement
    E. Extreme hunger

ANSWERS AND EXPLANATIONS

1. **Answer A.** The temporal sequence of EKG morphologies in acute MI is generally hyperacute T waves, ST elevation, T-wave inversion, and Q waves. Hyperacute T waves may also be seen in hyperkalemia and (along with ST elevation) in benign early repolarization, acute pericarditis, and left ventricular hypertrophy. ST elevation may also be seen in bundle branch block and ventricular aneurysms. The evolution in the preceding sequence in the appropriate clinical setting usually points to ST-elevation myocardial infarction (STEMI). This is a strong argument for performing repeated EKGs in the evaluation of acute coronary syndrome in the ED.

2. **Answer C.** Given the hyperacute onset of swelling and the location, the patient likely has a parotid gland stone. Sudden blockage of the Stensen duct can cause almost immediate swelling. CT imaging is the best modality for evaluation of the stone and exclusion of other etiologies, though imaging is not always needed in clear-cut cases. X-ray imaging, with or without contrast misses many parotid gland stones and are not useful in the clinical setting. MRI does not visualize salivary gland stones well. PET scans are generally used to detect cancer and the sudden onset of symptoms in the case doesn't warrant an evaluation for this. Theoretically, an existing parotid mass could undergo sudden hemorrhage and cause hyperacute swelling, but parotid cancers are quite rare and occur less commonly than other salivary gland cancers. (Figure from Sherman SC, Ross C, Nordquist E, et al., eds. *Atlas of Clinical Emergency Medicine.* 1st ed. Philadelphia, PA: Wolters Kluwer; 2015.)

3. **Answer C.** The patient has primary herpetic gingivostomatis due to HSV-1. The lesions are concentrated on the hard palate and gums, rather than the soft palate more posteriorly (which would be a sign of herpangina due to coxsackievirus). In most cases, supportive care is all that is required. However, in cases where oral intake is limited due to pain, treatment with valacyclovir is indicated. Nystatin is used for candidal therapy and would not be appropriate here. No abscess exists to perform incision and drainage. Immune-suppressants such as methotrexate or prednisone are not indicated for this primary viral infection. (Figure from Gehrig JS, Willmann DE, eds. *Foundations of Periodontics for the Dental Hygienist.* Philadelphia, PA: Wolters Kluwer; 2011.)

4. **Answer C.** The most common cause of bacterial meningitis in middle-aged and older adults is pneumococcus. Group B streptococcus is common among neonates, *Listeria* in extremes of age, and meningococcus in young adults. *H. influenzae* used to be a very common cause of bacterial meningitis among children, but the introduction of the HiB vaccine has drastically reduced the frequency of this pathogen.

5. **Answer B.** Zika virus is a flavivirus, the same genus as dengue, West Nile, and yellow fever. It is associated with fetal *microcephaly*, rather than macrocephaly, in babies of infected mothers, as well as Guillain–Barre syndrome in the patients themselves. Characteristic symptoms include fever, myalgias, and rash, although many patients are completely asymptomatic. The 2015 outbreak of Zika started in Brazil and spread throughout the Americas. Mortality is extremely low and as of mid-2016, no vaccine or pharmacotherapy has been established.

6. **Answer A.** Lipase and amylase have roughly the same sensitivity for diagnosing acute pancreatitis, although their sensitivity depends on the threshold value above normal used to establish the diagnosis (most authors suggest a cutoff of three times the upper limit of normal). Lipase is almost certainly more specific than amylase, because almost all lipase originates from the pancreas. However, there is a small amount of gastric lipase, and lipase levels may be elevated in the setting of a gastric or duodenal ulcer, severe renal insufficiency, or in some cases of bowel obstruction. Although both enzymes tend to rise at approximately the same rate, lipase remains elevated for a longer period of time (lipase remains elevated for 8 to 14 days, although amylase returns to normal after 5 to 7 days). The degree of elevation of amylase or lipase does not correlate with disease severity. The ratio of amylase to lipase has not proven to be useful.

7. **Answer B.** The CT scan shows a right-sided epidural hematoma. While the patient is initially awake and alert, this may be indicative of the lucid interval that is often seen in patients with epidural hematoma (although it is neither sensitive nor specific for the diagnosis). Acute worsening of the clinical status mandates returning to the ABCs of trauma evaluation. Although burr hole placement is the most important definitive management, control of the airway is the most important initial action. CT and Focused Assessment with Sonography in Trauma (FAST) scans have largely replaced DPL in the ED. In an unstable patient with a suspected intraperitoneal source of bleeding despite a negative FAST scan, DPL may be performed if the patient is too unstable for CT scan (e.g., persistent, severe hypotension). However, in solitary head trauma, such a scenario is unlikely. Thoracotomy is indicated in patients with penetrating trauma to the chest who arrest in the ED or shortly beforehand. Nasogastric tube placement is contraindicated

in patients with severe head and facial trauma as damage to the inferior portion of the skull may allow the tube to pass from the nose into the cranium. (Figure courtesy of Robert Hendrickson, MD. In: Greenberg MI, Hendrickson RG, Silverberg M, et al., eds. *Greenberg's Text-Atlas of Emergency Medicine.* Philadelphia, PA: Lippincott Williams & Wilkins; 2004:51, reprinted with permission.)

8. **Answer B.** The majority of completed suicides among both men and women involve firearms. The presence of a firearm in the house is an independent risk factor for completed suicide and the patient should be directly asked about this on history. Drug ingestion, usually with antidepressants, is the most common method of suicide attempts, and the second most common method of completed suicide by women. Carbon monoxide poisoning is employed less often. Hanging is the second most common method of completed suicide by men. Wrist cutting almost never results in completed suicide.

9. **Answer D.** Iron toxicity can be life threatening. Ingestion of large quantities of iron overwhelms the body's iron-binding capacity and causes GI, cardiac, CNS, hepatic, and renal damage. Nausea, vomiting, diarrhea, and GI bleeding are the most common symptoms. Diagnosis involves serial serum iron levels and plain abdominal radiographs to demonstrate passage of the radiopaque iron pills. Treatment involves whole bowel irrigation with polyethylene glycol, deferoxamine chelation in patients with severe overdoses (defined as rising iron levels, absolute level >500 μg/dL, or worsening clinical course), and dialysis of the chelated iron when renal failure is present. Activated charcoal does not adequately bind heavy metals. Gastric lavage is rarely indicated for any overdose, except in certain cases when patients present within 30 minutes of overdosing. Ipecac is almost never indicated for any overdose. Hemodialysis is only necessary when renal failure limits the body's ability to clear chelated iron.

10. **Answer E.** The decision about when to resume feeding and what patients should be allowed to eat is a matter of ongoing controversy. In the past, all patients underwent continuous NG suctioning or were kept NPO. Currently, the only indication for NG suctioning is intractable vomiting or ileus. Some studies suggest that early enteral nutrition may actually improve outcomes. Laboratory and radiographic evidence of pancreatitis is likely to persist until patient discharge, so these are not useful guides for resuming feeding. Many authors now recommend that enteral feeds should be started as soon as a patient is able to tolerate them. Although there is a dearth of evidence regarding the composition of feeds, it is known that pancreatic secretions decrease as carbohydrate composition exceeds 50% of the caloric content of the diet. Therefore, it makes sense to start with a low

calorie, carbohydrate-rich diet, and steadily increase both the caloric and the fat content of the diet over a period of days.

11. **Answer E.** The anterior circulation refers to the region of brain tissue served by the internal carotid arteries. Approximately 80% of cerebral blood flow is derived from the carotid arteries. This includes the anterior cerebral artery, the middle cerebral artery, and the ophthalmic artery (branch of the internal carotid artery just before joining the circle of Willis). Hemiparesis and hemisensory loss of the leg is a result of anterior cerebral artery ischemia. Transient monocular blindness (amaurosis fugax) is a result of ischemia in the ophthalmic artery. Aphasia and hemiparesis are due to ischemia in the middle cerebral artery. Ataxia and vertigo along with nausea and vomiting are caused by posterior circulation ischemia (to the cerebellum). The posterior circulation originates in the vertebral arteries (which originate from the subclavian arteries), which join to form the basilar artery and then bifurcate to form the two posterior cerebral arteries. This system supplies the remaining 20% of cerebral blood flow, delivering blood to the cerebellum and brainstem as well as to the visual occipital lobe and medial aspect of the temporal lobe.

12. **Answer D.** Rheumatic fever occurs several weeks after untreated streptococcal pharyngitis. The diagnosis is made by the Jones criteria—either two major (polyarthritis, erythema marginatum, chorea, carditis, subcutaneous nodules) or one major and two minor (arthralgias, fever, increased erythrocyte sedimentation rate (ESR) or C-reactive protein (CRP), prolonged PR interval). Migratory arthritis of major joints is the most common symptom, followed by carditis. Chorea and erythema marginatum are uncommon but fairly specific given a history of antecedent pharyngitis. Fever is neither sensitive nor specific.

13. **Answer B.** The patient has temporal arteritis. Steroids are the mainstay of management and should be initiated even before temporal artery biopsy is done. Once significant visual loss has occurred, only one out of three patients who receive IV steroids will improve in the affected eye. However, steroids will nearly eliminate contralateral eye involvement. Patients have a significantly higher risk of thoracic aorta aneurysms, and a slightly higher risk of abdominal aorta aneurysms. Women are five times more likely to be affected than men. Patients younger than 50 years are rarely affected.

14. **Answer D.** In a young healthy female with acute-onset debilitating abdominal pain, the time-sensitive diagnosis is ovarian torsion. Delays of even several hours can result in irreversible ovarian necrosis and potential infertility. Evaluation with pelvic ultrasound and gynecologic consultation is indicated. CT studies produce

unacceptable delays in the evaluation of ovarian torsion. The other major diagnosis in the differential in this case is ureteral colic from kidney stone. Although kidney stone also can be an emergent issue, immediate operative management is rarely required when concomitant urinary tract infection is not present. Torsion occurs more commonly about 2 weeks into the menstrual cycle when ovulation is occurring. An enlarged ovary (due to tumor, cyst, or abscess) is the strongest risk factor. Ovarian torsion risk is also increased during pregnancy.

15. **Answer B.** Wounds >5 cm in length, in locations other than the head and neck, in patients with diabetes are most likely to be infected. Interestingly, the 6 and 12 hour time windows that are often used to determine infection risk do not actually predict higher infection risk. Wounds with visible contamination also increase wound infection rates, but not as much as the other factors above, and this risk is mitigated through appropriate wound irrigation with tap water or saline.

16. **Answer E.** The patient has evidence of uncomplicated urinary tract infection (UTI). The most common cause is *E. coli,* followed by other gram-negative bacilli, then streptococci. Treatment in cases of uncomplicated UTI is for 3 days with either TMP-SMX or a fluoroquinolone, or 5 days with nitrofurantoin, depending on local resistance patterns. The overuse of levofloxacin for respiratory infections has fostered fluoroquinolone resistance among a significant number of urinary *E. coli* isolates, making it useless for empiric treatment of UTIs in many communities. Regardless, the patient has allergies to both sulfa drugs and fluoroquinolones. Doxycycline and azithromycin have better coverage against gram-positive organisms and atypicals and often lack effectiveness against gram-negative bacilli. In some communities, *E. coli* also remains sensitive to cephalexin, amoxicillin, or amoxicillin–clavulanic acid.

17. **Answer C.** The patient most likely has myocarditis, which in the United States is usually because of viruses, most commonly Coxsackie B. A viral prodrome usually precedes overt signs of cardiac involvement, such as chest pain or signs of heart failure. No common ED laboratory or imaging study is helpful in making the diagnosis of myocarditis—antimyosin scintigraphy or more invasive endomyocardial biopsy is indicated. Coronary artery disease is uncommon in patients of this age in the absence of risk factors. Aortic dissection is uncommon in the absence of trauma or history of hypertension or Marfan disease. Stroke is not suggested by the symptoms, and diabetic ketoacidosis (DKA) is unlikely with normal glucose and bicarbonate.

18. **Answer B.** *Carpal tunnel syndrome* refers to median neuropathy due to compression at the wrist. Common conditions associated with carpal tunnel syndrome include diabetes, hypothyroidism, pregnancy, and rheumatoid arthritis. Findings include pain and paresthesias in the thumb, index, and long fingers. Phalen test (pain from holding the wrists flexed for 60 seconds) is more sensitive than Tinel test (pain from tapping the volar wrist), but neither is reliable enough to exclude or prove the diagnosis and nerve conduction studies are the gold standard. Treatment involves wrist splinting, with surgery reserved for refractory cases.

19. **Answer E.** This patient has evidence of bilateral facial nerve paresis. Bilateral facial nerve paresis or paralysis is rare in the setting of Bell palsy and its presence should prompt a search for alternative diagnoses. In general, patients with bilateral facial nerve paresis should be considered to have Lyme disease until proved otherwise. This patient's recent camping trip suggests the possibility of a remote tick bite, which led to infection with the spirochete *Borrelia burgdorferi*. Ten percent of patients with erythema migrans, who are not treated, will develop neurologic manifestations, the most common of which is facial nerve palsy. Interestingly, patients with facial nerve paralysis due to Lyme disease typically have other constitutional symptoms or neurologic findings that point toward the diagnosis. Other causes of bilateral facial nerve palsy include myasthenia gravis, lymphoma, sarcoidosis, brainstem tumors, and GBS.

20. **Answer D.** Historically, the diagnosis of a concussion has been based on a history of loss of consciousness or a change in cognition that may also be associated with amnesia. While all of these symptoms may be present in patients with concussions, very few patients with symptoms suggestive of a concussion have amnesia or have lost consciousness. Instead, the diagnosis of concussion is based on a constellation of symptoms in after head trauma. Headache and dizziness or unsteadiness are the most common symptoms of concussion. Other symptoms include trouble concentrating, light or sound sensitivity, drowsiness, and irritability or personality changes. Neuroimaging studies are not helpful unless there is a strong suspicion for skull fracture or intracranial hemorrhage. Patients with a concussion should undergo physical and cognitive rest until all their symptoms are completely resolved, after which they may return to participate in regular activities in a graded fashion.

21. **Answer E.** The patient has both clinical and radiographic evidence of CAP. Treatment with antibiotics should be initiated as soon as possible. Routine blood cultures and sputum Gram stain in immunocompetent patients with CAP are not helpful and rarely change management. CT scan of chest is not indicated unless PE is suspected or the chest x-ray does not show consolidation despite the presence of strong clinical signs of

pneumonia. Arterial blood gas is not helpful in the routine evaluation of pneumonia in the absence of suspicion of hypercarbia.

22. **Answer A.** Management of hydrocarbon toxicity is generally supportive. Hydrocarbons most commonly cause pulmonary toxicity and cardiac dysrhythmias. The most common scenarios are inhalation through "huffing" paint or glue cans and oral ingestion of hydrocarbons, followed by nausea, vomiting, and pulmonary aspiration. There is no evidence that antibiotics, steroids, or diuretics improve outcomes in hydrocarbon aspiration. Activated charcoal does not bind hydrocarbons and should not be used.

23. **Answer E.** Though it is not rare, osteomyelitis is a relatively uncommon infection among normal hosts. However, it occurs with increased frequency in patients with sickle cell disease, HIV, and in dialysis patients or other chronically ill patients with indwelling catheters. In contrast to adults, osteomyelitis most commonly occurs due to hematogenous spread in pediatric patients. *Staphylococcus aureus* accounts for 50% of infections, though *Salmonella* is the most common isolate in patients with sickle cell disease. The long tubular bones are most frequently affected (tibia > femur > humerus), while the vertebrae are most commonly affected in adults. X-rays are frequently nonspecific, or normal in the early phase of illness, as are the WBC count, erythrocyte sedimentation rate, and CRP. The illness typically begins gradually with symptoms of fever and malaise. However, as the infection intensifies in the affected bone, patients complain of focal bone pain, and there may be some associated soft-tissue swelling. This should lead to imaging of the area which yields the diagnosis.

24. **Answer D.** The head impulse test (or sometimes the head thrust test), is a bedside test used to distinguish central versus peripheral pathology in patients who present with a vestibular syndrome. It is most effective in testing patients with unremitting rather than transient symptoms. The test assesses the patient's vestibule–ocular reflex (VOR). Patients with a normal VOR are able to maintain their fixed gaze when their head is turned to the left and right. Testing patients with a vestibular lesion demonstrates that their eyes are "dragged" off target before marching back to the target in a saccadic fashion. Counterintuitively, a "normal" test in which the patient demonstrates normal fixation is more concerning for a central lesion and those patients should receive an urgent MRI. Abnormal tests indicate a peripheral lesion affecting vestibular nerve (cranial nerve VIII) which is more reassuring. Answers A–C are all essentially similar with respect to being central lesions. Oculomotor nerve palsies create diplopia and would reveal an eye that is displaced "down and out" compared to normal.

25. **Answer B.** The patient likely has toxic shock syndrome (TSS), given the preceding skin infection, sunburn-like diffuse rash, hypotension, and fever. TSS is a toxin-mediated disease, either due to staphylococcal TSS toxin-1 or *S. pyogenes* exotoxins A and B. Staphylococcal TSS used to occur secondary to superabsorbent tampons in menstruating women, but now, like streptococcal TSS, it is largely because of systemic and postsurgical infections. Multiorgan failure is characteristic of both processes. Blood cultures are usually negative in staphylococcal TSS and positive in approximately half of the cases of streptococcal TSS. Mortality for staphylococcal and streptococcal TSS is 5% and 30%, respectively. Management involves removal of any foreign bodies, antibiotics directed at streptococci and staphylococci, vasopressors, intravenous fluids, and intensive care monitoring.

26. **Answer D.** Pemphigus vulgaris is the most common form of pemphigus, although it is a rare disease. It most commonly affects older individuals in the sixth decade. Nikolsky sign, which occurs when pressure applied to the margin of a blistered or ulcerated lesion expands the lesion into the adjacent apparently normal skin, is the clinical hallmark of the disease. Although antibiotics are important in cases of secondary infection, corticosteroids are the mainstay of therapy. Most patients have oral lesions that start as blisters, which then spontaneously rupture to leave painful oral ulcers that are slow to heal. Oral ulcers may precede cutaneous disease by several months. The cause of the disease is unknown, although there is a genetic predisposition and an autoimmune mechanism involving circulating IgG antibodies to keratinocytes.

27. **Answer D.** Patients with acute decompensated CHF (ADHF) and severe hypertension benefit from afterload and preload reduction and intravenous nitroglycerin (NTG) achieves this goal. Sublingual nitroglycerin is rapidly absorbed and provides a dose equivalent to more than 50 mcg/minute for a brief period. Thus, it should be used while an IV infusion is being prepared. In addition, oxygen combined with noninvasive positive pressure ventilation with BiPAP or continuous positive airway pressure (CPAP) helps recruit alveoli (from positive end expiratory pressure) and is a critical component of initial therapy. While many patients ultimately need diuresis, intravenous loop diuretics such as furosemide offer limited benefit in the hyperacute setting of ADHF. In particular, furosemide induces some degree of arteriolar constriction resulting in increased systemic vascular resistance and mean arterial pressure which undermines the goals of treatment. Finally, as shown by Gheorghiade M et al., there is negative correlation between hypertension and mortality in the setting of ADHF. This may be because patients with severe long-standing hypertension typically have diastolic

heart failure which is easy to address in an acute exacerbation while normotensive or hypotensive patients have systolic heart failure.

28. **Answer B.** The large majority of kidney stones <5 mm will pass spontaneously without the need for lithotripsy or surgical extraction. The large majority of stones >5 mm will *not* pass spontaneously. Stones may become stuck in several areas along the urinary tract—renal calyx, ureteropelvic junction, midureter at the iliac vessels, ureterovesicular junction, and vesical opening. Urologic management of kidney stones is through extracorporeal shock wave lithotripsy, percutaneous nephrolithotomy, or surgical extraction. Pain and nausea are potential indications for admission of patients with kidney stones but are not independently associated with low passage rate. Age of the patient and composition of the stone are not directly associated with passage of the stone.

29. **Answer B.** The patient has central retinal artery occlusion (CRAO), probably caused by a thromboembolus from atrial fibrillation or carotid atherosclerosis. The conditions listed in her past medical history are all risk factors for CRAO. Intermittent globe massage is indicated to increase ocular carbon dioxide content, which leads to vasodilation of the retinal arteries. Lateral canthotomy is used to treat retrobulbar hematoma and has no role in management here. Aspirin, heparin, and TPA have not been shown to improve outcomes in CRAO.

30. **Answer A.** Malignant neoplasms account for more than half of all cases of large bowel obstruction. Volvulus and diverticulitis (either through stricture, abscess, or phlegmon formation) are the second and third most common causes.

31. **Answer A.** The chest x-ray shows an enlarged, boot-shaped heart, consistent with tetralogy of Fallot. Patients with suspected tetralogy of Fallot should be managed in a step-wise manner—oxygen, fluid resuscitation, morphine, and α-agonist therapy. Prostaglandin E_1 may be indicated in neonatal patients to prevent closure of the ductus arteriosus and ensure enough shunting of blood to the pulmonary vasculature. The major adverse effects of prostaglandin E_1 are apnea and hypotension. Albuterol is useful in cases of reactive airway disease but does not benefit with congenital heart disease. Indomethacin promotes closure of the ductus and would be detrimental. Aspirin is never indicated in pediatric patients except in the setting of Kawasaki disease. Ribavirin is indicated in select patients with RSV bronchiolitis. (Figure courtesy of Mark Silverberg, MD. From Silverberg M. *Hurst's the Heart.* 11th ed. McGraw-Hill; 2004:602.)

32. **Answer B.** The most dangerous cause of neonatal conjunctivitis is *N. gonorrhoeae*. It is less often seen in Western countries due to chemoprophylaxis but is still an important cause of ophthalmia neonatorum due to its potential for invading the intact corneal epithelium and causing blindness. Treatment should be prompt with topical and parenteral antibiotics. Choices A and C occur more often in slightly older infants and cause less severe sequelae. Choices D and E may be more common given the practice of prophylaxis of all neonates with erythromycin ointment, but both processes are easily halted by removing the erythromycin and cause no long-lasting sequelae.

33. **Answer B.** *C. trachomatis* is the most common bacterial cause of STD in the United States. Most women infected with *C. trachomatis* are asymptomatic (as many as 85%), although up to one-third of women will have *signs* of infection upon physical examination. *C. trachomatis* takes up residence in the endocervix and causes an intense inflammatory reaction resulting in mucopurulent cervicitis. Treatment consists of a single 1-g dose of azithromycin or 7 days of 100 mg of doxycycline given twice daily. In the setting of more severe infection (pelvic inflammatory disease), doxycycline should be given for 14 days and combined with empiric treatment for *N. gonorrhoeae* and probably *Trichomonas* as well.

34. **Answer D.** Conductive problems such as cerumen impaction and foreign body impaction are the most common causes of acute-onset hearing loss in the absence of trauma. Cerumen impaction is more common than foreign body impaction, since many foreign bodies are oddly shaped and do not completely obstruct the external auditory canal, which allows for continued, if suboptimal, hearing.

35. **Answer E.** This patient has tinea capitis, which is a fungal infection of the scalp usually caused by *Trichophyton tonsurans*. Tinea capitis should be suspected in all prepubescent children with hair loss, particularly if the hair loss is focal and incomplete, or is associated with scale and lymphadenopathy. There may be scattered hairs that are broken near the base within a generalized area of alopecia, resulting in the appearance of black dots on the scalp surface ("black dot" ringworm). Although topical agents such as selenium sulfide and topical ketoconazole may reduce infectivity, they are insufficient as monotherapy. In all cases, oral therapy with griseofulvin (either micronized or ultramicronized) is required. Transmission from person to person is common, and *Trichophyton* remains infectious in combs and hairbrushes for long periods. (Figure from Fleisher GR, Ludwig S, Baskin MN. *Atlas of Pediatric Emergency Medicine.* Philadelphia, PA: Lippincott Williams & Wilkins, 2004.)

36. **Answer B.** Central cord syndrome is the most common incomplete spinal cord syndrome. Unlike anterior cord syndrome, central cord syndrome typically results from forced *hyperextension* injuries in arthritic middle-aged and older adults. The posterior ligamentum flavum is thought to buckle and compress the cord against anterior osteophytes, resulting in a contusion to the central aspects of the cord. Due to the topography of the spinal cord, extension injuries occurring at the level of the cervical spine result *primarily* in flaccid paralysis of the *upper* limbs; to a lesser extent, spastic paralysis or paresis of the lower extremities occurs in the setting of large cord lesions. Furthermore, distal muscles are affected more than proximal muscles. There is variable sensory dysfunction, but because most sensory neurons are located peripherally, sensory findings tend to be less prevalent. Finally, there should be preserved perianal sensation, voluntary rectal motor function, big toe flexor activity, and preservation of the bulbocavernosus reflex. Together, the presence of these functions is referred to as *sacral sparing*.

37. **Answer E.** The CT reveals the classic "teardrop" sign associated with orbital floor fracture. Direct trauma to the orbit causes an immediate rise in intraorbital pressure fracturing the weakest borders of the orbit. This most commonly results in fractures of the orbital floor and medial orbital wall. Due to swelling and stretching of the infraorbital nerve, there is often transient hypoesthesia in its distribution lasting for 1 to 2 weeks. In addition, the inferior rectus muscle may become entrapped in the orbital floor defect; effectively tethering the globe such that upward gaze is limited or not possible. Patients may complain of diplopia if partial upward gaze is possible. Enophthalmos results from loss of orbital volume and supporting structures. It may not be visible acutely because of the swelling associated with the injury. However, delayed repair is required if it is present 2 weeks after the injury. Periorbital emphysema results from communication of the orbit with the sinus, an air-filled structure. It is important to note that exophthalmos resulting from a retroorbital hematoma can also occur. This is a true emergency that may require immediate lateral canthotomy. (Figure from Harris JH, Harris WH. *The Radiology of Emergency Medicine.* 4th ed. Lippincott Williams & Wilkins; 1999:70, with permission.)

38. **Answer E.** Migraine headaches usually respond to early administration of NSAIDs or acetaminophen. When these do not work, however, the serotonin receptor ($5\text{-HT}_{1B/1D}$) agonists (e.g., sumatriptan and dihydroergotamine) can be used to abort the migraine. Parenteral metoclopramide (D_2 antagonist, 5-HT_3 antagonist, 5-HT_4 agonist) has been shown to be superior to opioid therapy in several studies of migraine treatment. It should be used in conjunction with an anticholinergic agent to prevent significant akathisia. Lorazepam and other benzodiazepines appear to be less effective at treating the pain of a migraine attack, though they can be used to reduce anxiety and provide mild sedation in these patients.

39. **Answer C.** Major depression is a type of mood disorder, which requires either depressed mood or anhedonia (loss of interest or pleasure in pleasurable activities) for the diagnosis. According to the Diagnostic and Statistical Manual of Mental Disorders, Fourth Edition (DSM-IV) criteria, symptoms need to be present for 2 or more weeks for formal diagnosis. Symptoms include disturbances in appetite, sleep, concentration, activity, and energy and thoughts of guilt or suicide. The symptoms should not be caused by a thought disorder, medical condition, or substance abuse. Delusions and visual hallucinations are more characteristic of thought disorders than major depression. Major depression is almost 10 times as common as bipolar disorder. It is extremely difficult to distinguish dementia from depression in the elderly on clinical grounds alone. Sometimes a trial of antidepressant therapy may be necessary to make the diagnosis—major depression is extremely responsive to pharmacotherapy whereas dementia is not.

40. **Answer B.** Acute gastroenteritis is most commonly caused by viruses, but bacteria account for an important subset of cases. In the absence of severe electrolyte abnormalities, seizures associated with diarrhea are often because of *Shigella* species, which are the most common bacterial causes of acute gastroenteritis overall. *Salmonella* is not typically associated with seizures. *Campylobacter* and *Yersinia* species may cause an illness that mimics appendicitis. *Vibrio* species usually cause a typical, nonspecific gastroenteritis.

41. **Answer B.** Generally, pediatric patients with oral burns can be safely discharged home with minimal or no ancillary testing. Delayed labial artery bleeding occurs 7 to 14 days after the initial injury, when the eschar falls off the wound. It typically responds to local, direct pressure, although patients will occasionally require a figure-8 suture to control bleeding. Otherwise, the most serious complication of burns to the oral commissure is a cosmetic facial deformity. Therefore, patients should be urgently referred to a facial or oral surgeon for further evaluation and possible oral splinting. There is no correlation between an isolated oral burn and cardiac injury or myoglobinuria. However, the patient should receive a thorough examination to ensure that there are no other contact wounds indicating a more extensive electrical path.

42. **Answer C.** Though most hospital flow meters are only demarcated to 15 L/minute, most of them can achieve

flow rates well beyond this rate. FiO_2 levels greater than or equal to 90% are achievable with flow rates of 30 to 60 L/minute while using a conventional reservoir face mask (commonly called a nonrebreather even though most such masks are actually rebreather masks). Spontaneously breathing patients achieve a maximal reservoir of oxygen and denitrogenation after about 3 minutes of normal breathing or after eight vital capacity breaths. Noninvasive positive pressure ventilation is an excellent adjunct for patients who can't achieve adequate oxygen saturation levels with a standard reservoir mask as above. "Blow by" oxygen provides only ambient FiO_2 levels, while nasal cannulas and venturi masks don't provide adequate oxygen levels to maximize preoxygenation.

43. **Answer C.** The patient likely has a moderate grade lateral ankle sprain. A stirrup-style ankle brace restricts only inversion and eversion but allows for dorsiflexion and plantarflexion, which is important in optimal recovery from ankle sprains. Gentle range-of-motion exercises (such as tracing letters with toes) along with standard rest–ice–compression–elevation management are also indicated. A lace-up style brace can work as well, but restricts all range of motion in the ankle joint, potentially slowing recovery. Non-weight-bearing or toe-touch ambulation for ankle sprains is not typically indicated unless there are accompanying signs of occult fracture. Recommending direct force trauma to the joint soon after the ankle sprain is suboptimal.

44. **Answer A.** The radiograph demonstrates an anterior shoulder dislocation, with the humeral head displaced anteriorly relative to the glenoid. Common complications include (in order of decreasing frequency) axillary nerve injury (causing deltoid anesthesia), humeral head fracture (Hillman–Sachs deformity), and glenoid rim disruption (Bankart lesion). Vascular compromise in shoulder dislocations is rare. Acromioclavicular separation and clavicular fractures are rarely associated with shoulder dislocations because of different mechanisms. The mechanism of an anterior dislocation is trauma to the abducted and externally rotated upper extremity. Clavicle fractures and acromioclavicular separations tend to occur with trauma to the adducted arm. (Figure courtesy of Shoma Desai, MD. In: Greenberg MI, Hendrickson RG, Silverberg M, et al., eds. *Greenberg's Text-Atlas of Emergency Medicine.* Philadelphia, PA: Lippincott Williams & Wilkins; 2004:497, with permission.)

45. **Answer B.** The term "lupus anticoagulant" is a frustratingly confusing misnomer. Most patients with lupus anticoagulant do not have SLE, and most patients with SLE do not have lupus anticoagulant. Additionally, lupus anticoagulant is actually a *pro*thrombotic process, causing an increased risk of clotting rather than bleeding. Lupus anticoagulant binds to the prothrombin activator complex and prolongs the partial thromboplastin time (PTT), which is not corrected in a mixing study with normal blood. Treatment for thrombotic complications usually involves anticoagulation with heparins, Coumadin, or direct factor Xa inhibitors. The term "lupus anticoagulant" is used because (1) SLE patients with lupus anticoagulant are more likely to have clinically significant disease compared to the general population and (2) in vitro, the lupus anticoagulant does act as a clotting inhibitor (as opposed to the in vivo thrombotic effect).

46. **Answer E.** The EKG demonstrates Wenckebach phenomenon or Mobitz type I AV block. The PR interval progressively increases in length and predictably drops a QRS beat after the second prolongation. In the absence of symptoms of other serious cardiac disease, management involves outpatient follow-up. Pacemaker placement would be required for patients with Mobitz type II second-degree or third-degree AV block. Atropine is used to treat hemodynamically unstable bradydysrhythmias. Amiodarone may be used to treat a variety of tachydysrhythmias but is not indicated for patients with AV blocks. Adenosine is used to abort supraventricular tachycardias.

47. **Answer A.** The large majority of kidney stones <5 mm will pass spontaneously without the need for lithotripsy or surgical extraction. The large majority of stones >5 mm will *not* pass spontaneously. Urinalysis in patients with kidney stones most often shows microscopic hematuria, although 10% to 20% of cases will have completely normal urinalyses. The narrowest portion of the ureter, and one of the most common sites of obstruction, is the ureterovesicular junction at the distal-most point of the ureter. Medical management of kidney stones involves aggressive pain and nausea treatment, copious fluid intake, and stone analysis to assess for risk factors to prevent recurrence. The most common stone types are in decreasing order of frequency: calcium, struvite, uric acid, and cystine.

48. **Answer E.** Aneurysms are most often asymptomatic and diagnosed incidentally on routine examination or imaging studies. Most symptomatic patients complain of vague abdominal pain or abdominal distension, although urinary retention and constipation may occur. Nausea occurs only in the setting of other symptoms pointing to the diagnosis. Acute abdominal pain or distension in patients at risk for AAA indicates rapid expansion or rupture.

49. **Answer D.** Nearly 90% of newborns with a dislocated hip or reduced hip that can be dislocated on examination (Barlow test) most often have normal hips by 2 months of age, provided those with a dislocated hip have the hip reduced upon examination (which allows

for normal development). Testing of the hips is a two-stage process. Barlow test determines whether a reduced hip can be dislocated or subluxed from the joint. The hips are flexed to 90 degrees, the thighs are adducted, and posterior pressure is applied in line with the femoral shaft to dislocate the hips posteriorly. A positive test occurs when dislocation is felt or heard as a click. Ortolani test confirms that the hips are dislocated or subluxed. Once the hip is posteriorly displaced, the thigh is abducted, which reduces the femoral head with a palpable clunk. Infants with a positive test warrant close follow-up with repeat examinations and ultrasound at 4 to 6 weeks. However, most infants continue to develop normally. The cause is not known, but it is more common in the left hip and in female infants. While patients with Down syndrome and Ehlers–Danlos syndrome more frequently have congenital dislocation (now called developmental dysplasia or developmental dislocation), it is most common in otherwise normal infants. In untreated patients, a leg-length discrepancy and the Trendelenburg gait pattern (in which weakness of the ipsilateral hip abductors causes the pelvis to drop to the unaffected side while walking) often develop.

50. **Answer A.** Standard treatment for pediatric patients with acute gastroenteritis is ORT. Standard solutions are available and consist of hypotonic fluid and essential electrolytes. Administration of ORT may occur in the ED, hospital floor, or at home. Patients may continue to have vomiting and/or diarrhea and still be candidates for ORT. Contraindications to ORT include shock, lethargy, severe abdominal tenderness or rebound, bowel obstruction, and severe underlying medical illness. Failure of ORT should necessitate intravenous fluid hydration. Treatment of acute gastroenteritis with ORT observed in the ED is cost-effective and clinically efficacious. Hospital admission may be prevented by this ED observation of parent-administered ORT.

51. **Answer C.** Myocarditis is most commonly postviral, including Coxsackie B, adenovirus, and influenza. Bacterial and protozoal pathogens are less common etiologies. More than half the number of patients report an antecedent nonspecific viral syndrome. Acute symptoms include myalgias, fever, fatigue, chest pain, and shortness of breath, but none of these is present in most cases. Myocarditis may lead to dilated cardiomyopathy, causing overt heart failure. Leukocytosis is uncommon, EKG findings are nonspecific, and echocardiogram may show evidence of global hypokinesis. The gold standard for diagnosis is endomyocardial biopsy, but there are many false negatives due to the patchy nature of the inflammation.

52. **Answer B.** Button batteries lodged in the esophagus or trachea can cause obstruction, necrosis, and perforation. Esophageal button batteries should be removed urgently

with upper endoscopy. Any button battery distal to the esophagus may be managed expectantly and will likely pass without any specific treatment. Ipecac is rarely indicated for any ingestion anymore. Activated charcoal is not indicated for foreign body ingestions. Whole bowel irrigation may be useful to help speed passage of post-esophageal button battery that has been slow to progress with expectant management alone.

53. **Answer A.** Ethylene glycol is metabolized to glycoaldehyde by alcohol dehydrogenase, and glycoaldehyde is converted to glycolic acid by aldehyde dehydrogenase. Glycolic acid is then converted to glyoxylic acid, which is converted to oxalic acid. Oxalic acid binds calcium and forms calcium oxalate crystals, which can precipitate in the renal tubules, brain, and lungs, causing necrosis. Approximately one-third of patients with ethylene glycol poisoning have hypocalcemia, which can lead to QT prolongation and seizures. Hyperkalemia is more common than hypokalemia, probably due to the metabolic acidosis caused by ethylene glycol poisoning. Anemia, thrombocytopenia, and hypermagnesemia do not usually occur in patients with ethylene glycol poisoning.

54. **Answer C.** Tumor lysis syndrome (TLS) describes the constellation of problems that arises from massive cell death that occurs in the setting of chemotherapy of rapidly growing, highly chemo-sensitive malignancies. The tumors most commonly associated with TLS are high-grade lymphomas (such as Burkitt lymphoma and other high-grade non-Hodgkin lymphomas) and acute myeloid leukemia (AML). However, TLS can occur in the setting of chemotherapy for any cancer and is in part dependent on the total cancer burden, as well as pre-existing renal disease, patient hydration status, and the acidity of a patient's urine.

55. **Answer C.** The patient presents with findings consistent with infectious mononucleosis (bilateral tonsillar exudates, posterior cervical lymphadenopathy) as well as a generalized rash after starting antibiotic. Amoxicillin and ampicillin are the classic agents responsible for the rash, though it has been associated with other antibiotics. As the patient has Epstein-Barr virus (EBV), there is no indication to change the antibiotic. The patient does not have scarlet fever, which is the rash associated with group A strep pharyngitis. Pastia lines are confluent lines of petechiae found in the skin creases of patients with scarlet fever.

56. **Answer D.** The foundation of treatment for rhabdomyolysis is the administration of large volumes of normal saline early in the course of the disease. Urine output should be maintained between 200 and 300 mL/hour and patients may require as much as 20 L of fluid in the first 24 hours to achieve such a flow rate. Mannitol is an osmotic diuretic that may help maintain urine output,

especially in cases of oliguric renal failure. Bicarbonate causes urine alkalinization, which helps to keep myoglobin soluble, and may therefore enhance its clearance. The goal is to keep the urine pH above 6.5. Deferoxamine is an iron chelator that may have a protective role as it inhibits lipid peroxidation, which may shield myocyte membranes. Furosemide has also been used in cases of oliguric renal failure. However, furosemide causes urine acidification and may therefore enhance myoglobin precipitation into casts worsening renal function.

57. **Answer D.** The CT reveals an epidural hematoma, as shown by its biconcave (sometimes called lentiform) shape. Children are more prone to forming epidural hematomas because the dura is less tightly attached to the skull than it is in adults. This patient's CT demonstrates a right-sided parietal epidural hematoma. This applies superior and lateral pressure to the entire right brain, pushing the brain toward the midline and toward the tentorium cerebelli. This latter pressure squeezes the oculomotor nerve against the temporal bone, resulting in partial oculomotor nerve (cranial nerve III) palsy and ipsilateral pupillary dilation. Complete third nerve palsies, in which the affected eye is deviated laterally and inferiorly ("down and out") may also occur but are a late finding. Contralateral palsies can also occur but also indicate more severe trauma and are a late finding. Bitemporal hemianopsia, in which there are bilateral temporal visual field cuts, are caused by pressure on the optic chiasm, classically due to a pituitary tumor.

58. **Answer D.** Both bacteriuria and urinary tract infection (UTI) should be treated aggressively in pregnant women, as they can cause serious complications with delivery. The prevalence of bacteriuria may be higher in pregnant women than in nonpregnant women, but UTI rates are comparable. Symptoms are identical between the two groups. Gram-negative enteric bacteria cause the vast majority of UTIs in pregnant women, but a crucial organism to consider is Group B *Streptococcus*, which can cause serious neonatal infection. Nitrofurantoin, penicillins, and cephalosporins are the drugs of choice. Sulfonamides are not safe during the third trimester because of the possibility of neonatal hemolysis. Fluoroquinolones cause various congenital defects. Although amoxicillin would be a reasonable choice in most patients, the allergy to penicillin is an obvious contraindication.

59. **Answer E.** Diverticuli are most common in the left colon, particularly the sigmoid colon, among patients from the Western world. Japanese patients most commonly have diverticula in the right colon. Even among Japanese who have immigrated to the United States and who consume a low-fiber, high-fat Western diet, diverticula are typically limited to the right colon. However, such patients have a significantly higher incidence of disease than their counterparts in Japan. The most common treatment for diverticular disease (in the absence of diverticulitis) is a high-fiber diet. Fiber bulks the stools theoretically preventing stools from getting caught in existing diverticuli while also helping to prevent the development of further diverticuli. Diverticulosis is the most common cause of massive lower GI bleeding. It usually occurs due to diverticuli in the right colon.

60. **Answer B.** The patient has tetralogy of Fallot (TOF), and is experiencing a "tet spell" which is a hypercyanotic episode due to near complete right ventricular outflow tract (RVOT) obstruction resulting in severe right to left shunting and cyanosis. Though mild episodes are often self-limited, they can be life threatening. Typically, oxygen has already been applied to a cyanotic infant. Thus, the first step is to place the neonate into a knee to chest position to increase systemic vascular resistance and decrease right to left shunting. If the spell fails to resolve, morphine is infused at 0.1 mg/kg along with IV fluids (20 mL/kg). If the spell continues, intravenous beta-blockers (such as esmolol or propranolol) are used followed by phenylephrine

61. **Answer D.** Clavicular fracture is extremely common with shoulder trauma. The vast majority of clavicular fractures are treated conservatively with shoulder sling and orthopedic follow-up. Operative repair is almost never indicated in nondisplaced, closed fractures, because conservative management results in excellent functional outcomes. There is no proven advantage of the figure-of-eight brace over simple sling, and it may actually cause skin necrosis if applied too tightly. Emergent MRI is almost never indicated in acute injuries, and clavicle fracture with concomitant rotator cuff injury is rare. Shoulder arthrocentesis is indicated only in cases of suspected septic arthritis and has little role in acute trauma.

62. **Answer C.** The superior lid contains a hordeolum (or stye) with surrounding blepharitis. A hordeolum refers to localized infection of a meibomian gland in the lid, usually because of *S. aureus*. Treatment involves warm compresses, with topical erythromycin ointment applied to the lid if there is a surrounding blepharitis. Systemic antibiotics are rarely indicated in patients with hordeolum. Eyelid culture is unlikely to be helpful or easy to obtain. Aspiration of the area is strictly contraindicated given the proximity to the globe. Topical antivirals are indicated only in patients with herpes keratitis. The lower lid has a chalazion, which is a subacute, granulomatous lesion also treated with warm compresses. (Figure from Tasman W, Jaeger EA, eds. *The Wills Eye Hospital Atlas of Clinical Ophthalmology.* 2nd ed. Philadelphia, PA: Lippincott Williams & Wilkins; 2001, with permission.)

63. **Answer B.** With the possible exception of elderly patients older than 75 to 80 years, the annual incidence of pneumonia in children under 5 years is higher than at any other time of life. *M. pneumoniae* is the most common cause of CAP in "school-aged children," 5- to 15-year olds, as well as in young adults. Increasingly, *Chlamydia pneumoniae* is thought to be a common cause of pneumonia in children aged 5 to 15 years, although *Mycoplasma* remains the chief cause of pneumonia in this group. The most common causes of pneumonia in the neonate, from birth to 3 weeks, are group B *Streptococcus*, gram-negative enterobacteria (e.g., *E. coli*), and *Listeria monocytogenes*. Such infections are uncommon but can be severe when present. Between the ages of 3 weeks and 3 months, *Chlamydia trachomatis* is most common (i.e., not *C. pneumoniae*) followed by *S. pneumoniae*. Between 4 months and 4 years, viruses (e.g., respiratory syncytial virus [RSV], parainfluenza virus, influenza, adenovirus, rhinovirus) are the most common cause. *S. pneumoniae* remains an important cause of bacterial pneumonia in this age-group, but the use of the pneumococcal conjugate vaccine has reduced its role as well as the morbidity associated with CAP caused by *S. pneumoniae*. It is no easier to differentiate between typical and atypical pneumonia in a pediatric population than in adults. Studies have demonstrated that the presence of symptoms that may suggest a viral etiology to pneumonia such as rhinorrhea, myalgias, or an illness in a family member do not help to determine the cause of pneumonia.

64. **Answer A.** The most common etiology of subarachnoid hemorrhage is berry aneurysm, representing about 80% of cases. The second most common cause is arteriovenous malformation. Neoplasia, mycotic aneurysm, moyamoya, and amyloid angiopathy are far less commonly seen (though the incidence of amyloid angiopathy is increased in the geriatric population).

65. **Answer C.** Clinicians should maintain a high degree of suspicion for an open globe rupture when patients present with marked decreased visual acuity after orbital trauma, which is a common manifestation of globe rupture. Hyphema and subconjunctival hemorrhage most commonly occur without concomitant globe rupture but are often present in the setting of globe rupture as well. While subconjunctival hemorrhage does not typically affect visual acuity, patients can experience profound subconjunctival hemorrhage, termed bullous subconjunctival hemorrhage, in which the degree of subconjunctival bleeding and subsequent conjunctival swelling is so severe that it prevents direct visual inspection of the underlying ocular structures and completely impedes vision. Patients with hyphema may have normal vision or may only have light perception, also depending on the severity of bleeding. However, when such patients are placed in a seated position, the blood

in the anterior chamber slowly forms a layer at the bottom of the chamber, and vision often improves. Blowout fractures are common in patients with globe rupture but most commonly occur without associated globe rupture or changes in acuity. Bloody chemosis refers to hemorrhagic swelling to the conjunctiva, which is what results in severe subconjunctival hemorrhage, as detailed above.

66. **Answer D.** "Hamman crunch" refers to the crunching sound heard during cardiac auscultation in the setting of pneumomediastinum. Radiographic abnormalities are present in up to 90% of patients with esophageal perforation, and include pneumomediastinum, subcutaneous emphysema, pleural effusion, and pulmonary infiltrate. Pleural effusions may occur and are usually right sided if the perforation occurs in the midesophagus, but left sided if the perforation occurs in the distal esophagus. Pneumoperitoneum may also occur if the patient has a rupture of the intra-abdominal esophagus. (Figure from Swischuk L. *Emergency Radiology of the Acutely Ill or Injured Child.* 2nd ed. Philadelphia, PA: Lippincott Williams & Wilkins; 1986:63, 77, 79, with permission.)

67. **Answer A.** Unlike cases of spontaneous bacterial peritonitis (SBP), where gram-negative enteric organisms predominate, patients with peritoneal dialysis catheters tend to develop peritonitis from gram-positive organisms, most commonly *Staphylococcus* species. Clinical signs and symptoms of infection can be extremely mild and asymptomatic infection is common. Diagnosis is through analysis of the peritoneal fluid—100 or more WBC per mm^3 with a predominance of neutrophils or a positive Gram stain makes the diagnosis. Most cases can be treated on an outpatient basis with intraperitoneally administered antibiotics. The antibiotics of choice are vancomycin plus any antibiotic with good gram-negative coverage, such as a fluoroquinolone, third-generation cephalosporin, aminoglycoside, or aztreonam.

68. **Answer D.** This patient has erythema multiforme (EM) minor (no mucosal involvement), which is a relatively benign disease that results from a host immune response to antigenic exposure. EM minor is at the benign end of a clinical spectrum that includes EM major, Stevens Johnson syndrome (SJS), and toxic epidermal necrolysis (TEN). The classic rash is typically symmetric and involves the extremities, palms, and soles. The archetypal lesion is a "target" lesion measuring <3 cm and consisting of two concentric rings around a dusky, central disk. Mucosal involvement never occurs in EM minor, whereas it is very common in EM major and is almost exclusively limited to the oral cavity. Nikolsky sign describes the tendency for the top layer of skin to rub off when it is touched. It is classically associated with pemphigus vulgaris. Corticosteroids are sometimes used for treatment but their benefit has not been proved. Immunoglobulin plays no

role in treatment. The lesions resolve without intervention within 1 to 3 weeks. Although almost 50% of cases of EM minor are idiopathic, HSV is the most common infectious agent triggering the disease. EM is typically caused by infection, whereas SJS and TEN are typically due to drug exposure. (Figure courtesy of Lawrence B Stack, MD. In: Plantz SH, Huecker M, eds. *Step-Up to Emergency Medicine*. Philadelphia, PA: Wolters Kluwer; 2015.)

69. **Answer E.** Umbilical cord prolapse occurs in association with fetal malpresentation approximately 50% of the time (e.g., footling breech). However, the remaining 50% of cases occur in normal cephalic presentations. The overall incidence is roughly 1 in 160 to 1 in 600 births. Steps to arrange immediate cesarean delivery should be taken without delay. In the interim, the goal of the ED physician is to preserve umbilical circulation by relieving pressure upon the umbilical cord. All of the procedures listed may be helpful in the setting of umbilical cord prolapse. If cesarean delivery is not available, the umbilical cord should be placed back into the uterus (funic reduction) and the fetus should be delivered vaginally as soon as possible. Umbilical cord entanglement is a common complication of funic reduction.

70. **Answer C.** The patient has a kerion, which is an inflammatory lesion caused by an immune response to tinea capitis (due to *Trichophyton* or *Microsporum* species infection). The lesion can appear similar to an abscess, but kerions are more broad-based and often covered by scales. Incision, drainage, and oral antibacterials are not indicated, as no bacterial infection commonly exists. Oral antifungal therapy (with griseofulvin or newer antifungals such as itraconazole) is superior to topical antifungal therapy. Oral therapy must be continued for 6 weeks, as is common with many fungal infections. Kerions are often diagnosed when patients return to seek care for lesions which were incised and drained and exhibit no improvement. (Figure courtesy of Robert Hendrickson, MD. In: Greenberg MI, Hendrickson RG, Silverberg M, et al., eds. *Greenberg's Text-Atlas of Emergency Medicine*. Philadelphia, PA: Lippincott Williams & Wilkins; 2004:51, with permission.)

71. **Answer A.** The image shows sigmoid volvulus. Sigmoid volvulus is primarily a disease of the elderly as well as patients in long-term care facilities and patients with neurologic or psychiatric disease. It is thought that medications used to treat psychiatric and neurologic disease may have detrimental effects on colonic motility predisposing to volvulus. It is also frequently associated with chronic constipation. Patients with small bowel obstruction usually have a history of vomiting, and plain films would reveal circumferential plica circularis instead of noncircumferential haustrae of the large bowel. Intussusception is rare in adults and x-ray

findings are neither sensitive nor specific. Diabetic gastroparesis would demonstrate a large gastric bubble or dilation rather than colonic dilation. Almost all patients with Hirshsprung disease are diagnosed before the age of 2. (Figure from Harris JH, Harris WH. *The Radiology of Emergency Medicine*. 4th ed. Philadelphia, PA: Lippincott Williams & Wilkins; 1999, with permission.)

72. **Answer C.** Epinephrine dosing remains a confusing topic, largely because guidelines vary in their nomenclature. To make things simple, it is easy to remember that 1:1,000 doses are always given SQ or IM, whereas 1:10,000 doses (which are *less* concentrated) are given intravenously. The concentration of a 1:1,000 solution of epinephrine is 1 mg/mL, whereas the concentration of a 1:10,000 solution is 0.1 mg/mL (i.e., 10 times less concentrated). Therefore, 0.3 mL of a 1:1,000 solution is 0.3 mg. Delivery of 0.2 to 0.5 mg of epinephrine IM is the preferred dose and method of delivery in the setting of anaphylaxis. Subcutaneous delivery, which was favored in the past, results in slower and more erratic absorption. IM delivery is quick, effective, and extremely easy (and is the basis for the commercially available EpiPen, so IM delivery can be demonstrated to patients who may later need to self-administer the medication). It is critical to administer epinephrine early in the course of anaphylaxis. Epinephrine functions better as a front-line treatment than as "rescue" therapy late in the course. This dose may be repeated every 5 to 15 minutes.

73. **Answer A.** Octreotide is a longer lasting, synthetic analog of somatostatin. It inhibits the release of several vasodilatory hormones such as glucagon, and has direct effects on vascular smooth muscle. The end result of its effects is selective vasoconstriction of the splanchnic vasculature, thereby decreasing pressure and bleeding in existing esophageal varices. Propranolol is useful as a prophylactic adjunct to prevent rebleeding. Vasopressin has been used in the past to control variceal hemorrhage but it has prohibitive side effects, including myocardial ischemia. Therefore, it is currently not recommended for routine use.

74. **Answer D.** Patients with acute ureterolithiasis usually (sensitivity of 71% to 95%) have hematuria on urinalysis. Importantly, the absence of hematuria does not rule out stone, nor does the presence rule it in. Black race has traditionally been associated with lower likelihood of kidney stones although more recent research suggests that there is no correlation (either higher or lower likelihood) with black race. Hypotension argues against the possibility of a kidney stone and may suggest a vascular process, hemorrhage, or sepsis. Fever can certainly occur in the setting of a kidney stone, but it does not significantly increase the likelihood of diagnosis, especially relative to pyelonephritis or sepsis. An abnormal

Rovsing sign (eliciting pain in the right lower quadrant when the left lower quadrant is palpated) is sometimes seen in patients with acute appendicitis. Abdominal and even flank tenderness are usually absent in patients with acute ureterolithiasis. (Annals Apr 2016)

75. **Answer C.** The PSI is a scoring system which was first developed in a retrospective, observational study by Fine et al. in 1997. The aim of the study was to develop a rule to identify patients with low 30-day mortality from community-acquired pneumonia. Calculating the PSI is a two-step process. In step one, the physician determines if a patient has any "high-risk" criteria, the presence of which is independently associated with mortality. These criteria include patients older than 50, any of five comorbid diseases (neoplastic disease, congestive heart failure, cerebrovascular disease, renal disease, and liver disease), and five physical examination findings (altered mental status, pulse ≥125 per minute, respiratory rate ≥30 per minute, systolic blood pressure <90 mm Hg, and temperature, <35°C or ≥40°C). Patients without any of these criteria are classified as risk class I. All other patients are assigned to risk classes II, III, IV, or V based on the number of points calculated in step 2 of the PSI. In step 2, patients are assigned points for each risk factor that they have. Of all factors, age is the most heavily weighted in calculating the PSI.

76. **Answer C.** In addition to age-related decreases in creatinine clearance, NSAID therapy carries a high risk of renal injury as well as atrial fibrillation and cardiovascular ischemia. Oral NSAID therapy should not be used for routine pain management in geriatric patients. Amlodipine, metoprolol, hydrocodone, and gabapentin are far less nephrotoxic than NSAIDs. Hydrocodone can certainly cause delirium and constipation, which can indirectly lead to renal toxicity, but this effect is not as pronounced as NSAID-associated renal injury.

77. **Answer D.** For a given voltage, AC is thought to be three times more dangerous than DC. This is due to the fact that AC current causes repetitive muscle contraction or tetany once the "let-go current" is exceeded. This results in prolonged exposure and more severe injury. High-voltage electrical injuries should be treated like crush injuries, because there is often a large amount of tissue damage underneath normal appearing skin. It is impossible to predict the degree of underlying damage from the extent of cutaneous burns. Fewer than 10% of patients experiencing low-voltage electrical injury develop a cardiac dysrhythmia. In those patients who do suffer cardiac arrest due to an arrhythmia, ventricular fibrillation is most common. Triage priorities are different in cases of high-voltage electrical injury or lightning strikes. Patients with obvious signs of life tend to do well and can afford a small delay in definitive care.

Furthermore, due to the possibility of a good outcome with cardiopulmonary resuscitation (CPR), patients without signs of life should receive immediate care.

78. **Answer A.** The patient has necrotizing (malignant) otitis externa. This condition is seen almost exclusively in the elderly, the immunocompromised, and diabetic patients. It is far more serious than simple otitis externa due to the risk of spread of infection to the mastoid bone, the dural sinuses, and the meninges. Early, mild cases may be treated with outpatient fluoroquinolones active against *Pseudomonas*, but most cases will require admission and possible surgical debridement. *Pseudomonas* and *Staphylococcus aureus* are the most common bacterial pathogens implicated. The facial nerve is the most commonly affected cranial nerve in otitis externa. CT scan, rather than x-rays, is indicated for evaluation of spread of disease. Antivirals have no role in management.

79. **Answer C.** Group A streptococcal (GAS) pharyngitis carries the risk of acute rheumatic fever and acute glomerulonephritis. Treatment with antibiotics may decrease the risk of rheumatic fever, but has no effect on the development of glomerulonephritis. In the Western world, antibiotics are controversial due to the low rate of rheumatic fever and the greater risk of side effects from antibiotics. No strains of GAS pharyngitis have been shown to be resistant to penicillins. Cephalosporins are the preferred alternative if penicillins are contraindicated as resistance to macrolides has been exhibited. Intramuscular therapy is an excellent alternative to oral therapy and is the preferred treatment modality when compliance issues are suspected.

80. **Answer D.** Any patient with acute agitation and the potential for violence either to self or others must be physically and chemically restrained. Rapid tranquilization is ideally accomplished with a combination of haloperidol and benzodiazepine. Benztropine could also be given to reduce the incidence of acute dystonic reactions that may accompany administration of the antipsychotic medication. Observing the patient in an agitated state struggling against restraints is contraindicated, as the patient may cause harm to himself while fighting. The diagnosis of NMS is a clinical one based on the presence of fever, altered mental status, muscular rigidity, and frequent autonomic instability. While affected patients often have significant creatine kinase elevations, the test is no diagnostic for NMS. Trying to perform a CT scan with the patient in an acutely agitated, violent state will be impossible and just put the patient and staff at risk for injury. Rapid sequence intubation is not indicated unless rapid tranquilization is unsuccessful and serious morbidity is suspected in the patient, necessitating emergent workup for acute medical or traumatic cause for the psychosis.

81. **Answer C.** The most common causes of acute otitis media are *S. pneumoniae* and *M. catarrhalis. M. pneumoniae* is an uncommon cause of otitis media, especially in this age-group. The incidence of infections due to *H. influenzae* has decreased since the introduction of the HiB vaccine. Viruses as a group account for up to one out of every six cases of otitis media—RSV is the single most common viral cause of otitis media. Group A *streptococcus* is the least common of the bacterial pathogens listed.

82. **Answer C.** The patient has an inflammatory, monoarticular arthritis. The differential diagnosis includes septic arthritis, gout, and rheumatoid arthritis. Clinical differentiation between these three entities can be very difficult. Fever is present in most but not all patients with septic arthritis. Only 50% of patients with septic arthritis will have an abnormal blood WBC count, and only 50% will have positive blood cultures. The diagnosis rests on knee arthrocentesis and synovial fluid analysis. Fluid indices suggestive of septic arthritis include elevated fluid WBC count (>5,000 cells per mm^3), neutrophilic predominance (>75%), decreased glucose, positive Gram stain, and negative crystal assessment. It is important to recognize that only about two-thirds of patients with septic arthritis will have a positive Gram stain. Patients with acute monoarticular arthritis without a pre-existing condition of rheumatoid arthritis or gout should never be discharged without evaluation for septic arthritis. MRI of the knee should rarely, if ever, be performed in the ED for any indication. Serum uric acid levels are unreliable markers for acute gouty arthritis and should never be used to rule out septic arthritis.

83. **Answer C.** Anterior cord syndromes cause bilateral deficits in motor function and pain/temperature sensation below the level of injury. The lateral spinothalamic and the corticospinal tracts carry pain/temperature and motor fibers, respectively. The dorsal columns, carrying vibration, position, and fine touch sensation, are commonly spared. Cranial nerves arise directly out of the brainstem and are not commonly injured in cord syndromes except in rare circumstances. Causes of anterior cord syndrome include anterior spinal artery injury or infarction, spinal cord trauma, and intervertebral disk herniation. Prognosis is not as good as other causes of incomplete cord injuries.

84. **Answer E.** Due to the large distribution of vestibular pathways in the brain, there are many possible centrally located lesions that result in vertigo. The most important of these for emergency room physicians is vertebrobasilar insufficiency (transient ischemic attacks (TIA) of the vertebrobasilar arterial circulation) or frank cerebellar stroke. Vertebrobasilar arterial ischemia is especially common in elderly patients with typical risk factors for vascular disease (e.g., diabetes, hypertension, hyperlipidemia, and smoking). It is important to recognize these patients because they require admission and possible monitoring in an ICU setting (depending on their syndrome). Cerebellar infarctions are known for an unpredictable clinical course and sudden deterioration of previously alert, stable patients. Neurosurgical intervention is typically required when the cerebellar infarct results in impingement on the fourth ventricle with subsequent hydrocephalus. The optimal time of intervention, however, has yet to be determined.

85. **Answer B.** The degree of retropharyngeal (also known as prevertebral) soft-tissue swelling indicates that the patient has a retropharyngeal abscess or developing abscess (phlegmon) (Fig. 12-17). A good rule of thumb is to recall that the soft-tissue width at the level of C2 should be no greater than half the width of the C2 vertebral body. In this patient's case, the width of the soft tissue is approximately the same as the adjacent vertebral body. The CT also clearly demonstrates that the area of swelling extends several levels, though the normal width of the prevertebral tissues increases in the lower cervical spine, such that at C5, the normal width is up to the width of the adjacent vertebral body.

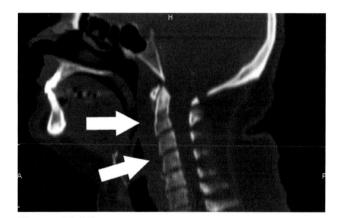

Figure 12-17

86. **Answer E.** This patient is at risk for aspiration pneumonia by virtue of his decreased airway protection and tube feeds. Although there is no definitive way to diagnose aspiration pneumonia, this patient's history of witnessed vomiting with choking in the setting of a patient at risk for aspiration is virtually diagnostic for aspiration. Aspiration pneumonitis is caused by an inflammatory response in the lungs after the aspiration of low pH gastric contents. Aspiration pneumonitis develops within hours of aspiration, and its severity is directly related to the volume and pH of the aspirated material. Treatment is supportive, and antibiotics and

steroids are not useful. However, episodes of aspiration pneumonitis may become secondarily infected, resulting in aspiration pneumonia. More commonly, aspiration pneumonia develops without significant preceding pneumonitis. Such infections are due to the aspiration of oropharyngeal flora and are most commonly polymicrobial. While anaerobes have classically been implicated in cases of aspiration, anaerobic antibiotic coverage may actually only be needed in patients with very poor oral hygiene, putrid sputum, or evidence of necrotizing pneumonia or lung abscess chest x-ray. Metronidazole is a specific therapy for anaerobic infections, but its use as monotherapy in aspiration pneumonia is associated with a high failure rate. The fluoroquinolones are broad-spectrum agents and they achieve good tissue levels. However, they do not need to be combined with corticosteroids, for which there is no role in the setting of aspiration, despite their wide use. Aztreonam does not have any gram-positive coverage, so it should not be used as monotherapy. First-line antibiotic therapy in nursing home residents with aspiration pneumonia may include piperacillin–tazobactam, levofloxacin, or ceftazidime.

87. **Answer C.** Corneal ulcers in the setting of contact lens use are frequently caused by *Pseudomonas* infections and require aggressive treatment with antipseudomonal antibiotics such as ciprofloxacin. Erythromycin and trimethoprim–polymyxin B are inadequate to treat *Pseudomonas* infections. While irrigation may help transiently reduce surface bacterial counts, this patient needs antibiotic treatment. Patching corneal ulcers should be avoided, particularly when an infection is present as bacteria may thrive in the warm, dark environment created by patching.

88. **Answer C.** Although retinal hemorrhage is a well-known marker for child abuse (shaken baby syndrome), it is present in almost half of all neonates, due to normal birth trauma. Resolution tends to occur in 1 month.

89. **Answer C.** The patient has nearly complete opacification of the left lung. In trauma patients who are usually supine, this indicates a large hemothorax, as blood will layer through gravity throughout the entire lung field. Treatment involves tube thoracostomy drainage and possible thoracotomy if the exsanguination is rapid or severe. Pneumothorax may be concomitant but is not evident on this chest x-ray. Pericardial tamponade is best diagnosed by FAST scan. Pneumoperitoneum is not evident—air under the left diaphragm is much more likely to be a physiologic gastric bubble. Diaphragmatic rupture would be indicated by abdominal organ herniation into the thorax which is not evident. (Figure courtesy of Mark Silverberg, MD. In: Greenberg MI, Hendrickson RG, Silverberg M, et al., eds. *Greenberg's Text-Atlas of*

Emergency Medicine. Philadelphia, PA: Lippincott Williams & Wilkins; 2004:637, with permission.)

90. **Answer B.** Though WNV continues to receive substantial media coverage, it remains an uncommon cause of severe encephalitis. Herpes simplex virus is the most common cause of severe encephalitis. WNV is almost wholly transmitted by mosquito bites, though wild birds serve as a reservoir for viral amplification. The majority of patients are symptomatic. Among patients who have symptoms, West Nile fever is the most common presentation, consisting of constitutional symptoms that are indistinguishable from other viral illness, including common infections such as influenza. Due to the lack of specific symptoms in such patients, they will not likely be diagnosed with WNV. Fortunately, the disease is most often self-limited, so making a firm diagnosis is not imperative. Among patients with neuroinvasive disease, encephalitis, meningitis, or flaccid paralysis are the most common presenting symptoms. Such patients can be diagnosed by the detection of IgM and IgG antibodies due to the rapid seroconversion that occurs among infected patients. While treatment adjuncts are being studied for patients with severe disease, treatment remains supportive.

91. **Answer B.** More than three-fourths of all patients with AIDS will develop PCP at some point in their lifetimes. It is also the most common identifiable cause of death in AIDS patients. *Pneumocystis* is classified as a protozoan, but has many characteristics of a fungus. Symptoms of PCP, like all pneumonias, include fever, cough, and shortness of breath, but a subacute or mild course is characteristic. Chest radiography classically demonstrates diffuse, bilateral interstitial infiltrates, but can be completely normal up to 20% of the time. First-line therapy is with TMP-SMX. Corticosteroids are indicated in patients who have significant hypoxia. Pentamidine, dapsone, or clindamycin plus primaquine may be used as alternatives. The other answer choices are all common opportunistic infections in AIDS patients, but occur less often than *Pneumocystis*.

92. **Answer E.** Left ventricular assist devices (LVADs) are associated with a host of complications. All patients require anticoagulation to reduce the risk of pump thrombosis. While the use of anticoagulants increases bleeding risk, the risk is further increased because patients with LVADs develop an acquired von Willebrand syndrome because the pump machinery breaks the normally long vWF chains into shorter, less effective segments. The driveline connects the extracorporeal electronic controller to the motor which is attached to the heart. As with any foreign body, drivelines are susceptible to infection and are covered with a sterile dressing. Right heart failure is a frequent complication

either secondary to the increased right heart workload or to a malignant rhythm such as ventricular tachycardia or fibrillation (which has less effect on the left heart because it is device dependent).

93. **Answer A.** TB is a chronic, progressive, multisystem illness caused by *Mycobacterium tuberculosis*, an aerobic, acid-fast bacillus. Initial infection occurs through respiratory particles from infected individuals. TB is characterized by primary infection, during which the positive pressure differential (PPD) skin test turns positive, followed by reactivation disease, when the clinical manifestations and pathology become evident. The overall most common symptom of pulmonary TB is cough, followed by weight loss, night sweats, chest pain, dyspnea, and hemoptysis. Patients rarely present to the ED until they develop hemoptysis. Initial evaluation includes a chest x-ray, which has excellent negative predictive value except in HIV patients. Findings on chest x-ray of primary TB can be indistinguishable from any lobar pulmonary infiltrate combined with hilar lymphadenopathy. Reactivation TB characteristically demonstrates an apical infiltrate which may be cavitary. Sputum samples for acid-fast bacilli analysis should be obtained in the ED before any antimicrobial therapy is given. If the patient is not producing sputum, inpatient gastric aspiration of swallowed sputum or bronchoscopic sampling is indicated. Given the indolent, chronic nature of pulmonary TB infection, antimycobacterial agents need not be started in the ED.

94. **Answer C.** Although some patients with pontine hemorrhage may have only very small areas of involvement and only moderate symptomatology, pontine hemorrhagic stroke typically involves the entire anterior aspect of the pons, resulting in coma, miosis (pinpoint pupils), horizontal gaze palsy, and erratic breathing requiring intubation and mechanical ventilation. Miosis results from disruption of ascending sympathetic fibers that innervate the pupillary dilator apparatus. Horizontal gaze palsy results from involvement of the abducens nucleus (CN VI), which is located in the central pons. Lateral medullary syndrome is due to occlusion of the posterior inferior cerebellar artery (PICA), whereas locked-in syndrome is due to occlusion of the basilar artery. Neither syndrome involves miosis and patients with locked-in syndrome retain normal eye movement. Pseudobulbar palsy is due to the bilateral lesions of the corticobulbar tracts to lower cranial nerves and may result in dysphagia, dysarthria, and dysphonia. It spares the cranial nerves controlling the extraocular muscles (CN III, IV, and VI).

95. **Answer C.** TAI occurs most commonly from high-speed motor vehicle collisions (MVCs) causing blunt thoracic trauma. Most traumatic aortic ruptures are immediately fatal, but patients who survive to ED evaluation are usually successfully treated. The descending aorta just distal to the subclavian artery is the most commonly injured site. Chest and back pain are the most common symptoms. The initial screening test is plain chest x-ray—however, the sensitivity of plain films is only up to 85%. In cases where suspicion for TAI is high, confirmatory CT aortography should be performed, as it has close to 100% sensitivity. Transesophageal echocardiography may be used in select cases where CT scan is not possible, but transthoracic echocardiography is much less accurate and should be used only to evaluate for pericardial effusion or tamponade, not TAI. Management of TAI involves operative repair, but blood pressure and heart rate control with β-blockers is essential to prevent further damage to the aorta from shear forces.

96. **Answer E.** Koplik spots are irregularly shaped bright red macules that contain a central, punctate, bluish-white spot. Their presence is pathognomonic for measles. They are most commonly found on the buccal mucosa and are classically located opposite the second molars.

97. **Answer B.** *Y. pestis,* the etiologic agent of bubonic plague, is a gram-negative coccobacillus which can cause a number of different clinical syndromes. In this country, it is endemic in the southwestern United States but it has gained notoriety along with anthrax and tularemia because of its potential use as a possible biologic weapon. Pneumonic plague is caused by the inhalation of infective droplets from animals or *persons.* Rodents are the natural hosts but pets can "bring the disease home." After an incubation period of 1 to 6 days, pneumonic plague is an aggressive disease and many patients progress rapidly to septic shock and death without early treatment. Initially, patients may complain of typical symptoms of pneumonia, and their chest x-rays frequently show alveolar infiltrates. Chest x-rays may also reveal a picture consistent with acute respiratory distress syndrome (ARDS), with diffuse bilateral patchy infiltrates and cavitation. None of the other agents demonstrate person-to-person transmission.

98. **Answer A.** Traumatic diaphragmatic injuries are almost equally caused by blunt and penetrating mechanisms. They much more commonly occur on the left side, because the liver serves as excellent protection against both injury and post-traumatic herniation. Once the diaphragm is injured, the defect remains without spontaneous healing due to the constant pressure subjected to the diaphragm by normal respiratory forces. The main problem with missed diagnosis is the high rate of delayed herniation of abdominal contents into the thorax, which can occur months or even years after the initial injury. None of the standard diagnostic tests for trauma (FAST, CT scan, DPL, radiography) is sensitive

or specific enough to accurately evaluate for diaphragmatic injury. Direct visualization with thoracoscopy or laparoscopy in suspected cases is required.

99. **Answer E.** The most commonly cited abnormality is QTc shortening, but any of the listed changes may occur.

100. **Answer A.** Migratory pain from the periumbilical region to the right lower quadrant has moderately high specificity for appendicitis. Radiation of pain to the scapula is more suggestive of biliary pathology. Pain from appendicitis is usually less than 24 hours in duration, but sometimes patients present later if there is temporary relief of the pain (immediately after perforation). Movement and coughing usually exacerbate the pain of appendicitis and other causes of peritoneal irritation. Anorexia is very sensitive for the diagnosis of appendicitis.

Index

Note: Page number followed by f indicates figure only.